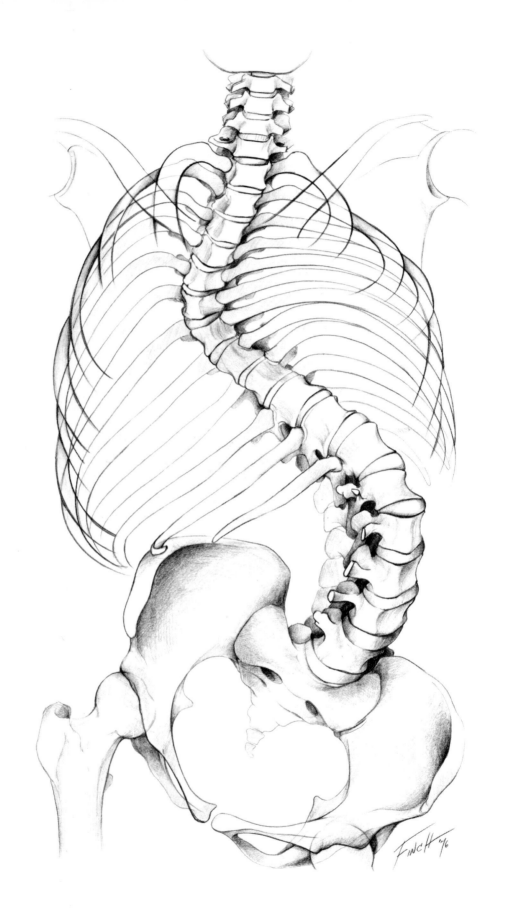

# SCOLIOSIS
## and Other Spinal Deformities

JOHN H. MOE, M.D.          ROBERT B. WINTER, M.D.

DAVID S. BRADFORD, M.D.          JOHN E. LONSTEIN, M.D.

*Illustrated by*
MARTIN E. FINCH

1978
W. B. SAUNDERS COMPANY
Philadelphia • London • Toronto

W. B. Saunders Company: West Washington Square
Philadelphia, PA   19105

1 St. Anne's Road
Eastbourne, East Sussex BN21 3UN, England

1 Goldthorne Avenue
Toronto, Ontario M8Z 5T9, Canada

**Library of Congress Cataloging in Publication Data**

Main entry under title:

Scoliosis and other spinal deformities.

1. Spine — Abnormalities.    2. Scoliosis.    I. Moe, John H.
[DNLM: 1. Scoliosis.    2. Spine — Abnormalities.
3. Spinal diseases. WE735 S423]

RD768.S33      617'.375      76–50153

ISBN 0–7216–6427–X

Scoliosis and Other Spinal Deformities                    ISBN   0-7216-6427-X

Last digit is the print number:     9     8     7     6     5     4     3     2     1

This book is dedicated to those who have suffered most by the many hours we have spent writing this book, our wives and children. May they somehow forgive us for that irretrievable time.

# DAVID S. BRADFORD, M.D.

Professor, Orthopaedic Surgery. Department of Orthopaedic Surgery,
University of Minnesota. Director of Resident Education,
University of Minnesota. Attending Staff, Fairview-St. Mary's Hospital.
Scoliosis Service, Twin Cities Scoliosis Center.

# JOHN E. LONSTEIN, M.D.

Assistant Professor, Orthopaedic Surgery. Department of Orthopaedic Surgery,
University of Minnesota. Attending Staff, Fairview-St. Mary's and
Gillette Children's Hospitals. Scoliosis Service, Twin Cities Scoliosis Center.

# JOHN H. MOE, M.D.

Professor Emeritus, Orthopaedic Surgery. Department of Orthopaedic Surgery,
University of Minnesota. Attending Staff, Fairview-St. Mary's Hospital.
Director, Twin Cities Scoliosis Center.

# ROBERT B. WINTER, M.D.

Professor, Orthopaedic Surgery. Department of Orthopaedic Surgery,
University of Minnesota. Director of Orthopaedic Education,
Fairview-St. Mary's Hospital. Director of Medical Education,
Gillette Children's Hospital. Scoliosis Service, Twin Cities Scoliosis Center.

*Illustrated by*

# MARTIN FINCH

Assistant Professor and Director, Biomedical Graphic
Communications, Health Science Center,
University of Minnesota

# FOREWORD

In 1955, Dr. George Eggers, then president of the Southern Medical Society, invited me to present a paper on scoliosis before the orthopaedic section of that society.

I presented a series of 128 patients with paralytic curvatures treated by cast correction and spine fusion between 1948 and 1954. In retrospect, the results were only moderately good. The presentation was honest and showed an over-all pseudarthrosis incidence of 60 per cent, but it also showed that some loss of correction could be improved by cast correction when the pseudarthrosis was repaired. This was an advance when compared with other reported results. Dr. Eggers was impressed and urged me to write a much needed book on scoliosis treatment. I did not feel that my experience at that time justified such an attempt.

During the following years, many orthopaedic surgeons have urged me to publish such a volume. Now, after 28 years of learning, we will do so. This book is written with the major assistance of men who have gained basic knowledge of scoliosis treatment from working with me at Gillette Children's Hospital in St. Paul, the University of Minnesota Hospitals, and Fairview Hospital in Minneapolis. These men have advanced far beyond my early teaching and have attained national and international renown as authorities in all fields of scoliosis, kyphosis, and other spine deformities.

With the formation of the Scoliosis Research Society, founded in 1966 at the University of Minnesota, there has been an upsurge of interest in all aspects of thought and treatment of scoliosis throughout this country and in Canada, Mexico, South America, and Europe. No longer is scoliosis the cinderella of orthopaedic surgery.

The scoliosis service in the Twin Cities has always been cognizant of the need for adopting all modalities of treatment that will benefit the patient. The frank admission of errors in management and the avoidance of their repetition has been another dictum that has promoted improved results.

To John Cobb, whose scoliosis service at the hospital for special surgery in New York attained international renown by 1947, I owe deep gratitude and respect for the help he so freely gave to me in my early years of endeavor in scoliosis. He gave unstintingly of his time in analyzing and helping me to overcome the problems that were encountered.

Another pillar of strength and encouragement has been Walter Blount of Milwaukee, whose friendship, keen mind, and sound judgment have been a constant source of inspiration to me. His Milwaukee brace represents a major advance in treatment. Together we have improved the brace to its present form.

Joseph Risser of Pasadena, California, taught me how to apply and to use the localizer cast in 1952. This proved to be a great improvement over the hinged body cast, as taught to me by John Cobb, for the curve correction was as good or better, and the patient's comfort was immeasurably greater.

I have borrowed freely from Yves Cotrel of Berck-Plage, France, in adopting his overhead suspension strap instead of the fixed localizer of Risser.

Paul Harrington of Houston, Texas, gave us the first effectual and safe method of internally correcting and stabilizing curvatures of the spine. The Harrington instrumentation of spinal curvatures has been a mainstay of our operative treatment of scoliosis since 1960.

Arthur Hodgson of Hong Kong demonstrated the effectiveness of anterior excision and bone grafting of tuberculous lesions of the spine in 1956. In 1965 he demonstrated the value and safety of the anterior approach to the spine in severely angulated congenital kyphoscoliosis. Since 1966, we gradually became knowledgeable in this surgical approach, and it is now a common and essential method of treatment in selected spine problems.

The early diagnosis and treatment of all spine deformities have not been appreciated by most orthopaedic surgeons until recently. A school survey program was first instituted by MacEwen and Shands in Delaware, Brooks in California, and sometime later by Winter, Lonstein, Bradford, and Moe in Minnesota. In the absence of knowledge of the etiology of idiopathic scoliosis, the early recognition of a curvature by trained school personnel has proved eminently successful. Lack of cooperation by general practitioners and pediatricians has diminished rapidly, and the public is now recognizing the importance of early diagnosis and is lending enthusiastic support to the school survey program.

We are deeply indebted to the splendid teamwork that has been amply demonstrated by the administrative, medical, and paramedical personnel who have made it possible for us to develop the Twin Cities Scoliosis Center. We pay tribute to the entire hospital staff involved in this service:

—The floor nursing staff, whose professional competence makes the surgical treatment a success and whose personal involvement allays the fears that are so prevalent in families of scoliosis patients.

—The efficient operating room nursing staff, as well as those in the recovery room and the postoperative areas.

—The intensely interested physical therapy staff and the cooperative roentgenologists and their staff of technicians.

—The department of anesthesiology and its staff of anesthetists, for without their intense interest, loyalty, and sound knowledge, our efforts would indeed be under a great handicap.

—The efficient thoracic surgeons who so willingly, effectively, and enthusiastically expose the spine anteriorly, making our anterior spine corrections and decompressions so very much easier and lessening our burdens.

—A special tribute must go to the dedicated and loyal office staff, without whose help no scoliosis center could function.

—My colleagues, Robert B. Winter, David S. Bradford, and John E. Lonstein, who collaborated with me in preparing this volume, are to me a constant source of pride. From the original scoliosis service at Gillette Children's Hospital, initiated in 1948, has evolved the Twin Cities Scoliosis Center, composed of Gillette Children's Hospital, the University of Minnesota Hospitals, and Fairview Hospital. This is now a large scoliosis center, and its development has been due to the store of knowledge accumulated by the combined efforts of all who have worked together and shared knowledge. It is our desire to share this knowledge with you, the reader.

JOHN H. MOE

# ACKNOWLEDGMENT

We, the authors of this volume, know how many hours of toil our secretarial staff endured in typing and retyping its contents. We wish to acknowledge their most important contribution and to thank them sincerely for their efforts and patience.

| | |
|---|---|
| Ruby Bauer | Mary Lou Moe |
| Kristi Coffin | Susan Myhre |
| Glenda Davis | Jenell Phillips |
| Terre Frelix | Norma Reberg |
| Kari Graham | Janet Schneider |
| Linda Lovejoy | Phyllis Weigum |
| Christine Mazurkiewicz | |

In a like manner, the Photography Departments of Fairview Hospital and Gillette Children's Hospital spent many hours in obtaining the best prints possible. We are proud of them and thank them as well.

| | |
|---|---|
| Tom Cooley | Peggy Habermaier |
| Gordon Dunn | Ken Jandl |
| Ned Gardner | Becky Schmidt |

To the W. B. Saunders Company and particularly to Brian Decker, Medical Editor, for his patience in waiting for the chapters to come in one by one, we owe a debt of gratitude.

To Martin Finch, the illustrator from the University of Minnesota, Department of Photography and Art, we are also deeply indebted. His superb skill in providing illustrations adds a great deal to the teaching value of this volume.

# CONTENTS

# Chapter 1

# HISTORICAL ASPECTS OF SCOLIOSIS

Scoliosis is derived from the Greek word meaning curvature. As used in medical literature, it signifies lateral curvature of the spine. The normal spine has curves when viewed from the side, but there is no lateral deviation when viewed from the front or back.

Scoliosis is a deformity recognized since ancient times. In "De Articulationes" of the *Corpus Hippocraticum*, there is a description of normal and abnormal spinal curves. One passage states, "There are many varieties of curvatures of the spine even in persons who are in good health, for it takes place from natural conformation and from habit, and the spine is liable to be bent from old age and from pains." The possible relationship between spinal deformity and pulmonary disease was also mentioned. Treatment was recognized to be difficult and ineffective. The poor prognosis in patients with early onset of spine deformity was described. No distinction was made between deformity of infection and true scoliosis. Treatment of spine deformities was by forcible traction, both horizontal and with underarm and leg distraction in suspension (Fig. 1–1).[1]

Galen (131–201 A.D.) coined the words kyphosis, lordosis, and scoliosis.[13] His treatment of spine deformities followed that of Hippocrates.

From the fifth to the fifteenth centuries, little progress was made in treatment of spine deformities. Paul of Aegina (625–690 A.D.)[35] wrote a treatise of "Seven Books," which was a bright light in a dark period. During the middle ages, deformed individuals were objects of scorn and derision. Their handicaps were considered a form of divine punishment, although the hunchback and the dwarf were in demand as court jesters.

Ambroise Paré (1410–1590)[34] thought that poor posture was a probable cause of scoliosis. He described congenital scoliosis and recognized cord compression as a cause of paraplegia. His treatment of scoliosis adhered closely to the hippocratic method, but he added a steel corset made by armorers.

André, who was the first to use the word orthopedia, in 1741,[3] wrote about spine curvatures, giving special attention to postural and sitting habits as a preventive measure and to corsets and exercise as methods of treatment.

The "jury mast" for sustained head traction during ambulation was developed by Levacher in 1764.[29] Myotomies were advocated by Guérin in 1839.[17, 18] Volkmann resected protruding ribs in 1889.[19] Royle[8] reported a resected hemivertebra in 1928,[9] following a suggestion made by Codivilla in 1901.[9]

Postural habits continued to be considered the cause of scoliosis throughout the nineteenth century. Exercises and body bracing were the recommended treatment, and distraction in bed or on a frame was used to correct the spine deformity. Hare[19] demonstrated startling improvement using plaster replicas of his patients' torsos in his book published in 1849 (Fig. 1–2). The flagrant dishonesty of his allegations is very evident.

Ingenious vertical distraction frames with corrective pressure pads appeared under the name of Hoffa and others in Germany, and

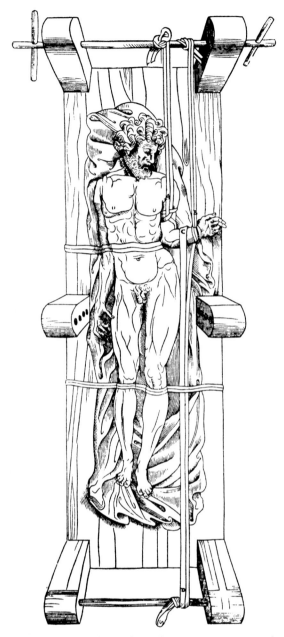

**Figure 1–1** The Machine of Hippocrates. It was used in a like manner for torso distraction.

Louis Sayre applied plaster torso casts in vertical suspension. Brackett and Bradford in 1895 devised a horizontal distraction frame with a "localizer" attachment, very similar to that used by Risser in 1952 (Fig. 1–3).

With the discovery of roentgen rays in 1895 by Wilhelm Konrad Roentgen, professor of physics in Strassburg, Würtzburg, and later in Munich, the etiologic factors involved in scoliosis became increasingly evident. Although Calot[36] performed a fusion for tuberculosis of the spine prior to Hibbs, he abandoned the procedure as unsuccessful.

De Quervain[10] published a description of his method of spine fusion in 1917, but the successful surgical treatment of scoliosis began with Hibbs. He described his method of spine fusion for tuberculosis of the spine in 1911.[22] In this article he suggested its possible use in scoliosis, and later (in 1914) performed the first fusion for scoliosis. He reported 59 scoliosis fusions in 1924.[23] With Risser and Ferguson he published an end result study of 360 fusions for scoliosis.[24] In this same article, the use of the turnbuckle corrective cast was described, to which the name of Risser is commonly ascribed. Hibbs's relatively many failures were mainly due to inability to recognize fusion defects and to an inadequate period of immobilization after fusion.

Others attempting to correct and fuse scoliotic spines met with a high percentage of failures. During the decade of 1930 to 1940, treatment by fusion fell into disrepute because of the poor results. Steindler's fusion results were so poor that he gave up the idea entirely and again resorted to exercises, bracing, and attempts to establish better compensation and balance.[37]

In 1941, a group of 425 cases of idiopathic scoliosis was studied by a committee of the American Orthopaedic Association.[2] This was a very dismal report, giving the following conclusions: 60 per cent of cases treated by exercise and bracing progressed, and 40 per cent were unchanged. Correction and fusion in 180 cases showed pseudarthroses in 54. Of 214 patients treated by fusion, 29 per cent lost all correction. Of the entire group, 69 per cent had an end result rated poor or fair and 31 per cent good and excellent.

Fusion with cast correction provided fairly good results in the hands of the few orthopedic surgeons who chose to study the problem thoroughly and to pay close attention to meticulous details of cast correction, technique of fusion, and protection of the fusion until graft maturation. Through the efforts of these men—Cobb, Risser, and a very few others—surgical treatment of scolio-

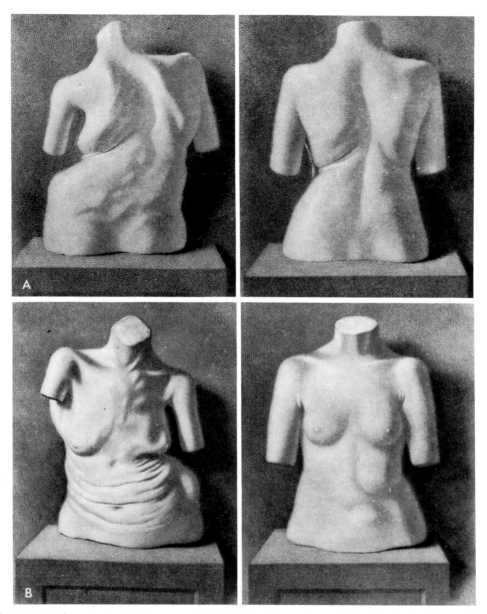

**Figure 1–2** "The patient, age 18 years, was treated in lateral recumbency with traction to shoulders and feet, on a specially designed inclined plane of the author's design for 12 months." From "Practical Observations on the Prevention, Causes, and Treatment of Curvatures of the Spine." Samuel Hare, Surgeon, London, 1849.

sis began slowly to regain its proper status. In 1946, Blount and Schmidt devised a distraction brace, combined with lateral pressure pads. This early Milwaukee brace was at first used only in the operative treatment of scoliosis. Its success in curve correction led to increasing enthusiasm for its improvement, both in fit and construction. Such changes led to greater correction of the curvature and ultimately to use of the appliance as an ambulatory brace in the nonoperative treatment of lesser curves. It has proved successful in a high percentage of properly selected patients.[4, 5, 6, 7]

Surgical treatment by spinal fusion has made great advances in recent decades. Through improved fusion techniques and the addition of abundant autogenous bone, the pseudarthrosis rate has been lowered to an acceptable percentage. Graft defects are now

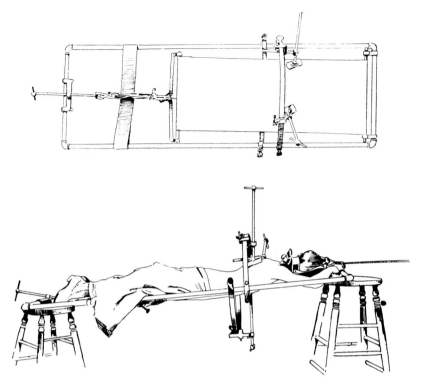

**Figure 1–3**   The horizontal distraction frame of Brackett and Bradford (1895).

recognized early, while external support is still being worn. Repair is then successfully performed without significant loss of correction. Harrington instrumentation, first successfully used in 1960,[20, 21] has added internal stability to the fused spine and permitted ambulation in a well-fitted cast or Milwaukee brace soon after surgery without loss of correction.

The advent of Harrington instrumentation marks a milestone in the surgical fusion of the scoliotic spine. Its early use was not successful because many inexperienced orthopedic surgeons considered it as the answer to all scoliosis problems and forgot the importance of meticulous fusion and cast techniques. Our own experience with several hundred scoliotic spines treated by cast correction and fusion proved of great benefit when Harrington instrumentation was added to the armamentarium. Harrington instrumentation has now withstood the test of time and is a mainstay in the surgical treatment of scoliosis.[28, 30, 31, 32]

In 1956, A. R. Hodgson of Hong Kong described the anterior approach to the spine for treatment of tuberculous spondylitis.[26] The operation consisted of exposure and re-

moval of the tuberculous debris and insertion of rib grafts. Although the results appeared satisfactory, the procedure did not gain immediate acceptance by tuberculosis experts, and its popularity did not become widespread for some time.

In 1965, Hodgson described his first case of anterior opening wedge osteotomy for a congenital kyphosis.[25] The result was satisfactory, with 25 degrees of final correction. Since that time, the anterior approach for spine deformities has become increasingly recognized as a necessary procedure for most patients with a sharply angulated kyphosis or kyphoscoliosis and for the release of cord impingement in paraplegia. Our experience, coupled with that of Hall, Leatherman, Simmons, and others, has established this approach as a vital and necessary addition to the surgical treatment of spinal deformities.

The use of the "halo" for distraction of the spinal column was developed at Rancho Los Amigos, in Downey, California, by Nickel, Perry, and Garrett.[4] The halo was originally connected to a body cast to provide stable spine distraction in paralytic spines. With a tracheostomy and mechanical breathing assistance, surgical fusion of the collapsing spine became a relatively safe procedure in patients with severe respiratory depletion. Later, at our Scoliosis Service, we added femoral traction, which became a common method of correcting all severe forms of scoliosis.[27]

In 1969, A. F. Dwyer of Australia reported a new method of correcting lateral curvatures of the spine by anterior disc excision combined with the insertion of special screws and compression of the vertebral bodies with a fixed cable.[12] Excellent correction was obtained, and the method has gained wide acceptance for use in selected cases of severe deformity.

The halopelvic hoop was developed by Dewald[11] in Chicago. It was popularized in Hong Kong by Hodgson, Yau, and O'Brien, and it has become an accepted form of correction in certain severe spine deformities.[33] Another form of spine distraction, using the halo in a wheelchair with an overhead suspension, was devised by Pierre Stagnara of Lyon, France.

The founding of the Scoliosis Research Society at the University of Minnesota in 1966 must be considered a landmark in progress of scoliosis treatment. For the first time, a large group of enthusiastic orthopedic surgeons came together in the United States and Canada for the express purpose of standardizing scoliosis treatment and solving the many problems brought about by divergent opinions. No organization has created such worldwide stimulation toward progress in scoliosis treatment.

Treatment of scoliosis has come of age and is no longer haphazard. Centers for study and treatment of scoliosis are being formed in increasing numbers. Scoliosis research societies are being organized all over the world, and information of value is being given international attention. Highly motivated orthopedic surgeons whose main interest is scoliosis are freely exchanging opinions with their fellows. Their motive is the development of the best possible treatment of scoliosis.

Understanding of the principles of scoliosis treatment is the basic requirement for good results. The varieties of treatment modalities have become numerous. Experience and judgment are of primary importance. Reliable surgical techniques have developed, and mishaps seldom occur in skilled hands. The need for young orthopedic surgeons to train in the best centers and to continue the good work already begun has never been greater.

## References

1. Adams, F.: The Genuine Works of Hippocrates. New York, William Wood and Company.
2. American Orthopaedic Association Research Committee: End result study of the treatment of idiopathic scoliosis. J. Bone Joint Surg., 23:963, 1941.
3. Andre, N.: L'orthopaedia, ou l'art de prevenir et de corriger dans les enfants deformite a du corps. Paris, 1741.
4. Blount, W. P.: Scoliosis and the Milwaukee brace. Bull. Hosp. Joint Dis., 19:(2), 152–165, 1958.
5. Blount, W. P.: Non-operative treatment of scoliosis. A.A.O.S. Symposium on the Spine, Nov., 1967. St. Louis, C. V. Mosby, pp. 188–195.
6. Blount, W. P.: Use of the Milwaukee brace. Orthop. Clin. North Am., 3:3–16, 1972.
7. Blount, W. P., and Schmidt, A. C.: The Milwaukee brace in the treatment of scoliosis. Proc. Am. Acad. Orthop. Surg., J. Bone Joint Surg., 39A:693, 1957.
8. Calot, F.: L'ortopedie indispensible aux practiciens. Paris, Meloine, 1923.
9. Codivilla, A.: Sulla scoliosi congenita. Arch. di Ortop. 18:65, 1901.
10. De Quervain, E., and Hoessly, H.: Operative immobilization of the spine, Surg. Gynecol. Obstet., 24:428, 1917.
11. Dewald, R. L., and Ray, R. D.: Skeletal traction for the treatment of severe scoliosis. J. Bone Joint Surg., 52A:233–238, March, 1970.
12. Dwyer, A. F.: An anterior approach in scoliosis. A preliminary report. Clin. Orthop., 62:192, 1969.
13. Galen: De Moto Maerculorum.
14. Garrett, A., Perry, J., and Nickel, V.: Stabilization of the collapsing spine. J. Bone Joint Surg., 43A:4, 1961.
15. Goldstein, L. A.: Surgical management of scoliosis. J. Bone Joint Surg., 48A:167–196, 1966.
16. Goldstein, L. A.: Treatment of idiopathic scoliosis by Harrington instrumentation and fusion with fresh autogenous iliac bone grafts. Results in 80 cases. J. Bone Joint Surg., 51A:209–222, 1969.
17. Guérin, J.: Memoire sur les deviations simulees de l'epine et les moyens. Gaz. Med. de Paris, 7:241–247, 1839.
18. Guérin, J.: Remarques preliminaires sur le traitement des deviations de l'epine par la section des muscles du dos. Gaz. Med. de Paris, 10:1–6, 1842.
19. Hare, S.: Practical Observations on the Prevention, Causes and Treatment of Curvatures of the Spine. London, 1849.
20. Harrington, P. R.: Treatment of scoliosis. Correction and internal fixation by spine instrumentation. J. Bone Joint Surg., 44A:591–610, 1962.
21. Harrington, P. R.: Technical data in relation to the successful use of instrumentation in scoliosis. Orthop. Clin. North Am., 3(1):49–67, 1972.
22. Hibbs, R. A.: An operation for progressive spinal deformities. N.Y. Med. J., 93:1013, May 27, 1911.

23. Hibbs, R. A.: A report of fifty-nine cases of scoliosis treated by the fusion of ration. J. Bone Joint Surg., 6:3, 1924.

24. Hibbs, R. A., Risser, J. C., and Ferguson, A. B.: Scoliosis treated by the fusion operation. An end result study of three hundred and sixty cases. J. Bone Joint Surg., 13:91, 1931.

25. Hodgson, A. R.: Correction of fixed spinal curves. J. Bone Joint Surg., 46A:1221–1227, 1965.

26. Hodgson, A. R., and Stack, F. E.: Anterior spine fusion. Br. J. Surg. 44:266, 1956.

27. Kane, W., Moe, J., and Lai, C.: Halo-femoral pin distraction in treatment of scoliosis. J. Bone Joint Surg., 49A:1018, 1967.

28. Leider, L. L., Moe, J. H., and Winter, R.: Early ambulation after surgical treatment of idiopathic scoliosis. J. Bone Joint Surg., 55A:5, 1973.

29. Levacher, A. F. T.: Nouveau moyen de prevenir et de guerir la courbure de l'epine. Mem. Acad. R. Chir., 4:596, 1768.

30. Moe, J. H.: Methods and techniques of evaluating idiopathic scoliosis. A.A.O.S. Symposium on the Spine, Nov. 1967, pp. 196–240. St. Louis, C. V. Mosby.

31. Moe, J. H.: Methods of correction and surgical techniques in scoliosis. Orthop. Clin. North Am., 3(1):17–48, 1972.

32. Moe, J. H., and Valuska, J.: Evaluation of treatment of scoliosis by Harrington instrumentation. J. Bone Joint Surg., 48A:1656–1657, 1966. In proceedings of the American Orthopedic Association.

33. O'Brien, J.: Halo-pelvic traction. Acta Scand. Orthop., Suppl. 163, 1975.

34. Paré, A.: Collected Works. Translated by Th. Johnson, London, 1634.

35. Paul of Aegina. Collected Works. Translated for Sydenham Society by F. Adams, London, 1834, et seq.

36. Royle, N. D.: The operative removal of an accessory vertebra. Med. J., Aust., 1:467, 1928.

37. Steindler, A.: Diseases and Deformities of the Spine and Thorax. St. Louis, C. V. Mosby, 1929.

38. Tambornino, J., Armburst, E., and Moe, J. H.: Harrington instrumentation in correction of scoliosis. A comparison with cast correction. J. Bone Joint Surg., 44A:(2)313–321, 1969.

39. Volkmann, R.: Resektion von Rippendtucker bei Scoliose. Berl. Klin. Wehnsehr., 50, 1889.

# Chapter 2

# CLASSIFICATION AND TERMINOLOGY

## INTRODUCTION

In any scientific field, it is important to have a basic language. Without this language, we cannot communicate accurately. In the field of spinal deformity, a standardized language has developed, largely due to the efforts of the Scoliosis Research Society. Throughout this book we shall adhere to this standard terminology, deviating only when absolutely necessary.

## CLASSIFICATION

There are three basic types of spine deformity: scoliosis, kyphosis, and lordosis. These may occur singly or in combination. Deformities are also classified according to magnitude, location, direction, and etiology. Thus, a patient may be described as having a "30 degree right thoracic scoliosis due to cerebral palsy." Another patient might be described as having a "110 degree thoracolumbar congenital kyphosis." With such verbal description, an accurate portrayal of the deformity can be communicated.

Classification of spinal deformities by etiology is presented below.

### Structural Scoliosis

I. Idiopathic
  A. Infantile (0–3 years)
    1. Resolving
    2. Progressive
  B. Juvenile (3–10 years)
  C. Adolescent (> 10 years)
II. Neuromuscular
  A. Neuropathic
    1. Upper motor neuron
      a. Cerebral palsy
      b. Spinocerebellar degeneration
        i. Friedreich's disease
        ii. Charcot-Marie-Tooth disease
        iii. Roussy-Lévy disease
      c. Syringomyelia
      d. Spinal cord tumor
      e. Spinal cord trauma
      f. Other
    2. Lower motor neuron
      a. Poliomyelitis
      b. Other viral myelitides
      c. Traumatic
      d. Spinal muscular atrophy
        i. Werdnig-Hoffmann
        ii. Kugelberg-Welander
      e. Myelomeningocoele (paralytic)
    3. Dysautonomia (Riley-Day)
    4. Other
  B. Myopathic
    1. Arthrogryposis
    2. Muscular dystrophy
      a. Duchenne (pseudohypertrophic)
      b. Limb-girdle
      c. Facioscapulohumeral
    3. Fiber type disproportion
    4. Congenital hypotonia
    5. Myotonia dystrophica
    6. Other

III. Congenital
    A. Failure of formation
        1. Wedge vertebra
        2. Hemivertebra
    B. Failure of segmentation
        1. Unilateral (unsegmented bar)
        2. Bilateral
    C. Mixed
IV. Neurofibromatosis
V. Mesenchymal disorders
    A. Marfan's
    B. Ehlers-Danlos
    C. Others
VI. Rheumatoid disease
VII. Trauma
    A. Fracture
    B. Surgical
        1. Post-laminectomy
        2. Post-thoracoplasty
    C. Irradiation
VIII. Extraspinal contractures
    A. Postempyema
    B. Post-burns
IX. Osteochondrodystrophies
    A. Diastrophic dwarfism
    B. Mucopolysaccharidoses (e.g., Morquio's syndrome)
    C. Spondyloepiphyseal dysplasia
    D. Multiple epiphyseal dysplasia
    E. Other
X. Infection of bone
    A. Acute
    B. Chronic
XI. Metabolic disorders
    A. Rickets
    B. Osteogenesis imperfecta
    C. Homocystinuria
    D. Others
XII. Related to lumbosacral joint
    A. Spondylolysis and spondylolisthesis
    B. Congenital anomalies of lumbo-sacral region
XIII. Tumors
    A. Vertebral column
        1. Osteoid osteoma
        2. Histiocytosis X
        3. Other
    B. Spinal cord (see neuromuscular)

## Nonstructural Scoliosis

I. Postural scoliosis
II. Hysterical scoliosis
III. Nerve root irritation
    A. Herniation of nucleus pulposus
    B. Tumors

IV. Inflammatory (e.g., appendicitis)
V. Related to leg length discrepancy
VI. Related to contractures about the hip

## Kyphosis

I. Postural
II. Scheuermann's disease
III. Congenital
    A. Defect of formation
    B. Defect of segmentation
    C. Mixed
IV. Neuromuscular
V. Myelomeningocele
    A. Developmental (late paralytic)
    B. Congenital (present at birth)
VI. Traumatic
    A. Due to bone and/or ligament damage without cord injury
    B. Due to bone and/or ligament damage with cord injury
VII. Post-surgical
    A. Post-laminectomy
    B. Following excision of vertebral body
IX. Post-irradiation
X. Metabolic
    A. Osteoporosis
        1. Senile
        2. Juvenile
    B. Osteomalacia
    C. Osteogenesis imperfecta
    D. Other
XI. Skeletal dysplasias
    A. Achondroplasia
    B. Mucopolysaccharidoses
    C. Neurofibromatosis
    D. Other
XII. Collagen disease
    A. Marie-Strümpell
    B. Other
XIII. Tumor
    A. Benign
    B. Malignant
        1. Primary
        2. Metastatic
XIV. Inflammatory

## Lordosis

I. Postural
II. Congenital
III. Neuromuscular
IV. Post-laminectomy
V. Secondary to hip flexion contracture
VI. Other

## Classification by Anatomic Area

Curvatures are described by the area of the spine in which the *apex* of the curve is located.

Cervical curve: apex between C1–C6.
Cervicothoracic curve: apex at C7–T1.
Thoracic curve: apex between T2–T11.
Thoracolumbar curve: apex at T12–L1.
Lumbar curve: apex between L2–L4.
Lumbosacral curve: apex at L5–S1.

*Note:* The word dorsal is not used for curve description. Dorsal is the opposite of ventral. All vertebrae have a dorsal aspect (i.e., the laminae and spinous processes).

## TERMINOLOGY

The terms listed in the preceding sections and the ones defined in the glossary below have been compiled by the terminology committee of the Scoliosis Research Society. This is an ongoing committee, and both the classification and terminology are revised periodically to incorporate advances in knowledge.

## A GLOSSARY OF SCOLIOSIS TERMS

**Adolescent scoliosis.** Spinal curvature presenting at or about the onset of puberty and before maturity.

**Adult scoliosis.** Spinal curvature existing after skeletal maturity.

**Angle of thoracic inclination.** With the trunk flexed 90 degrees at the hips, the angle between the horizontal and a plane across the posterior rib cage at the greatest prominence of a rib hump.

**Apical vertebra.** The most rotated vertebra in a curve; the most deviated vertebra from the vertical axis of the patient.

**Body alignment, balance, compensation.** 1) The alignment of the midpoint of the occiput over the sacrum in the same vertical plane as the shoulders over hips. 2) In roentgenology, when the sum of the angular deviations of the spine in one direction is equal to that in the opposite direction.

**Café au lait spots.** Light brown irregular areas of skin pigmentation. If sufficient in number and with smooth margins, they suggest neurofibromatosis.

**Compensatory curve.** A curve, which can be structural, above or below a major curve that tends to maintain normal body alignment.

**Congenital scoliosis.** Scoliosis due to congenitally anomalous vertebral development.

**Curve measurement.** Cobb method: Select the upper and lower end vertebrae. Erect perpendiculars to their transverse axes. They intersect to form the angle of the curve. If the vertebral end-plates are poorly visualized, a line through the bottom or top of the pedicles may be used.

**Double major scoliosis.** A scoliosis with two structural curves.

**Double thoracic curves (scoliosis).** Two structural curves within the thoracic spine.

**End vertebra.** 1) The most cephalad vertebra of a curve, whose superior surface tilts maximally toward the concavity of the curve. 2) The most caudad vertebra whose inferior surface tilts maximally toward the concavity of the curve.

**Fractional curve.** A compensatory curve that is incomplete because it returns to the erect. Its only horizontal vertebra is its caudad or cephalad one.

**Full curve.** A curve in which the only horizontal vertebra is at the apex.

**Nonstructural curve.** A curve that has no structural component and that corrects or overcorrects on recumbent side-bending roentgenograms.

**Gibbus.** A sharply angular kyphos.

**Hysterical scoliosis.** A nonstructural deformity of the spine that develops as a manifestation of a conversion reaction.

**Idiopathic scoliosis.** A structural spinal curvature for which no cause is established.

**Iliac epiphysis, iliac apophysis.** The epiphysis along the wing of an ilium.

**Inclinometer.** An instrument used to measure the angle of thoracic inclination or rib hump.

**Infantile scoliosis.** Spinal curvature developing during the first three years of life.

**Juvenile scoliosis.** Spinal curvature developing between skeletal age of three years and the onset of puberty.

**Kyphos.** A change in alignment of a segment of the spine in the sagittal plane that increases the posterior convex angulation.

**Kyphoscoliosis.** Lateral curvature of the spine associated with either increased posterior or decreased anterior angulation in the sagittal plane in excess of the accepted norm for that region. In the thoracic region 20 to 40 degrees of kyphosis is considered normal.

**Lordoscoliosis.** Lateral curvature of the spine associated with an increase in anterior curvature or a decrease in posterior angulation in the sagittal plane in excess of normal for that region. In the thoracic spine, where posterior angulation is normally present, less than 20 degrees' curvature constitutes lordoscoliosis.

**Major curve.** Term used to designate the largest structural curve.

**Minor curve.** Term used to refer to the smallest curve, which is always more flexible than the major curve.

**Pelvic obliquity.** Deviation of the pelvis from the horizontal in the frontal plane. Fixed pelvic obliquities can be attributable to contractures either above or below the pelvis.

**Primary curve.** The first or earliest of several curves to appear, if identifiable.

**Rib hump.** The prominence of the ribs on the convexity of a spinal curvature, usually due to vertebral rotation best exhibited on forward bending.

**Skeletal age, bone age.** The age obtained by comparing an anteroposterior roentgenogram of the left hand and wrist with the standards of the Gruelich and Pyle Atlas.

**Structural curve.** A segment of the spine with a lateral curvature that lacks normal flexibility. Radiographically, it is identified in supine lateral side-bending films by the failure to correct fully. They may be multiple.

**Vertebral end-plates.** The superior and inferior plates of cortical bone of the vertebral body adjacent to the intervertebral disc.

**Vertebral growth plate.** The cartilaginous surface covering the top and bottom of a vertebral body which is responsible for the linear growth of the vertebra.

**Vertebral ring apophyses.** The most reliable index of vertebral immaturity, seen best in lateral roentgenograms or in the lumbar region in side-bending anteroposterior views.

In the above glossary, several terms are used to describe curves. These terms have often been used interchangeably. It seems desirable to comment further at this time in order to avoid confusion for the reader later in this book. The terms causing confusion are as follows: primary curve, secondary curve, compensatory curve, major curve, minor curve, structural curve, and nonstructural curve.

A structural curve is "a segment of the spine with a lateral curvature having lack of normal flexibility. Radiographically, it is identified in supine bending films by the failure to correct." The key phrase here is "lack of normal flexibility." There is a segment or area of the spine that does not have normal mobility. By definition, then, a nonstructural curve has normal flexibility. A good example of a nonstructural curve is that seen in the lumbar spine of a patient with inequality of leg length. When the leg length is corrected by a lift, the curve disappears. In the sitting or supine position, the curve disappears. On bending films, the spine bends equally to the right and left, with no area of fixation. Leg length inequality, even if existing for many years, does not cause a structural curve.

A compensatory curve is "a curve above or below a major curve that tends to maintain normal body alignment. It may be structural or nonstructural." When a patient has a single structural curve, regardless of etiology, there must be a curve above and/or below that structural curve in order to keep the head above the pelvis. At first, the compensatory curve is fully flexible and thus nonstructural. However, over the course of time, because it is constantly present, the tissues develop "fixation" in this curved position, and the compensatory curve becomes structural. Even though it develops structural qualities, it is still a compensatory curve.

The term secondary curve is synonymous with compensatory curve. It is used in conjunction with the term primary curve, which describes the original structural curve of the patient.

A primary curve is "the first or earliest of

several curves to appear, if identifiable." Often the patient comes to the physician at the age of sixteen with two structural curves, both quite significant, both about equal in magnitude, and both having structural qualities. It can be quite difficult or even impossible to know whether the patient has one primary curve and one secondary curve with highly structural qualities or two primary curves. Double or even triple primary curves are well-recognized entities.

Because of the frequent impossibility of defining a "primary" curve, many physicians have abandoned that term and use instead the term major curve. A major curve is "the larger curve, always structural," as distinguished from a minor curve, which is "the lesser curve, which may be partially structural or nonstructural."

Thus, the patient presenting with two curves, both large and both structural, might be called a "double primary curve pattern" by one physician and a "double major curve pattern" by another. Neither physician is necessarily incorrect.

In this book, we will use the terms primary, compensatory, and major. We will not use the terms secondary or minor. We will use the term primary only when we know for sure that a curve was indeed the first curve. Figure 2–1 shows a patient who came to us with a double structural curve problem, both curves of large magnitude and quite structural. Is this a double primary pattern?

When radiographs were found that had been taken nine years previously (at age 3), it was obvious that the thoracic curve was "primary" and the lumbar curve "second-

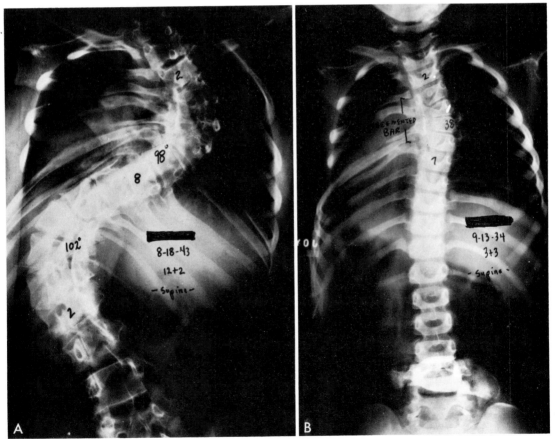

**Figure 2–1** A, Demonstrates a patient who came to us with a double structural curve problem, both curves of large magnitude and quite structural. Is this a "double primary pattern"? B, Radiographs were found that had been taken nine years previously at age 3. It was obvious that the thoracic curve was "primary" and the lumbar curve "secondary," but by age 12, the patient had a "double major" curve problem.

ary"; but by age 12, the patient had a "double major" curve problem.

## Bibliography

McAlister, W. H., and Shackelford, G. D.: Classification of spinal curvatures. Radiol. Clin. North Am., *13*:93–112, 1975.

Terminology Committee, Scoliosis Research Society: A glossary of scoliosis terms. Spine, *1*:57–58, 1976.

Cobb, J. R.: Outline for the Study of Scoliosis. Instructional Course Lectures, The American Academy of Orthopaedic Surgeons. Ann Arbor, J. W. Edwards, *5*:261, 1948.

Goldstein, L. A., and Waugh, T. R.: Classification and terminology of scoliosis, Clin. Orthop., *93*:10–22, 1973.

# Chapter 3

# PATIENT EVALUATION

When a patient with a spine deformity is first seen by the orthopedic surgeon, accurate evaluation and documentation of all findings are imperative. When the evaluation of the patient and of the deformity has been made, correct diagnosis of the etiology of the deformity can be made. The presence of any complications resulting from the deformity, such as pain, cardiopulmonary insufficiency, or neurologic loss, is sought and documented.

## HISTORY

A complete history is essential. It should include information concerning the spine deformity, the patient's general condition and health, family history, and the patient's age and maturity.

### Spine Deformity

The examining physician inquires as to how the deformity was first noted—routine school screening, routine physical examination by a family practitioner, or by a parent while fitting clothes. Has any increase in the deformity occurred since it was initially noted? If there has been any previous treatment, was it nonoperative or operative? Was a brace fitted? If so, what kind, by whom, and how long was it worn? Was it worn full-time or part-time? If previous surgical treatment has been performed, by whom, and what was the extent of postoperative immobilization? Is there any evidence of complications of the deformity, for example back pain? If so, what is the location, when does it occur, and is there any radiation of the pain? Is there any

evidence of cardiopulmonary decompensation? Are there any neurologic symptoms suggesting either a cause or a complication of the deformity?

### Patient History

The general health of the patient is evaluated. Have there been any previous illnesses, operations, or severe injuries? In cases where young children are seen with spine deformities, a prenatal and postnatal history is necessary. This includes the health of the mother during pregnancy, history of drugs taken during the first trimester, and the presence of complications during pregnancy or delivery or in the immediate postnatal period. Information with regard to general health and milestones of development during infantile and juvenile years is reviewed.

### Family History

A family history is taken concerning other family members with a spine deformity. The age of all the siblings is documented, and if possible, they are all examined briefly with the forward bending test to evaluate the presence of a spine deformity (see page 17). In certain familial neuromuscular diseases, a family history is especially important.

### Maturity

In the adolescent years, assessment of the maturity of the patient is very important.

**13**

This evaluation includes the onset of the rapid growth spurt in early adolescence, of menarche in girls, and of voice change in boys. The critical point is the onset of breast development and pubic hair development, as this marks the beginning of the early adolescent growth spurt. The menarche indicates a point at which approximately two thirds of the adolescent growth spurt has been completed. This information is used in the comparison of physiologic and skeletal age with chronologic age.

## PHYSICAL EXAMINATION

After the history has been taken, the patient is examined. There are three important areas to be documented—deformity, etiology, and complications. The patient should be examined undraped except for a small pair of underpants (Fig. 3–1A). In adolescent girls, who are often shy and withdrawn, it is permissible to use an examination gown open at the back. However, even if a gown is used, the chest must be examined at some stage

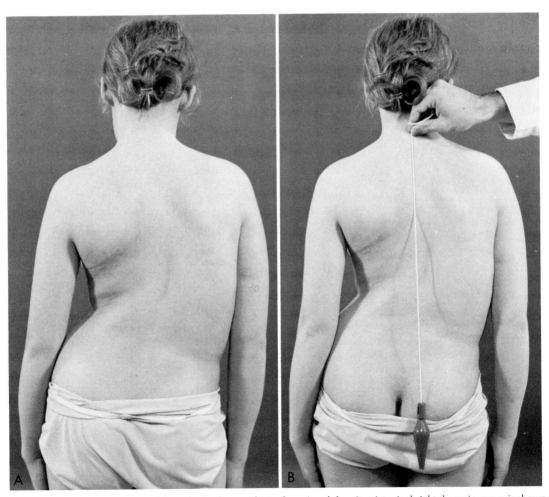

**Figure 3–1** A, Patient viewed from the back to evaluate the spine deformity. A typical right thoracic curve is shown. The left shoulder is lower and the right scapula more prominent. Note the decreased distance between the right arm and the thorax, with the shift of the thorax to the right. The left iliac crest appears higher, but this is due to the shift of the thorax with fullness on the right and elimination of the waistline. The "high" hip is thus only apparent, not real. B, Plumbline dropped from the prominent vertebra of C7 (vertebra prominens) measures the decompensation of the upper thorax over the pelvis. The distance from the vertical plumbline to the gluteal cleft is measured in centimeters and is recorded noting the direction of deviation. In this example, the deviation is to the right. When there is a cervical or cervicothoracic curve, the plumb should fall from the occipital protuberance (inion).

during the procedure. The patient is evaluated generally for body habitus and facies. The sitting and standing height, arm span, and weight are measured and recorded. In the general evaluation, the presence of dwarfism and other generalized diseases is noted.

Depending on the findings of the general evaluation, additional examination will focus on the suspected diagnosis; e.g., examine the cornea for clouding (mucopolysaccharidosis), palate for arching (Marfan's syndrome), ear for deformity (congenital deformity), neck for webbing (Turner's syndrome). A plumbline is used to measure the compensation of the trunk as related to the pelvis (Fig. 3–1B). The plumbline is made using a plumb-bob, the simplest plumb-bob being a weight tied to a piece of string. The string is held over the prominent spinous process of the seventh cervical vertebra (vertebra prominens) and a vertical line obtained with the weighted plumb. The distance from the vertical string to the gluteal cleft is measured in centimeters and noted as being a deviation to the right or the left. When cervical or cervicothoracic scoliosis is present, the plumb should fall from the inion (occipital protuberance).

The most dependable spot to use to compare the shoulder levels is the acromioclavicular joint, which can be seen both anteriorly and posteriorly. The distance from the level to the higher shoulder is measured in centimeters and charted (Fig. 3–2). Prominence of the trapezius neckline is also noted. Continuing to view the patient from behind, the level of the pelvis is noted. As the curve is often accompanied by decompensation of the torso over the pelvis, the level of the iliac crest may be difficult to feel. A more accurate evaluation is the comparison of the levels of the posterior or anterior superior iliac spines, the difference being approximated in centimeters.

The range of motion of the spine is noted on flexion, extension, and side bending. This side bending, especially side bending aided by the examiner, will indicate the flexibility of a curve (Fig. 3–3A). In paralytic patients with very severe deformities, the flexibility can be tested by grasping the head at the area of the mastoids and lifting the patient either from a sitting or standing position. This will demonstrate the flexibility of the curve and whether compensation can be obtained (Fig. 3–3B). Where pain is present, the exact area of ten-

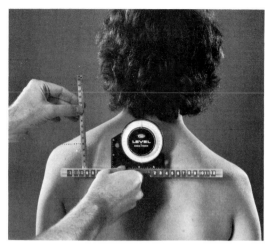

**Figure 3–2** Measurement of shoulder level using a level. Note the difference in the trapezius neck line and elevation of the left shoulder with a high left thoracic curve. The level is made horizontal and placed at the level of the acromioclavicular joint on the right. The vertical distance from the level to the high left shoulder is measured in centimeters. An elevation of the left shoulder of 4 centimeters is shown.

derness must be sought by careful palpation both in a standing and prone position.

One of the most important tests in the physical examination is the forward bending test, which permits evaluation of scoliosis, kyphosis, and lordosis. The patient bends forward at the waist, standing with the feet together and knees straight. The arms are dependent and do not rest on the legs. The hands are held together, fingers and palms opposed (Fig. 3–4). It is important to use a standardized position. If one knee is flexed, one arm held lower than the other, or the arms resting on the thighs, the back is not straight, and the presence of a prominence is impossible to evaluate. The patient is viewed from both the front and back. The examiner looks at the trunk with his eyes level with the back. The two sides—from the upper thoracic to the lumbosacral area—are compared, to see whether one side is higher than the other (Fig. 3–4B). A spirit level is placed over the area or areas of maximal prominence with the spirit level centered on the palpable spinous processes. The level is made horizontal and the distance from the zero mark to the highest point of the prominence measured. The same distance is then taken from the midline to the "valley" on the opposite side, and the perpendicular distance from the spirit level to

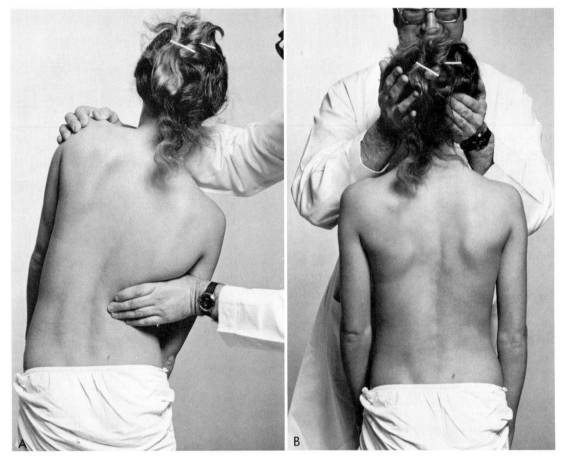

**Figure 3–3**   Evaluation of spine flexibility. *A,* Side bending to the right aided by the examiner demonstrates the flexibility of a right thoracic curve. *B,* In patients with severe or paralytic deformities, the flexibility is tested by grasping the head in the area of the mastoid processes and lifting the patient.

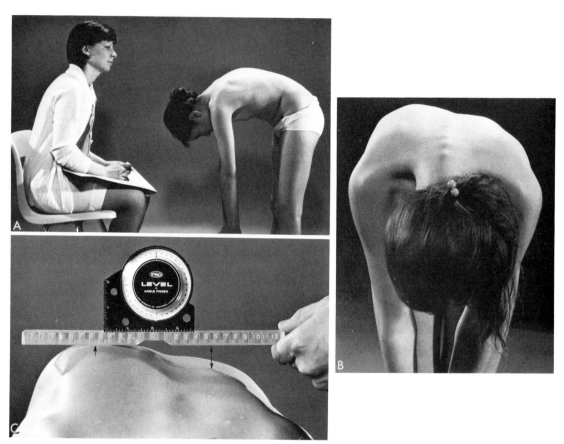

**Figure 3–4**   Forward bending test. *A,* The patient stands with feet together and knees straight and bends at the waist. The arms are dependent and held with fingers and palms opposed. The examiner looks down the back to view the thoracic and lumbar areas. (From Lonstein, J. E., et al: Minn. Med., 59:51, 1976; reprinted with permission.) *B,* The two sides are compared. Note the presence of a right thoracic prominence. *C,* Measurement of the prominence. The spirit level is positioned with the zero mark over the palpable spinous process in the area of maximal prominence. The level is made horizontal and the distance to the apex of the deformity (5 to 6 centimeters) noted. The perpendicular distance from the level to the valley is measured at the same distance from the midline. A 2.4 centimeter right thoracic prominence is shown.

the back is measured in millimeters (Fig. 3–4C).

When more than one prominence is present, each one is evaluated in a similar manner, and the side and site of the prominence (thoracic, high or low, thoracolumbar, or lumbar) are noted. When patients are unable to stand, an accurate determination cannot be made, but even in the sitting position, forward bending is still possible, and the size and site of the rotational problems can still be evaluated. It also should be noted whether the prominence is gentle or very sharp due to marked angulation of the ribs.

With the forward bending test, the correction of lordosis is noted. In the forward bending position, the patient is also viewed from the side to determine the lateral contour of the spine, i.e., gentle contour versus a sharp angular gibbus, indicating an area of structural kyphosis (Fig. 3–5).

During the forward bending test, attention is also paid to the manner in which the patient bends forward. With very tight hamstrings (as in spondylolisthesis), there is inability to bend forward or severe restriction

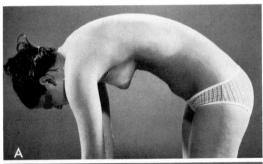
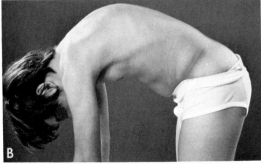

**Figure 3–5** Side view in forward bending position to view kyphosis. A, Normal thoracic roundness is demonstrated with a gentle curve to the whole spine. B, An area of increased bending is seen in the thoracic spine, indicating structural changes—Scheuermann's disease, in this example.

of forward bending (Fig. 3–6A). Occasionally a minimal curve is noted, which, on forward bending, shows a large rotational prominence, with the patient deviating to one side. This is indicative of an irritative lesion, especially a spinal cord tumor, osteoid osteoma, or herniated disc (Fig. 3–6B and C). Full neurologic evaluation and myelography are indicated in these patients.

The skin is examined for any evidence of café-au-lait spots or subcutaneous soft tumors to indicate neurofibromatosis (Fig. 3–7A). In addition, the skin of the back is inspected for any hair patches, dimples, skin pigmentation, or midline tumors to suggest a spinal dysraphism (Fig. 3–7B). In myelodysplastics, the condition of the skin of the back, as well as the presence of a sac and previous method of sac closure, is noted. (The skin of the whole body is inspected when café-au-lait spots are being sought). Scars on the chest wall due to previous thoracotomies for congenital cardiac defects or tracheo-esophageal fistulae are noted.

The chest is also inspected, and the state of maturity of the child is noted in terms of breast development in girls and pubic hair development in both sexes. Presence of a pectus excavatum or pectus carinatum is recorded, as well as of an anterior rib prominence. In scoliosis, the anterior prominence is on the side opposite the posterior rib prominence and is due to distortion and rotational deformity of the spine. The ears are inspected for evidence of preauricular ear tags or dimples (there is a correlation between the latter and congenital scoliosis). Joint flexibility is evaluated by thumb-to-wrist approximation, finger hyperextension, and knee and elbow recurvation (Fig. 3–7C).

The lower extremities are examined for the presence of hip or knee flexion contractures (Fig. 3–7D). In examining the feet, compare foot size and note any deformity (Fig. 3–7E and F).

A brief neurologic examination of the lower extremities is performed in all patients to test tone and reflexes (Fig. 3–7G). The distance between the anterior superior iliac spines and medial malleoli is used to compare leg lengths (Fig. 3–7I). In patients with neurologic disease, a complete neurologic evaluation with full sensory and motor testing is necessary. During the examination, an assessment is made of the patient's intelligence and mental status.

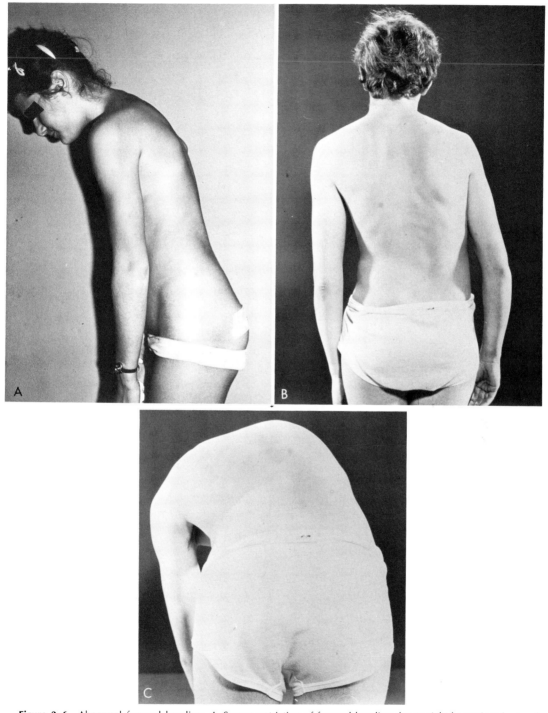

**Figure 3–6**  Abnormal forward bending. *A*, Severe restriction of forward bending due to tight hamstrings is seen in this patient with spondylolisthesis. *B*, A 16 year old boy with back pain shows trunk deviation to the left when viewed from the back. *C*, On forward bending, the trunk deviates to the left instead of forward, indicating a "spasm" curve. X-rays revealed an osteoid osteoma of the second lumbar vertebra.

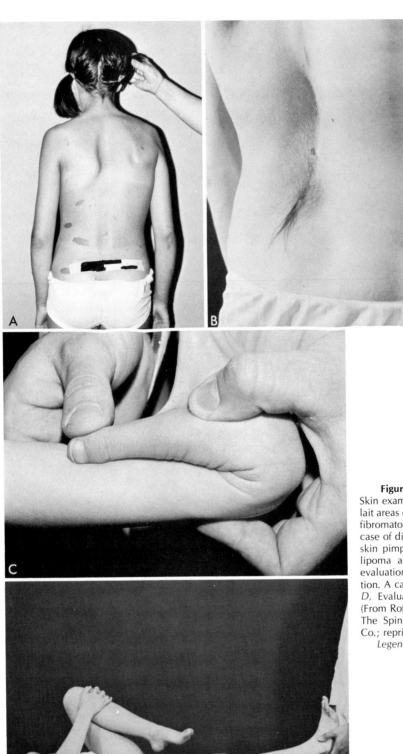

**Figure 3–7** Physical examination. *A,* Skin examination shows numerous café-au-lait areas of pigmentation, indicating neurofibromatosis. *B,* Lumbar hair patch seen in a case of diastematomyelia. In this condition, skin pimples, midline pigmentation, and a lipoma are also seen. *C,* Joint flexibility evaluation using thumb or wrist approximation. A case of extreme flexibility is shown. *D,* Evaluation of hip flexion contracture. (From Rothman, R. H., and Simeone, F. A.: The Spine, Philadelphia, W. B. Saunders Co.; reprinted with permission.)

*Legend continued on the opposite page*

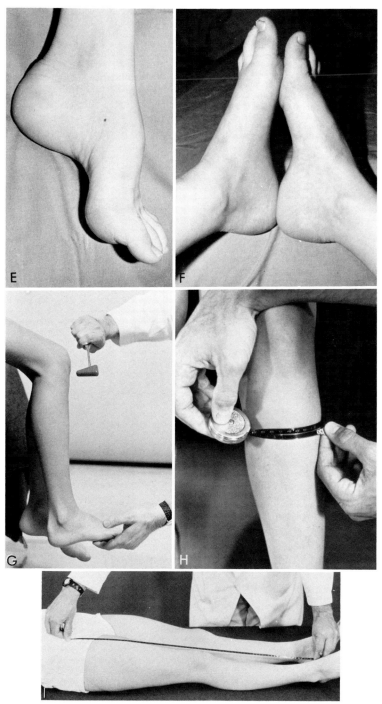

**Figure 3-7** *Continued* E, Foot deformities seen with spinal dysraphism. Note the marked cavus. F, Marked difference in foot size alerts the examining physician to the possibility of spinal dysraphism. G, Neurologic evaluation is mandatory for all patients. H, Measurement of thigh and calf circumference to evaluate hypertrophy or wasting. (From Rothman and Simeone; reprinted with permission.) I, Leg length accurately measured from the anterior superior iliac spine to the medial malleolus. (From Rothman and Simeone; reprinted with permission.)

## School Screening

The forward bending test (see Fig. 3–4) is used in the early detection of scoliosis by school screening. Schoolchildren are checked annually using this test.[57,106] The school nurses and the school physical education teachers are instructed in the basics of school screening and the mechanism of the foward bending test at regional workshops organized by the state health or education department aided by an orthopedic surgeon. With the forward bending test, very minor differences in the two sides can be appreciated. Once the deformity has been detected, the child is referred to the family physician. The forward bending test is repeated, and when necessary, a standing x-ray is taken to evaluate the deformity. If scoliosis is diagnosed, the child is referred to an orthopedic surgeon or crippled children's clinic for full evaluation and treatment.

## RADIOGRAPHIC EVALUATION[108]

After a complete history and physical examination have been performed, accurate assessment of the spine deformity is necessary to plan the course of therapy. The radiographic evaluation of the deformity is the most valuable diagnostic tool available to the orthopedic surgeon. With the aid of the radiographs, a diagnosis of the etiology and type of spine deformity is made. This documentation involves evaluation of the curvatures in terms of site, magnitude, and flexibility, as well as an assessment of the patient's maturity, which is an important factor in the choice of therapy. Additional specialized radiographic examinations, including myelography, angiography, laminography, and intravenous pyelography, are occasionally necessary.

One of the most important aspects of radiographic evaluation of the spine deformity is correct labeling and marking of each radiograph. The spine films are all viewed as if viewing the patient from the back; that is, the right side of the patient is viewed on the right side of the radiograph. All radiographs should be marked with the patient's name, institution where the radiograph was taken, the date, patient's age in years and months, and the patient's position (i.e., standing or supine) (Fig. 3–8A).[9] Where special distances (such as

6 feet, or 2 meters) are used, this fact should be noted on the radiograph, as should additional information, such as bending to the left, bending to the right, or oblique view. Since the radiograph is viewed opposite to all other radiographs, appropriate adjustment to the labeling is necessary so that with the radiograph in the viewing position, all the marking and labeling can be read. All the markings should be placed either at the top, in a corner, or along the side of the radiograph, where they will not interfere with the evaluation and measurement of the spine deformity. In addition, the side (right or left) should be labeled appropriately (Figs. 3–8 and 3–9).

This documentation is invaluable, as when these films are viewed later, the exact date, position, and manner of evaluation are easily available and cannot be erased from the film. It is far better to have the information photographically printed on the film than to write it there.

## Routine Radiographic Evaluation of Spine Deformity

For the accurate assessment of spine deformities, a standard series of radiographic projections are used. With scoliosis, upright anteroposterior (AP) and lateral views plus supine right and left bending views are taken (see Fig. 3–8). A kyphosis routine includes upright AP and lateral views and a supine hyperextension lateral view for flexibility. In addition, a radiograph of the left hand and wrist for evaluation of bone age is taken if the patient is under age 20.

### UPRIGHT EVALUATION

Upright x-ray films are obtained on all patients able to sit or stand. Standing anteroposterior and lateral views are taken, and sitting films are used in patients unable to stand. Such patients include the very young and those with paralysis or weakness of the lower extremities with inability to stand unaided or with a leg length difference that causes problems in standing erect. All upright radiographs are taken at a six-foot (two-meter) distance to standardize the evaluation and to allow accurate measurement of spine growth. The radiograph is taken using either a 14 × 36 inch (36 × 91 cm.) film or (where the latter

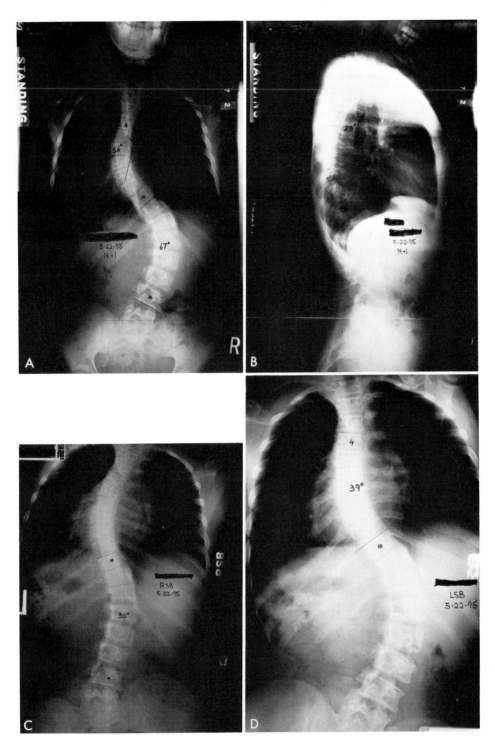

**Figure 3–8**  The series of radiographs for evaluation of scoliosis consists of: A, a standing anteroposterior view, B, standing lateral view, C, supine right side bending view, and D, supine left side bending view.

In the upper left corner the hospital name, date of evaluation, and patient's name should appear. The right and left sides are marked. On the standing x-ray the position (standing) and distance, 72 inches (2 meters) are recorded on the film, as are the name and age of the patient and the date.

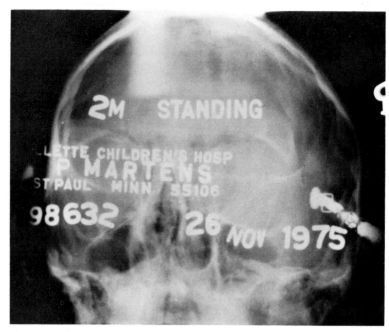

**Figure 3–9** Alternate method of x-ray marking—all the information is imprinted on the film radiographically.

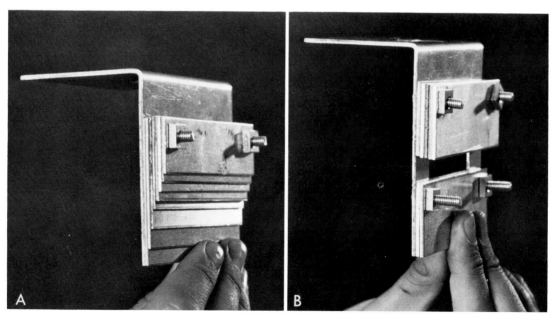

**Figure 3–10** Aluminum filters used to screen out a portion of the x-ray beam to give uniform density of the spine on the x-ray film. *A,* The anteroposterior filter consists of 1 mm. thick layers of aluminum, with the thickest portion in the region of the occiput and cervical spine. The filter gets progressively thinner and terminates opposite Ll. *B,* The lateral wedge filter has a thick portion in the area of the occiput and cervical spine. There is no filter in the area of the shoulder, a small filter in the thoracic area, and no filter in the lumbar area.

is not available) a 14 × 17 inch (36 × 43 cm.) film. The smaller film is positioned with the upper end just above the shoulders, allowing all or most of the spine to be viewed on one radiograph. This smaller film is all that is necessary to visualize the whole spine in infants and small children.

The larger (36 in., or 91 cm.) film is valuable for the complete assessment of older children and adults. With this film, the *whole* spine is seen on the radiograph. High thoracic or cervical curves are missed when the smaller (17 in., or 43 cm.) film is used. The relationship of the head and shoulders to the pelvis can be appreciated.

To make the radiographic density of the vertebral column uniform, an aluminum filter is used to screen out a portion of the radiation beam. The filters are placed on the x-ray tube in the path of the radiation beam. The anteroposterior filter is shown in Figure 3–10*A*. The thicker portion is in the region of the occiput and cervical spine, and the filter gets thinner and terminates opposite L1. The lateral wedge filter also consists of aluminum layers 1 millimeter thick, with the thicker portion again used in the region of the occiput and cervical spine. In the area of the shoulder and lumbar spine, there is no filter because of the large amount of radiation necessary to obtain an adequate x-ray film in these areas (Fig. 3–10*B*).

In the upright view, the spine is centered on the middle of the Bucky, and the special wedge filters are used for each projection. The top of the 14 × 36 inch cassette is placed at the level of the external auditory meatus, and both radiographs are taken on deep inspiration. In both views, the patient stands as upright as possible with no rotation present, with feet together and knees completely straight (Fig. 3–11). Shoes are not worn unless a lift is used in one shoe to correct leg length discrepancy.[10] In this case, an additional film may be taken without the lift. In patients unable to stand, an unsupported sitting view is taken. No hand support is used to stabilize the trunk and decrease the deformity; thus the full effects of gravity on the deformity are shown.

In the lateral projection, a standard position is used with the arms held at 90 degrees flexion of the shoulder and supported with the use of an IV (intravenous) standard. This can be raised and lowered and thus posi-

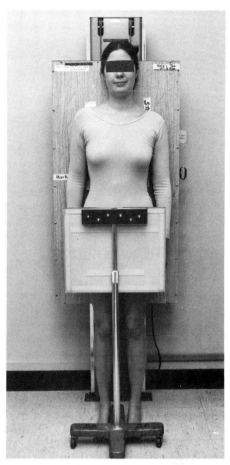

**Figure 3–11** Position for anteroposterior standing x-ray. The patient stands fully erect with feet together and knees straight. The 14 × 36 in. (36 × 91 cm.) cassette is positioned with the top at the external auditory meatus. Note the gonadal screen with the top at the level of the anterior superior iliac spines. This is used in all films except the initial series.

tioned at the correct height for each patient. The base must be stable (Fig. 3–12). In patients who stand with the aid of crutches, both standing and unsupported sitting x-ray films should be obtained. The latter shows the true status of the spine deformity without the suspension effects of the crutches.

On the initial AP upright evaluation, no screening of the gonadal area is used, since it is necessary to see the pelvis and hip joints. On all subsequent studies, a gonadal screen is used. The one found to be most effective is a lead screen of appropriate thickness fixed to an IV stand, which can be raised and lowered, and the shield is positioned over the

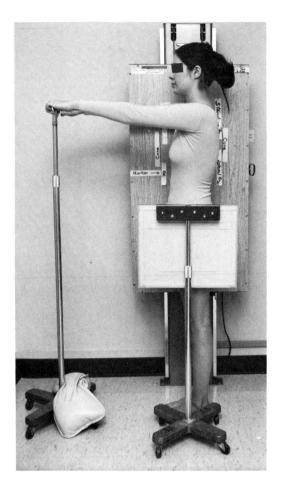

**Figure 3–12** Position for lateral standing x-ray. The erect position and cassette placement are the same as in Figure 3–11. The arms are positioned at shoulder height and are resting on an IV standard, which can be adjusted to the patient's height. Note the gonadal screen positioned with the top at the level of the anterior superior iliac spine. If it is positioned too high, the sacroiliac joint will be obscured. Note the film markers on the cassette holder.

lower abdomen. The upper end of this shield should be just below the iliac crest, allowing evaluation of the iliac crest epiphyses (see Figs. 3–11 and 3–12).

In patients wearing a cast or brace, appropriate adjustments in the exposure are necessary to adequately demonstrate the spine.

### SUPINE EVALUATION

Supine radiographs are taken in selected cases to show the status of the deformity with the effect of gravity eliminated. In patients unable to sit (the severely paralyzed or the very young), these supine films form the basis of the evaluation. Supine x-ray films are also used in the course of treatment, for example in monitoring of the effect of traction, postoperatively, and in the assessment of the fusion. The supine radiograph is made on a 14 × 17 inch (36 × 43 cm.) film at a standard

40 inch (102 cm.) distance without the use of filters. As this film usually gives better bone detail than the standing view, it is valuable for the assessment of congenital anomalies and other lesions.

### FLEXIBILITY EVALUATION (Fig. 3–13)

After assessing the magnitude of the deformity in the upright position, knowledge of the flexibility of the curves is important. Flexibility views consist of active side bending x-ray films in scoliosis, hyperextension films[10] in kyphosis, and flexion views in lordosis. These radiographs are all taken with the patient in a supine position, and they involve active muscle power for correction of the deformity. In patients with large curves (over 90 degrees) or neuromuscular scoliosis, a traction film is often used, as there is inadequate muscle power for active correction of the deformities. In some centers the traction film is used in all cases to show the correctability of the deformity.

**Side Bending View.** Once the curve pattern has been determined on a standing film, side bending views are taken to demonstrate the flexibility of each curve. The patient is supine with maximal voluntary side bending toward the convexity of the curve, using a 14 × 17 inch film (Fig. 3–13A). For example, if there is a left high thoracic, right thoracic, left lumbar curve pattern, side bending films are taken showing the high left thoracic area bending to the left, the right thoracic area bending to the right, and the left lumbar area bending to the left. Sometimes separate exposures are necessary for each curve evaluation. In small children, left and right side bending films will show the whole spine on the radiograph and are all that is necessary. In positioning the radiograph, an attempt is made to make the pelvis parallel to the bottom of the Bucky. If obliquity of the lumbosacral area is demonstrated in the upright evaluation, a side bending view of the lumbosacral junction is necessary to evaluate the flexibility of this fractional or partial curve. Each film has to be marked accurately to show that the evaluation is supine and marked as LSB (left side bending) or RSB (right side bending).

**Hyperextension.** Flexibility of kyphosis is shown with a hyperextension x-ray film. This is taken with the patient supine and lying on a styrofoam block centered at the apex of the kyphosis. A lead arrow is placed in the center of the styrofoam block to show where the maximum correcting force is situated. A cross-table lateral view shows the flexibility of the kyphosis (Fig. 3–13B).

**Lordosis.** When lordosis is present, its flexibility is determined with a forward flexion x-ray film. As lordosis is usually in the lumbar or thoracolumbar area, flexibility can be seen with a lateral radiograph taken in the knee-chest position, that is, with the knees maximally flexed on the abdomen. This view can be obtained with the patient supine, on the side, or sitting and flexed forward over the knees (Fig. 3–13C, D, and E).

**Traction Radiograph.** In neuromuscular diseases, the patient is often unable to actively correct the deformity, and either a passive side bending film or a traction film is necessary. A supine AP radiograph is taken with two technicians giving maximum distraction, one by grasping the head at the mastoid processes or using a disposable head halter, and the other pulling the legs, with maximum force being applied as the radiograph is taken (Fig. 3–13F).

All these flexibility views are then compared with the standing and supine views to show the maximum correctability of the curves.

## EVALUATION OF MATURITY

A spot AP radiograph of the left hand and wrist is taken in all patients under 20. This is compared with the standard views in the Greulich and Pyle Atlas.[42] It demonstrates the skeletal age of the patient, which is compared with the chronologic age and is used in conjunction with the evaluation of the iliac epiphyses and vertebral ring apophyses. Because knowledge of bone maturity is invaluable in planning a treatment program, skeletal age is of more benefit than chronologic age, as it gives a true representation of bone maturity.

## SPECIAL VIEWS

In certain instances, special views are necessary to demonstrate the spine anatomy. The commonest are the oblique films of the fusion area to demonstrate the incorporation of the bone graft and adequacy of the fusion mass. These are taken supine in the right and left oblique planes to present the fusion mass in profile. Oblique views are also used in the lumbosacral area to demonstrate the presence of a pars interarticularis defect in spondylolisthesis. In addition, a spot lateral standing radiograph is sometimes necessary to show the anatomy of the lumbosacral junction, as this might not be adequately seen on the standing 36 inch (92 cm.) film.

With abnormalities at the lumbosacral junction, a Ferguson view is necessary. This is a radiograph taken with the tube tilted cephalad 30 degrees in a male and 35 degrees in a female. The x-ray beam in this view goes through the lumbosacral intervertebral disc and demonstrates the anatomy of this junction, eliminating the effects of lordosis (Fig. 3–14).

A similar view can be obtained if a supine AP radiograph is taken with the hips flexed approximately 90 degrees. This position also eliminates lumbar lordosis. The

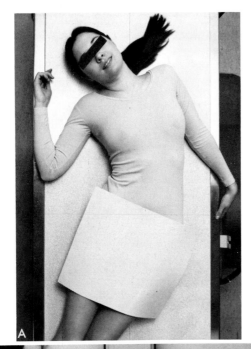

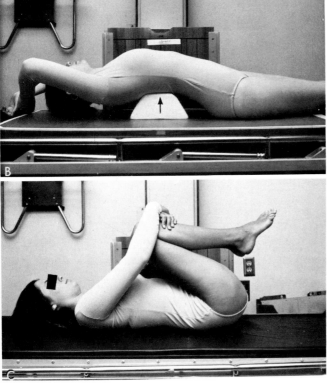

**Figure 3–13** Flexibility evaluation. *A,* Supine right side bending position to evaluate the flexibility of a right thoracic curve. The patient bends actively to the right with maximal bending as the exposure is taken. Note the gonadal screen. *B,* Hyperextension position to evaluate the flexibility of kyphosis. The patient lies on a styrofoam block, which is positioned under the apex of the kyphosis. A lead arrow in the block indicates the apex of the hyperextension force on the film. *C,* Flexion position for flexibility evaluation of lordosis. Patient is either supine or sitting, and the x-ray is taken in maximum flexion, with knees drawn up to the chest (knee-chest position).

*Legend continued on the opposite page*

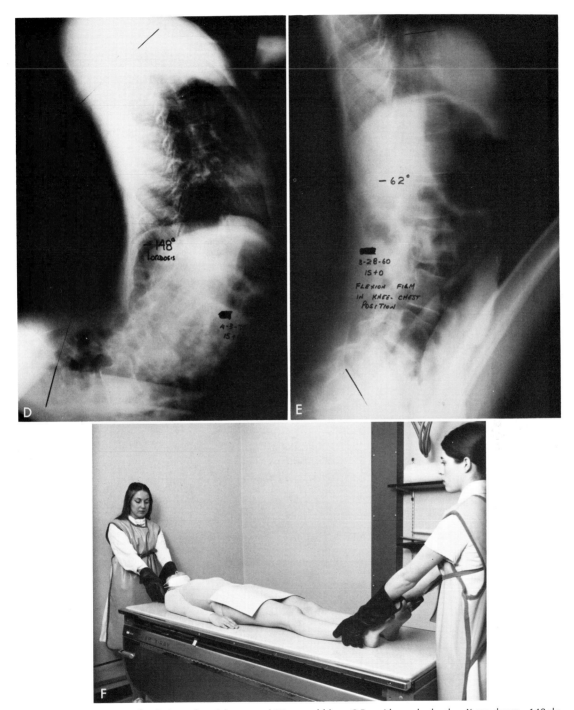

**Figure 3–13** *Continued.* *D,* Lateral upright x-ray of 15 year old boy, S.B., with cerebral palsy. X-ray shows −148 degrees of lordosis. *E,* Flexion film of S.B. taken in knee-chest position, showing correction to −62 degrees of lordosis. *F,* Traction film. This is used in patients with large curves (over 90 degrees) or in patients with neuromuscular scoliosis. Traction is applied by a disposable head halter and leg traction.

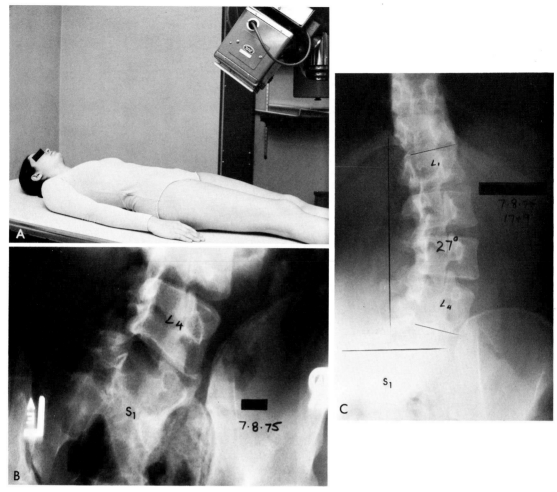

**Figure 3–14**   Ferguson view. *A,* Position for Ferguson view. The patient is supine, and the tube is tilted cephalad so that the x-ray beam goes through the lumbosacral joint. *B,* Anteroposterior view shows a right lumbar curve, but the lumbosacral joint cannot be seen, a shift to the right being obvious. *C,* In the Ferguson view the anatomy of the lumbosacral area is seen. The sacrum is normal, and there is a hemivertebra at L5 causing an acute tilt of L4.

Ferguson view should not be used routinely, as the gonadal irradiation from this one view is equal to the total irradiation of a routine scoliosis series.

**Curve Evaluation**

When a complete series of radiographs has been obtained, they are reviewed by the orthopedic surgeon to evaluate the curve pattern, magnitude and flexibility, and the patient's maturity. The important films for the initial evaluation are the upright anteroposterior and lateral views, as the curve pattern and measurements are determined on these.

In fact, one or both of these standing views is all that is necessary to determine the presence of a curve, and if one is present, the remainder of the routine views are taken.

*GENERAL EVALUATION*

General evaluation of the radiograph is performed to help determine the etiology of the spine deformity. The presence of congenital anomalies is sought, such as hemivertebra, wedge vertebra, failure of segmentation, unsegmented bar, or "block" vertebra. The length of the curve is observed. A short angular curve raises the suspicion of neurofibromatosis; a long sweeping C curve suggests neuromuscular disease.

In addition to the vertebrae, other structures appearing on the radiograph are examined. In paralytic spine deformities, there may be rib drooping, owing to intercostal paralysis (Fig. 3–15). In neurofibromatosis, there is scalloping of the vertebral bodies as well as thin spindly ribs (Fig. 3–16). Rib synostosis is often found accompanying congenital scoliosis. The humeral heads, scapulae, lung fields, heart, pelvis, and proximal femurs must also be examined. In congenital spine deformities and when a suspicion of spinal dysraphism or spine tumor exists, the distance between the pedicles is measured (interpediculate distance), and the midline bony spur of a diastematomyelia is sought (Fig. 3–17).

## CURVE PATTERN

Once the diagnosis has been made and congenital anomalies sought, the curve pat-

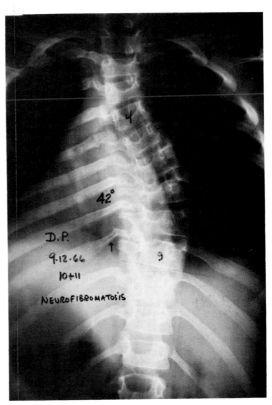

**Figure 3–16** Standing x-ray of a 10 year, 11 month old boy, showing a 42 degree right thoracic curve. Note the thinning of the neck of the ribs on the left side. The head of the rib is deformed in the area of the concavity of the curve. Mild vertebral scalloping is seen on the right. These features are hallmarks of neurofibromatosis.

tern, seen on the upright anteroposterior radiograph, is evaluated. The curve site is classified according to the position of the apical vertebra—cervical, thoracic, or lumbar. In a junctional curve (cervicothoracic or thoracolumbar), the apex is at the junction of the two areas, e.g., for a thoracolumbar curve the apex of the curve is at T12, between T12 and L1, or at L1.

Note that the term dorsal is not used interchangeably with thoracic. This is because anatomically all the vertebrae are dorsal with reference to the body, dorsal being the opposite of ventral. The correct anatomic term is thus thoracic.

## CURVE MEASUREMENT

Once the curve pattern has been noted, the magnitude and extent of each curve is de-

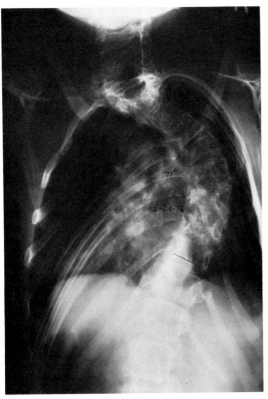

**Figure 3–15** Rib droop due to intercostal paralysis. This is a radiographic indication of neuromuscular scoliosis.

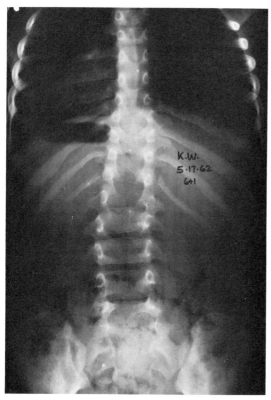

**Figure 3–17** In diastematomyelia the distance between the pedicles in the lumbar spine is increased. This is especially obvious at L2. A midline bony spur is visible at the upper part of the body of L2.

vexity of a curve. The disc space next to the end vertebra is usually parallel to the vertebra, as this is a transitional area between two curves.

After the cranial and caudal end vertebrae of *each* curve have been identified, the curves are measured. A line is drawn at the upper end of the cranial end vertebra along the end-plate, or by marking the upper or lower edges of the pedicle shadows (use the most clearly defined line). A line is drawn at the lower end of the caudal vertebra at the inferior end-plate of the body or the lower end of the pedicle shadows. Note that the pedicles are used only if they are clearly visible and symmetrical. It is the angle formed by these two lines that is measured. Lines are drawn at right angles to the two end vertebral lines, and the angle formed is the one measured. This is called the Cobb-Lippman technique of measurement.[18]

When the first curve has been measured, the remainder of the curves are measured in a similar manner. Theoretically a new line is necessary to include the end vertebra in each curve. However, if vertebral wedging is not present, this is not necessary, as the lower and upper bony plates of the vertebral body are parallel. Thus, the lines marking the ends of the first measured curve are used to measure the adjacent curves. It is important to note that the end vertebra is shared by two curves. Thus, the curves are described as, for example, T4–T12 right thoracic curve or T12–L4 left lumbar curve.

*Vertebral Rotation.* The shadows of the pedicles demonstrate the degree of vertebral rotation present. This system was described by Nash and Moe[73] and classified into four grades (Fig. 3–19). Zero rotation is when the pedicle shadows are symmetrical and equidistant from the sides of the vertebral bodies. Grade I rotation is when the pedicle shadow has moved away from the side of the ver-

termined (Fig. 3–18). The first step is identification of the end vertebrae. They are identified by the following characteristics:

1) The end vertebra is the last vertebra that is tilted into the concavity of the curvature being measured. When there are parallel vertebrae at the end of a curve, the one farthest from the apex is the end vertebra.

2) The disc spaces are normally narrower on the concavity and wider on the con-

**Figure 3–18** Curve measurement. *A,* The first step is identification of the end vertebrae of a curve. The end vertebrae are the last vertebrae tilted into the concavity of the curve being measured. The next vertebrae tilt away from the concavity of the curve. *B,* The disc spaces are narrower on the concavity of the curve and wider on the convexity. The disc spaces next to the end vertebrae are parallel. The next disc space is wedged in the opposite direction, being narrower on the concavity of the adjacent curve. *C,* The end vertebrae are T6 and T12. A line is drawn at the lower end-plate of T12 and a perpendicular drawn to this line. An alternate line at the lower end of the pedicles is shown. *D,* The procedure is repeated by drawing a line at the upper end-plate of T6, and the angle between the two perpendiculars is measured with a protractor. The lower end of the pedicles can also be used to mark the end vertebrae when the pedicles are well defined.

*Illustration continued on the opposite page*

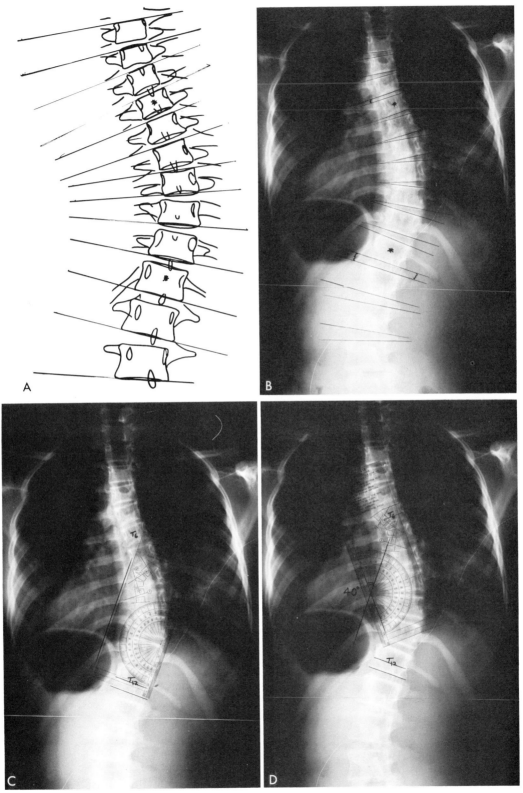

**Figure 3–18**  *See opposite page for legend.*

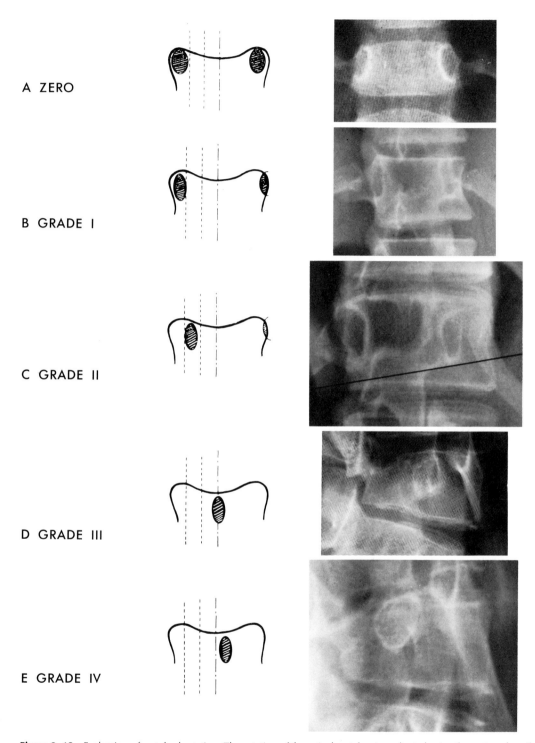

**Figure 3–19** Evaluation of vertebral rotation. The rotation of the apical vertebra is evaluated using the system described by Nash and Moe.[73] A, Zero rotation. The pedicle shadows are equidistant from the sides of the vertebral bodies. B, Grade I rotation. The pedicle shadow on the convexity has moved from the edge of the vertebral body. C, Grade II rotation. Rotation intermediate between Grade I and III. D, Grade III rotation. The pedicle shadow is close to the center of the vertebral body. E, Grade IV rotation. The pedicle shadow is past the center of the vertebral body. (From Nash and Moe, 1969.)

tebral body. In Grade III rotation, the pedicle shadow is in the center of the vertebral body. Grade II is intermediate between Grades I and III. Grade IV rotation is when the pedicle shadow is past the center of the vertebral body and is closer to the side of the concavity of the curve. The end vertebra commonly has neutral rotation. Sometimes rotation, especially in long thoracic or thoracolumbar curves, continues beyond the end vertebra of the major curve into the compensatory curve below.

After the curves have been measured, they are marked on the radiograph, with care being taken to label the vertebrae. These have to be counted to identify the vertebral bodies correctly, as there are often 11 or 13 ribs and an extra lumbar vertebra. In addition to marking the magnitude of the curves and the end vertebrae with a soft-tip lead pencil that is easily erasable from the radiograph (alcohol sponges are used for this), the patient's name, date of examination, chronologic age, and position of examination are marked in an area where they are easily seen—usually in the upper abdomen, where the radiograph is lighter.

The same technique is used on the lateral projection. End vertebrae are identified according to the criteria just described, and any kyphosis or lordosis is measured. On this radiograph the best method for finding the end vertebra is to look for the vertebra that is tilted into the concavity of the curve and that when measured would give the largest curve (Fig. 3–20). With the identification of the amount of kyphosis or lordosis, a simple system for documenting these is to call all kyphotic angles positive (+) and all lordotic curves negative (−), zero degrees being a straight spine. In this manner, the curves can be evaluated and documented using a standard nomenclature.

In congenital spine anomalies the description of the site of the anomaly is very important, especially with reference to failure of vertebral body formation (hemivertebra). All the vertebrae and hemivertebrae are numbered, from the cranial to the caudal extremity (Fig. 3–21). In addition, all the hemivertebrae are numbered. Thus the anomaly associated with a midthoracic hemivertebra is described as follows: "A hemivertebra is situated at T6 on the right with an associated 45 degree curve from T5 to T7." The incorrect

way to describe the hemivertebra is to say, "A hemivertebra is situated between T5 and T6 on the right." In addition to counting the vertebrae, the ribs need to be carefully examined and counted, as commonly a hemivertebra has an associated rib. Areas of failure of vertebral body segmentation usually have associated defects of rib segmentation.

When all the curves have been identified, marked, and measured on the upright views, the flexibility films—that is, the side bending, flexion and hyperextension views—are measured. The end vertebrae, having been identified on the upright film, are now constant for the remainder of the radiographic evaluation. They are usually constant for the remainder of the patient's course of treatment. When brace treatment shortens the length of the curve, the new curve is measured. With the flexibility radiographs, the end vertebrae are identified and the curve measured. Often the central portion is more rigid on side bending, and if this central area were measured, a lesser degree of flexibility would be found. It is important to measure the same curve on the upright and flexibility radiographs. Lack of flexibility can be noted as follows: "The standing x-ray shows a 30 degree T5–T12 right thoracic curve, which on side bending corrects to 8 degrees, but the central apical portion shows more rigidity." With flexible curves, there is overcorrection of the curve, which is documented as a negative amount; for example, a 20 degree curve corrects to −5 degrees. When measuring flexibility, only the side bending film to show correction is measured, for example, a right side bending film of a right-sided curve. The left side bending film of that curve is not measured.

The same procedure is followed for the hyperextension lateral radiograph of a kyphotic curvature or a forward bending film of a lordotic curve to document the flexibility of these deformities.

### MATURITY

In determining a patient's maturity, a number of radiographic factors are used.

**Bone Age.** Bone age is evaluated using the radiograph of the left hand. This film is taken on all patients under the age of 20 and is compared to the standards found in the Greulich and Pyle Atlas.[42]

**Iliac Epiphyses.** The ossification of the

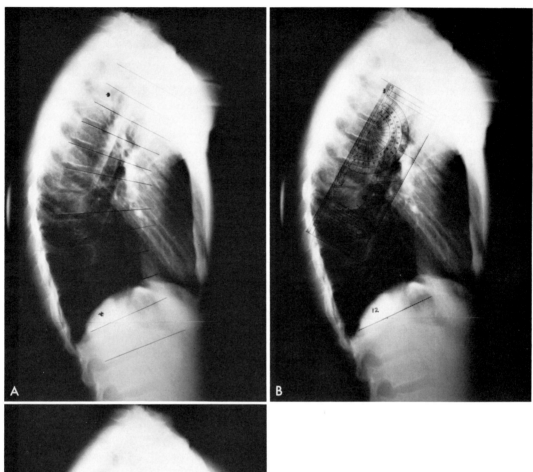

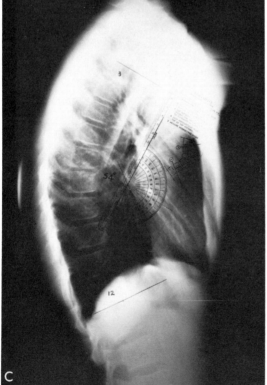

**Figure 3–20** Kyphosis measurement. *A,* The end vertebrae are identified. These vertebrae are the last vertebrae tilted *into* the concavity of the kyphosis. The next vertebrae tilt away from this concavity. *B,* The end vertebrae are T3 and T12. A line is drawn at the upper end-plate of T3 and a perpendicular drawn to this line. *C,* The procedure is repeated by drawing a line at the lower end-plate of T12. The angle between these two perpendiculars is measured using a protractor, indicating kyphosis with a + (positive) sign, +54 in this example. A similar method is used to measure lordosis, indicating lordosis with a − (negative) sign.

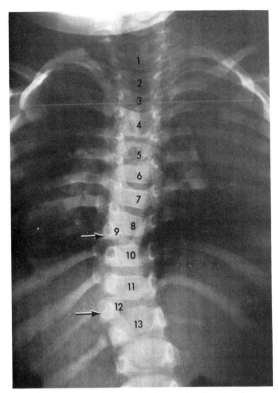

**Figure 3–21** Anteroposterior projection to demonstrate numbering of hemivertebrae. There are two hemivertebrae on the left, and the vertebrae are numbered from cranial to caudal, *each* hemivertebra being numbered.

iliac crests as originally described by Risser[84] is evaluated. This is especially important in brace patients, as the effectiveness of the orthosis and the wearing schedule depend on bone maturity.[9, 70] Normally, ossification starts at the anterior superior iliac spine and progresses posteriorly to the posterior superior iliac spine, but it may appear in a fragmented manner. Once complete ossification has occurred, fusion of the epiphysis with the ilium takes place. Risser divided the iliac crest into four quarters and thus designated the excursion as 1+ with 25 per cent of the excursion completed, 2+ with 50 per cent, 3+ with 75 per cent, 4+ for complete excursion, and 5+ when the excursion and the fusion to the ilium were complete (Fig. 3–22).

A study by Green and Anderson[1] has shown a correlation with Risser's 5+ sign and cessation of height increase.

***Vertebral Ring Apophyses.*** The vertebral ring apophyses lie at the upper and lower margins of the body overlying the cartilage growth plate. These initially appear as a separate ossified area (Fig. 3–23) and form a complete ring, which fuses with the vertebral bodies. They are seen most clearly on the lateral x-ray film but with experience can be easily identified on the anteroposterior projection. Fusion of the apophysis with the body coincides with complete cessation of spine growth.

### Special Radiographic Studies

Certain radiographic studies are used in special cases in the evaluation of spine deformity. These studies are the laminogram, myelogram, intravenous pyelogram, derotated view of curve, "rib hump" view, angiogram, and upper gastrointestinal evaluation.

### LAMINOGRAM

A laminogram, or tomogram, is a radiologic technique for visualization of difficult areas. An anatomic visualization is obtained of an anomaly or other deformity as if the bone had been sliced and each slice separately examined. This effect is obtained by having both the x-ray source and x-ray plate moving while the film is being taken. This in effect puts only a specific area into focus, with the remainder of the body out of focus. This area is varied to obtain a series of radiographs (Fig. 3–24).

***Indications.*** The laminogram is used in cases of congenital spine anomalies where the actual pathology is obscure on the plain radiographs. It is used in congenital scoliosis and kyphosis to evaluate the true anatomy of the deformity, in anterior fusions to evaluate the incorporation of the bone graft, and for special lesions such as osteoid osteoma.

### MYELOGRAM (SPINOGRAM)

***Indications.*** A myelogram is *not* a routine investigation performed on all patients with spine deformity. It is used on special occasions with specific indications. Where widening of the interpediculate distance is found, a myelogram should be performed. With careful study of the radiograph for a bony spur in the midline, the myelogram permits diagnosis of spinal dysraphism and diastematomyelia (Fig. 3–25). In syringomyelia

*Text continued on page 42*

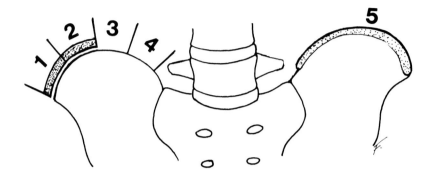

A

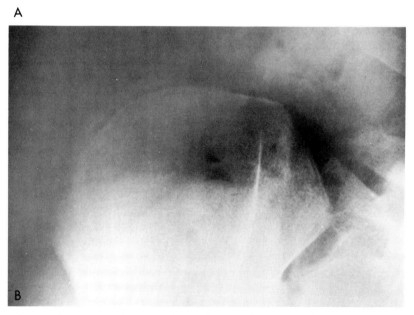

B

**Figure 3-22**   Iliac epiphysis. *A,* Ossification of the epiphysis usually starts at the anterior superior iliac spine and progresses posteriorly. The iliac crest is divided into four quarters, and the excursion or stage of maturity is designated as the amount of progression. In the example shown, the excursion is 50 per cent complete, and the Risser sign is thus 2+. On the right, the excursion is complete *and* the epiphysis has fused with the iliac crest—a Risser 5+sign. *B,* A Risser 2+excursion.

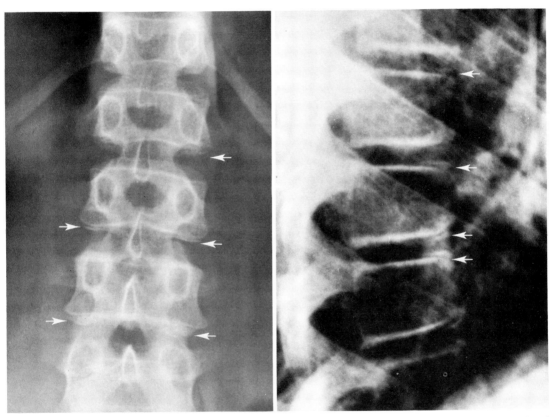

**Figure 3–23** Anteroposterior and lateral x-ray films showing ring apophysis ossification adjacent to the vertebral end-plates. The ossification is more easily seen on the lateral view.

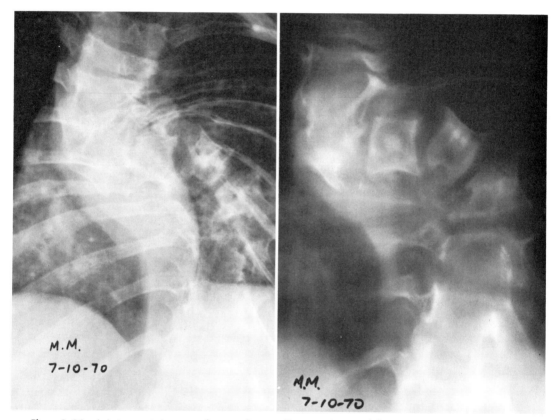

**Figure 3–24**   *A,* Anteroposterior x-ray of a case of a neurofibromatosis spine deformity. The vertebral anatomy is poorly visualized. *B,* Anteroposterior laminogram demonstrates the severe vertebral dysplasia caused by the neurofibromatosis.

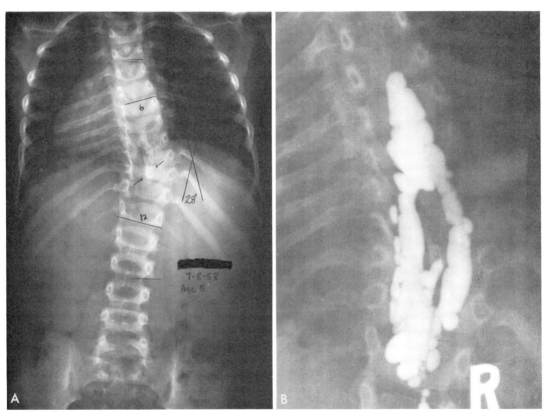

**Figure 3–25** Myelogram. A, Diastematomyelia seen on a standing x-ray film, with widened interpediculate distance and midline bony spur well visualized. B, Myelogram showing a filling defect in the area of the bony spur where the dural sac is divided in two.

and spinal cord tumors, the widening is associated with thinning and erosion of the pedicles.

In cases where compression of the spinal cord is present, a myelogram is mandatory. Here the kyphosis is associated with neurologic deficits, and the level of the obstruction and the presence of any intradural pathology must be assessed. In any case where the presence of spinal cord tumor or other intradural pathology is suspected, a myelogram should be performed.

In cases where a wedge excision of a vertebral body or excision of a hemivertebra is planned, a myelogram should be performed to obtain a thorough knowledge of the anatomy of the dural sac at the level of the planned osteotomy. Knowledge of the size and shape of the canal is necessary for the planning of the operative procedure.

*Technique.* The technique differs from that normally used for evaluation of lumbar or cervical nerve root compression. Because information about the spine deformity, dural sac obstruction, or intraspinal pathology is being sought, more dye than usual is necessary. The technique employed is that of Gold and Leach;[40] using a large volume myelography. Here, large amounts — up to 90 ml. — of dye (Hypaque or Pantopaque) are used. The volume used should be sufficient to fill the subarachnoid space so that adequate visualization of the pathologic condition is obtained.

During the myelogram it is often necessary to rotate the patient so that a true anteroposterior or lateral view is seen and rotation caused by the deformity is eliminated. This procedure permits an accurate anatomic assessment of the subarachnoid space and is especially important in the evaluation of spinal dysraphism or intradural space-occupying lesions. In addition to this rotation, it may be necessary to remove the needle after the dye has been introduced so that the patient can be turned to a supine position, allowing visualization of the dural sac in the area of a kyphosis. In kyphosis, if the myelogram is performed with the patient in a prone position, it is impossible to get the dye to pool at the apex of the kyphosis; the only way this can be done is by turning the patient supine after removing the needle. Using this maneuver, any obstruction at the apex of the kyphosis can be visualized. Occasionally, in heavy or obese patients or where difficulty is experienced in obtaining an accurate picture of the myelogram, it is necessary to use laminography with the dye in place to visualize the dye column. Air myelography is performed at some centers and is a very safe procedure that provides excellent visualization of the dural sac. We have little experience with this technique.

Water-soluble dyes, used for lumbar myelograms, cannot be used above the L1 level, as the dye is too irritating to the spinal cord.[65]

*Intravenous Pyelogram (Urogram).* Because of the high frequency of renal anomalies associated with congenital spine deformities (see Chapter 7), an intravenous pyelogram is mandatory for all patients with congenital spine anomalies. It should be performed when the diagnosis of a congenital anomaly is made. The intravenous pyelogram is performed in a routine manner. Light anesthesia (Ketamine) should be used in small children and infants.

An intravenous pyelogram is also used in cases of myelodysplasia and other paraplegic disorders for evaluation of the renal tract. The presence of any obstruction is documented, and the anatomy of the kidneys, renal calyces, and ureters is assessed (Fig. 3–26).

*Derotated View of Spine*[93] *(Plan d'election of Stagnara).* In kyphoscoliotic curves (usually over 100 degrees), the anteroposterior radiograph does not represent the true magnitude of the curvature. The lateral deviation of the spine is accompanied by vertebral rotation. If the "rotational kyphosis" and perhaps the true kyphosis were eliminated, the curve would be larger. To achieve this effect radiographically, the rotation is eliminated by taking an oblique view and measuring the curve. The ideal would be to examine the spine with the aid of fluoroscopy, rotating the patient until the maximal curve is seen, and then take a radiograph. In practice, the rotation of the thorax is used to take this radiograph. The cassette is positioned parallel to the medial aspect of the rib prominence, and the film is taken with the x-ray beam at right angles to the plate (Fig. 3–27). This method throws the curve in profile, giving the true scoliosis. This view is also useful in the evaluation of congenital anomalies and suspected diastematomyelia. With the derotation of the

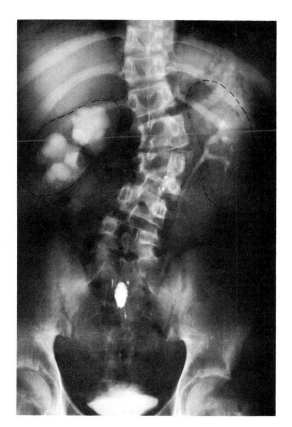

**Figure 3–26**  Sixteen year old boy diagnosed as having scoliosis on a routine school screening examination. The hemivertebra at L3 is seen. A routine intravenous pyelogram was performed and demonstrates the marked hydronephrosis on the right due to a uterovesical obstruction. This congenital obstruction was treated surgically. The reduction of renal parenchyma on the right is also seen. (From Lonstein, J. E., et al.: Minn. Med., 59:51, 1976; reprinted with permission.)

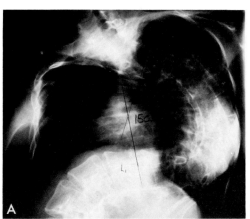

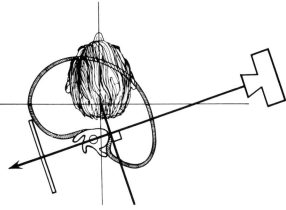

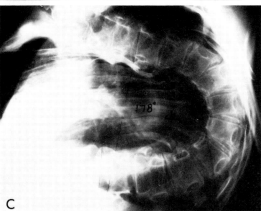

**Figure 3–27**  Derotated view of the spine. A, Antero-posterior standing x-ray of a severe 150 degree right thoracic curve. Note that the anatomy of the curve is not visible, and it appears as if there is a bar on the concavity of the curve, i.e., a congenital scoliosis. B, Diagram to demonstrate derotation view. The cassette is positioned parallel to the medial aspect of the rib prominence and the x-ray beam is at right angles to this plate. C, This view eliminates the effect of rotation. The apical vertebrae are well seen and the anatomy clearly visualized. There is no congenital unsegmented bar. This is an example of paralytic scoliosis following poliomyelitis. Note that with the rotation eliminated, the scoliotic curve is larger (178 degrees).

spine, a true anteroposterior view of the vertebral bodies is obtained and the vertebral anatomy appreciated.

***Tangential ("Rib Hump") View of the Rib Deformity.*** Occasionally, surgery is performed on the rib prominence directly to reduce it and improve the cosmetic appearance of the back. A tangential view demonstrates this prominence radiographically, showing the relationship of the vertebral bodies to the ribs. This view is taken with the patient bending forward and the x-ray beam directed tangentially across the back (Fig. 3–28).

***Angiogram.*** INDICATIONS. In scoliosis, a spinal cord angiogram has been used in very special cases. In the past, its use has been recommended for evaluation of the site of the main blood supply of the spinal cord (artery of Adamkiewicz).[50] It has been used in cases where obstruction of the vascular supply of the cord is suspected; for example, tuberculosis, intraspinal space-occupying lesions, or compression of the spinal cord due

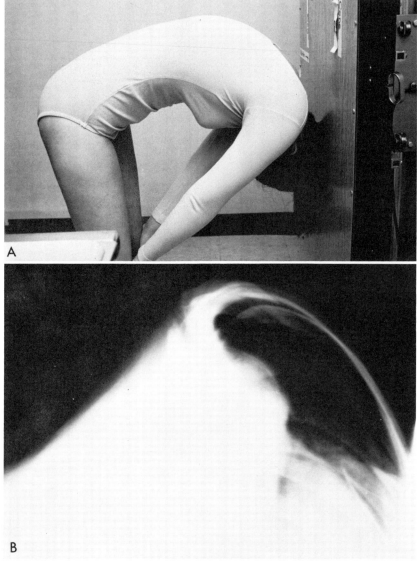

**Figure 3–28**   Tangential view of rib deformity. *A,* The patient bends forward and leans against the x-ray cassette. The x-ray beam directed tangentially across the back. *B,* Tangential view of a severe rib prominence. Note the marked upward slope of the head of the rib.

to a kyphotic deformity. Because of the difficulty of the procedure and the inherent dangers, we feel that the procedure has few indications. It might prove helpful in cases of an intraspinal vascular anomaly or tumor, where exact knowledge of the feeding vessels is necessary (arteriovenous malformation). There is a wide variation in the blood supply of the cord, and the single feeding artery has been shown by Dommisse to be less important than the anastomosis at each level.[27]

TECHNIQUE. The technique for evaluation of the blood supply of the spinal cord or intraspinal pathology is very exacting. A transfemoral approach is used, with retrograde catheterization of the aorta and cannulation of each individual intercostal artery. Dye is injected at each level, and appropriate radiographs are taken. This careful technique involves the intercostal arteries bilaterally in the area under evaluation. The dangers are damage to the intercostal artery or the main femoral artery due to the repeated manipulations of the intra-arterial catheter (Fig. 3–29).

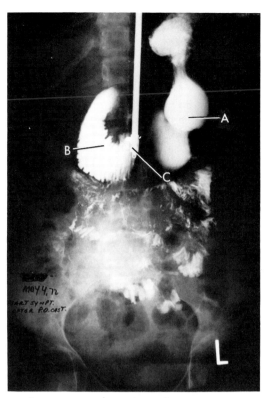

**Figure 3–30** Gastrografin swallow in a 16 year old girl with vascular obstruction of the duodenum. One week postoperatively, after being placed in a postoperative cast and ambulated, she had nausea and vomiting. A Gastrografin swallow shows the slight distention of the stomach (A) and the marked distention of the duodenum (B). The obstruction is partial, and at the third part of the duodenum (C). The cast was removed and the patient kept supine. A nasogastric tube was used to decompress the stomach, and resolution of the obstruction followed.

*Upper Gastrointestinal Evaluation.* The use of an upper GI radiographic evaluation is sometimes necessary in patients with vascular obstruction of the duodenum (see Chapter 16). A Gastrografin (not barium) swallow is used with visualization of the radiopaque substance in the stomach to evaluate the outflow obstruction at the second part of the duodenum. This test confirms a suspected diagnosis of vascular obstruction of the duodenum, or cast syndrome, and differentiates between complete and partial obstruction of the duodenum (Fig. 3–30).

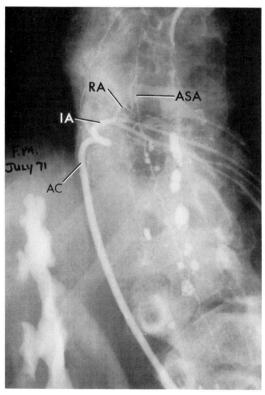

**Figure 3–29** Anterior spinal artery angiogram. Retrograde arterial catheter (AC) is positioned in an intercostal artery, which is well visualized (IA). The radicular artery (RA) is a branch of the intercostal artery and supplies the anterior spinal artery (ASA).

## LABORATORY TESTS

In the evaluation of a patient with a spine deformity, the laboratory plays a role in general evaluation of the patient and in some cases aids in the diagnosis of the etiology of the deformity.

Every surgical case needs a hemoglobin and hematocrit determination, white cell count, and urinalysis for preoperative evaluation. For adults, in addition, a BUN, creatinine, glucose test, and cardiogram are ordered when necessary. In myelodysplastics and patients with spinal cord trauma, knowledge of the status of kidney function is essential. A BUN, creatinine levels, creatinine clearance test, and culturing of a urine sample are minimal baseline tests to be performed. In cases where infection is suspected, a white cell count and differential count and a sedimentation rate determination are necessary. In postoperative infections, serial tests are necessary, since these results may be high as a result of the surgical trauma alone.

The laboratory plays a minor role in the diagnosis of the etiology of spine deformity. If mucopolysaccharidosis or homocystinuria is suspected, evaluation of mucopolysaccharide metabolites and homocystine levels in urine will aid in the diagnosis of these more unusual causes of spine deformity.

## PULMONARY FUNCTION EVALUATION

And in these cases where the gibbosity is above the diaphragm, the ribs do not expand properly in width, but forward, and the chest becomes sharp, pointed and not broad, and they become affected with difficulty of breathing and hoarseness, for the cavities which inspire and expire the breath do not attain their proper capacity. ·

This description of cardiopulmonary failure was written by Hippocrates in *On the Articulations.*[47] Since the time of Hippocrates the effect of scoliosis on the respiratory system—dyspnea and early death—has been well documented. A complete understanding of pulmonary physiology and function tests is essential for anyone caring for patients with scoliosis.

After Hippocrates' classic description of pulmonary insufficiency in scoliosis few reports of this association appeared in the literature until the late 1700s. The earliest reports of Cullen (1787)[22] and Sauvages (1768)[86] attributed the dyspnea entirely to compression of the lungs. Other reports appeared in the German and French literature in the 1800s.[14, 16, 22, 24, 25, 61, 63, 74, 77, 78, 79, 81, 96]   In 1854, Schneevogt used the first spirometer to demonstrate reduced vital capacity with spinal deformities.[87] The first reports in the English literature were written after the turn of the century and dealt mainly with the clinical syndromes and autopsy findings of these patients.[11, 20] These studies first reported the pulmonary changes and associated cardiac hypertrophy, especially of the right ventricle. Flagstad and Kollman, in 1928, evaluated paralytic and nonparalytic scoliosis and showed a correlation of reduced vital capacity with poor muscle function and with curvature of the thoracic spine.[30] Chapman et al.[17] in an excellent review in 1939, first coined the term pulmonocardiac failure. They demonstrated that the initial effects of the deformity are on the lungs (pulmonary failure), and subsequently the heart is affected (right heart failure).

Chapman et al.[17] were also the first to state that this series of events leads to a reduced longevity with death from cor pulmonale. Subsequent long-term studies by Nilsonne and Lundgren[75] and Nachemson[72] have demonstrated the higher mortality in patients with scoliosis when compared to the general population. Cardiac and pulmonary failure was the most common cause of death in the scoliotic group and occurred in the fifth decade. Zorab has emphasized this fact and also stated that death in children with severe scoliosis is due to acute respiratory infection.[111]

To this knowledge of the mortality associated with untreated scoliosis must be added the knowledge of the morbidity from respiratory problems that can occur during treatment.[3, 7, 85, 90] It is thus mandatory that the physician caring for the scoliotic patient have a thorough understanding of the pathophysiology of the pulmonary changes in these patients. He should be familiar with pulmonary function evaluation, the effects of scoliosis on these parameters, and the effects of surgery both immediately postoperatively and in the long term.

### Pulmonary Function Tests

Pulmonary function tests allow determination of the pretreatment risk of patients with spine deformities and help in prevention of postoperative complications. The tests can be divided into four groups: 1) static values, 2) dynamic values, 3) functional efficiency values, and 4) radioactive xenon studies. The first three tests are used routinely in scoliosis, but the xenon studies are used only for special cases.

## STATIC VALUES

The static values represent the volume of air in the respiratory tree broken down into functional components. The values of importance are the vital capacity, total lung capacity, and residual volume. The total lung capacity is the volume of air a person can voluntarily trap in his lungs. It is made up of two parts: the portion that can be exhaled after a maximum inspiratory effort (vital capacity) and the portion remaining in the bronchial tree after this maximum expiration (residual volume) (Fig. 3–31).

The vital capacity is measured using a spirometer and expressed as a percentage of predicted normal values. The predicted normal value in subjects without spine deformities is based on the subject's age and height. There is normally a large error inherent in this estimate of predicted "normal vital capacity." A ±20 per cent deviation of vital capacity is "normal." A vital capacity between 60 and 80 per cent is categorized as moderate restriction, and below 40 per cent is considered severe restriction.

In patients with spine deformities, the curvature has reduced the patient's height. If the standing height is taken to calculate the predicted normal vital capacity, an incorrect value will be obtained, with a reduced vital capacity appearing normal. Traction or surgery adds to the inaccuracy; it lengthens the spine and thus raises the predicted vital capacity. Since the observed vital capacity is expressed as a percentage of the predicted value, surgery or traction may falsely appear to have caused pulmonary function deterioration.

Alternate methods have thus been devised to calculate nondeformed height in scoliotic patients. These include calculations using body surface area,[103] geometric measurements from spine radiographs,[98] calculations of "straightened" spine length,[5] tibial height,[109] and arm span.[48] The most accurate and easiest to use has been the arm span as first described by Hepper et al.[46] The arm-span/height ratio was calculated as 1.03:1 for men and 1.1:1 for women, with a standard deviation of ± 0.02. Johnson and Westgate extended these studies and found the differences among sex and age groupings to be insignificant.[48] They arrived at a ratio of 1.03:1 with a standard deviation of ± 0.02, which can be applied to all patients when calculating height from arm span.

## DYNAMIC VALUES

Dynamic values are those relating to a patient's function within a limited time period. The most important value is the one-second timed vital capacity (also called forced expiratory volume in one second, $FEV_1$), and it is compared with the total vital capacity. The normal value is 80 per cent. In obstructive lung disease, the value is reduced proportionately. Maximal inspiratory and expiratory flow rates and maximum breathing capacity also provide data relating to dynamic values.[23]

## FUNCTIONAL EFFICIENCY VALUES

The functional efficiency of the lung is tested by comparing the volume of dead space with the total lung volume, the normal value being 35 per cent. In addition, the ef-

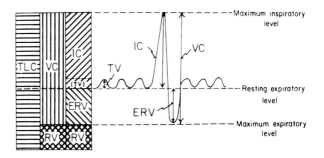

**Figure 3–31** Pulmonary function. Relationship of the vital capacity (VC), residual volume (RV), tidal volume (TV), expiratory and inspiratory reserve volumes (ERV and IRV), and total lung capacity (TLC). (Adapted with permission from Comroe, J. H., Jr., et al. (eds.): The Lung. Clinical Physiology and Pulmonary Function Tests. Chicago, Year Book Medical Publishers, 1962, p. 8.)

ficiency is tested by evaluation of the alveolar-arterial oxygen gradient. Normally all the oxygen in the alveoli is not taken up by the arterial blood. The normal gradient between alveolar and arterial oxygen pressure ($PAO_2$) is 10 mm. in the normal adult. If an increased $PAO_2/PaO_2$ gradient exists, blood is being shunted through the lungs without being oxygenated.

### RADIOACTIVE XENON[133]

Xenon is an insoluble gas with a short half-life of five days. It is forced into solution and then is injected into the superior vena cava. The xenon[133] passes out of the blood into the alveoli and can be measured by means of radioactive counters that are placed over the chest, giving information relating to venous perfusion of the lungs. The patient then breathes xenon, and using the same counters, information relating to aeration of the lungs is obtained. Using these tests, data are obtained regarding the aeration/perfusion ratios of the whole lung, lobes of the lung, and of the lung volumes. In the supine position, there is a relatively even distribution of aeration and perfusion in all lobes of the lung. In the erect position, there is a decrease in perfusion from the base to the apex, while with greater activity there is increased perfusion until the apices themselves are perfused.

Radioactive xenon studies are used in experimental studies of the pathophysiology of respiration in scoliosis. They are rarely used for the clinical evaluation and care of these patients.[88]

### Effects of Scoliosis on Pulmonary Function

In patients with significant scoliosis, it has been well established that pulmonary functions are inhibited, with reduction of total lung capacity and vital capacity.[3, 14, 101] The residual volumes are normal until late in the pathologic process. The reduction of pulmonary functions, especially of vital capacity, is significantly correlated with the severity of the curvature,[12, 30, 32, 39, 43, 52, 59, 60, 104] with consistent decrease being seen with curves over 60 degrees.[89, 110] With curves greater than 90 degrees, the vital capacity is reduced by a much greater amount than the total lung capacity.

Several factors have been proposed to explain the reduced pulmonary functions. Muscle function has been shown to be important, as patients with poor muscle function (as in poliomyelitis) have a much greater reduction in vital capacity than patients with similar curves and normal muscle function. The chest deformity may be a factor by causing simple compression of normal lung tissue and limiting expansion and thus lung volume. Thoracic lordosis also plays a role, as shown in a report by Winter, Lovell, and Moe, where marked reduction in pulmonary functions was seen with thoracic lordosis.[107] Lordosis has a more profound effect on pulmonary functions than scoliosis or kyphosis. A third factor concerns the distensibility of the thoracic cage. Simple strapping of the thorax in normal individuals has been shown by Caro and Dubois to decrease the maximum expiratory flow rate, maximum breathing capacity, and vital capacity.[15] Makley et al. demonstrated similar changes after application of a preoperative Risser localizer cast.[59] Bergofsky et al. emphasized the importance of this decreased distensibility or compliance of the respiratory system and found the work of breathing increased five times in adults with scoliosis when compared with normal adults.[3] These findings of decreased compliance and increased work of breathing have since been confirmed by numerous papers.[29, 49, 95]

Functional pulmonary values provide minimal help in evaluating patients with scoliosis. The timed vital capacity is usually of little value; although the vital capacity is reduced, since there is little obstructive component, the reduced volume is exhaled at a normal rate. On the other hand, the reduced vital capacity results in a reduction of maximum breathing capacity, a reduction that also is directly proportional to the severity of the curvature.[12, 30, 32, 39, 44, 52, 59, 80, 84] Although there is no obstructive pulmonary disease, the maximum expiratory flow rate is reduced. Dayman[23] and Fry and Hyatt[33] have shown that in normal subjects, the gas flow rate changes proportionately with the degree of inflation of the lung. Since the vital capacity and thus inflation capacity may be reduced in thoracic scoliosis, a decrease in flow rates may also be expected.

Arterial hypoxemia is noted in patients with severe curves.[67, 101, 103] There is altered regional perfusion, with venoarterial shunting. Lung tissue adjacent to the convex portion of the curvature is small with atelectatic areas.[30] In addition, the dead space is increased. Bjure et al.[6] noted that in some patients, the alveoli and airways started to close at lung volumes greater than the functional residual capacity. This process creates alveoli that are not ventilated, and thus the blood perfusing them is not oxygenated. Increased shunting has been shown to occur, especially with curves over 55 to 65 degrees. Riseborough and Shannon[83] and Westgate[102] found the lung on the convex side to be affected more, while Dollery et al.[26] and Littler et al.[55] found no significant difference in perfusion and ventilation between the two lungs.

## Effects of Surgical Correction

### IMMEDIATELY POSTOPERATIVE

Immediately after surgery, lung volumes and flow rates may be reduced by 10 to 30 per cent, from pain, drugs, and metabolic alterations. In addition, pulmonary secretion production is reduced, with reduced bronchial drainage.[85] The reduced pulmonary function will jeopardize any patient with severe reduction in resting vital capacity. A 40 per cent reduction in vital capacity and maximum breathing capacity has been shown by Westgate to greatly increase the risk of postoperative complications and respiratory failure.[48, 105] Patients with borderline pulmonary functions, therefore, require preoperative therapy, consisting of intermittent positive pressure breathing, (IPPB), use of blow bottles, coughing, respiratory physiotherapy, and occasionally, postoperative ventilatory support.[105] If respiratory failure or right heart failure is unrelieved or precipitated by traction, surgery is impossible.

### LATE CHANGES

Numerous investigations have been undertaken to evaluate the effects of surgical correction on pulmonary physiology with tests of pre- and post-fusion functions. The results are varied and sometimes difficult to compare, as in some papers the corrected height is not used to calculate predicted normal values.

One would expect, excluding permanent defects in lung tissues, that correction of the spinal curvature would increase the size of the thoracic cavity, improve rib movements, and make possible an increase in lung volumes. Some studies show this increase; others show decreased volumes, and still others report no change. Cotrel et al.[21] found an improvement in vital capacity of 30 to 40 per cent with his EDF (elongation derotation flexion) method of casting and fusion, but this improvement was not calculated with a corrected height. Gazioglu et al.[36] obtained a gain of 17 per cent in vital capacity one year after surgery. The results were not influenced by the preoperative degree of curvature, and arm span measurements were used in the calculation of predicted normal values. Meznik et al.[69] showed a mean increase of 10 per cent in the majority of cases reported but provided no information on the method of predicting normal values.

Mazoyer[64] evaluated 70 cases seven to eight years postoperatively and found an increase in the vital capacity, but this was not correlated with height or predicted normal values. Boyer[13] evaluated the improvement in severe adult idiopathic scoliosis (curves averaging 159 degrees). All cases showed improvement of 35 to 60 per cent, with greater increase being found in those with greater restriction of functions preoperatively. In 28 cases of post-poliomyelitis scoliosis, 14 showed an increased vital capacity of 28 per cent, and 9 showed a reduction of 20 per cent. Similar large increases were found by Winter et al.[107] in cases of severe thoracic lordosis and moderate (30 to 47 degrees) scoliosis. Vital capacity was reduced from 57 to 36 per cent of predicted normal. After surgical correction, only one of the five patients had decreased vital capacity, one was unchanged, and four had vital capacity increased from 773 to 2120 cc. In an excellent article by Lindh and Bjure,[54] a significant increase was found in all cases, with a 10 per cent improvement in vital capacity, total lung capacity, functional reserve capacity, and residual volume. The height correction was calculated geometrically, with the use of a flexible rule to obtain the spine length from the radiograph. The improvement was greater for the larger curves.

Opposite results wre found in a few series. Westgate and Moe[103] found a decrease in vital capacity up to five years postoperatively. The preoperative height was used when predicting normal values of lung volume, the patients were kept recumbent, and there was no chest window or routine pulmonary exercises. Henche et al,[45] using predicted height, showed a decrease in vital capacity one year after surgery for both idiopathic and paralytic scoliosis.

No significant improvement in pulmonary physiology was found by Makley et al.[59] after spine fusion. Cook et al.[19] and Gucker[43] had similar results and even showed a tendency to further decrease in lung volumes after fusion. Meister and Heine[67] reported no change in vital capacity one year after surgery, with normal values being calculated from preoperative and postoperative heights. Vallbona et al.[98] used a corrected height for predicting vital capacity and reported no significant change in lung volumes one year after surgery.

There is only one pulmonary function that increased in all patients after surgical correction of scoliosis. The $PaO_2$ is consistently increased if it was reduced preoperatively. Shannon et al.[89] investigated changes in gas exchange following fusion. The dead space was reduced, with no change in the regional ventilation perfusion or lung volumes. Gas exchange is thus improved because there is a reduction of the preoperative shunting. Their results suggest that permanent vascular changes occur with curves over 60 degrees.

The preoperative and postoperative treatment routines probably influence the changes in lung volumes. Lindh and Nachemson[53] showed that breathing exercises are important for obtaining a quicker return to preoperative vital capacities after the decrease that occurs immediately after surgery. This difference was shown by comparing a group trained in breathing exercises with one untrained in these exercises. However, the difference between the two groups decreased so that no significant variation was found in long-term follow-up. In addition to exercises, Sinha and Bergofsky have shown that routine treatment with the IPPB method causes early improvement in lung function.

Postoperative immobilization has been shown to be a factor in the early reduction of postoperative pulmonary function. Minimal restriction of chest expansion must be present, as in a Milwaukee brace or in a cast with adequate plaster removed to allow full chest expansion. Makeley et al.[59] and Caro and Dubois[15] have shown the restrictive effect of the original Risser cast and chest strapping. The influence of early postoperative ambulation and activities in the cast on pulmonary function changes has not been evaluated, but early return to the preoperative functional level can be anticipated to have a beneficial effect on pulmonary function.

In summary, the surgical correction of scoliosis improves lung volumes, a greater improvement being found with the larger preoperative restrictions and larger curvatures. Gas exchange is also improved, with an increase in the $PaO_2$ valve. These changes are dependent on postoperative breathing exercises, the use of IPPB, and an external support with minimal restriction of chest expansion.

## DOCUMENTATION

The accurate recording of all findings in the care of a patient with scoliosis is of utmost importance. Such documentation permits evaluation of the various treatment modalities available.

All pertinent findings on initial evaluation must be recorded accurately. All measurable physical findings should be noted. Documentation of findings such as "a little decompensation," "a moderately large rib prominence," or "right shoulder slightly elevated" is worthless without numerical amounts. It is impossible to compare the effect of treatment unless values are given to all measurable entities and the results recorded.

Dr. Paul Harrington has developed a data storage and retrieval system utilizing electronic data processing (computer). The system stores the data about the patient's history, physical examination, radiologic evaluation, surgical treatment, and response to surgery. Programs to evaluate these data have been developed. This system has been adopted by the Scoliosis Research Society for use by its members and others. In this way, the combined experience of these physicians can be pooled and evaluated.

This system has been expanded at the Twin Cities Scoliosis Center to include patients treated nonoperatively. Information about all patients treated by the authors has been placed on coding forms (Fig. 3–32) and stored for evaluation and retrieval utilizing electronic data processing. With the addition of the current status of the surgical, brace, and nontreated patients, a long-term evaluation of these groups will be possible.

The radiograph forms the basis for the treatment of all spine deformities. All films should be marked with the patient's name, date of examination, and position of evaluation (See Fig. 3–8). In addition, the curves should be measured and the result recorded on the radiograph. These figures should also be recorded on the treatment chart, eliminating ambiguities such as "slight improvement", "a little loss of correction," or "a few degrees' change." In addition, we place the

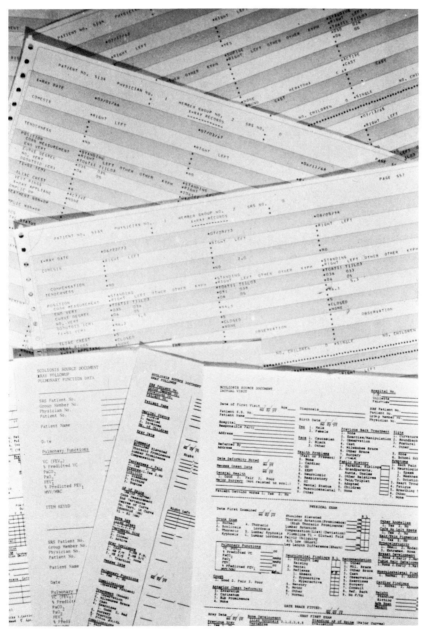

**Figure 3–32** Documentation forms used at the Twin Cities Scoliosis Center.

**TWIN CITIES SCOLIOSIS CENTER**

F.V.
U.H.
G.C.H.

## X-RAY SUMMARY FOLDER

Name: ______
Birth Date: ______ Hospital Number ______
Etiology: ______

Age of Onset of Menses: ______
Date Curve First Noted: ______
Symptoms: ______

Family: ______

Previous Treatment: ______

Major 1 ______
2 ______
3 ______
Compensatory ______
Other ______
Rib Prominences (CM) ______
Lumbar Prominences (CM) ______

Cast: L.C. ______ ☐
Risser ______ ☐
Halo ______ ☐
Other ______ ☐
Harrington Instruments: ______
Distraction 1 ______
2 ______
3 ______
Contraction ______
Trans Sacal Bar ______
Rib Resection ______ ☐
Transverse Process Osteotomies ______ ☐
Dates/Type of Surgery: ______

Complication: ______

| | Date | Bone Age | Chron. Age | Iliac Epiphyses | Vertebral Rings | Position of Patient | Curves | | | | Extent of Rotation |
|---|---|---|---|---|---|---|---|---|---|---|---|
| 1 | | | | | | | | | | | |
| 2 | | | | | | | | | | | |
| 3 | | | | | | | | | | | |
| 4 | | | | | | | | | | | |
| 5 | | | | | | | | | | | |
| 6 | | | | | | | | | | | |
| 7 | | | | | | | | | | | |
| 8 | | | | | | | | | | | |
| 9 | | | | | | | | | | | |
| 10 | | | | | | | | | | | |
| 11 | | | | | | | | | | | |
| 12 | | | | | | | | | | | |
| 13 | | | | | | | | | | | |
| 14 | | | | | | | | | | | |
| 15 | | | | | | | | | | | |
| 16 | | | | | | | | | | | |
| 17 | | | | | | | | | | | |
| 18 | | | | | | | | | | | |
| 19 | | | | | | | | | | | |
| 20 | | | | | | | | | | | |
| 21 | | | | | | | | | | | |
| 22 | | | | | | | | | | | |
| 23 | | | | | | | | | | | |
| 24 | | | | | | | | | | | |
| 25 | | | | | | | | | | | |

SMEAD'S 3-5 SP69917

**Figure 3–33** X-ray summary folder used at the Twin Cities Scoliosis Center for storing of selected x-rays to demonstrate the changes in the curves with treatment.

pertinent radiographs of each patient in a special summary folder (Fig. 3–33). This facilitates storage and retrieval of the important radiographs and allows easy comparison of current radiographs with the original presenting deformity so that progression or the effect of therapy, bracing, or surgery may be evaluated. Radiographs should never be destroyed or transferred to microfilm.

## References

1. Anderson, M., Hwan, S., and Green, W. T.: Growth of the normal trunk in boys and girls during the second decade of life. J. Bone Joint Surg., *47A*: 1554, 1965.
2. Bachmann, M.: Die Varanderugen des Innern Organe Bei Hochgradiger Skoliosen and Kyphoskoliosen. Stuttgart, 1899.
3. Bergofsky, E. H., Turino, G. M., and Fishman, A. P.: Cardiorespiratory failure in kyphoscoliosis. Medicine, *38*:263, 1959.
4. Björk, L.: Transverse tomography in determination of lung volumes in kyphoscoliosis. Acta Radiol. Diag., *14*:412, 1973.
5. Bjure, J., Grimby, G., and Nachemson, A.: Correction of body height in predicting spirometric values in scoliotic patients. Scand. J. Clin. Lab. Invest., *21*:189, 1968.
6. Bjure, J., Grimby, G., Kasalicky, J., Lindh, M., and Nachemson, A.: Respiratory impairment and airway closure in patients with untreated idiopathic scoliosis. Thorax, *25*:451, 1970.
7. Block, A. J., Wexler, J., and McDonnell, E. J.: Cardiopulmonary failure of the hunchback. JAMA, *212*:1520, 1970.
8. Block, A. J., and Olsen, G. N.: Preoperative pulmonary function testing. JAMA, *235*:257, 1976.
9. Blount, W., and Mellencamp, D.: Scoliosis treatment. Minn. Med., *56*:382, 1973.
10. Board, R.: Radiography of the scoliotic spine. Radiol. Technol., *38*:219, 1967.
11. Boas, E.: The cardiovascular complications of kyphoscoliosis, with report of a case of paroxysmal auricular fibrillation. Am. J. Med. Sci., *166*:89, 1923.
12. Böhmer, D.: Lungenfunktion, Skoliose and Operation Eine Statistiche Analyse. Z. Orthop. *111*:822, 1973.
13. Boyer, A.: Etude de la restriction ventilatoire des scolioses adultes avant et apres traitement chirurgical. M.D. Thesis Claude Bernard University, Lyon, 1973.
14. Calumette, M.: Bull. Soc. Anat., 1868.
15. Caro, C., and Dubois, A.: Pulmonary function in kyphoscoliosis. Thorax, *16*:282, 1961.
16. Castex, M. R.: Insuficiencia Cardiaca en una Cifoescoliotica. La Prensa Med. Buenos Aires, Supp. 13, 1916.
17. Chapman, E., Dill, D. B., and Graybiel, A.: Decreased functional capacity of the lungs and heart resulting from deformities of the chest. Medicine, *18*:167, 1939.
18. Cobb, J. R.: Outline for the study of scoliosis. In instructional course lectures, the American Academy of Orthopaedic Surgeons, vol. 5. Ann Arbor, Mich., J. W. Edwards Co., 1948.
19. Cook, C. D., Barrie, H., Deforest, S. A., and Helliesen, P. J.: Pulmonary physiology in children. III, Lung volumes, mechanics of respiration and respiratory muscle strength in scoliosis. J. Pediatr., *25*:766, 1960.
20. Coombs, C.: Fatal cardiac failure occurring in persons with angular deformity of the chest. Br. J. Surg., *18*:326, 1930.
21. Cotrel, Y., Morel, G., and Rey, J. C.: La scoliose idiopathique. Acta. Orthop. Belg., *31*:795, 1975.
22. Cullen's Nosologia (John Thomson, 1820 translation), 108, 1787.
23. Dayman, H.: The expiratory spirogram. Am. Rev. Resp. Dis., *83*:842, 1961.
24. De Sottas, E.: De l'influence des deviations vertebrale sur les functions de la respiration et de la circulation. Paris, 1865.
25. De Vesian, F.: Etude sur la pathologie des poumons et du coeur chez les bossus. These fac. de Paris, Nov. 20, 1884.
26. Dollery, C., Gillam, P. M. S., Hugh-Jones, P., and Zorab, P.: Regional lung function in kyphoscoliosis. Thorax, *20*:175, 1965.
27. Dommisse, G. F.: The blood supply of the spinal cord. J. Bone Joint Surg., *56B*:225, 1974.
28. Fishman, A.: Pulmonary aspects of scoliosis. In Zorab, P. A. (ed.): Proceedings of Symposium on Scoliosis, Published by the National Fund for Research into Poliomyelitis and Other Crippling Diseases, Vincent House, London. 1965, p. 52.
29. Fishman, A.: The syndrome of chronic alveolar hypoventilation. Bull. Physiopath. Resp., *8*:971, 1972.
30. Flagstad, A., and Kollman, S.: Vital capacity and muscle study in one hundred cases of scoliosis. J. Bone Joint Surg., *10*:724, 1928.
31. Forget: Jour. Hebdomadaire, 1836.
32. Freyschuss, U., Nilsonne, U., and Lundgren, K. D.: Idiopathic scoliosis in old age. Acta Med. Scand., *184*:365, 1968.
33. Fry, D., and Hyatt, R.: Pulmonary mechanics, normal and diseased. Am. J. Med., *29*:672, 1960.
34. Fua, C.: Turbe cardiocircolatorie nelle malformazioni scheletriche del torace. Minerva Med., *64*:4861, 1973.
35. Gaskell, D.: Physiotherapy for scoliotic patients in respiratory failure. Physiotherapy, *60*:71, 1974.
36. Gazioglu, K., Goldstein, L. A., Femi-Pearse, D., and Yu, P. N.: Pulmonary function in idiopathic scoliosis. J. Bone Joint Surg., *50A*:1391, 1968.
37. Gazioglu, K.: Pulmonary function before and after orthopaedic correction of idiopathic scoliosis. Bull. Physiopath. Resp., *9*:711–713, 1973.
38. Gillam, P.: Regional blood flow in kyphoscoliosis. In Zorab, P. A. (ed.): Proceedings of Symposium on Scoliosis. Published by the National Fund for Research into Poliomyelitis and Other Crippling Diseases, Vincent House, London, 1965, p. 61.
39. Godfrey, S.: Respiratory and cardiovascular consequences of scoliosis. Respiration *27*:67, 1970.
40. Gold, L., Leach, C., Kieffer, S. A., Chou, S. N., and Peterson, H. O.: Large volume myelography. Radiology, *97*:531, 1970.
41. Gracey, D.: A perplexing problem in pulmonary therapy. Heart and Lung, *2*:915, 1973.

42. Greulich, W. W., and Pyle, S. I.: Radiographic Atlas of Skeletal Development of the Hand and Wrist, 2nd ed. Stanford, Calif., Stanford University Press, 1959.

43. Gucker, T., III: Changes in vital capacity in scoliosis. J. Bone Joint Surg., 44A:469, 1962.

44. Heine, J., and Meister, R.: Skoliose und Lungenfunktion. Z. Orthop. 111:669, 1973.

45. Henche, H. R., Morscher, E., and Weisser, K.: The effects of the Harrington instrumentation on pulmonary functions in the treatment of scoliosis. In Operative Treatment of Scoliosis. Fourth International Symposium, Nymegen, Netherlands, p. 89. Georg Thieme, Suttgart, 1973.

46. Hepper, N. E., Black, L. F., and Fowler, W. S.: Relationship of lung volume to height and arm span in normal subjects and in patients with spinal deformity. Am. Rev. Resp. Dis., 91:356, 1965.

47. Hippocrates: On the Articulations. In Adams, F. (trans.): The Genuine Works of Hippocrates, vol. 2. London, Sudenham Society, 1849.

48. Johnson, B., and Westgate, H.: Methods of predicting vital capacity in patients with thoracic scoliosis. J. Bone Joint Surg., 52A:1433, 1970.

49. Kafer, E.: Respiratory function in paralytic scoliosis. Am. Rev. Resp. Dis., 110:450, 1974.

50. Keim, H. A., and Hilal, S. K.: Spinal angiography in scoliosis patients. J. Bone Joint Surg., 53A:904, 1971.

51. Kittleson, A. C., and Lim, L. W.: Measurement of scoliosis. Am. J. Roentgenol., 108:775, 1970.

52. Lamarre, A., Hall, J., Weng, T., Aspin, N., and Levison, H.: Pulmonary functions in scoliosis one year after surgical correction. J. Bone Joint Surg., 53A:195, 1971.

53. Lindh, M., and Nachemson, A.: The effect of breathing exercises on the vital capacity in patients with scoliosis treated by surgical correction with the Harrington technique. Scand. Int. Rehab., Med. 2:1, 1970.

54. Lindh, M., and Bjure, J.: Lung volumes in scoliosis before and after correction by the Harrington instrumentation method. Acta Orthop. Scand., 46:934, 1975.

55. Littler, W., Brown, I. K., and Roaf, R.: Regional lung function in scoliosis. Thorax 27:420, 1972.

56. Littler, W.: Cardio-Respiratory Failure and Scoliosis. Physiotherapy, 60:69, 1974.

57. Lonstein, J. E., Winter, R. B., Moe, J. H., Bianco, A. J., Campbell, R. G., and Norval, M. A.: School screening for the early detection of spine deformities. Minn. Med., 59:51, 1976.

58. MacEwen, G., Winter, R., and Hardy, J.: Evaluation of kidney anomalies in congenital scoliosis. J. Bone Joint Surg., 54A:1451, 1972.

59. Makley, J., Herndron, C. H., Inkley, S., Doershuk, C., Matthews, L. W., Post, R. H., and Littell, A. S.: Pulmonary function in paralytic and non-paralytic scoliosis before and after treatment. J. Bone Joint Surg., 50A:1379, 1968.

60. Mankin, H., Graham, J., and Schack, J.: Cardiopulmonary function in mild and moderate idiopathic scoliosis. Journal of Bone and Joint Surgery, 46A:53, 1964.

61. Marfan: Arch Gen. Med., 1884.

62. Marra, A., and Micillo, E.: Fisiopatologia respiratoria nelle deformita della colonna vertebrale. Arch. Monaldi, 29:421, 1974.

63. May, R.: Zum situs Viscerum bei Skoliose. Dtsch. arch. Klin. Med., 50:389, 1892.

64. Mazoyer, D.: Seventy cases of scoliosis, late teenagers and adults, influence of treatment on breathing. Paper presented to Scoliosis Research Society, Lyon, France, Sept., 1973.

65. McAlister, W., and Shackelford, G.: Measurement of spinal curvatures. Radiol. Clin. North Am., 13: 113, 1975.

66. McNeill, T. W., Huncke, B., Kornblatt, I., Stiehl, J., and Khan, H. A.: A new advance in water soluble myelography. Spine, 1:72, 1976.

67. Meister, R., and Heine, J.: Vergleichende Untersuchungen der Lungenfunktion bei jugendlichen Skoliosepatienten vor und nach der Operation nach Harrington. Z. Orthop. 111:749, 1973.

68. Meister, R., Klempt, H. W., and Heine, J.: Pulmonalarterienmitteldruck und Lungenfunktion bei Skoliosepatienten. Med. Welt, 26:1397, 1975.

69. Meznik, F., Koller, H., and Kummer, F.: Die Entwicklung der Lung enfunktion nach Skolioseoperationen. Z. Orthop., 110:542, 1972.

70. Moe, J., and Kettleson, D.: Idiopathic scoliosis, analysis of curve patterns and the preliminary results of Milwaukee brace treatment in one hundred and sixty-nine patients. J. Bone Joint Surg., 52A:1509, 1970.

71. Moragrega, J., Galland, F., Alatriste, V. M., and Bonetti, P. F.: La Funcion Pulmonar en la Cifoescoliosis Acentuada. Arch. Inst. Cardiol. Mex., 43:392, 1973.

72. Nachemson, A.: A long term followup study of nontreated scoliosis. Acta Orthop. Scand., 39:466, 1968.

73. Nash, C., and Moe, J.: A Study of Vertebral Rotation. J. Bone Joint Surg., 51A:223, 1969.

74. Neidert, quoted by Bauer, J., and Bollinger, O.: Uber Idiopathische Herzuergrosserung. Fortschr. Univ. Munchen Pettenkofer, 1893.

75. Nilsonne, U., and Lundgren, K. D.: Long-term prognosis in idiopathic scoliosis. Acta Orthop. Scand., 39:456, 1968.

76. Paramelle, B., and Perdrix, A.: Traitement et surveillance des grandes insuffisances respiratoires chroniques. Sem. Hop. Paris, 49:2155, 1973.

77. Paul, C.: Diagnosis and Treatment of Heart Disease. Paris, 1883.

78. Pisani, A.: Sopra le al-teragioni cardio-pulmonari che si riscontrano nella cifoscollosi. Gazz degli Ospendali e dell Cliniche, 25:1436, 1904.

79. Pletneff, D.: Cardiac insufficiency in connection with curvature of the spine. Prakt. Vrach. S. Peterb., 8:405, 1908.

80. Prime, F.: Routine lung function studies in kyphoscoliosis. In Zorab, P. A. (ed.): Proceeding of Symposium on Scoliosis published by the National Fund for Research into Poliomyelitis and Other Crippling Diseases, Vincent House, London, 1965, p. 57.

81. Reid, L.: Autopsy studies of the lungs in kyphosis. In Zorab, P. A. (ed.): Proceedings of Symposium on Scoliosis published by the National Fund for Research into Poliomyelitis and Other Crippling Diseases, Vincent House, London, 1966, p. 71.

82. Rieder, J.: Die Respiration and Circulationstorungen bei Kyphoscoliosis Dorsalis. Univ. Berlin, July, 1911.

83. Riseborough, E., and Shannon, D.: The effects of

scoliosis on pulmonary function and changes occurring in the lungs following surgical correction of idiopathic scoliosis. *In* Keim, H., (ed.): Second Annual Postgraduate Course on Management and Care of the Scoliosis Patient. Warsaw, Ind., Zimmer, 1970.

84. Risser, J. C.: The iliac apophysis: An invaluable sign in the management of scoliosis. Clin. Orthop., *11*: 111, 1958.

85. Ryberg, J.: Pulmonary function in scoliosis. Course on Scoliosis, Minneapolis, August 22, 1972.

86. Sauvages: Nosologica Methodica. Amsterdam, *1*:667, 1768.

87. Schneevogt, G.: Ueber den Praktischen werth der Spirometer. Z. Rationelle Med., *5*:9, 1854.

88. Shannon, D., Riseborough, E. J., Valenca, L. M., and Kazemi, H.: The distribution of abnormal lung function in kyphoscoliosis. J. Bone Joint Surg., *52A*:131, 1970.

89. Shannon, D., Riseborough, E., and Kazemi, H.: Ventilation perfusion relationships following correction of kyphoscoliosis. JAMA, *217*:579, 1971.

90. Shin, F.: Some anaesthetic problems in corrective spinal surgery in children in Hong Kong. Anaesth. Intens. Care, *1*:328, 1973.

91. Simon, G.: Lung vascularity and movements of the diaphragm. *In* Zorab, P. A. (ed.): Proceedings of a Symposium on Scoliosis published by the National Fund for Research into Poliomyelitis and Other Crippling Diseases, Vincent House, London, 1965, p. 65.

92. Sinha, R., and Bergofsky, E.: Prolonged alteration of lung mechanics in kyphoscoliosis by positive pressure hyperinflation. Am. Rev. Resp. Dis., *106*:47, 1972.

93. Stagnara, P.: Examen du scoliotique, *In* Deviations Laterales du Rachis: Scolioses. Encyclopedie Medicochirurgicale (Paris), Appareil Locomoteur, 7, 1974.

94. Stoboy, H., and Speierer, B.: Lungenfunktionswerte und Spiroergometrische Parameter Wahrend der Rehabilitation von Patienten mit idiopathischer Skoliose. Arch. Orthop. Unfallchir., *81*:247, 1975.

95. Ting, E. Y., and Lyons, H. A.: The relation of pressure and volume of the total respiratory system and its components in kyphoscoliosis. Am. Rev. Resp. Dis., *89*:379, 1964.

96. Traube: Beitr. Phys. Path., *3*:354, 1879.

97. Turino, G. M., Goldring, R. M., and Fishman, A. P.: Cor pulmonale in musculoskeletal abnormalities of the thorax. Bull. N. Y. Acad. Med., *41*:959, 1965.

98. Vallbona, C., Harrington, P. R., Harrison, G. M., Freire, R. M., and Reese, W. O.: Pitfalls in the interpretation of pulmonary function studies in scoliotic patients. Arch. Phys. Med. Rehabil., *50*:68, 1969.

99. Vitko, R., Cass, A., and Winter, R.: Anomalies of the genitourinary tract associated with congenital scoliosis and congenital kyphosis. J. Urol., *108*: 655, 1972.

100. Wanderman, K. L., Goldstein, M. S., and Faber, J.: Cor pulmonale secondary to severe kyphoscoliosis in Marfan's syndrome. Chest, *67*:250, 1975.

101. Weber, B., Smith, J. P., Briscoe, W. A., Friedman, S. A., and King, T. K.: Pulmonary function in asymptomatic adolescents with idiopathic scoliosis. Am. Rev. Resp. Dis., *111*:389, 1975.

102. Westgate, H.: Hemi-lung ventilation and perfusion changes secondary to thoracic scoliosis. J. Bone Joint Surg., *50A*:845, 1968.

103. Westgate, J., and Moe, J.: Pulmonary function in kyphoscoliosis before and after correction by the Harrington instrumentation method. J. Bone Joint Surg., *51A*:935, 1969.

104. Westgate, H.: Pulmonary function in thoracic scoliosis, before and after corrective surgery. Minn. Med., *53*:839, 1970.

105. Westgate, H., and Johnson, B.: Pre-operative pulmonary evaluation and post-operative respiratory management of patients with severe thoracic scoliosis. J. Bone Joint Surg., *53A*:195, 1971.

106. Winter, R. B., and Moe, J. H.: A plea for the routine school examination of children for spinal deformity. Minn. Med., *57*:419, 1974.

107. Winter, R., Lovell, W., and Moe, J.: Excessive thoracic lordosis and loss of pulmonary function in patients with idiopathic scoliosis. J. Bone Joint Surg., *57A*:972, 1975.

108. Young, L. W., Oestreich, A. E., and Goldstein, L. A.: Roentgenology in scoliosis: Contribution to evaluation and management. Am. J. Roentgenol., *108*:778, April, 1970.

109. Zorab, P. A., and Prime, F.: Estimation of height from tibial length. Lancet, *1*:195, 1963.

110. Zorab, P. A.: Assessment of cardio-respiratory function. *In* Zorab, P. A. (ed.): Proceedings of a Symposium on Scoliosis. Published by the National Fund for Research into Poliomyelitis and Other Crippling Diseases, Vincent House, London, 1965, p. 54.

111. Zorab, P. A.: Prognosis for life in childhood scoliosis. Arch. Dis. Child., *48*:824, 1973.

# Chapter 4

# NATURAL HISTORY OF SPINAL DEFORMITY

## INTRODUCTION

One cannot begin to study the treatment of any medical condition without knowledge of its natural history. If diabetes mellitus were, for example, only a problem of elevated blood and urine glucose levels and were not associated with any morbid problems related to this chemical abnormality, treatment with insulin would not be necessary. It is necessary to detect diabetes early and to institute prompt and appropriate treatment, for it has been well demonstrated that survival is longer and complications such as blindness can be reduced or minimized with appropriate treatment.

Such is also the case with scoliosis. The 10 year old child with a 30 degree thoracic curve has no complaints. She is not aware of the existence of her condition so she has no psychologic problem. She has no pain. She has no signs of spinal cord compression. She has no loss yet of vital capacity, so she has no dyspnea. Nevertheless, we treat such a child because we must *prevent* these secondary effects and not wait for them to happen. By waiting, it is then too late to accomplish the ideal result.

How do we know what is going to happen? We can learn only by studying those who have not been treated. In some situations, the outcome without treatment is obvious, clear-cut, and inevitable. In these circumstances, the recommendations for treatment are easy. We speak from a position of firm knowledge. In other circumstances, the basis of knowledge is less firm, and our recommendations must be tempered. It is the purpose of this chapter to outline the major studies that have been made of natural history of scoliosis, especially idiopathic scoliosis, as we know it today. It is hoped that knowledge will grow steadily in this area, for it is the vital heart of treatment.

## STUDIES OF THE PREVALENCE OF SCOLIOSIS

The prevalence of any condition can be determined only on the basis of mass screening techniques applied to unselected large population groups. Figures based only on patients who seek medical care are quite unreliable.

Two types of prevalence studies have been performed—those based on chest x-rays taken for tuberculosis screening and those based on school screening. Shands and Eiseberg[42] reviewed minifilms of 50,000 people and noted scoliosis of 10 degrees or more in 1.9 per cent of those over age 14. Scoliosis of 20 degrees or more was observed in 0.5 per cent. There were 3.5 females to 1.0 males in their study.

Duhaime, Archambault, and Poitras[16] noted scoliosis in 1.1 per cent of 14,886 people seen in minifilms. The mean age was 14.

Of the 164 patients detected, 108 were personally interviewed by the authors. Of these, 107 had idiopathic scoliosis. (The other was congenital.) Eight patients had curves over 40 degrees, and 16 had curves between 20 and 40 degrees. The remaining 84 had curves between 5 and 20 degrees. Strayer[43] reviewed the chest x-rays of 928 women entering a hospital for childbirth. Sixty-five, or 7 per cent, had scoliosis. Forty-five had curves of 10 to 19 degrees, 12 had curves of 20 to 29 degrees, and 7 had curves of 30 degrees or more. Tulit[44] noted 337 cases of scoliosis (0.47 per cent) in 22,089 x-ray films of persons over age 14. Minifilm chest x-rays have three disadvantages—small size, underpenetration of the spine, and lack of visualization of the lumbar spine.

Studies of the prevalence of scoliosis based on mass screening of schoolchildren is a relatively recent advance. This technique provides more accurate analysis, since true spine films can be obtained of all suspect cases. Orthopedic screening of schoolchildren was started in 1962 in North America in the state of Delaware.[13] Hensinger et al. reviewed the 10-year experience in Delaware.[22] In this program, which included screening for other orthopedic problems as well as spine deformity, 316,000 students (grades 1 through 12) were examined. Of these, 3061 were referred by the initial examiner to a physician for final screening. Of the 3061, 1109 were referred because of a spinal problem. Of the 1109 with possible spinal abnormality, 599 were sent for further evaluation. Of this 599, 475 had scoliosis, 47 kyphosis, 15 lordosis, 18 poor posture, 17 back pain, and 27 torticollis.

Wynne-Davies,[46] in a survey of 10,000 schoolchildren in Edinburgh, noted scoliosis in 1.3/1000 under age 8 and 1.8/1000 over age 8. In children under age 8, the incidence was equal in males and females, but over age 8, males had an incidence of 0.2/1000 and females 4.6/1000. Lezberg[30] reviewed 6000 students, kindergarten through twelfth grade, in the Falmouth, Massachusetts, school system. Eighty children (1.2 per cent) were found to have curvatures. The highest incidence was found in the fifth through ninth grades.

Sells and May[40] screened 3064 students in the seventh, eighth, and ninth grades at the Shoreline public schools near Seattle, Washington. There was an equal number of boys and girls. Forty-eight (1.6 per cent) had confirmed scoliosis. Findings were positive in 1.1 per cent of males and 2.1 per cent of females. Of the 48 discovered, 41 had been previously undetected.

Golomb and Taylor[20] reviewed 3299 female students in Sydney, Australia, 197 (5.9 per cent) of whom had at least minimal signs of scoliosis. In 84 (2.5 per cent) of these cases, the problem was significant enough to notify the parents.

Segil[41] reviewed both Caucasian and African (black) students in Johannesburg, South Africa. Curves of 10 degrees or more with clinically significant rotation were considered serious enough to make a positive diagnosis. Based on this criterion, 2.5 per cent of the Caucasians reviewed (929 students), and 0.03 per cent of the Africans (1016 students) had scoliosis. This is the only known study of different racial groups. The difference in prevalence is highly significant.

Lonstein and co-workers[31] reviewed 80,000 schoolchildren in Minnesota in the 1973–74 school year and expanded this to 250,000 students in the 1974–75 school year. Of these, 5.5 per cent were found to have a positive rib hump on the forward bending test. Accurate figures are not available as to how many of these students had positive findings on spine x-ray films. This study is of interest because it can be compared to a study by Kane and Moe[25] in which the prevalence of scoliosis in Minnesota was analyzed[25] by determining the number of patients who came to orthopedists for treatment. By their criteria, there was a prevalence of 0.013 per cent and a ratio of 5.1 females per male patient.

Brooks and associates have done detailed screening of schoolchildren in Los Angeles.[5, 6] In their studies 3492 children were reviewed, with the following results: 624 had positive physical signs suggestive of scoliosis, and 474 had scoliosis of 5 degrees or more on a standing radiograph. Of the 474, 188 were male and 286 were female. The prevalence was thus determined to be 13.6 per cent, the highest reported figure. In their review, the commonest curve was thoracolumbar. Spontaneous improvement was noted in 22 per cent. Brown et al. noted an incidence of 10.8 per cent out of 4723 children screened (fifth through eighth grade) in a suburb of Los Angeles.[7]

Drummond, Rogala, and Gurr[15] examined 14,900 students in Montreal, Canada. The initial screeners (school nurses) felt that 1252 merited more detailed evaluation. Of the 1252, 821 (5.5 per cent of the 14,900 screened) were believed to have a definite scoliosis. Detailed evaluation of the 821 revealed that 610 had structural scoliosis of 5 degrees or more with a rotational deformity. Idiopathic scoliosis was found in 603 of the 610. Five patients had spine deformity (kyphosis) due to Scheuermann's disease, 57 were found on radiographic examination to have a rib hump but not scoliosis, 16 had nonstructural scoliosis due to leg length discrepancy, and 4 had spine deformity due to spondylolisthesis. The incidence of spine deformity was 4.6 per cent and that of scoliosis, 4.1 per cent. Curves of 5 to 10 degrees were found in 305 children. In this group, there was an equal number of males and females. There were 244 children with curves of 11 to 20 degrees. In this group there were 1.6 females to 1.0 male. Fifty-four patients had curves greater than 20 degrees. In this group there were 6.4 females to 1.0 male. Curves under 30 degrees were initially not treated but were periodically re-examined by radiograph. As a group, progression occurred in 13.6 per cent. By sex, there was progression in 19.3 per cent of the females and only 9.2 per cent of the males.

Of the 14,900 children, 40 (or 2.7 per 1000 screened) required treatment, 37 by bracing and 3 by surgery. The authors concluded that 4 per cent of 12 to 14 year old students have scoliosis. The sex incidence was equal in small curves but was 80 per cent female for curves needing treatment.

Cost accounting was done on this study, and the cost was calculated to be $1684 per 400 students screened. Assuming that there would be one child requiring surgical treatment out of 400, if no early detection was carried out, the cost would be $5500. Thus, early detection is advantageous not only because it prevents surgery but also because it is economical.

## STUDIES OF UNTREATED CURVES DURING GROWTH

From the previous studies, it is reasonable to assume that about four to five per cent of North American school children aged 12 to 14 have scoliosis, which can be defined as a visible rotational deformity on forward bending and a measurable curve of 5 degrees or more on a standing radiographic projection. Of this group, the sex ratio is about even for small and early curves of 10 degrees or less.

As these children grow, some curves resolve spontaneously, some remain unchanged, and some progress. Progression is far more likely in girls than in boys.[37] Only about 3 per 1000, or 0.3 per cent, will require some form of treatment, either bracing or surgery.

Clarisse[9] presented a review of 110 patients with idiopathic scoliosis curvatures of 10 to 29 degrees presenting to physicians during growth. These were followed without treatment unless they progressed beyond 30 degrees. Of those patients presenting between ages 3 and 11, 53 per cent showed an increase. Of those presenting after the onset of menses, only 15 per cent showed an increase. Curves were classified by area. In prepubertal patients, thoracic curves increased in 50 per cent of patients, thoracolumbar curves increased in 70 per cent, lumbar curves in 30 per cent, and double major curves in 75 per cent.

Heine and Reher[21] reviewed 146 idiopathic scoliosis patients followed one or more years during growth and 110 for two years or more. Progression always coincided with growth spurts, and the degree of progression depended on the site of the curve. Thoracic curves and double curves showed the most progression and lumbar and thoracolumbar curves the least. One patient with a thoracic curve progressed from 16 to 84 degrees between age 12 and age 14.

Ponseti and Friedman[36] reviewed 394 patients, 335 of whom were followed to skeletal maturity with no treatment except for exercises. Table 4–1 summarizes their analysis. The more severe progressions were also related to age at onset; the earlier the onset, the worse the prognosis. It was noted that early onset cases tended to progress slowly for a while and then "fall apart."

James[23] also reviewed a large number of untreated patients. His conclusions were similar to those of Ponseti and Friedman—that thoracic curves progressed the most and that the earlier the onset, the worse the prognosis.

Duval-Beaupere[17] reviewed 560 untreated patients, 500 of whom were paralytic and 60 idiopathic. The average final curve at the end of growth for the whole group was

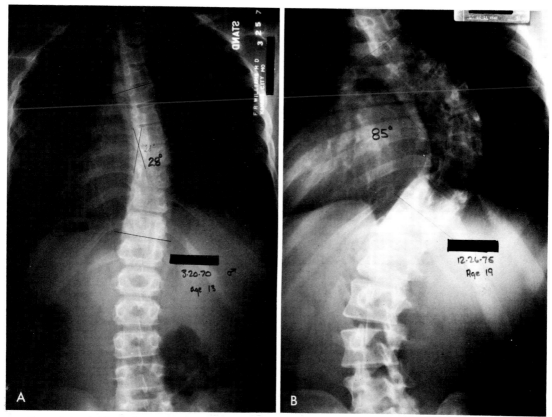

**Figure 4–1**  *A,* AP standing x-ray of a 13 year old boy. A 28 degree right thoracic T5–T11 curve is noted. No treatment was given. *B,* The same patient 5½ years later, at age 19. The curvature has now increased to 85 degrees. There has been a significant loss of pulmonary function.

100 degrees, and for those with idiopathic scoliosis was 82 degrees. The average curve for the whole group was 25 degrees at the onset of puberty (first appearance of breast development and/or pubic hair development, which occurred at chronologic age 10, on the average). The end of growth was at chrono-logic age 15. Thus the average progression from onset of puberty to end of growth was 75 degrees, or *15 degrees per year.*

Roaf,[39] James[24] and others[11, 34, 38] have also published reports of the natural history of paralytic curves. On the average, paralytic curves tend to progress more rapidly and

**TABLE 4–1  Progression of Curves**

| Area of Curve | No. of Patients | | Degree of Curve at End of Study Period | | | | Average Curve at Maturity |
|---|---|---|---|---|---|---|---|
| | | | <40° | 40°–60° | 60°–80° | >80° | |
| Lumbar | 88 | | 52 | 29 | 5 | 2 | 37° |
| Thoracolumbar | 54 | | 27 | 12 | 12 | 3 | 43° |
| Double | 117 | Thoracic | 28 | 53 | 24 | 12 | 52° |
| | | Lumbar | 58 | 42 | 11 | 6 | 41° |
| Thoracic | 71 | | 5 | 13 | 18 | 35 | 81° |
| Cervicothoracic | 5 | | 3 | 2 | 0 | 0 | 35° |

reach more severe levels than do those found in idiopathic scoliosis.

## STUDIES OF THE NATURAL HISTORY OF SCOLIOSIS IN ADULT YEARS

Hippocrates described clearly the respiratory handicap of severely scoliotic patients. Many authors since then have substantiated the problem of cardiorespiratory failure in the "hunchback" and severely scoliotic. The reader is referred to the classic papers of Chapman et al.[8] and Bergofsky et al.[3] Severe limitation of vital capacity eventually leads to right heart failure. Right heart failure responds poorly to medical treatment, and death usually occurs within 18 to 36 months of the onset of heart failure.

It was not until the past 10 to 15 years that more detailed information has been available about the frequency of such complications as well as the relationship of heart failure to the location, pattern, and degree of scoliosis. Furthermore, little attention had previously been given to the other complications of scoliosis, e.g., psychologic disturbance, degenerative arthritis, and spinal cord and nerve root compression.

In 1968, two very significant studies appeared. Nilsonne and Lundgren[33] traced 113 patients who presented originally in the years 1913 to 1918. No treatment had been given to those patients. Paralytic and congenital scolioses were excluded from the study, thus making it a study of the long-term prognosis of idiopathic scoliosis. Of the 113 patients, 88 were female and 25 male. The average age at which the child was first seen was 15.9 years. The study was performed in 1963, thus making available follow-ups of up to 50 years. Only 11 of the 113 patients could not be traced. Of those who could be traced, 56 were alive and 46 had died. The mean age of death was 46.6 years. Mortality was noted to be particularly high after the age of 45. There were 31 actual deaths compared with 9.6 expected deaths for the Swedish population at that time. In other words, the mortality rate was twice as high as for the general population. The causes of death were analyzed. Cardiac or pulmonary disease accounted for about 60 per cent of the deaths. Sixteen of the deaths were specifically diagnosed as right heart failure.

In addition to mortality, social and sociomedical aspects were analyzed. It was noted that patients with idiopathic scoliosis had a reduced physical work capacity, particularly in severe cases. Of the women studied, 76 per cent were unmarried. All the living patients were studied as to their work function and any subjective back trouble. Back symptoms were reported by 90 per cent of the patients, mostly in the form of a feeling of tiredness or pains in the thoracic or lumbar spine on exertion. Many of the patients had used some type of corset most of their lives. Thirty per cent had received a disability pension for their back trouble, while a further 17 per cent felt they were unable to work and had apparently managed by living with parents or relatives most of their lives. Altogether 47 per cent of the living patients were disabled.

In a second study reported in the same journal, Nachemson[32] analyzed 130 scoliotic patients first seen during the years 1927 to 1936. No treatment had been given to these patients. Diagnoses included poliomyelitis, congenital and idiopathic scoliosis, and miscellaneous causes. Of the group, 75 per cent were female, and 25 per cent were male. The average age of the patients at their first visit was 14 years. Of the 130 patients, 117 were traced in 1966. Of these, 20 were dead, 16 having died from cardiopulmonary diseases that were probably related to the curvature of the spine. A statistical analysis of the average Swedish population was compared to the study group. Like Nilsonne and Lundgren, Nachemson found the mortality rate to be twice the normal. The 97 living patients were also surveyed as to disability and back pain. In regard to disability compensation, 28 patients (30 per cent of the living patients) claimed disability compensation. Four of the 28 received their compensation for causes other than the scoliosis. The average age at which disability was claimed was 36. Another 15 patients reported serious heart and lung troubles, and 10 of these were on constant medication with digitalis or other similar drugs. Of those engaged in full-time work, 48 were engaged in some kind of light occupation, and 21 had moderately active work. No one was occupied in hard manual labor. Pain in the back was a relatively constant finding in 39 of the 97 patients. A brace or corset of some kind was used by 24 patients. It was the author's opinion that 1) the mortality rate was twice the normal, 2) there was a decreased ability to perform ordinary work, and 3) pain in the back was a relatively constant symptom in 39 of the 97 patients. The author stated, "This is probably due to the severe degree of osteoarthritic changes that always will occur in these patients."

The third major study focusing on long-term follow-up of nontreated patients was reported in 1969 by Collis and Ponseti.[10] During 1968, these authors attempted to find the 358 patients with idiopathic scoliosis studied in 1950 by Ponseti and Friedman.[36] They were able to trace 245 of the 358 patients. Some of the patients refused to answer questionnaires, and others were excluded because of previous incorrect diagnoses. Thus 215 of the original 358 patients (60 per cent) were actually reviewed. This, unfortunately, is a much smaller percentage of follow-up than was obtained in the Swedish studies. Of the 215 patients, 3 had already undergone spine fusion in adult life, and 17 had died between 1948 and 1968. The authors actually examined 106 patients (30 per cent), and information about the remainder was obtained by questionnaire and mailed x-ray films. The average age at follow-up was 42 years, and the average follow-up period was 24 years. There were 165 female patients (85 per cent) and thirty (15 per cent) male patients. Twenty patients (10 per cent) had never married. Contrary to the Swedish studies, in which early x-ray films were not available, this study contains the original radiographs as well as recent films. The recent x-ray films showed curves of less than 50 degrees in 28 per cent of the patients, between 50 and 74 degrees in 34 per cent, between 75 and 99 degrees in 22 per cent, and more than 100 degrees in 16 per cent. All of the patients were either housewives or gainfully employed except four who were mentally retarded and one who was receiving welfare payments. Because of their back problems, 32 patients (16 per cent) restricted occupational or recreational activities or avoided heavy housework.

In regard to back symptoms, 22 per cent of the patients had no back symptoms, 16 per cent had rare back pain, 31 per cent had occasional back pain, 16 per cent had frequent back pain, and 15 per cent had daily back pain. Twenty-five per cent of the patients had

sought medical care because of back symptoms at least once in the interval. Hospitalization for back pain had been a rare occurrence. Compared to a control group, the amount of back pain, visits to doctors, and hospitalizations for back pain were the same. Fifteen per cent of the patients complained of shortness of breath that occasionally limited their activities.

On physical examination, 52 patients had no back tenderness, and 54 had tenderness in one or more areas. Vital capacity was measured and was more than 2 liters in all except 10 patients. Per cent of normal was obtained using the patient's actual height, and therefore the figures are not valid. Pulmonary symptoms were noted to correlate directly with diminished vital capacity. It was observed that 66 per cent of patients with thoracic curves greater than 60 degrees had diminished vital capacities.

In 134 patients, x-ray films made in 1968 could be compared to the last available films, taken 20 or more years previously. The major curve increased an average of 15 degrees. Comparison was made of the progression seen radiographically according to the state of maturity at the time of the earlier x-ray film. Three groups were compared: those in whom the iliac epiphyses had begun their excursion but had not completed excursion; those in whom the iliac epiphyses had completed excursion but had not fused to the ilium; and those in whom the iliac epiphyses were fused. In the first group, there was an average increase of 25 degrees in the curve; in the second group, a 15 degree average increase; and in the third group, only a 10 degree average increase.

Different curve patterns were analyzed separately. For thoracic curves, 27 per cent of the patients had a curve measuring under 75 degrees, 34 per cent had a curve between 75 and 100 degrees, and 39 per cent had a curve greater than 100 degrees. The degree of curve increase varied according to the size of the curve at completion of iliac crest ossification. Curves under 60 degrees increased an average of only 6 degrees and none more than 15 degrees. Curves greater than 80 degrees increased an average of 9 degrees and only one more than 15 degrees. However, the curves between 60 and 80 degrees increased most (an average of 28 degrees, ranging from 17 to 92 degrees). The most severe cardiopulmonary symptoms were observed in this group of patients. Diminished vital capacity was found in 68 per cent and was directly correlated with degree of curvature. The vital capacity of patients with curves between 80 and 89 degrees averaged 80 per cent, whereas those with curves greater than 140 degrees averaged only 36 per cent of normal.

Double major thoracic and lumbar curves caused less obvious cosmetic deformity, owing to the balanced patterns of the curves. These patients had fewer pulmonary symptoms and better vital capacities than those with thoracic curves. Following ossification of the iliac crest, the thoracic curves increased an average of 11 degrees and the lumbar curves an average of 9 degrees.

For thoracolumbar curves, five measured between 45 and 75 degrees, six were between 75 and 99 degrees, and three curves were greater than 100 degrees. Curves increased an average of 17 degrees betweeen 1948 and 1968. A translatory shift between spinal segments was observed in 33 per cent of these patients, far above the proportions seen in the overall group.

Lumbar curves ranged from 15 to 85 degrees. Only 13 had curves greater than 50 degrees. The average curve increase was 9 degrees after skeletal maturity. Curves greater than 31 degrees increased an average of 18 degrees, and curves of less than 31 degrees did not increase. Mild arthritic spurring was seen in 15 patients.

This study provides valuable information, since it contained radiographic follow-up not available in the previous studies. Unfortunately, the percentage of follow-up was not as good. There appeared to be much less back disability and much less sociopsychologic disturbance in the Iowa study.

Of the 245 patients located, seven per cent died in the intervening period. The age of death ranged from 18 to 77. In no patient was cor pulmonale secondary to scoliosis implicated as the cause of death. Certainly the mortality in the Iowa study was much lower than in the Swedish studies. However, it must be remembered that that the duration of follow-up was much shorter, and, as noted by Nilsonne and Lundgren, patients tend to do fairly well until the age of 45, at which time the mortality rate seems to increase suddenly. A further study of the Iowa group is

being planned by Ponseti and should materially add to knowledge about the natural history of scoliosis.

We have considerable reservations about the implications of the Iowa study, because we have seen a large number of patients previously seen and "nontreated" at Iowa City. Most of these patients have come to us with severe curvatures, severely disabling back pain, dyspnea, and a multitude of other problems. Many of these patients have required extensive reconstructive spinal surgery in adulthood. (See Figure 17-1, for an example of a patient seen in Iowa City at the age of 17 and subsequently seen at the University of Minnesota at the age of 39. Her curvature had increased from 65 to 101 degrees, and she was severely disabled by back pain.)

Further studies by Bjure and Nachemson[4] of the material from Sweden have included more detailed pulmonary function evaluation as well as psychologic evaluation. It is Nachemson's opinion that a 50 year old woman with a 90 degree thoracic scoliosis has a mortality rate three times greater than normal, a twenty times greater chance of working disability, a chance of marriage one quarter that of the normal population, and definite psychologic (but not psychiatric) disturbances.

Fowles et al[18] traced 221 patients in Canada, 117 of whom had been untreated. They were able to locate 55 patients who were alive and 10 who were dead. Of those living, 40 per cent had intermittent pain, and 24 per cent had constant pain. The pain was correlated with the size of the curve. Those with little or no rotational deformity had minimal pain. There was a greater amount of pain after the age of 30. Of the group, 22 per cent were unemployed, 15 per cent had never worked, and none was doing heavy work. Nine per cent received pensions specifically for scoliosis. Sixty-seven per cent of the patients were psychologically embarrassed by their curve. There were fewer marriages in the scoliotic group as compared to normal, and the curvature had a very profound effect on self-image.

Of the ten dead, four had idiopathic, three congenital, and three paralytic scoliosis. Five of the deaths were cardiopulmonary, four were unrelated to scoliosis, and one was not determined.

Rather than study a specific group of scoliosis patients from adolescence into adulthood, Ghavamian[19] reviewed 3050 patients presenting to an orthopaedic surgeon during adult life with back pain. The purpose of the study was to determine the incidence of scoliosis within this group. Of the 3050, 852, or 28 per cent, had minor scoliosis (under 15 degrees). Curvatures due to discogenic muscle spasm and leg length inequality were not included. Of the 852, 50 per cent had spina bifida occulta (which is present in 5 per cent or less of the normal general population). Pain usually began after age 30. In patients with a single curve, the pain was at the center of the curve. In double curves, pain was at the junction of the two curves. The pain was on the convex side in one quarter of the patients, on the concave side in one quarter, and on both sides in the remainder. Cervical curves were noted in 24 per cent of the patients. These were due to disc disease at either C5–C6 or C6–C7. Eleven per cent of the patients exhibited a thoracic curve, and 57 per cent had a lumbar curve. Only 8 per cent had a cervicothoracic curve. Right-sided curves were more common than left-sided curves. There was an equal number of males and females. It was the conclusion of the author that minor curves often led to pain. The pain seemed to be discogenic at the apex of the curve. Of the total group, 60 per cent of the symptomatic curves were in the lumbar spine, and 24 per cent were in the cervical spine.

## SUMMARY

What can be said about the natural history of scoliosis? The preceding studies are in some ways complementary and in other ways conflicting. The final answer is far from apparent. Furthermore, it is going to be difficult in the future to obtain any series of untreated patients, since treatment has become far more aggressive during the past 25 years.

Other information as to the natural history of curvatures can be gleaned from studies of patients undergoing treatment in adulthood.[12, 14, 26, 27, 28, 35] If patients did not have trouble as adults, they would not require surgical treatment. Such is not the case. The reader is referred to Chapter 17 for further details regarding the problem of the adult presenting with a scoliosis problem.

On the basis of the patients seen by the authors at this Center, we cannot help but feel that there are a large number of adults with truly symptomatic scoliosis. Many of these patients present to us primarily with dypsnea, some even with cor pulmonale. Some of these patients do not have pain, but the majority are significantly limited in their functional capacity.

Other patients present to us with pain as the major complaint. This is far more likely with thoracolumbar or lumbar curves either in isolation or in a double major curve pattern. It has been stated that "scoliotic adults have no more back pain than the population as a whole" and "arthritic troubles in the adult scoliosis population are a myth." We cannot agree with these statements. *Hundreds* of adult scoliosis patients have come to us with significantly painful arthritic problems. Their lives have been made miserable by their difficulties. Surgical correction and fusion of their curves has in the majority of cases produced a lasting and very pleasant improvement.

We therefore cannot agree with Ponseti and Nachemson, who imply that in the adult scoliotic pain is a minimal problem. We do agree with Nilsonne and Lundgren[33] and Nachemson[32] that thoracic scoliosis produces a significant deleterious effect on pulmonary function, particularly in curves greater than 60 degrees. We thus support some of the findings of these studies but do not agree with others.

There can be no question that the adult with a curve of 60 degrees or more stands a great risk for the development of increasing curvature and increasing loss of pulmonary function. It cannot be assumed that curvature in the adult will not progress. It is our opinion that the adult with a thoracolumbar curve of 60 degrees or more has a high risk of progression and a high risk of painful arthritic complications.

Most workers agree that the natural history of curves of less than 40 degrees is one of a rather benign condition. Most do not progress or progress only minimally. Most do not become significantly symptomatic or bothersome. On the other hand, curves of greater than sixty degrees have such a high likelihood of adult problems that fusion of the adolescent with a curve of sixty degrees or greater can be justified on a prophylactic basis.

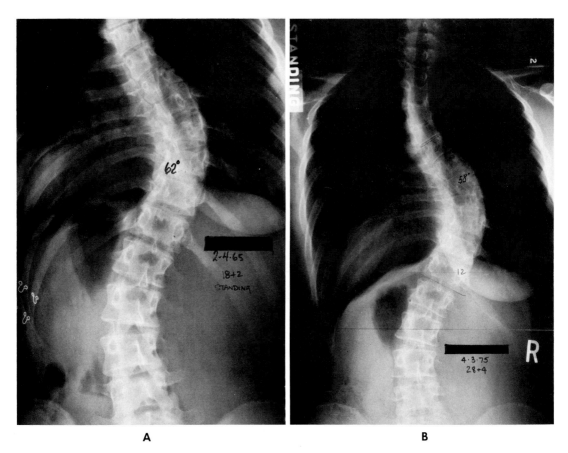

**A**                                    **B**

**Figure 4–2** *A,* An 18 year old girl with a 62 degree right thoracic idiopathic scoliosis. She had no pain, no dypsnea, and was not psychologically bothered by her curve. Her pulmonary functions were tested and were within normal limits. The iliac epiphyses had fused to the sacrum. Because of the benign nature of her curve, no treatment was considered necessary. She was advised to return periodically for evaluation. *B,* The same patient 10 years later (age 28). Her curve measures 58 degrees; there has been no loss of correction since the age of 18. She continues to have no pain, no dyspnea, normal pulmonary functions. She is now married and has two children and accepts her curve. No treatment continues to be our recommendation for this patient.

Curves between 40 and 60 degrees cause a treatment dilemma. Each case must be considered individually. If a patient presents at age 30 with a significantly painful 50 degree curve, it must be duly investigated and treated. If a patient presents at the age of 30 with a 50 degree thoracic curve which is nonprogressive, not painful, and nondebilitating from a psychologic point of view, there really is no justification for surgical treatment. Such a patient is portrayed in Figure 4–2.

## References

1. Bake, B., Bjure, J., Kasalichy, J., and Nachemson, A.: Regional pulmonary ventilation and perfusion distribution in patients with untreated idiopathic scoliosis. Thorax, *27*:703–712, 1972.

2. Bengtsson, G., Fallstrom, K., Jansson, B., and Nachemson, A.: A psychological and psychiatric investigation of the adjustment of female scoliosis patients. Acta Psychiatr. Scand., *50*:50–59, 1974.

3. Bergofsky, E. H., Turino, G. M., and Fishman, A. P.: Cardiorespiratory failure in kyphoscoliosis. Medicine, *38*:263–317, 1959.

4. Bjure, J., and Nachemson, A.: Non-treated scoliosis. Clin. Orthop., *93*:44, 1973.

5. Brooks, H. L., Azen, S. P., Gerberg, E., Brooks, R., and Chan, L.: Scoliosis: a prospective epidemiologic study. J. Bone Joint Surg., *57A*:968–972, 1975.

6. Brooks, H. L., Gerger, E., Mazur, H., Brooks, R., and Nickel, V. L.: The epidemiology of scoliosis—a prospective study. Orthop. Rev., *1*:17–23, 1972.

7. Brown, J., Bonnett, C., and Miller, M. J.: Scoliosis detection clinic. Orthop. Digest, March, 1975, pp. 14–16.

8. Chapman, E. M., Dill, D. B., and Graybiel, A.: The decrease in function capacity of the lungs and heart resulting from deformities of the chest: Pulmonocardiac failure. Medicine *18*:167–202, 1939.

9. Clarisse, P.: Prognostic Evolutif des Scolioses Idiopathiques Mineures de 10° to 29° en Periode de Croissance. Doctoral thesis, Univ. Claude Bernard, Lyon, 1974.

10. Collis, D. K., and Ponseti, I. V.: Long-term followup of patients with idiopathic scoliosis not treated surgically. J. Bone Joint Surg., 51A:425–445, 1969.

11. Colonna, P. C., and Vom Saal, F.: A Study of paralytic scoliosis based on 500 cases of poliomyelitis. J. Bone Joint Surg., 23:335–353, 1941.

12. Coonrad, R. W., and Feierstein, M. S.: Progression of scoliosis in the adult. J. Bone Joint Surg., 58A:156, 1976.

13. Cronis, A., and Russell, A. Y.: Orthopaedic screening of children in Delaware public schools. Del. Med. J., 37:89–92, 1965.

14. Dawson, E. G., Caron, A., and Moe, J. H.: Surgical management of scoliosis in the adult. J. Bone Joint Surg., 55A:437, 1973.

15. Drummond, D., Rogala, E., and Gurr, J.: School screening, a community project. Paper presented at the Quebec Scoliosis Society Meeting, Montreal, June, 1976.

16. Duhaime, M., Archambault, J., and Poitras, B.: School screening for scoliosis. Paper presented at the Quebec Scoliosis Society, Montreal, June, 1976.

17. Duval-Beaupere, G.: Pathogenic relationship between scoliosis and growth. In Zorab, P. A. (ed.): Proceedings of 3rd Symposium held at the Institute of Diseases of the Chest, London. Scoliosis and Growth, 1971.

18. Fowles, J. V., Drummond, D. S., Ecoyer, S., Roy, L., and Kerner, M.: The prognosis of untreated scoliosis in the adult. Paper presented at Scoliosis Research Society, Louisville, 1975. J. Bone Joint Surg., 58A:156, 1976.

19. Ghavamian, T.: The Future of minor scoliotic curves of the spine. Exhibit, AAOS, Washington, D.C., 1972.

20. Golomb, M., and Taylor, T. K. F.: Screening adolescent school children for scoliosis. Med. J. Aust., June 14, 1975, pp. 761–762.

21. Heine, J., and Reher, H.: Die Progredienz der unbehandelten idiopathischen Skoliose bis Wachstumsabschluss. Z. Orthop., 113:87–96, 1975.

22. Hensinger, R. N., Cowell, H. R., MacEwen, G. D., Shands, A. R., and Cronis, S.: Orthopaedic screening of school age children: Review of a 10-year experience. Orthop. Rev., 4:23–28, 1975.

23. James, J. I. P.: Idiopathic scoliosis: The prognosis, diagnosis and operative indications related to curve patterns and the age of onset. J. Bone Joint Surg., 36B:36–49, 1954.

24. James, J. I. P.: Paralytic scoliosis. J. Bone Joint Surg., 38B:660–685, 1956.

25. Kane, W. J., and Moe, J. H.: A scoliosis prevalence survey in Minnesota. Clin. Orthop., 69:216–218, 1970.

26. Keim, H. A.: Scoliosis can progress in the adult. Orthop. Rev., 3:28, 1974.

27. Kostiuk, J. P., Israel, J., and Hall, J. E.: Scoliosis surgery in adults. Clin. Orthop., 93:225–234, 1973.

28. Leatherman, K. D.: Changing concepts in the treatment of adult scoliosis. Paper presented at AAOS, New Orleans, 1976.

29. Leidholt, J., and Ballard, A.: The disability of lumbar curves in adulthood. J. Bone Joint Surg., 56A:444, 1974.

30. Lezberg, S. F.: Screening for scoliosis (preventive medicine in a public school). Phys. Ther., 54:371–372, 1974.

31. Lonstein, J. E., Winter, R. B., Moe, J. H., Bianco, A. J., Campbell, R. G., and Norval, M. A.: School screening for the early detection of spine deformities. Minn. Med., 59:51–57, 1976.

32. Nachemson, A.: A long term followup study of nontreated scoliosis. Acta. Orthop. Scand., 39:466–476, 1968.

33. Nilsonne, U., and Lundgren, K. D.: Long-term prognosis in idiopathic scoliosis. Acta Orthop. Scand., 39:456, 1968.

34. Permin, W.: Treatment of poliomyelitis. J. Bone Joint Surg., 57A:508, 1953.

35. Ponder, R. C., Dickson, J. H., Harrington, P. R., and Irwin, W. D.: Results of Harrington instrumentation and fusion in the adult idiopathic scoliosis patient. J. Bone Joint Surg., 57A:797–801, 1975.

36. Ponseti, I. V., and Friedman, B.: Prognosis in idiopathic scoliosis. J. Bone Joint Surg., 32A:381–395, 1950.

37. Report of the Research Committee of the American Orthopaedic Association: End result study of the treatment of idiopathic scoliosis. J. Bone Joint Surg., 23:963–977, 1941.

38. Risser, J. C., and Ferguson, A. B.: Scoliosis: Its Prognosis. J. Bone Joint Surg., 18:667–670, 1936.

39. Roaf, R.: Paralytic scoliosis. J. Bone Joint Surg., 38B:640–659, 1956.

40. Sells, C. J., and May, E. A.: Scoliosis screening in public schools. Am. J. Nurs., 74:60–62, 1974.

41. Segil, C. M.: The incidence of idiopathic scoliosis in the Bantu and white population groups in Johannesburg. J. Bone Joint Surg., 56B:393, 1974.

42. Shands, A. R., Jr., and Eisberg, H. B.: The incidence of scoliosis in the state of Delaware. A study of 50,000 minifilms of the chest made during a survey for tuberculosis. J. Bone Joint Surg., 37A:1243, 1955.

43. Strayer, L.: The incidence of scoliosis in the post partum female on Cape Cod. Paper presented at the SRS, Wilmington, 1972.

44. Tulit, A.: Screening of vertebral scoliosis by mass x-ray pictures. Tuberk: Tudobet 22:44–45, 1969.

45. Turrini, P., Frigo, G.: Valutazione Critica del Tratlamento Incruento in Rapporto all Evoluzione della Scoliosi Idiopatica. Miner. Orthoped., 20:382–388, 1969.

46. Wynne-Davies, R.: The Aetiology of Infantile Idiopathic Scoliosis. J. Bone Joint Surg., 568:565, 1974.

# Chapter 5

# THE NORMAL SPINE: ANATOMY, EMBRYOLOGY, AND GROWTH

## ANATOMY

The routine anatomy of the bones, muscles, and ligaments of the spine is so well covered in textbooks of anatomy that repetition here would be useless. Attention will be directed to the less commonly discussed areas that have relevance to the spine surgeon.

### Blood Supply of the Spinal Cord

Arterial blood supply comes to the spinal cord via the main vessels, the anterior median longitudinal arterial trunk (frequently called the anterior spinal artery), and the two posterolateral longitudinal arterial trunks. These three vessels course the entire length of the spinal cord, from the medulla oblongata to the conus medullaris. They are supplied by the medullary feeder arteries, which occur at varying levels and in varying numbers. The location and frequency of these feeder arteries have been of great concern to spinal surgeons. The fear of creating paraplegia by the transection or ligation of the major feeder artery has haunted us all. The most significant study of the blood supply of the spinal cord has been done by Dommisse[4] (Fig. 5–1). Previous studies, particularly that by Suh and Alexander,[34] implied a rather constant occurrence of the artery of Adamkiewicz (the major medullary feeder of the cord) at the

T10 level on the left, and additional feeders at C3, T3, and L2 on the left and C5, T1, T5, and L5 on the right. The studies of Dommisse, however, showed the extreme inconsistency of these feeder vessels. In the 36 cadavers studied, no two had the same pattern. The artery of Adamkiewicz was on the right side in 17 per cent.

In embryologic development, the spinal cord is supplied by feeder vessels coming in via the foramina at every vertebral level. These gradually decrease, leaving the cord supplied by feeder vessels at the proximal and distal ends only, plus a few collaterals be-

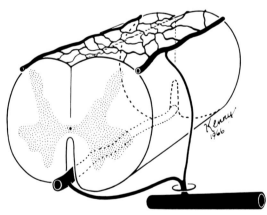

**Figure 5–1** A diagram illustrating the single anterior median longitudinal arterial trunk and the paired posterolateral longitudinal arterial trunks. A medullary feeder artery is also shown. (Reprinted from Doppman, J. L., DiChiro, G., and Ommaya, A. V.: *Selective Arteriography of the Spinal Cord.* St. Louis, W. H. Green, 1969.)

tween. In essence, the cervical and lumbar sections of the cord are richly supplied, and the thoracic cord is precariously supplied. The anterior longitudinal arterial trunk is smallest in the thoracic cord, and the collateral feeders are least numerous. In the anterior longitudinal trunk, the flow is downward from the cervical cord and upward from the thoracolumbar region with a "watershed" region at T1–T7 (Fig. 5–2).

The average number of anterior medullary feeder arteries is 8, with a range from 2 to 17. The posterior medullary feeders are smaller and more numerous, with an average of 12 and a range of 6 to 25. There are cross-communications between the posterolateral

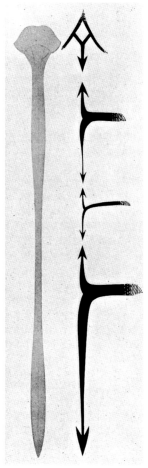

**Figure 5–2** A diagrammatic representation of the zones of blood supply to the cord. The richly supplied cervical and lumbar enlargements are shown as heavy arrows and the more meager thoracic supply by the smaller arrow. (Reprinted from Doppman, J. L., DiChiro, G., and Ommaya, A. V.: *Selective Arteriography of the Spinal Cord.* St. Louis, W. H. Green, 1969.)

longitudinal arterial trunks at almost every level. There are, however, no communications between the anterior and posterolateral longitudinal trunks.

Extradural intraspinal cross-linkages do occur frequently, and in addition, there are cross-linkages anterior to the vertebral bodies from one segmental vessel to another. There are also linkages from one segmental vessel to the next at the foraminal level outside the spinal canal. In summary, there are abundant collaterals external to the spinal canal as well as inside the canal and in the extradural area. Intradurally, however, there is meager collateral circulation for the anterior median longitudinal arterial trunk, especially in the thoracic cord.

In Dommisse's study, six cadavers had only one feeder vessel to the anterior spinal artery, the majority had either two or three, three had four feeder arteries, and one had five feeder arteries. The origin of the thoracic feeder vessels was found to be the corresponding thoracic aortic segmental vessel.

One of the major fears of spine surgeons in first doing the Dwyer procedure was that paraplegia would occasionally occur due to ligation of the segmental vessel that supplied the major feeder vessel of the thoracic cord (the artery of Adamkiewicz). Since statistically it was thought to be at T10 on the left, and since the left T10 segmental vessel was frequently ligated, this was a reasonable concern. In practice, however, no paraplegia has been reported from this cause. In performing the Dwyer procedure (or any anterior spine operation) the surgeon should be careful to ligate the segmental vessels in the mid-lateral area of the vertebral body rather than near the foramen, thus preserving the important collateral channels.

In analyzing paraplegias related to the treatment of spine deformities, one notes that *virtually all paraplegias are related to stretch*, either suddenly with Harrington rods, or gradually with skeletal traction. This problem is discussed in Chapter 16.

The Dwyer procedure has the distinct advantage of shortening the long side (convexity) of the curve rather than lengthening the short side (concavity) as does the Harrington distraction rod.

The blood supply of the spinal cord can be studied by specialized angiographic techniques. However, these are difficult tests, requiring sophisticated equipment and considerable expertise. Doppman, DiChiro, and Ommaya[5] published an excellent monograph on the subject. The technique has its greatest value in the study of arteriovenous malformations of the spinal canal and spinal cord.

Keim and Hilal[16] performed spinal angiography in 33 scoliosis patients. In two patients the blood supply was found to be so poor that surgical correction of the curves was canceled. This was probably an unwarranted fear, since one of these two patients was subsequently operated on by the senior author of this text (J.H.M.) without neurologic complications. Angiography is not a be-

nign procedure, since vascular spasm, allergies, and damage to the femoral artery can occur. At the present time, angiography of the spinal cord seems to have no practical value in either the evaluation or the management of the scoliosis patient.

Only one spinal angiogram for a scoliosis patient has been done at this center. Unfortunately, occlusion of the femoral artery resulted, and despite two attempts at thrombus removal, the femoral artery remained obstructed. Fortunately, the patient's age (nine years) permitted adequate collateral circulation, and the limb was not lost. Figure 5–3 shows the angiographic study of this patient.

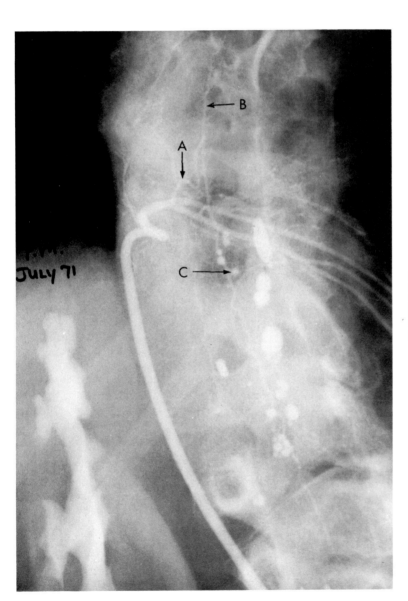

**Figure 5–3** Angiography of the spinal cord. Arrow A points to the artery of Adamkiewicz, Arrow B to the ascending anterior median longitudinal trunk, and Arrow C to the descending anterior median longitudinal trunk.

## EMBRYOLOGY

Understanding of the normal embryology of the vertebral column and spinal cord is necessary before one can appreciate some of the congenital anomalies that can occur. As many events in embryologic development occur at the same time, this description will be divided into three parts: 1) development of the somites, 2) development of the spinal cord, and 3) development of the vertebral column.

### Development of the Somites

In the earliest stages the embryonic disc has two layers—ectoderm on the future dorsal aspect, with the amniotic cavity on one side, and endoderm, which ventrally forms the roof of the yolk sac (day 12, gestational age). At the cranial end of the two-layered embryonic disc the layers are fused, forming the prechordal plate. Caudally the ectoderm forms the primitive streak. Just cranial to the primitive streak the cells thicken, forming the primitive knot or Hensen's node. In the center of this, the cells invaginate to form the primitive pit, which is equivalent to the blastopore of lower animals. From the primitive pit, cells migrate between the ectoderm and endoderm in a cranial direction, forming the notochordal process, which grows to meet the prechordal plate. At the same time, cells migrate from the primitive streak between the ectoderm and endoderm around the notochordal plate to cranially form the third embryonic layer, the mesoderm (day 18). The primitive pit deepens into the solid notochordal process, which now becomes tubular. The notochordal process comes to lie directly in contact with the yolk sac, forming a ridge in the roof of the yolk sac, the notochordal plate. Thus at this stage, there is a direct communication between the yolk sac and amniotic cavity through the notochordal process and the primitive pit. This connection is called the neurenteric canal. It may have relevance to the development of such conditions as diastematomyelia. The exact stage and site of closure of the primitive pit and disappearance of Hensen's node are unknown. The endoderm on each side of the notochordal plate curls under until it meets and reunites, producing the true notochord. This process starts cranially and extends caudally and is completed by the end of four weeks, or 4 mm. crown-rump (CR) length, 25-somite stage. The true notochord induces the thickening in the overlying ectoderm to form the neural plate.

When the notochord and neural tube develop, the intraembryonic mesoderm lies as a complete layer between the ectoderm and endoderm. This mesoderm thickens to form two longitudinal paramedian columns, called the paraxial mesoderm. Laterally the mesoderm differentiates into the intermediate mesoderm and lateral mesodermal plate. The intermediate mesoderm gives rise to the genitourinary system, and the lateral mesodermal plate is continuous with the mesoderm of the somatopleure lining the amniotic cavity, and the splanchnopleure lining the yolk sac.

Starting on the twentieth day of gestation, the cells of the paraxial mesoderm undergo a segmentation process. The somites are formed and are separated by intersegmental fissures. The first cranial somites appear in the middle portion of the embryo just caudal to the cranial end of the notochord. Because of the predominant cephalic development following this stage, the region where the first somites appear actually corresponds to the future occipital area. This segmentation process proceeds in a craniocaudal direction, and at the end of the fifth week, 42 somites are formed. On the external surface of the embryo, these somites are visible as a series of elevated "beads" along the dorsolateral surface of the embryo. On cross section, the somites are wedge-shaped with a central cavity, the myocoele.

During this somite stage, the older cranial somites show some internal specialization. The cells lying dorsolateral to the myocoele plus cells that are proliferating in this primitive cavity form the skin integuments. The more medial cells form the dorsal musculature. These cells migrate between the endoderm and the ectoderm to form the paravertebral muscles and combine with the somatopleure to form the muscles of the limbs and the abdominal wall. The ventromedial cell mass forms the sclerotome. These cells migrate medially toward the neural tube and notochord to form the vertebral column.

## Spinal Cord Embryology

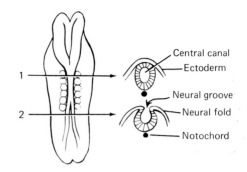

There are three stages of spinal cord development:

1) Neurulation, the formation of the majority of the spine cord and brain cranially
2) Canalization
3) Retrogressive differentiation.

### NEURULATION

At approximately the seventeenth to nineteenth day, the first differentiation toward the formation of a nervous system occurs. The midline cells of the ectoderm (neural plate) are specialized as neuroectoderm, and the process of neurulation separates these cells from the amniotic cavity, forming a complete covering of ectoderm. The neural plate sinks inward, becoming grooved, and its lateral margins curl over to join in the dorsal midline and form the neural tube. This tube is probably formed by a migration of cells in this area. The folding process proceeds cranially and caudally to a closed tube with cranial and caudal openings. The cells at the junction of the neural plate and ectoderm are specialized and become detached from both the neural tube and the ectoderm to form a mass of cells lying on the dorsal side of the neural tube; this is the neural crest. These cells are specialized and form the dorsal spinal ganglion cells.

Approximately three days after the neural tubes begin to fuse, the cranial portion of the neural tube differentiates to form the brain. The neural folds continue to close rostrally, the site of final closure being the anterior neuropore. This occurs at the 13 to 20 somite stage, and now the central canal of the neural tube is continuous with the amniotic cavity through the posterior neuropore.

The posterior neuropore closes two days later, at the 21 to 29 somite stage. This would locate the site of closure at about the first or second lumbar vertebra with variations two or more segments cranially or caudally, that is, T11 to L4. When the posterior neuropore closes, the initial stage of neural tube formation is complete, and the internal cavities of the nervous system are completely sealed. The communication between the central canal and the amniotic cavity is now absent (Fig. 5–4).

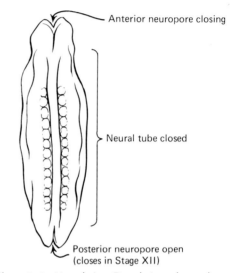

**Figure 5–4**   Neurulation. Dorsal view of an embryo at 22 days of gestation during initial fusion of the neural folds. On the right side are cross sections taken at the level of arrows 1 and 2. (Reprinted from Lamire et al.: Normal and Abnormal Development of the Human Nervous System. Hagerstown, Harper and Row Publishers, 1976.)

### CANALIZATION

With the complete closure of the neural tube, the lower lumbar, sacral, and coccygeal segments have not developed. The differentiation in this area is less well described than the process of neuralization. Recent studies suggest the process to be similar to that occurring in birds, which undergo canalization of the caudal cell mass and retrogressive differentiation.

At the caudal end of the neural tube and notochord, there is a large aggregate of undifferentiated cells extending into the primitive tail fold. At this stage, the only structures in this region are the mesonephros and hindgut. Some of the undifferentiated cells near the end of the neural tube orient themselves around small vacuoles (day 22 to 23). These undifferentiated cells around the vacuoles coalesce, and when this occurs two or three layers of cells take on the appearance of neural cells. These coalescing vacuoles make contact with the central canal of the neural tube into the tail. Studies of embryos at this stage of development show that the process of canalization lacks the precise changes of neurulation.

*Retrogressive Differentiation.* At this stage, there is regression of the structures formed during the canalization phase. This event occurs in a precise manner and is not a degenerative process but has been termed retrogressive differentiation by Streeter.[31, 32, 33]

Initial retrogressive differentiation occurs at the 11 mm. stage with disappearance of the embryonic tail. The regression of the neural tubes starts later, at the 13 to 18 mm. CR stage (48 days). The changes in the neural tube involve changes in the vertebral structures at the same time. During retrogressive differentiation, three structures are derived from the embryonic neural tube—the ventriculus terminalis, the filum terminale, and the coccygeal medullary vestige (Fig. 5–5). The lumen of the central canal decreases in size in its middle portion. The ventriculus terminalis remains throughout as an identifiable space. In most cases it is found within that portion of the spinal cord which will become the conus medullaris, but occasionally it is seen in the upper filum terminale. The ascent of the spinal cord is caused by differential growth that occurs in the embryo between the spinal cord and vertebral column. The vertebral column grows at a faster longitudinal rate than the spinal cord, causing the distal end of the spinal cord to "migrate" cranially. There is controversy as to exactly when the spinal cord reaches its adult position between L1 and L2, with estimates ranging from the embryonic period to the second year of life.

At the 3 mm. CR stage (60 days), the caudal neural tube atrophies, leaving a small ependymal rest at the tip of the coccygeal segments. This is known as the coccygeal medullary vestige. Between this vestige and the ventriculus terminalis, the neural tube atrophies into a fibrous band, the filum terminale. This structure persists throughout life and is divided into a cranial intradural subarachnoid part and a caudal part, which is fused with the dura.

## Vertebral Column Formation

Formation of the vertebral column occurs at the 3 mm. CR stage, or 23 days, with the formation of the somites and the sclerotome. As described, the somites are separated by intersegmental fissures, and the medial cells form the sclerotome. These cells migrate to form the first of three successive vertebral columns. Initially, there is the formation of a mesenchymal vertebral column, which becomes cartilaginous and then osseous.

### MEMBRANOUS PHASE

The initial migration of the mesenchyme from the sclerotome is toward the notochord, and it surrounds the notochord as a perichordal sheet. These cells around the notochord contribute to the bodies of the vertebrae and the intervertebral discs. They thus separate the notochord from the endoderm and the neural tube. This process starts initially in the cervical region on the twenty-third day at the 3 mm. CR stage and proceeds caudally. During the next 7 to 10 days, cells migrate in a dorsal direction to form the neural arch, and other cells move in a ventrolateral direction to form a primordia of the ribs. Thus, at the end of the membranous stage, cell migration in these three directions from the sclerotome

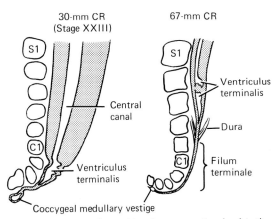

**Figure 5–5** Relationship of structures involved in the process of retrogressive differentiation. (Adapted from Streeter, 1919. Reprinted from Lamire et al.: Normal and Abnormal Development of the Human Nervous System. Hagerstown, Harper and Row Publishers, 1976.)

forms the membranous anlage of the definitive vertebral body.

Starting on approximately the twenty-fourth day, a resegmentation occurs in the membranous vertebral bodies. The cells of the somite divide into two cell masses, a cranial, less cellular portion and a caudal, more cellular portion. The division between these two halves is formed by the sclerotomic fissure of von Ebner. At the end of the membranous stage, some areas have both the intersegmental and the sclerotomic fissures. The dense caudal cells of one somite unite with the less dense cranial cells of the next caudal somite, forming the definitive vertebral body. The cells of the more dense section abutting on the sclerotomic fissure contribute the basic cells that form the annulus fibrosus and the enchondral growth plates of a cen-

trum. In addition, in the mesenchymal stage, the notochord, which up to this time has been of uniform thickness, shows a diameter change. The cells in the area of the future centrum become compressed and degenerate, whereas the cells in the area that will become the intervertebral disc proliferate to form the nucleus pulposus. Alternately, cells may migrate to the future disc region.

It is noted that with this resegmentation process, the somite, which was originally segmental (with a segmental muscle mass and spinal nerve and an artery lying between the segments), is converted into a definitive segment of the vertebral body. This segment is actually intersegmental and is spanned by the segmental muscle. The embryologic segmental spinal nerve now lies in an intersegmental position, while the embryologic intersegmen-

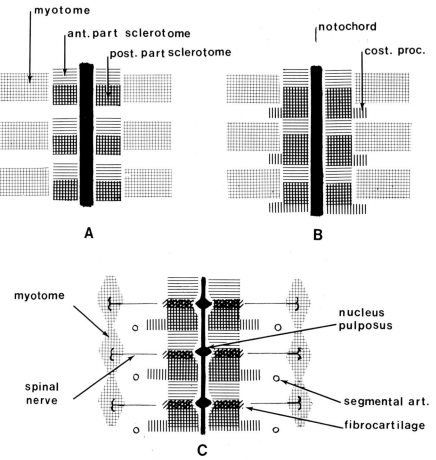

**Figure 5–6** *A,* Schematic representation of the development of the vertebrae. Initial stage of somite formation with a cranial less cellular and caudal more cellular portion. *B,* Cell migration with intersegmental and sclerotomic fissure shown. *C,* Final stage. (Reprinted from Parke, W. W.: Development of the Spine. *In* Rothman, J. R., and Simeone, F. A. (eds.) The Spine. Philadelphia, W. B. Saunders Co., 1975.)

tal vessel comes to lie across the center of the definitive vertebral body.

This resegmentation process probably starts in the lower cervical and upper thoracic areas and extends cranially and caudally (Fig. 5–6).

## CHONDRIFICATION

From the twentieth day of gestation (11 to 14 mm. CR length stage), centers of chondrification appear in the mesenchyme of the membranous vertebral column. In the centrum these centers appear initially on either side of the notochord before fusing. Two centers appear in the neural arches lateral to the neural tube, and their dorsal fusion establishes the neural arch and spinous process. Two additional centers appear at the union of the arch and the centrum, and these extend laterally into the transverse processes. The development of the neural arches starts at a stage later than that of the centrum, as the cells in this area are still proliferating to close the neural arch. The cells dorsal to the neural tube initially have two layers. The outer layer of the cells forms the arches by proliferation at the tips of the processes. This proliferation extends dorsally. The inner layer is called the closure membrane, and the inner cells form the dura mater by fusing across the midline, while the outer cells are continuous with the outer layer. At about the 50 mm. CR stage, these tips are almost united across the dorsal surface of the spinal cord in the upper cervical region, are in contact in the low cervical region, and are completely fused in the thoracic and lumbar regions.

During the seventh and eighth weeks, the anterior and posterior longitudinal ligaments form from the mesenchymal cells that surround the cartilaginous vertebrae. The relationship to the cartilaginous vertebrae is identical to the adult state; the anterior longitudinal ligament is strongly adherent to the anterior surface of the centrum, while the posterior longitudinal ligament is attached only to the edge of the disc.

Between the cartilaginous centra, a ring of cells establishes the annulus fibrosus around the portion of the notochord that will become the nucleus pulposus. With further chondrification on the centra, the notochord is destroyed in this area and remains in the vertebral disc area. Small remnants of the notochord remain in the centrum despite ossification as the mucoid streak.

## OSSIFICATION

The stage of ossification overlaps that of chondrification. In the vertebral arches this process follows a craniocaudal pattern, beginning in the cervical and thoracic regions from the 33 mm. CR stage and extending to the sacral region at the 52 mm. CR stage. In the vertebral bodies, ossification begins in the thoracolumbar region at the same time (34 mm. CR stage) and extends cranially and caudally, involving the sacral bodies at about 55 mm. CR stage and the cervical vertebral bodies at 70 mm. CR stage.

As with other bones, ossification of the vertebrae involves primary and secondary ossification centers. The primary centers in the vertebral body occur initially anterior and posterior to the vestigial mucoid streak. These two areas rapidly coalesce to form a center for the centrum, starting in the low thoracic and upper lumbar region at the 34 mm. CR stage. In the vertebral arches there are two ossification centers on each side. Although ossification starts in the arches in the cervical region, the laminae of the arches first unite in the lumbar region, and this subsequent union progresses cranially.

From the twentieth or twenty-fourth week, the enlargement of the ossification center for the centrum divides the vertebral body into two cartilaginous plates with endochondral ossification, which face the intervertebral discs. These discs are nourished by vascular tufts from the vertebral body, but these tufts do not extend into the annulus; all the nutrition is derived from diffusion. Around the ventral and lateral periphery of the centrum and disc interface, a C-shaped cartilaginous ring develops to form the ring apophyses, which ossify during the second postnatal decade. This ring firmly anchors the annulus to the body and, once ossified, receives the Sharpey's fibers of the annulus.

Secondary centers of ossification develop during the fifteenth to seventeenth years in the tips of the transverse processes and spinous processes and in the ring apophyses.

It must be remembered that the preced-

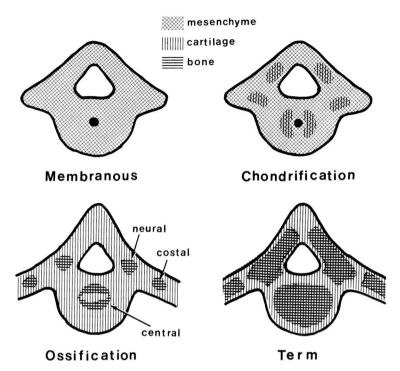

mesenchyme

cartilage

bone

**Membranous**

**Chondrification**

**Ossification**

neural

costal

central

**Term**

**Figure 5–7** Schematic representation of the development of the vertebrae, showing the stages of membranous development, chondrification, and ossification. (Reprinted from Parke, W. W.: Development of the spine. *In* Rothman, R. H., and Simeone, F. A.: The Spine. Philadelphia, W. B. Saunders Co., 1975.)

ing description applies to the typical vertebrae in the thoracic area. The exact site of the ossification centers is modified with the specialization of the vertebrae in different areas of the vertebral column. For example, in the lumbar area, secondary centers for the mamillary processes occur. It must be noted that throughout the vertebrae, the eventual fusion of the vertebral arches and the centrum occurs well anterior to the pedicles and occurs at the site of the neurocentral synchondrosis. Thus, the definitive vertebral body includes more than just the bone derived from the ossific center of the centrum, and the terms vertebral body and centrum are not interchangeable (Fig. 5–7).

## GROWTH OF THE SPINE

The majority of progressive spinal deformities of childhood have their most rapid increase during periods of growth acceleration. Thus, the student of spinal deformity has always been interested in spinal growth and its relationship to spinal curvature.

As shown by Tanner, normal longitudinal growth does *not* proceed in a uniform, linear pattern.[36] There are two periods of rapid growth, the first from birth to age three and the second at the adolescent growth spurt. The intervening period (i.e., from age three to the onset of puberty) is a period of quiet but steady growth. Contrary to popular thought, normal growth during this period is quite steady, without stops and starts. As measurements are made more precisely, growth during this period is shown to be linear (Fig. 5–8).

Total body height is composed of several regions or structures, including the head, cervical spine, thoracic spine, lumbar spine, femora, tibiae, and feet. All of these grow at different rates. The head is relatively large at birth and subsequently grows the least. The lower limbs are relatively short at birth and grow the most. The spine is intermediate between the head and legs in terms of quantity of growth. Normal growth can be plotted in two ways, either by height attained or by velocity (e.g., cm./year of growth) (Fig. 5–9).

The pubertal growth spurt is of particular interest to the spine surgeon and physician. The girl with a mild curve suddenly develops a severe curve. The patient doing well in a brace suddenly loses that response, and the brace "fails." A child solidly fused years before suddenly begins to develop either

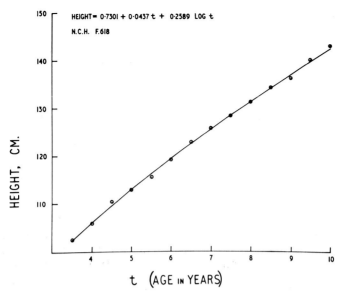

**Figure 5–8**  The carefully measured heights of a child from age 3 to age 10. This demonstrates the typical linear growth of this period. (Reprinted from Zorab, P. A. (ed.): Scoliosis and Growth. Proceedings of a Third Symposium held at the Institute of Diseases of the Chest, Brompton Hospital, London, on November 13, 1970. London, Churchill Livingstone, 1971.)

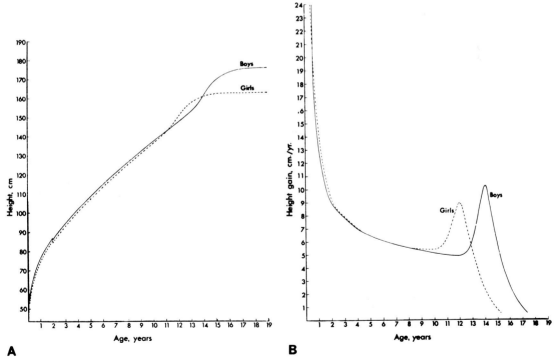

**Figure 5–9**  A, Growth charted from birth to maturity for both boys and girls. Height achieved is plotted against years. B, Growth velocity curves. This is the same material as in A but charted as growth gain (cm./year) against years. (Reprinted from Zorab, P. A. (ed.): Scoliosis and Growth. Proceedings of a Third Symposium held at the Institute of Diseases of the Chest, Brompton Hospital, London, on November 13, 1970. London, Churchill Livingstone, 1971.)

bending of the fusion mass or lengthening of the curve, or both. When exactly is this moment of crisis? How can we recognize its development?

In girls, the beginning of the growth spurt coincides with or is slightly before the start of breast and pubic hair development. This occurs at skeletal age 11 on the average (studies of Anglo-Saxon Caucasians). The peak velocity of the growth spurt is one year later, at age 12, and the spurt is over by age 14. The menarche occurs at age 13, two years after the onset of the growth spurt.

In boys, the peak height velocity occurs two years later than for girls. The adolescent growth spurt in boys is set later in their puberty than for girls, i.e., the growth spurt in boys starts slightly *after* the development of pubic hair, and in girls it starts slightly *before*. The average boy finishes the growth spurt at age 16 and all growth at age 17. It must be remembered that these are average values and there is a considerable range of normal. Similar studies of other races have not been done (Fig. 5–10).

The pathogenic relationship between scoliosis and growth has been extensively investigated by Duval-Beaupere.[7, 8] She studied 560 scoliosis patients, 500 paralytic (mostly poliomyelitis) and 60 idiopathic, as to the progression of their curves in relation to various aspects of growth and development. The curves increased at a steady rate until the onset of puberty (and the onset of the growth spurt). The curves then accelerated at a new rate. This new rate of curve increase continued until all growth ceased (approximately Risser 4+). It is of interest that the velocity of curve increase did not decrease as the velocity of spine growth began to slow down (Fig. 5–11).

What exactly is it about the adolescent growth spurt that makes a curvature increase? It is tempting to relate these growth changes to changes in growth of the vertebrae, but in actuality, most scolioses that are rapidly progressive at this time do not show alterations of bone growth. The curvatures are caused by deformation of the disc spaces and not by deformation of the vertebrae (Fig. 5–12).

Since the profound changes of puberty

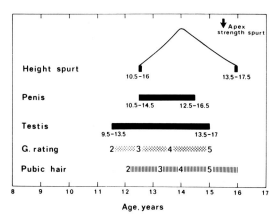

**Figure 5–10**   Peak velocity of growth as compared with various parameters of development. (Reprinted from Zorab, P. A. (ed.): Scoliosis and Growth. Proceedings of a Third Symposium held at the Institute of Diseases of the Chest, Brompton Hospital, London, on November 13, 1970. London, Churchill Livingstone, 1971.)

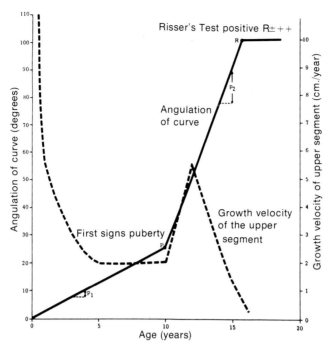

Longitudinal study of the development of scoliosis compared with growth velocity.
Key: - - - - - - - 53 Normal girls
500 Paralytic, 60 Idiopathic scoliotics

**Figure 5–11** Growth velocity (dotted line) plotted against angulation of the curve in 560 patients followed by Durar Beaupere. Note that the acceleration of curve increase occurs simultaneously with the accelerated growth. (Reprinted from Zorab, P. A. (ed.): Scoliosis and Growth. Proceedings of a Third Symposium held at the Institute of Diseases of the Chest, Brompton Hospital, London, on November 13, 1970. London, Churchill Livingstone, 1971.)

are hormonal, it is perhaps logical to think that the effects are due to hormonal influences on the soft tissues of the vertebral column. Although preliminary studies of hormonal factors have been started, our state of knowledge is so limited at this time that nothing of a concrete nature can be stated.

The effect of spine fusion on spine growth was a hotly debated topic for several years. Recently, however, it has been proved that the fused area does not grow longitudinally.[11, 13, 17, 19] Thus the question is: What is the optimal time for a spinal fusion? It should be obvious that there is no single best time for fusion. This varies with the diagnosis and the individual patient and will be discussed in subsequent chapters. Some general parameters are worthy of mention here.

Not all of the total body height is in the spine. Some is from the head, and a considerable amount is from the legs. The legs do not participate in the adolescent growth spurt. As shown by Anderson, Hwang, and Green,[1] the growth of the legs is a linear phenomenon. This makes estimates of leg length relatively easy when planning an epiphyseodesis for leg length inequality.

Charts of normal sitting heights as well as standing heights are available. The ratio of sitting height to standing height is about 63 per cent at age one, 60 per cent at age two, and finally 52 per cent in boys and 53 per cent in girls at the end of growth.[25]

Generally speaking, one's total height at the end of growth will be twice the height at age two. This is not merely an "old wives'

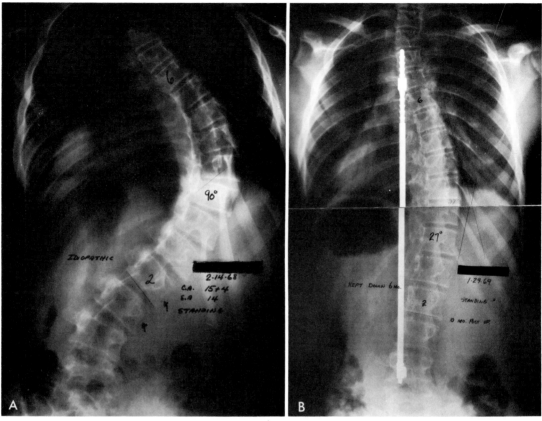

**Figure 5–12** *A,* A rapidly progressive adolescent scoliosis of 90 degrees. Note that the deformity occurs in the disc spaces, not in the vertebral bodies. *B,* The same patient, 10 months following correction and fusion. The correction has occurred in the disc spaces. The end-plates of each vertebra are parallel.

tale" but is confirmed by anthropomorphic tables. For example, consider an individual who is age two and 80 cm. in height. We know that his sitting height is 60 per cent of the total; thus his sitting height is 48 cm. and the leg portion 32 cm. At the end of growth, he will be 160 cm., and this about 50 per cent legs and 50 per cent upper segment, i.e., 80 cm. each. Thus, the lower segment will have grown from 32 cm. to 80 cm., or a 48 cm. gain, but the sitting segment, increased from 48 cm. to 80 cm., or only a 32 cm. gain.

What if we fused six segments of his spine at age two years? In a two year old, six segments of the spine account for $\frac{1}{6}$ of the sitting height. Thus, if six segments are fused at age two, $\frac{1}{6}$ of the amount of growth of the spine and head that would occur between age two and the end of growth will be lost. Since this total amount was 32 cm., the loss is equal to 5.3 cm. In summary, a six-segment fusion at age two will result in only a 5.3 cm.

loss of height at the end of growth. As a result, this individual's final total height will be 154.7 cm. instead of 160 cm., or a loss of 3.3 per cent. This, of course, assumes that this area of the spine would have grown normally and that all areas of the spine grow equally. Usually, however, we are dealing with pathologic spines in which normal vertical growth cannot occur. *Usually, the amount of shortening caused by the fusion is less than the amount of shortening that would have been caused by the progressive curve.*

From standard growth tables, we can determine that the average female spine grows 28.6 cm. between age 2 and age 16. Since there are 29 spinal segments, that is 1.0 cm./segment for 14 years, or 1.0/14 = 0.07 cm. per segment per year. From this number, the potential shortening caused by any spine fusion can be calculated as follows:[41] cm. of shortening = 0.07 × number of segments

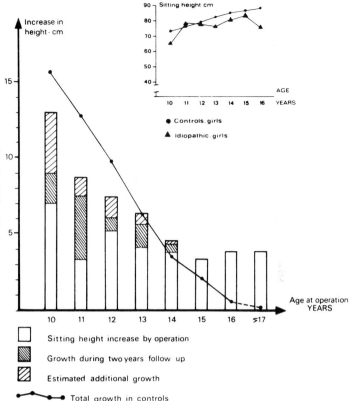

**Figure 5–13** Relationship of scoliosis surgery to body height. From age 13 on, the surgery always results in a taller child than if no surgery was done. Even at age 10, there is only 3 cm. difference between the fused child and the normal. (Reprinted from, Studies in idiopathic scoliosis. Nordwall, A.: Acta Orthop. Scand., Suppl. 150, 1973.)

fused × number of years of growth remaining.

The problem with this formula is that it assumes that all spinal segments have the same growth, but in fact lumbar segments grow more than thoracic segments. There will be a greater stunting effect if five lumbar vertebrae are fused than if five thoracic vertebrae are fused.

Nordwall[22] has graphed the effect not only of fusion on growth of the spine but also of the correction of the curve on total height. This also confirms the relatively small negative effect of spine fusion after age 10. At age 13, there is normal spine length, and beyond age 13, the correction effect far outweighs the stunting effect (Fig. 5–13).

# REFERENCES

1. Anderson, M., Hwang, S., Green, W. T.: Growth of the normal trunk in boys and girls during the second decade of life, related to age, maturity, and ossification of the iliac epiphyses. J. Bone Joint Surg., 47A:1554–1564, 1965.
2. Bick, . M., Copel, J. W., and Spector, S.: Longitudinal growth of the human vertebra. J. Bone Joint Surg., 32A:803–814, 1950.
3. Calvo, J. J.: Observations on the growth of the female adolescent spine and its relation to scoliosis. Clin. Orthop., 10:40, 1957.
4. Dommisse, G. F.: *The Arteries and Veins of the Human Spinal Cord from Birth.* Churchill Livingstone, Edinburgh, London, and New York, 1975.
5. Doppman, J. L., DiChiro, G., and Ommaya, A. V.: *Selective Arteriography of the Spinal Cord.* St. Louis, W. Green, 1969.
6. Duthie, R.: The significance of growth in orthopaedic surgery. Clin. Orthop., 14:7, 1959.
7. Duval-Beaupere, G.: Les Reperes de maturation dans la surveillance des scoliosis. Rev. Chir. Orthop., 56:56, 1970.
8. Duval-Beaupere, G.: The growth of scoliotic patients. Hypothesis and preliminary study. Acta Orthop. Belg., 38:365–376, 1972.
9. Ehrenhaft, J. L.: Development of the vertebral column as related to certain congenital and pathologic changes. Surg. Gynecol. Obstet., 76:282, 1943.
10. Epstein, B. S.: *The Spine — A Radiological Text and Atlas.* Philadelphia, Lea and Febiger, 1976.

11. Haas, S. L.: Influence of fusion of the spine on growth of the vertebrae. Arch. Surg., *41*:607, 1940.

12. James, C. C. M., and Lassman, L. P.: *Spinal Dysraphism — Spina Bifida Occulta*. London, Butterworth and Co., 1972.

13. Johnson, J. T. H., and Southwick, W. O.: Bone growth after spine fusion. J. Bone Joint Surg., *42A*:1396, 1960.

14. Karaharju, E. O.: Deformation of vertebrae in experimental scoliosis. The cause of bone adaptation and modeling in scoliosis with reference to the normal growth of the vertebra. Acta. Orthop. Scand., Suppl. 105, 1967.

15. Keim, H. A., and Hilal, S. K.: Spinal angiography in scoliosis patients. J. Bone Joint Surg., 904, 1971.

16. Lemire, R. J., Loeser, J. D., Leech, R. W., and Alvord, E. C.: *Normal and Abnormal Development of the Human Nervous System*. Hagerstown, Harper and Row, 1976.

17. Letts, R. M., and Bobechko, W. P.: Fusion of the scoliotic spine in young children. Clin. Orthop., *101*: 136–145, 1974.

18. Misol, S., Ponseti, J., Samaan, N., and Bradburg, J.: Growth hormone blood levels in patients with idiopathic scoliosis. Clin. Orthop., *81*:122, 1971.

19. Moe, J. H., Sundberg, A. B., and Gustilo, R.: A clinical study of spine fusion in the growing child. J. Bone Joint Surg., *46B*:784–785, 1964.

20. Nachlas, W., and Borden, J. N.: The cure of experimental scoliosis by directed growth control. J. Bone Joint Surg., *33A*:24, 1951.

21. Neugebauer, H.: Total estrogens in juvenile cases of scoliosis. Pediatrie und paedologie, *9*:5, 1974.

22. Nordwall, A.: Studies in idiopathic scoliosis. Acta Orthop. Scand., Suppl. 150, 1973.

23. Parke, W. W.: Development of the spine. *In* Rothman, R. H., and Simeone, F. A.: *The Spine*. Philadelphia, W. B. Saunders Co., 1975.

24. Rappaport, R., Forest, M., Bayard, F., Duval-Beaupere, G., Blizzard, R., and Migeon, C.: Plasma androgens and LH in scoliotic patients with premature pubarche. J. Clin. Endocrinol. Metab., *38*:401, 1974.

25. Risser, J., Agostini, S., Sampaio, J., and Garibaldi, C.: The sitting-standing height ratio as a method of evaluating early spine fusion in the growing child. Clin. Orthop., *24*:7, 1973.

26. Roaf, R.: Vertebral growth and its mechanical control. J. Bone Joint Surg., *42B*:40, 1960.

27. Schmorl, G., and Junghans, H.: *The Human Spine in Health and Disease*. New York and London, Grune and Stratton, 1971.

28. *Scoliosis and Growth*. Proceedings of a Third Symposium held at the Institute of Diseases of the Chest, Brompton Hospital, London, November 13, 1970. Ed.: P. A. Zorab, Churchill Livingstone, London, 1971.

29. Sensenig, E. C.: The early development of the human vertebral column. Contr. to Embryol., *33*:21–51, 1949.

30. Stillwell, D. L.: Structural deformities of vertebrae bone. Adaptation and modeling in experimental scoliosis and kyphosis. J. Bone Joint Surg., *44A*:611, 1962.

31. Streeter, G. L.: Factors involved in the formation of the filum terminale. Am. J. Anat., *25*:1–11, 1919.

32. Streeter, G. L.: Development horizons in human embryos. Description of age groups XI, 13 to 20 somites and age group XII, 21 to 29 somites. Contrib. Embryol., *30*:211–245, 1942.

33. Streeter, G. L.: Developmental horizons in human embryos. Description of age groups XIX, XX, XXI, XXII, and XXIII. Contrib. Embryol., *230*:167–196.

34. Suh, T. H., and Alexander, L.: Vascular system of the human spinal cord. Arch. Neurol. Psych., *41*:659, 1939.

35. Tanner, J. M.: *Growth at Adolescence*. 2nd Ed. London, Blackwell, 1962.

36. Tanner, J. M., Whitehouse, R. H., and Takaisni, M.: Standards from birth to maturity for height, weight, height velocity, and weight velocity: British Children, 1965. Arch. Dis. Child., *41*:454–471, 613–635, 1966.

37. Tuchmann-Suplesiss, H., David, G., and Haegel, P.: *Illustrated Human Embryology*. Vol. I., Embryogenesis. New York, Springer Verlag, 1972.

38. Veliskakis, K., and Levine, D.: Effects of posterior spine fusion on vertebral growth in dogs. J. Bone Joint Surg., *48A*:1367, 1967.

39. Willner, S., Nilsson, K. O., Kastrup, K., and Bergstrand, C.: Growth hormone and somatomedin A in girls with adolescent idiopathic scoliosis. Acta. Pediatr. Scand., *65*:547, 1976.

40. Willner, S.: The proportion of legs to trunk in girls with idiopathic structural scoliosis. Acta Orthop. Scand., *46*:84, 1975.

41. Winter, R. W.: Scoliosis and spinal growth. Orthop. Rev., *6*:17–20, 1977.

# Chapter 6

# IDIOPATHIC SCOLIOSIS

Idiopathic scoliosis is the most common of all forms of lateral deviation of the spine. As its name indicates, its etiology is unknown. It occurs during the growing years and is customarily divided into three types: infantile, juvenile, and adolescent. These are classified according to the age at which the deformity is first noted, which is not necessarily the same as the time the curvature first appears.

Idiopathic scoliosis develops in a previously normal straight spine and has been recognized as an entity for more than a century. Its relationship to scoliosis secondary to poliomyelitis has been disproved, as its incidence has remained the same since vaccines have virtually eliminated poliomyelitis. No relationship has been established to any form of scoliosis for which the etiology is known.

## ETIOLOGIC INVESTIGATIONS

Throughout the eighteenth and nineteenth centuries, scoliosis was believed to be caused by postural positioning of the body. During the past several decades investigations from many aspects have been described in innumerable publications. These include studies on alterations in connective tissue metabolism,[32] operative disturbance of bone and spinal ligaments,[16, 17] denervation procedures, metabolism of connective tissues, dietary factors, enzymatic factors, tendon and ligamentous elasticity, joint elasticity, the intervertebral disc, electromyography of the paravertebral muscles, vestibular function, vertebral rotation, and inheritance factors.[19, 42, 43, 44]

Of all these studies, none have shown any consistent abnormalities bearing on the etiology of idiopathic scoliosis, with the exception of investigations of the genetic aspects.

## GENETIC ASPECTS

It seems more than probable that idiopathic scoliosis is an inherited disease, the mode of inheritance being multifactorial. No chromosome anomalies have been found, but studies by DeGeorge and Fischer (1967),[10] Wynne-Davies (1968–1975),[43, 44, 45] Riseborough and Wynne-Davies (1973),[33] MacEwen and Cowell (1970),[19] and personal observations have borne out the fact that the disease is found in twins, families, and siblings more frequently than random distribution would suggest (Fig. 6–1). The degree and pattern of curvature are extremely variable. In our school survey program, which now comprises over 250,000 juvenile and early adolescent pupils, the incidence of persistent small flexible or structural curves is about five per cent, almost equally divided between boys and girls. A majority have a measurable rib hump. The majority of curves progress very little or not at all, but when progression does occur, it is found mainly in girls. Some curves improve spontaneously. Some curves progress but only by a small amount and may stop progressing in adolescence with final curves of 20 to 25 degrees.

Recent interest in the development of school survey programs may lead to further knowledge of the familial aspects of idiopathic scoliosis in its early development. The incidence of small curves in the general population and their relationship to the factors of inheritance and to large curves must still be investigated. (See Chapter 4.)

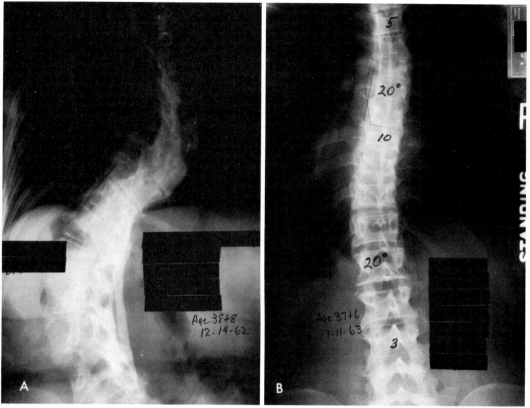

**Figure 6–1** *A,* An interesting study of two sisters, both with scoliosis, married to two brothers without scoliosis. No past history of scoliosis available in either family. Mrs. M.H., 38+8. Fused in adolescence. Analysis at present indicates that in Family, #1: C.H.: age 4 +3 to 13+0. The brace apparently corrected the high thoracic curve and was deemed necessary at that time. J.H., age 11+6 to 15+6, did not require treatment. D.H., son, age 9+3 to 17+3, was developing a progressive double major curve, thoracic and lumbar. *B,* Mrs. H.H., 37+6, sister of Mrs. M.H. (*A*). No treatment. Analysis of treatment program of children in this family shows: R.H., age 10+0 to 21+0, had definitely progressive double major curves, thoracic and lumbar, which needed the brace and responded very well in four years of bracing. C.H., age 6+2 to 12+0, spontaneously improved without treatment. L.H., age 6+6 to 17+0, had two 15 degree curves that decreased to 6 degrees without treatment.

## CURVE PATTERNS

Schulthess in 1905[37] published a classification of curve patterns in idiopathic scoliosis. In 1950, Ponseti and Friedman[31] reviewed 394 untreated adolescent patients with idiopathic scoliosis and classified them with modification from Schulthess. They divided curve patterns into five classes:

*Main Lumbar.* The apex is the first or second lumbar vertebra. The end vertebrae are T11 or T12 and L4 or L5. This pattern was found in 24 per cent of patients.

*Thoracolumbar.* The apex is T11 or T12. The end vertebrae are T6 or T7 to L1 or L2. This pattern was found in 16 per cent.

*Combined Thoracic and Lumbar.* The upper curve (thoracic) has its apex at T6 or T7. The lower curve (lumbar) has its apex at L2. The lower end vertebrae of the two curves were recognizable at onset, and the curves usually increased at the same rate, although the thoracic curve was usually the larger. This pattern was found in 37 per cent.

*Main Thoracic.* The apical vertebra is T8 or T9, the end vertebrae T6 and T11. This pattern was found in 22 per cent.

*Cervicothoracic.* The apex is T3. The upper end vertebra is found at C7 or T1 and the lower end vertebra at T4 or T5. This pattern was found in 1.3 per cent.

Since its publication, this classification has been used by most authors. While all forms of idiopathic scoliosis develop curve patterns, their importance increases with progression of the curvature in juvenile years and particularly during adolescent years.

In infantile idiopathic curves, most are left thoracic or thoracolumbar, although a few double thoracic and lumbar curves have been reported in Great Britain. Juvenile types are usually single major thoracic or double major thoracic and lumbar.

Confusion in terminology has been prevalent in the past. In the following description, all terms such as primary, secondary, and compensatory have been discarded in favor of Cobb's descriptive terms of major and minor curves.[6, 7] A major curve is the most deforming and the most structural. A minor curve is less deforming and less structural. Curves are described according to the location of the apical vertebra, vertebrae, or interspace.

In our experience, the following classification of curve patterns includes most types of curves and has been most helpful in outlining prognosis and treatment:

Single major thoracic
Single major thoracolumbar
Single major lumbar
Major thoracic and minor lumbar
Double major thoracic and lumbar
Double major thoracolumbar and thoracic
Double major thoracic
Multiple curve patterns

## Single Major Thoracic Curve Pattern
(Fig. 6–2)

The apex of the curve lies within the thoracic spine. The curve extends from T4, T5, or T6 to T11, T12, L1, or L2. The most common end vertebrae are T5 and T12. Nearly all have the convexity directed to the right. In magnitude and progression, these curves vary. When large, they are among the most deforming of all idiopathic spinal curvatures. The curve may have its onset during late juvenile years and not be discovered until early adolescence. The lumbar minor curve is nearly always flexible. On the lateral x-ray, the vertebral alignment is often minimally kyphotic or is flat. The thoracic spine may be actually lordotic, projecting anteriorly beyond the flat or neutral position. There is seldom a true kyphosis of significance. The term ky-

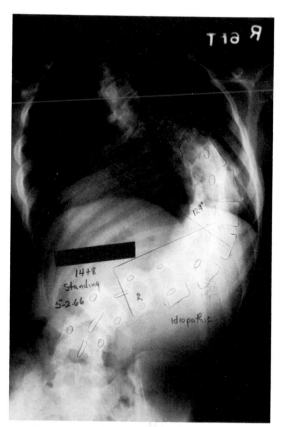

**Figure 6–2** A longer variety of the right thoracic major curve. Both upper thoracic and lower lumbar curves are nearly flexible and are minor.

phoscoliosis is seldom appropriate, because lordosis is most often present. Rib prominence does not constitute kyphosis. The lordosis of the thoracic spine may play a significant role in depletion of pulmonary function.[41]

Clinically, the rib prominence on the convexity varies in magnitude. These differences are not necessarily due to the size of the curves or to the rotation seen on the anteroposterior x-ray. On the forward bending test, a 40 degree curve may show only one centimeter of rib elevation, while some 25 or 30 degree curves may demonstrate rib elevation measuring four to five centimeters. We have seen straight spines and five degree curves with rib elevation of two to three centimeters and vertebral rotation present on the anteroposterior x-ray. Studies of idiopathic scoliosis have shown little correlation of the rib prominence, curve magnitude, vertebral rotation on anteroposterior roentgenograms, and rib vertebral angle.

## Single Major Thoracolumbar Curve Pattern
(Fig. 6–3)

This is a single curve in which the upper thoracic spine is straight or shows only a minimal flexible curve. The thoracolumbar curve is often very flexible. It extends from T8, T9, or T10 to L3, with the apex at the thoracolumbar junction. This curve pattern often displays a decompensation of the torso, with an offset of several centimeters. Below L3 there is a short compensatory fractional curve, which is usually flexible. The thoracolumbar curve is frequently seen as a small curve in school screening programs, but it is not a common pattern in surgical experience.

## Single Major Lumbar Curve Pattern
(Fig. 6–4)

This pattern is less common in adolescence, but it is frequently found as a small flexible curve in the early school screening program. The apex lies within the lumbar

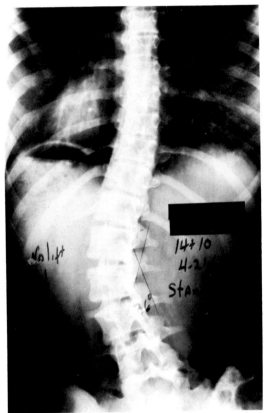

**Figure 6–4** D.T., age 14+10. Lumbar curve, 36 degrees, deforming. Note low pelvis on convexity—a not unusual occurrence. 4/21/61.

spine, usually at L2. The upper end vertebra may be T11 or T12, but it is most often L1. The lowest end vertebra most often is L5 but may be L4. There is a very short fractional curve between L4 or L5 and the sacrum. Lumbar curves are often accompanied by an uneven pelvic brim, which most often is lower on the convex side. This factor often contributes to the magnitude of the curve in the standing x-ray. Lumbar major curves seldom measure more than 60 degrees during adolescence, but they usually distort the waistline. Occasionally there is no noticeable deformity. The thoracic spine is seldom noticeably curved, but there is often a small fractional curve of two or three vertebrae directly above the upper end of the lumbar curve.

## Single Major High Thoracic Curve Pattern
(Fig. 6–5)

The high thoracic curve may occur without a lower thoracic curve or with a small

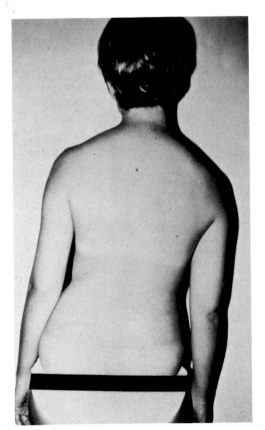

**Figure 6–3** D.D., age 24; severely decompensated single thoracolumbar pattern.

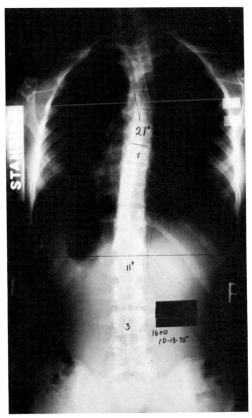

**Figure 6–5**  P.D., age 16+0. A single right high thoracic curve with neck deformity due to elevated right rib. Nearly all single high thoracic curves are left, making this an unusual curve. 10/13/75.

completely flexible curve below. The high thoracic curve is almost always convex to the left and produces a significant neck deformity. In the literature this type has been erroneously termed a cervicothoracic pattern, but the apex actually lies in the upper thoracic spine. The upper vertebra is nearly always T1 or T2 and rarely may be C7.

### Major Thoracic and Minor Lumbar Curve Pattern (Fig. 6–6)

This is a very common pattern, in which the right major thoracic curve is compensated by a lumbar curve that varies in its structural component. The thoracic curve remains larger and more structural. The lumbar curve may be of equal magnitude on upright x-ray measurement, but supine side-bending x-rays show a greater degree of flexibility.

With the passage of time and growth, the flexibility of the lumbar curve may decrease so that it also becomes a major curve. However, the thoracic curve remains the larger and is always more structural.

After the lumbar curve has become severely structural, the difference between this pattern and the double major thoracic and lumbar curve pattern becomes less distinct.

The thoracic curve is typically from T4 or T5 to T12 or L1. The lumbar curve usually extends to L4 or L5.

### Double Major Thoracic and Lumbar Curve Pattern (Fig. 6–7)

The thoracic curve is nearly always convex to the right and has its apex at T7 or

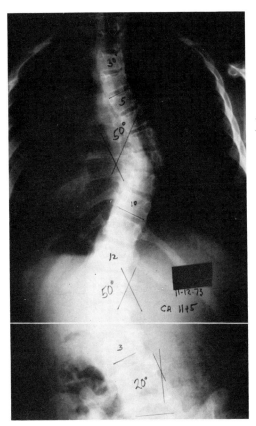

**Figure 6–6**  A right thoracic, left lumbar curve with a structural high left thoracic curve. The high left thoracic curve had its upper end at T2 and did not cause a rib elevation. At first evaluation, one might think this was a double major thoracic and lumbar curve. It is really a quadruple curve, although all curves are not major.

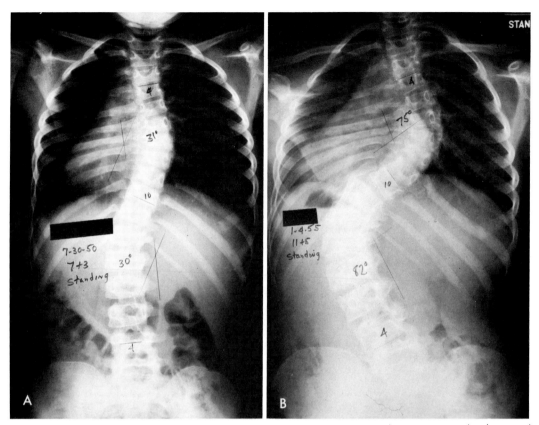

**Figure 6–7** *A,* J.P., age 7+3. A true double major thoracic and lumbar pattern. Both curves appeared at the same time and were equally structural from their onset. Right thoracic curve: T4–T10=31 degrees; standing left lumbar, T10–L4=30 degrees. No treatment. At this time there is a right thoracic, left lumbar major pattern. 7/30/50. *B,* J.P., age 11+5. Severe equal progression of curves: T4–T10=75 degrees; T10–L4=82 degrees standing. Lower curve apex at L1. 1/4/55.

T8. The upper end vertebra is T4, T5, or T6, and the lower end vertebra is T10, T11, or T12. The left lumbar curve has its apex at L1 or L2 and extends to L4 or L5.

Both curves appear simultaneously, usually during juvenile years, and are equally structural from the time of onset. They remain equally structural during their progression in the adolescent years. They are usually equal in magnitude and show little or no decompensation. Between the two curves there is always a neutrally rotated vertebra, which is sometimes called the transitional vertebra. This pattern usually progresses during adolescence.

**Double Major Thoracolumbar and Thoracic Curve Pattern** (Fig. 6–8)

The thoracic component is a short structural right curve. Usually the upper end vertebra is T4, and the lower end vertebra is T9 or T10. This type generally demonstrates little rib elevation. The apex is T6 or T7. The thoracolumbar left curve extends from T9 or T10 to L3, very seldom any lower. The apex is the interspace of T12–L1. The lower curve is more flexible than the thoracic curve above it but is more deforming. The curves may occasionally be reversed in direction. This pattern begins as two structural curves.

**Double Major Thoracic Curve Pattern** (Fig. 6–9)

This pattern was first recognized and described by Moe.[23] Its salient feature is the presence of two major curves, both occurring within the thoracic spine. The upper thoracic curve is virtually always to the left, with its apex at T3 or T4. The upper end of this curve

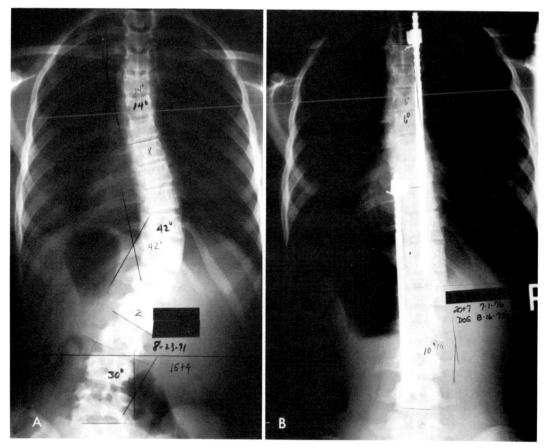

**Figure 6–8** *A,* K.R., age 15+4. A thoracolumbar idiopathic curve with a short lesser high thoracic curve above. The higher curve was less structural but would cause some neck asymmetry if not corrected. *B,* K.R., age 20+7. Both curves were fused with excellent correction. Note that a distraction strut bar was used for each curve and that the two bars were placed to overlap.

is either T1 or T2; the lower, T5 or T6. This curve is highly structural. The lower right curve has its apex within the thoracic spine and extends from T5 or T6 to T11 or as low as L2. This is also a major curve. In some cases, the lower thoracic curve is the less structural. The minor curve in the lumbar spine may be entirely flexible or minimally structural.

The time of appearance and the development of the structural changes are variable. The right thoracic curve may be the first to appear and to show structural fixation, but often the high thoracic curve is the most structural from the onset. The use of the Milwaukee brace, with its right thoracic pad, often promotes the increase of a slightly structural high thoracic left curve and causes it to become a major curve. The high left thoracic curve may in other instances be the

most obviously major curve from the onset. The double major thoracic curve pattern often makes its first appearance during the juvenile years (age four to the onset of puberty). Nearly all curves of this pattern are left high thoracic and right lower thoracic, but occasionally the reverse may be found.

It is especially important to recognize this curve pattern because of the deformity that may be produced by the high thoracic curve; for as it becomes increasingly structural, the first rib becomes elevated on the curve's convexity. This rib, with its overlying muscle, produces an obvious asymmetry of the base of the neck, made more noticeable by the lowering of the first rib on the opposite side. When the lower thoracic curve is large, the neck deformity is not so noticeable. If the lower curve alone is corrected and fused, the

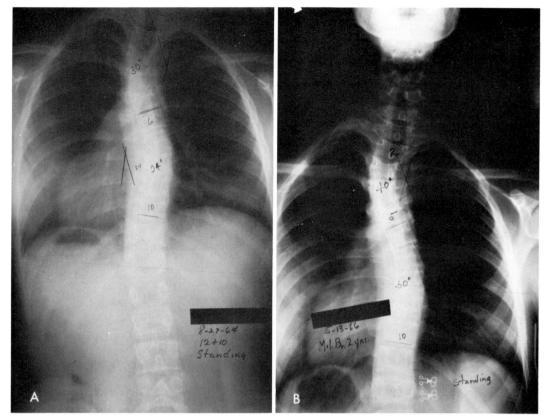

**Figure 6–9**  *A*, R.A., 8/27/64, age 12+10. A double thoracic major pattern. Treatment was Milwaukee brace. Upper thoracic, 30 degrees; lower thoracic, 24 degrees. Neck line slightly prominent on left. *B*, R.A., age 14+7. After two years in brace, curves still increasing: Upper, 40 degrees; lower, 30 degrees out of brace. Elevated left first rib is now more evident, and cosmetic appearance shows asymmetrical neck line. Decision made to correct surgically. 5/13/66.

deformity produced by the upper curve becomes very pronounced. This curve pattern is also of significance because it is so difficult to control by bracing. The upper curve rarely improves in a Milwaukee brace and often worsens.

If the upper end vertebra of the high thoracic curve is T2, the neck deformity is sometimes less pronounced than when the upper end vertebra is T1. If the upper curve is relatively flexible, the rib elevation and the neck deformity may not be increased by correcting only the lower curve. Occasionally, excellent cosmetic appearance is present with two moderate curves, and surgical correction is not indicated (see Fig. 6–13).

The deformity of the neckline is more evident when viewed from the front. It may be entirely overlooked because of long hair. The upper thoracic component of this pattern is commonly missed in the usual 14 × 17 inch x-ray, since it may not be included. Failure to include this area in the side bending films may also cause its structural nature to be overlooked.

### Multiple Curve Patterns (Fig. 6–10)

Although multiple curves have been noted by many, literature describing their occurrence has been almost nonexistent. Travaglini[39] gave the first detailed analysis of "multiple primary idiopathic scoliosis." One can take exception to his use of the word primary, for the curves do not all appear at once.

There are many forms of multiple curves, and they are not all necessarily major. The thoracic and lumbar major patterns always have small fractional curves above and below the two central curves. The double thoracic has a lumbar curve that is almost always flexible and with major curve characteristics seldom present. In rare instances, this type may become a triple major curve.

Multiple curves other than those previously described do occur, but they are usually short and nondeforming. Most are nonprogressive, but one or two may become major deforming curves and require specific treatment. It is axiomatic that the greater the number of curves and the shorter each curve, the less will be the total deformity. In some cases triple curves are all equally structural.

When a survey is made of the parents of children with idiopathic curves, it is not uncommon to find in one or both parents small multiple curves of which they were not aware. Such curves may also occur in adolescents, and unless one or more of the

curves are large, they are not deforming and often are not recognized.

Infrequently one curve (usually thoracolumbar) increases throughout adult life and requires correction and fusion because of pain and deformity.

### Lumbosacral Region

In all spinal curvatures involving the lumbar spine, the lumbosacral area including L5, L4, and sometimes L3 has been a region of dispute for many years. In idiopathic scoliosis the lower end vertebra of all lumbar curves is either L4 or L5. When the end vertebra is L5, there is a reversal of interspace wedging between L4 and L5, and similarly there is a convex wedging of the disc space

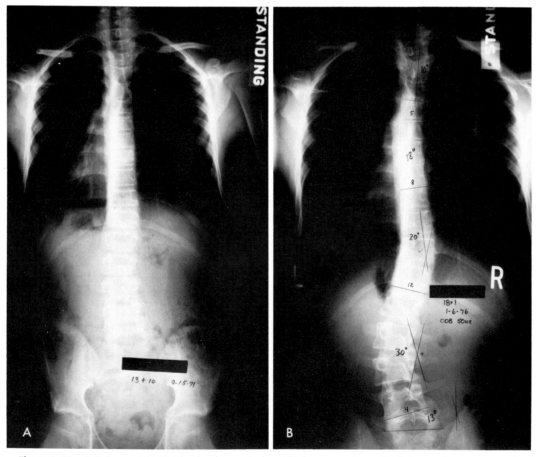

**Figure 6–10**   *A,* D.S., age 13+10. The development of a multiple curve pattern. The first curve to appear was a lumbar minor curve. 9/15/71. *B,* D.S., age 18+1. In another two years, the curve pattern remained the same, with a small increase in each curve. Brace now discontinued; its use did improve his roundback but had no effect on the multiple scoliosis.

between L5 and the horizontal sacrum. For this discussion, all congenital anomalies that give rise to an abnormal oblique upper surface of the sacrum must be eliminated, as must pars interarticularis defects, spondylolisthesis, and other lumbosacral abnormalities.

Not more than 25 years ago, there was a wide-spread belief among orthopedic leaders that the lumbosacral curve was the basis for curves above. Even thoracic curves were treated by lumbosacral fusion. Many orthopedic surgeons performed fusions from the third and fourth lumbar vertebrae to the sacrum using an obliquely placed tibial strut graft from the ilium to the convexity of the third lumbar vertebra. In addition, they performed a routine fusion of this area posteriorly. The strut graft was used as a corrective force to straighten the lumbar curve and secondarily, the thoracic curve. This procedure did not meet with success, although it was used in many patients.

The lumbosacral curve in idiopathic scoliosis is compensatory to curves above it. A study of 800 idiopathic curves by Fisk, Moe, and Winter[11] shows that this area is not the cause of either lumbar or thoracic curves. Nevertheless, it is an area that must be evaluated carefully.

If the end vertebra of the lumbar idiopathic curve is L5, there is only a one-segment fractional curve berween L5 and the horizontal sacrum. In recent years this has been called an "oblique take-off" from the sacrum. If both L4 and L5 are within the lumbosacral curve, the same entity exists. Whether it is a good descriptive term that conveys important and significant information remains a question.

The main significance of the lumbosacral curve is related to its flexibility as shown on side-bending x-rays of the area. In the young adolescent, these views usually show that L4 and L5 can be returned readily to a horizontal position over the sacrum. In older adolescents and in adults, this curve tends to become fixed, and only a partial return to the horizontal can be obtained. We do not feel that the entity "primary lumbosacral idiopathic scoliosis" exists.

## INFANTILE IDIOPATHIC SCOLIOSIS

Relatively rare in the United States and Canada, the entity of infantile idiopathic scoliosis has undergone extensive study in Great Britain and in France. It has long been recognized that these curves are different from those generally encountered and that a high percentage spontaneously resolve.

One of the first reports was that of Harrenstein of Amsterdam[12] in 1929. He reviewed his observations more fully in 1936,[13] noting the spontaneous disappearance of the curves in some infants. He treated most infants in a corrective plaster shell and reported that a majority of curves were progressive. Rickets was postulated as a cause in many. Based on cross section studies and noting the changes in the contour of the thorax in the developing infant from a square to an oval shape, he further postulated that any interference with growth and development of the rib epiphyses would produce inequality of the spine with development of a gibbus, which predisposed to scoliosis.

J. I. P. James of Edinburgh should be given credit for first recognizing infantile idiopathic scoliosis as an entity. In 1951[14] he reported on a study of 33 patients (21 boys and 12 girls). Four curves, all small, disappeared spontaneously. Eleven remained stationary during the period of observation. The remainder progressed severely.

The preliminary survey was followed by further reports by James and others. James, Lloyd-Roberts, and Pilcher[15] reviewed 212 infants in 1959, noting spontaneous resolution in 77 and progression in 135. These curves were all proved to be structural by clinical and x-ray evaluation with the infant held in vertical arm suspension. The sex distribution in 111 thoracic curves was 66 males and 45 females. Ninety curves were convex to the left and 21 to the right. Five were diagnosed at birth and the remainder during the second and third years. Progressive curves often became severe, reaching 100 degrees or more.

Scott and Morgan[38] analyzed 28 progressive infantile idiopathic curves and 7 resolving curves in 1955.

Lloyd-Roberts and Pilcher reviewed 100 infants in 1965[18] who had been diagnosed as having infantile idiopathic structural scoliosis by anteroposterior x-rays, in which the child was suspended by the arms. There were 67 males and 33 females. The curves were all thoracic, left in 85, right in 15. Plagiocephaly was present in 83. Diagnosis of scoliosis was made in most patients at age 3 to 6 months.

Complete resolution occurred without treatment in 92. The disorder resolved in 78 patients in one year and in 11 after three years, during which time a few progressed to as much as 35 degrees. Five progressed severely. No special features were noted to distinguish those who progressed from those who did not. Skull and rib cage moulding and pelvic obliquity were encountered, and these were suggested as possible contributing factors.

Walker, in 1967,[40] reviewed the use of the Denis Browne splint treatment in 49 infants with this form of scoliosis. Of this group, 40 resolved (81.7 per cent); 9 did not. In comparing this study with that of Lloyd-Roberts and Pilcher, it becomes obvious that the Denis Browne splint did not alter the natural course of the deformity.

All these investigators were unable to differentiate the progressive infantile idiopathic scolioses in their early form from those that were self-resolving. Mehta, in 1972,[20] reported a study of 361 patients with this disorder at the Royal National Orthopaedic Hospital in London. By contacting the mothers, 138 of these were returned for a follow-up study. Careful x-ray studies revealed a distinct difference in the relationship of the angle of the rib to the vertebral body in the infants with a progressive curvature from those with resolving curves. In normal infants, the ribs approach the bodies at the same angle bilaterally, but with curvatures they do not.

The rib-vertebral angle (R-V angle) measured at the apical vertebra (Fig. 6–11) is represented by a line drawn in the midvertebra vertically from the most clearly defined vertebral margin plus a line drawn from the midneck to the midpoint of the head of the rib. With no curvature these angles are equal bilaterally. To quote Mehta: "As the spine curves, there is increased downward obliquity of the ribs on the convex as compared with concave side, maximal at the apex of the curve."[20]

In the early stages of curvature, called Phase I by Mehta, a separation of the head of the rib from the body on both sides is seen radiographically. As the curve increases, the head of the rib on the convex side overlaps the upper corner of the corresponding vertebral body. This is termed Phase II by Mehta, and she did not find this to take place in any curve that spontaneously resolved.

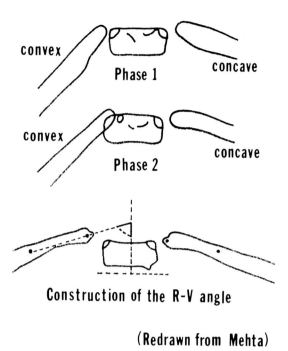

**Construction of the R-V angle**

**(Redrawn from Mehta)**

**Figure 6–11**   Phase 1, Phase 2, and method of measurement of R-V angle (see description in text).

In Phase I, the heads of the ribs are seen radiographically to be separated from the vertebral bodies. Here the R-V angle measurement difference was found to be smaller in the resolving curve. If the initial curve in Phase I was 20 degrees or more, it was regarded as a potentially progressive curve until proved otherwise by subsequent examination.

A definite differentiation could be made after a three-month period of observation. In resolving scoliosis, the R-V angle difference remained unchanged or decreased. Later observations by Mehta have shown that differentiation by the R-V angle comparison is 20 per cent inaccurate.[21]

A recent publication by Wynne-Davies[45] gives enlightening information on this mysterious deformity. She analyzed 134 infants with idiopathic scoliosis from a clinical, genetic, and epidemiologic standpoint. Of these, 97 developed a curve in the first six months of life. All of them had deformity of the head (plagiocephaly), and the flat side of the head always corresponded to the concave side of the curve. In normal infants, out of 223 examined, 28 per cent had varying degrees of plagiocephaly.

In the whole series, mental retardation was found in 13 per cent of the males with progressive scoliosis. Congenital dislocation of the hip occurred in 3.5 per cent and congenital heart disease in 2.5 per cent. Inguinal hernia was found in 7.4 per cent of the males, in 3 per cent of the parents, and in 3 per cent of the siblings. There was a greater than normal number of breech deliveries and of premature low birth weights in the males. A preponderance of curves appeared in births occurring during the winter months. Infants with progressive scoliosis usually had older mothers and came from poor families. Only three children in the series, all with resolving scoliosis, habitually lay prone in early infancy.

In this study by Wynne-Davies, the ratio of males to females was 3:2. There was a preponderance of left-side curves (76 per cent) and thoracic curves (98 per cent). Only 6 curves were present at birth; 91 developed between one and six months, and the remaining 37 were not proved. Of curves developing within the first six months, 64 per cent resolved. No reason for the low incidence of this deformity in the United States and Canada as compared to Great Britain was discovered.

Infantile idiopathic scoliosis appears to be a different entity from the adolescent type. Juvenile scoliosis is probably more closely related to the adolescent variety, since it is certain that many cases first noted in adolescence (or after the onset of puberty) have been present but unnoticed for some time during juvenile years. Progressive infantile idiopathic scoliosis also continues to progress throughout juvenile and adolescent years. In its severe form it shortens life through its severe depletion of pulmonary and cardiac function.

As an entity, the infantile variety lacks many of the characteristics of the adolescent type. It is more commonly found in the male, and it is often found associated with congenital abnormalities outside the spine. The spontaneous resolution of the curve in such a high percentage is found less often in juveniles and adolescent curves. Many curves appearing in juvenile years remain small and nonprogressive, and resolution of juvenile curves also occurs. Brooks[1] found resolution in 20 per cent of curves less than 25 degrees in young patients, and it is not uncommon to find a curve first noted in early juvenile or adoles-

cent years to remain unchanged during growth or at least to show only minor progression without treatment (see Fig. 6–19).

It appears that as little is known about the etiology of infantile idiopathic scoliosis as is known about the juvenile and adolescent varieties. Wynne-Davies wrote:[45]

The etiology of infantile idiopathic scoliosis must be multifactorial, with a genetic tendency to the deformity which can then be "triggered off" in different individuals by different factors, some medical, some genetic, and some social. The exact cause in each individual is likely to be different and the balance must vary from patient to patient; thus someone with a strong genetic tendency would need very little "triggering action." At the other end of the scale, scoliosis may possibly be produced in a child with no genetic tendency to the deformity, entirely by adverse environmental factors.

## Treatment

### NONOPERATIVE TREATMENT: THE SMALL AND MODERATE CURVE IN INFANCY (Fig. 6–12)

When a baby with infantile idiopathic scoliosis is first presented to the orthopedic surgeon, a careful analysis of all aspects of the condition must be made. The presence of plagiocephaly, congenital abnormalities of the extremities, and torticollis should be noted. The flexibility of the spine can be assessed clinically by carefully suspending the child by the arms. Radiography should be performed in both the supine and the suspended positions. These films must be of the highest quality, showing all vertebrae clearly in both the anteroposterior and the lateral views. A careful search is made for evidence of congenital abnormalities within the spine. The R-V angle of Mehta and the curve angle are measured in both the supine and the suspended positions.

Curves of less than 20 degrees in infants under six months of age should be observed and re-evaluated every two to three months. If the R-V angle of the convexity is suggestive of a potentially progressive curve and the curve measures more than 20 degrees when first seen, treatment should be instituted. If observation discloses an increase in the R-V angle or an increase in the curve angle and in structural fixation, immediate treatment must

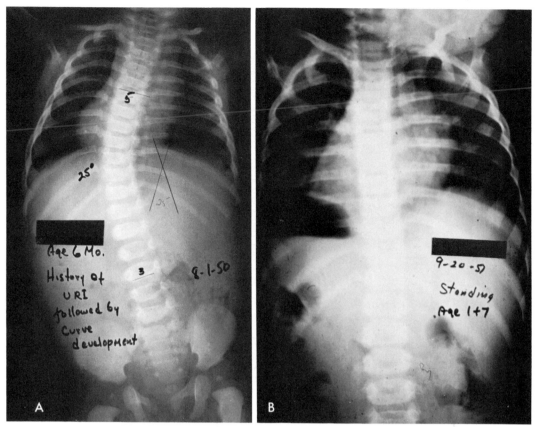

**Figure 6–12** *A*, M.D. A structural curve in a 6 month old female. Note the characteristic left thoracolumbar curve. 8/1/50. *B*, M.D., age 1+7. One year later without treatment, the curve had disappeared. This is a typical self-resolving infantile idiopathic curve. 9/20/51.

begin. If flexibility is satisfactory, the Kalabis splint (a three-point torso harness) may be used, but after six months of age the Milwaukee brace with a plastic pelvic girdle is usually more effective. A throat mold and occipital pads are not used in infants; instead, the neck ring is padded throughout. With a progressive curve in a child over one year, a series of casts, applied while the child is anesthetized with Ketamine, may restore correction, and the Milwaukee brace may again be used.

Curves that show no evidence of progression and that demonstrate a benign R–V angle should be watched, for these appear to be self-resolving.

Curves shown to be potentially progressive or that have demonstrated their progressive nature will nearly always respond to a vigorous early nonoperative regimen.

During the past few years an interesting observation has come from Morel of Berck-

Plage.[28] Infantile idiopathic curves of 40 to 60 degrees have been treated by a period of longitudinal Cotrel traction, followed by a series of E.D.F. (elongation, derotation, flexion) casts changed every two to three months. When curves are reduced to less than 10 degrees, the child is placed in a plastic corset or Milwaukee brace. Stable correction was obtained in a substantial percentage of these patients, permitting discontinuance of external support even in juvenile years. The changes that might take place during the rapid growth spurt of adolescence have not been substantially verified. The series to date indicates that this method may provide permanent correction in a formerly progressive curve.

We have observed such stabilization in a four year old boy with a 60 degree right thoracic curve that had been present in infancy and was progressing (Fig. 6–13). The

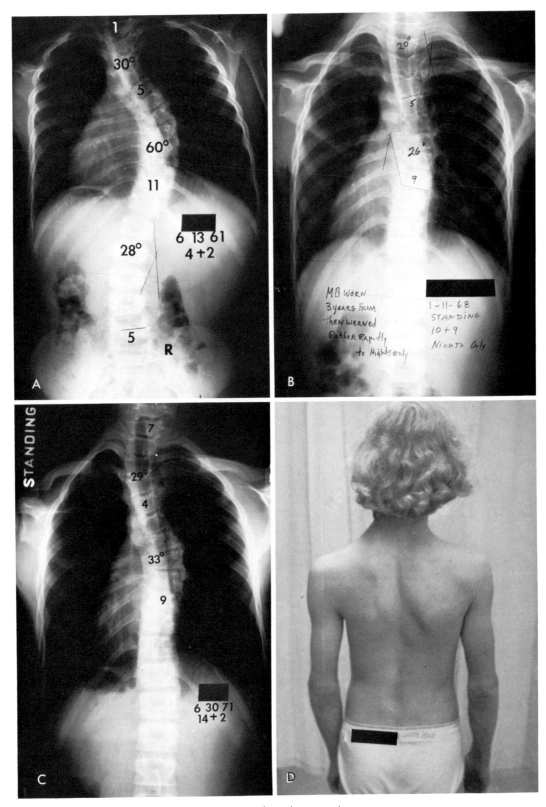

**Figure 6–13**  *See legend on opposite page.*

Milwaukee brace proved effective in correcting this curve to 20 degrees during bracing for two years, followed by night use only. The patient voluntarily discontinued use of the brace entirely at age 10 years. During the growth spurt that followed, the curve became a double thoracic pattern. Both curves were 38 degrees at age 17 years and were cosmetically very acceptable.

Since so few infantile idiopathic curves have come to our attention early, our observation of the results of treatment must be guarded. The axiom "Do not allow progression to occur" must be strictly observed. The few patients treated early by the regimen outlined have done well. The repeated cast treatment, as carried out in Berck-Plage, has not yet been instituted at our center.

## TREATMENT OF SEVERE CURVES
(Fig. 6–14)

The problem patients are those who have been seen after the curves have already progressed. Most have been seen with curves of more than 100 degrees (Fig. 6–15). These we have treated by halofemoral distraction, cast correction, a trial of a Milwaukee brace, and finally recorrection in a cast and spinal fusion. Correction after fusion has often been difficult to maintain, and osteotomies to regain correction have often been performed. One patient with a curve of 150 degrees at age eight developed neurologic complications both in halofemoral traction and after Harrington strut bar correction (Fig. 6–16). Fortunately, recovery occurred, but correction was unsatisfactory.

In dealing with severe untreated curves that began in infancy and have progressed, several conclusions were reached:

1) These curves were not responsive to any brace, including the Milwaukee. At first it was felt that with good correction in halofemoral distraction and a well-fitted cast to maintain correction for a period of six months, the Milwaukee brace could then satisfactorily control the curve until a better age for fusion was attained. This treatment proved inadequate in all instances, for great loss of correction occurred almost at once after bracing. Recorrection in a cast and another trial of the brace also failed. Early fusion of the central three-fourths of the curve following good cast correction and maintenance of correction in the cast for eight months followed by bracing also failed to maintain correction.

2) The best correction was attained when the initial halofemoral distraction and cast correction were immediately followed by a fusion of the entire curve and prolonged cast maintenance for a year. In our experience unilateral posterior fusions of the convex side did not maintain correction. One should avoid prolonged and excessive rib pressure by turnbuckle casts because of the thoracic cage deformity that may be produced.

3) Following fusion in the young, exploration and addition of bone combined with a search for a pseudarthrosis at six months postoperatively are often indicated in children under the age of eight years when there is x-ray evidence of an inadequate graft or loss of correction. X-rays do not demonstrate the fusion mass adequately in the young. X-ray demonstration of a solid graft is more readily visualized after the age of ten years. All fusions in the young should have external protection until they are close to maturity.

4) The Milwaukee brace often helps to maintain correction achieved but does not necessarily prevent loss of correction. The fusion mass in the young is plastic and malleable, and a solid fusion will bend under stress. Pseudarthroses must be diagnosed and repaired. Short fusions may need to be extended. Osteotomies and recorrection, using Harrington instruments as necessary, must be done early rather than delayed until loss is great. Close observation and institution of indicated treatment is mandatory throughout growth.

*Text continued on page 101*

**Figure 6–13** *A,* P.G., age 4+2. Curvature noted at age 2. T5–T11, right thoracic, 60 degrees, structural right side bending; T1–T5, left thoracic, 30 degrees, mildly structural left side bending; T11–L5, left lumbar, 28 degrees, nonstructural left side bending. Milwaukee brace ordered and worn full-time. 6/13/61. *B,* P.G., age 10+9. Wearing brace irregularly nights only. Correction maintained. 1/11/68. *C,* P.G., age 14+2. New brace ordered and instructed to wear full-time. Was uncooperative and wore it only sporadically at night during rest of adolescence. Has now lost correction but curves not visible cosmetically. T4–T9 (note shortening of this curve), 33 degrees; C7–T4, 29 degrees. Lumbar spine straight. 6/30/71. *D,* P.G., end result at age 15+8. Infantile idiopathic. There are now two thoracic curves, each measuring 38 degrees. Their balance is good, and the patient is cosmetically acceptable with a good result.

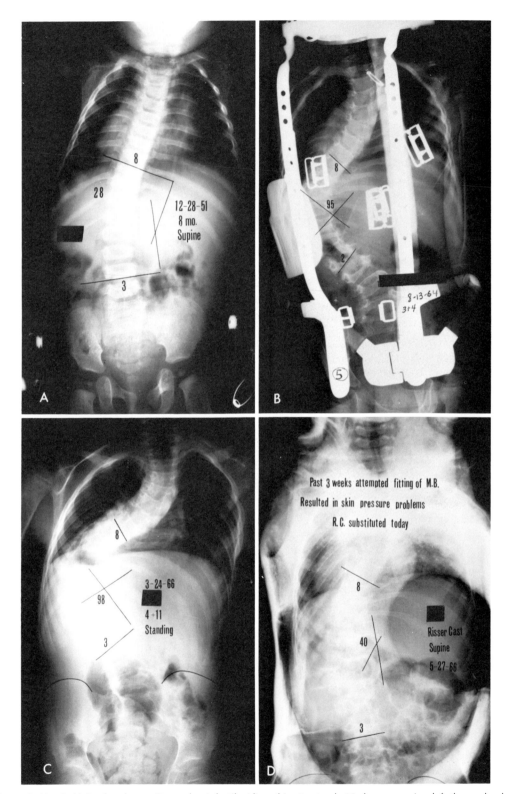

**Figure 6–14**  *A*, N.O., female age 8 months. Infantile idiopathic structural, 28 degrees supine left thoracolumbar.
*Legend and illustration continued on opposite page*

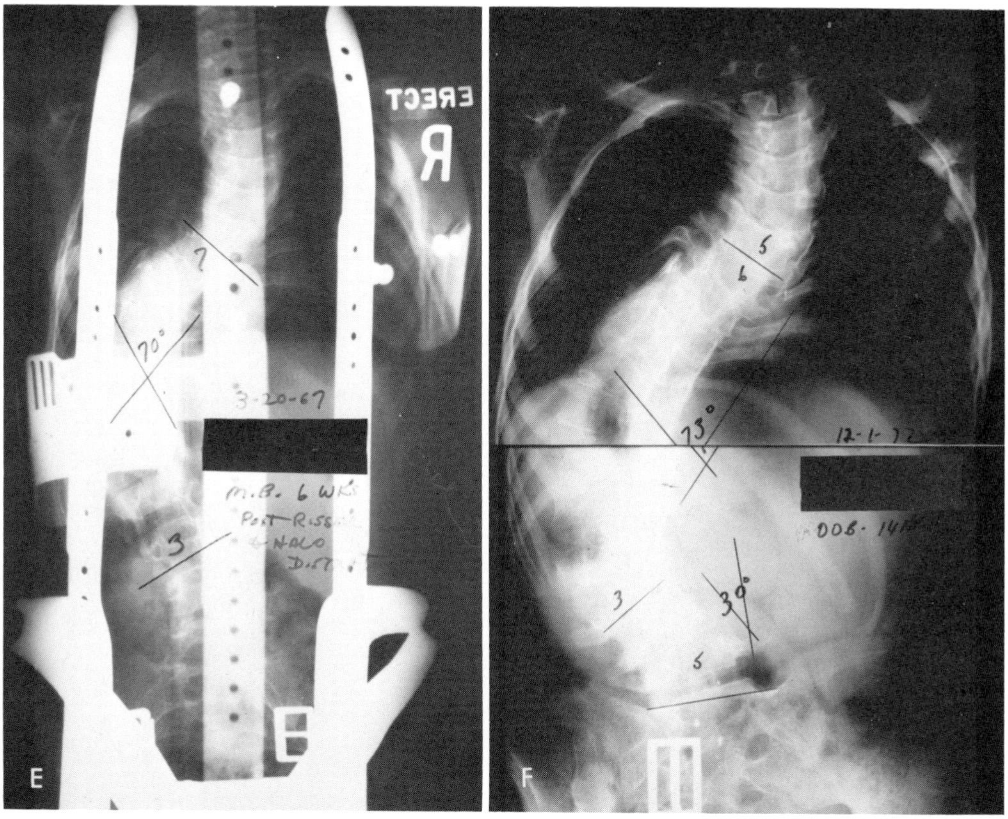

**Figure 6–14**  *Continued*
*B,* N.O., age 3+4. Severe progression. Unsuccessful correction in Milwaukee brace. *C,* N.O., age 4+11. Progression of curve to 98 degrees, standing. *D,* N.O., 5+1. Best cast correction (Risser localizer) was to 40 degrees. Patient sent home in cast with instructions to fit with Milwaukee brace in six months. *E,* N.O., age 5+11. Milwaukee brace again proved unsuccessful in maintaining good cast correction. *F,* N.O., 11+8. Fusion carried out in cast. Correction at 60 degrees by local original orthopedic surgeon. Loss of correction followed to 73 degrees. No further loss reported since 1972. Lesson learned: Best correction must be fused immediately. Milwaukee brace and cast correction do not maintain correction in severe infantile idiopathic curves. After early fusion of entire curve or curves in best correction, re-explore fusion to verify solidarity and keep patient in Milwaukee brace until mid or late adolescence.

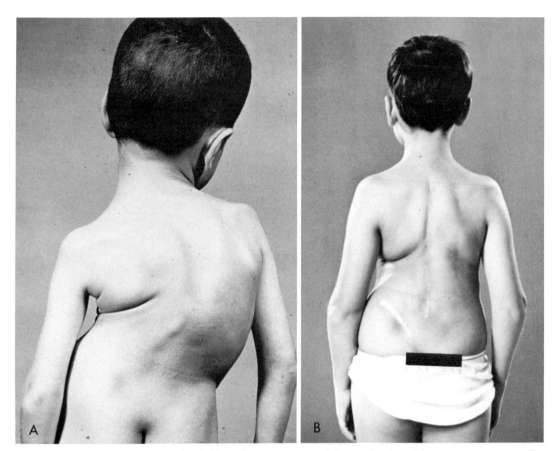

**Figure 6–15**  *A,* M.K., age 5+0. Infantile idiopathic curve untreated. Progressive since infancy; now very severe. Curve measured 115 degrees. *B,* M.K., age 14+6. Patient was held in a cast correction for nine months postoperatively, then transferred to a Milwaukee brace, which he wore for two years. This photograph, taken in 1975, represents an end result with a solid fusion and no further loss of correction. He has good balance and a reasonably satisfactory result. Total treatment program consisted of:

1. Halofemoral distraction
2. Cast for 6 mo.—correction at 40 degrees
3. Milwaukee brace with loss of correction
4. Cast correction with wedging
5. Fusion unilateral (convexity) with Milwaukee brace
6. Loss correction—bilateral fusion with osteotomy and wedging cast
7. Continued loss. Osteotomy fusion with Harrington distraction bar. Cast for 9 mo.
8. Milwaukee brace 2 years
9. Final correction: 52 degrees

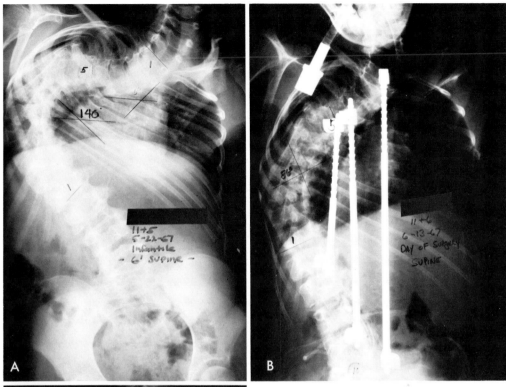

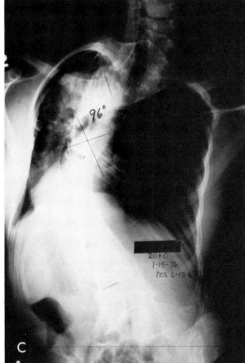

**Figure 6–16** *A,* K.F., age 11+5; supine x-ray. A neglected infantile idiopathic curve treated sporadically in underarm casts and poorly constructed Milwaukee braces. The standing x-ray taken when the patient was first seen at the University of Minnesota Scoliosis Service in 1967 has been lost. This supine x-ray measures approximately 140 degrees. The standing x-ray was 155 degrees. 5/22/67. *B,* K.F., age 11+6. Halo femoral traction resulted in correction to 88 degrees but also resulted in left brachial plexus paresis and was discontinued. The patient was taken to surgery, and three Harrington strut bars were inserted. No "wake-up" test was used (1967). The patient was not paraplegic immediately but developed complete paraplegia during the afternoon. She was taken at once to the operating room. The central rod was removed, and a complete unilateral laminectomy was done on the concave side. The remaining strut bars were loosened. She made a rather rapid and complete recovery from the paraplegia. 6/13/67. *C,* K.F., age 20+0. She developed a deep wound infection with draining sinuses. With removal of rods, the infection cleared up. The fusion on the convex side was solid. She has had no further trouble but still has a very severe deformity. This x-ray was taken nine years later. She is working and is not severely disabled, although her pulmonary function is rather severely depleted. 1/15/76.

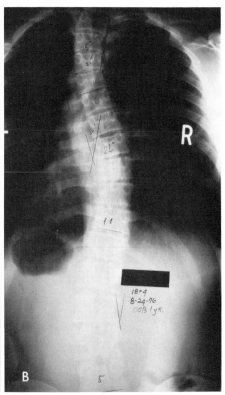

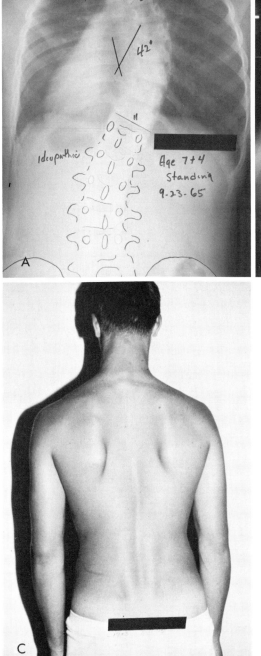

**Figure 6–17** *A,* T.E., 7+4. Juvenile idiopathic scoliosis in a male. There is a right thoracic curve of 42 degrees, T5–T11; the high thoracic curve is barely discernible. *B,* T.E., 18+4. The Milwaukee brace was worn full-time from age 7 to 16—then the patient gradually was weaned. At 18+4 he had been out of the brace completely for a year. His curves remained stable: 25 degrees above; 26 degrees below. *C,* T.E., 17+3. The patient's clinical appearance was excellent, with no sign of a curvature and no rib deformity.

The door is still open for the best treatment of the severe curves of infantile idiopathic scoliosis. Prevention of progression in the infant and young child is the best treatment. We must depend on our knowledgeable colleagues abroad, who are frequently exposed to this problem, for we here on the North American continent seldom encounter this entity. A program of treatment based on wide personal experience is needed.

## JUVENILE IDIOPATHIC SCOLIOSIS

These curves are "discovered" during the time from age four to onset of puberty, which is not necessarily the age of onset. A small curve may be present prior to discovery.

As reported worldwide, the sex incidence appears to be evenly divided in juvenile years. It is distinctly familial, and small nonprogressive curves are very common. Some of these are completely flexible, remain small, and lose little of the normal side-bending flexibility.

Progression in juvenile years is variable. Curves that have progressed to a severe structural condition in early juvenile years may in some instances be residuals of the progressive infantile variety, but most of these children reach the chronologic age of six or seven years with curves still 40 degrees or less (Fig. 6–17). These will usually respond well to Milwaukee brace treatment. The double major (thoracic and lumbar) type usually progresses slowly until mid or late adolescence (Fig. 6–18). The single thoracic pattern may remain static for a variable period. With the approach of adolescence, these curves usually begin to progress rapidly (Fig. 6–19). School survey programs are giving us much deeper insight into the behavior of curves in these preadolescent years.

### Nonoperative Treatment

The treatment of juvenile idiopathic scoliosis should consist of observation of flexible curves less than 25 degrees and the institution of brace treatment when progression is noted clinically and on x-ray. In evaluating x-rays, one may be easily misled by a patient's posture while the film is being taken. If in doubt, repeat the film under personal observation. Both unequal weight bearing and torso rotation may give a false impression of curve increase.

A study of many small curves in the juvenile years demonstrated the frequency with which they are found to remain unchanged or even improve without treatment (Fig. 6–20). The Milwaukee brace remains the best orthosis for thoracic or double major and lumbar patterns. The TLSO (see Chapter 15) has been shown to control the single flexible lumbar and thoracolumbar patterns of less than 40 degrees.

### Surgical Treatment

Prevailing orthopedic opinion in the past has strongly urged a delay of surgical spine fusion "until the end of growth." No greater error in judgment has ever been made in the overall treatment of scoliosis. Many patients have been allowed to progress to a large and more rigid curve or curves that no longer correct to a satisfactory degree. Most curves are surgically correctable to a varying degree even if they have become inflexible.

Operative treatment must be carefully considered in the juvenile years in cases where stable correction cannot be achieved within a reasonable time. It is discouraging to the patient and the family when a Milwaukee brace has been prescribed and worn for several years, only to be informed that correction is unsatisfactory and a fusion must be performed.

It has been established that a solidly fused spine does not lengthen during growth; therefore, fusion should be avoided if possible in earlier juvenile years. Moe, Sundberg, and Gustilo[26] reviewed 78 spine fusions after a period of several years in patients with an average age at fusion of 7.5 years. They found that in x-rays taken at a six-foot distance, almost none showed an increase in length of the fusion mass. A few showed a decrease in length and a few a slight increase, with a maximum increase of 0.6 cm. Only those showing no increase in the scoliosis angle were included in the study of increase in length of the fusion. They found as much as 1 cm. difference in length when the lateral views were compared with the anteroposterior views, the lateral views showing a longer fusion mass. This was ascribed to the magnification of the spine caused by increasing the

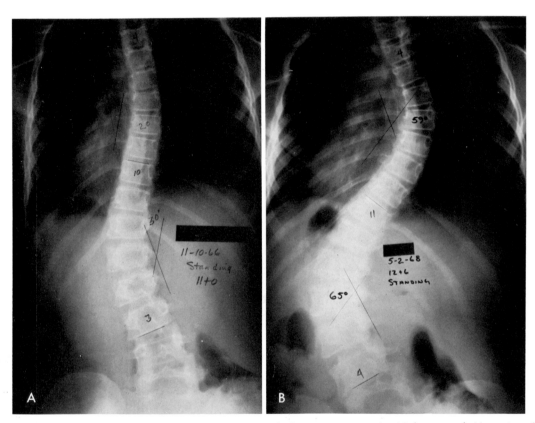

**Figure 6–18**   *A,* P.H., 11+0. At age 7, this female patient had two curves measuring 10 degrees each. Now, at age 11, both had increased, to 20 degrees T4–10 and 30 degrees T10–L3. No treatment had been instituted. *B,* P.H., 12+6. One year and six months later there was further increase: T4–10 is 59 degrees, and T10–L4 is 65 degrees. Still no treatment was given.
*Legend and illustration continued on opposite page*

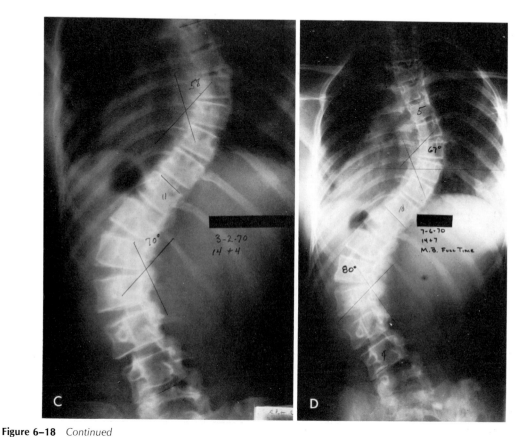

**Figure 6–18** *Continued*

*C*, P.H., 14+4. Another year and 10 months without treatment showed further increase. The upper curve was the same; the lower increased by only 5 degrees. At this late date, one could not expect the Milwaukee brace to accomplish correction in such severe curves. The brace should have been used at age 11 or before, when the curves were small. A Milwaukee brace was fitted at this time. *D*, P.H., 14+7. The patient was now wearing a Milwaukee brace. During the past four months, while in the brace full-time, both curves had increased. Upper curve now 67 degrees; lower, 80 degrees. This demonstrates the futility of Milwaukee brace treatment in severe curves.

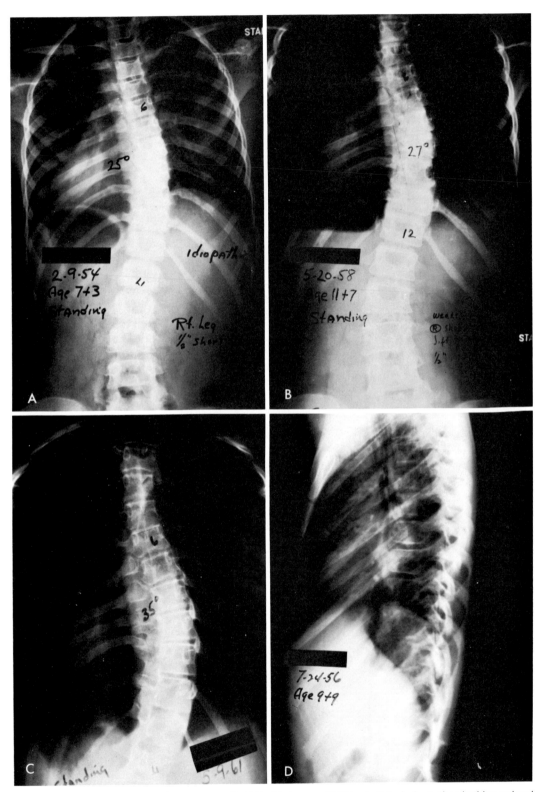

**Figure 6–19**  *A,* P.G., 7+3. Right thoracic curve T6–T12, 25 degrees. Right leg is ½ inch short. Shoe buildup ordered.

*Legend and illustration continued on opposite page*

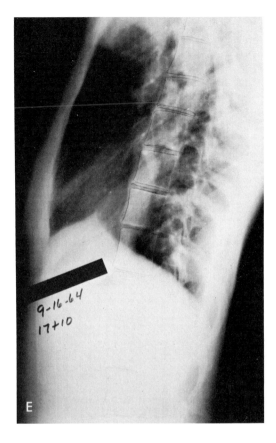

**Figure 6–19** *Continued*

*B,* P.G., 11+7. Slight change in curve: T6–12 now 27 degrees. Milwaukee brace ordered. *C,* P.G., 14+7. After three years in brace, curve worsened. Decompensated T6–L1, 35 degrees. Surgery considered. Patient grew over 12 inches in height during this period. This patient had developed a fairly severe thoracic lordosis during the period of wearing the brace. This x-ray taken three years prior to surgery. Final presurgical x-ray showed curve further progressed to 55 degrees. Surgical correction improved it to 20 degrees. *D,* P.G., 9+9. Normal lateral view. *E,* P.G., 17+10. After three years in brace, a definite thoracic lordosis had developed. X-ray taken just prior to surgery.

distance of the spine from the x-ray film. It was felt that increases in length of the fusion mass could likewise be ascribed to increase in size of the thorax.

Winter[42] reviewed the same group of patients with a much longer follow-up and came to the same conclusion, namely, that a solidly fused spine does not show elongation of the fusion area during growing years. Since it is better to have a fused, shorter but relatively straight spine than a scoliotic spine made much shorter by the curvature, early fusion should not be avoided. Early fusions have not produced severe lordosis except in a very few instances. Thoracic lordosis after fusion has usually been present prior to surgery. The studies showed only one patient who demonstrated a normal thoracic lateral view and who had a rather severe lordosis

after fusion. Her vital capacity was 60 per cent of predicted normal several years after fusion.

The fusion area in the juvenile patient must include all of the major curve, and it is wise to extend the fusion length at least two segments above and below the end vertebrae. The Harrington strut bar may be used if the bone is firm. Prior to the advent of the Harrington instrumentation, Risser cast correction with fusion proved very satisfactory and is still a good method of treatment for the juvenile patient. Fortunately most juvenile curves are of less than 50 degrees and are good brace candidates.

Younger juvenile patients with curves of 50 degrees or even more may be given brace treatment in order to help prevent progression while awaiting a more optimal age for fusion.

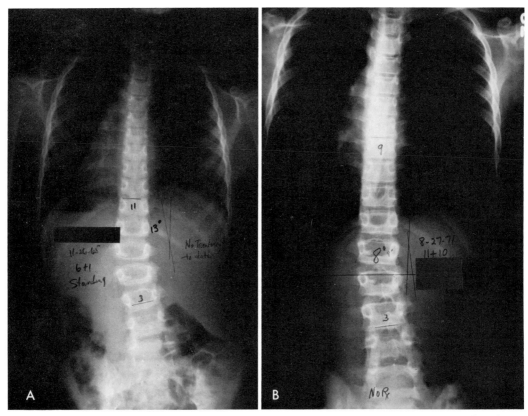

**Figure 6–20** *A,* C.H., age 6+1. A 13 degree flexible curve. This female patient was one of a family with scoliosis. The mother and three siblings all had curvatures. *B,* C.H., age 11+10. No treatment. Curves decreased; still flexible. Subsequent x-rays showed no change.

Few curvatures of 50 degrees or more are without disfigurement, and a few show satisfactory permanent correction by brace treatment.

The neglected severe juvenile curve of 70 degrees or more should be given the benefits of every corrective modality, including early fusion in the best possible correction. Halofemoral distraction is sometimes indicated preoperatively. Recorrections of fusions by osteotomies are often necessary.

In juvenile patients it is important to watch the curve carefully as they approach adolescence and the rapid growth spurt occurs (see Fig. 6–19). In the event of surgical fusion, external protection by the Milwaukee brace is essential during growing years. This will help to prevent loss of correction in the fusion area and also prevent minor curves from increasing.

We are unable to forecast accurately which curves in the young juvenile patient will progress. Small curves of 20 degrees or less should be carefully watched, and as long as they do not progress, no treatment is necessary. Progression during late juvenile years or early adolescence is common, and patients of this age must be given close, frequent observation. Bracing is mandatory for progressive curves in the young, and deterioration in the curve while being braced must be treated surgically.

## ADOLESCENT IDIOPATHIC SCOLIOSIS

It is during adolescence that most patients with idiopathic scoliosis are presented for diagnosis and treatment, some with small nonprogressive curves, others with curves of considerable magnitude. It is during early adolescence that all growth centers become unusually active, and a rapid increase in height may be expected. In progressive moderately structural curves, a rapid increase in curve magnitude can also be expected. Such increases, once begun, will nearly always continue throughout the adolescent years. On the other hand, there are many small curves in adolescence that do not increase.

The variation in behavior of adolescent idiopathic curvature creates many difficulties in judgment for the attending physician. Unless the orthopedic surgeon is knowledgeable in this special field, it is best for him to refer the family to a scoliosis center for decisions and treatment. School survey programs, as well as prior observations, have brought into sharp focus the unpredictability of idiopathic scoliosis. Many questions remain unanswered. How can one foresee the outcome of a small slightly structural curve in a preadolescent or early adolescent? Does the curve pattern serve as a guideline in evaluation? Clarisse,[5] in a study of the behavior of curves under 30 degrees in adolescence, showed that they progress very little if at all. He found that of 36 patients seen after menses began, only 1 progressed. Of 59 patients seen before onset of menses, progression was as follows: 92 per cent of double major curves, 70 per cent of thoracolumbar curves, 58 per cent of thoracic curves, and 29 per cent of lumbar curves.

## Determination of Maturation of the Spine

Since 1936, Risser[33] has advocated close attention to the ossification of the iliac epiphyses as indicative of spine growth activity. As he pointed out, ossification is usually first visible near the anterior spine and makes a slow excursion across the top of the ilium to the posterior spine area, where it makes first contact with the bony ilium. He postulated that with such contact, spinal growth activity ceased and thereafter idiopathic curves would not worsen. However, he now agrees that adult progression does occur, averaging two degrees per year. While the Risser sign should not be disregarded, it is now a proven fact that spine growth activity and curve progression do not necessarily cease with completion of excursion of the iliac epiphysis. Completion of ossification and union to the bony ilium remains a certain sign that growth is complete, but it still may not indicate that curve progression will stop during adult life.

Since the Milwaukee brace and other orthoses have been used to correct idiopathic curves during adolescent growth immaturity the issue of termination of growth activity in the spine has been brought into sharp focus. Other factors found in the child and on the spine roentgenogram assume greater importance than the Risser sign alone. In order of their importance, these are:

1. Incomplete ossification of the vertebral ring. This is the raised margin of cartilage that surrounds the outer margin of both the upper and the lower surfaces of each vertebral body. It overlies the cartilaginous end-plate, which, by the process of enchondral growth, vertically elongates the vertebral body. Visible ossification does not occur in this plate but is demonstrated in the vertebral rings. The function of the ring apophyses is not to provide longitudinal vertebral growth; they are traction apophyses that provide attachment for the annulus fibrosus and other ligamentous structures binding the bodies over the intervertebral disc. They are the only visible indicators of growth activity of the end-plates. They begin to show ossification centers just prior to adolescence; and with completion of their ossification, the end-plates are ossified also, and vertebral growth is complete. Incomplete ossification within the rings is a sign of incomplete vertebral growth. The activity of such ossification is often best seen in side-bending roentgenograms of the spine.

2. Risser's sign of excursion of the ossification of the iliac epiphyses.

3. The physiologic signs of maturation.

4. Cessation of increase in height of the patient.

5. Comparison of the bone age film of the left hand and wrist with films shown in the atlas of Greulich and Pyle.

6. The chronologic age of the patient.

## Stability of Correction

Milwaukee brace treatment is most successful in improving or maintaining mildly structural curves between 20 and 40 degrees. Many will correct rapidly and stabilize during growth, requiring only night use of the brace. This is the period for very careful analysis of such stability, for laxity in brace wearing may result in a rapidly progressive curve. It is wrong to state that the Milwaukee brace produces or achieves stability. The spine achieves stability of its own accord, and we do not know why some become stable in correction while others do not.

The test for stability of correction must be carried out before one allows increased time out of the brace during growth. A 10 year old patient may demonstrate rapid and excellent correction from 50 degrees to 0 degrees within one year. A radiograph taken immediately after the brace is removed may show only a 5 degree loss, but after several hours out of the brace, the loss of correction will be 25 degrees or more. The amount of time permitted out of the brace must be based on the measurement of the curve after trial periods of brace removal. A 5 degree loss in one hour will do no harm, but a 30 degree loss over a period of several hours must not be allowed. The patient who demonstrates such instability must continue full-time brace wearing, and the test should be repeated every four to six months. In many patients the spine does not become stable for several years during adolescence or may never show stable correction.

Early idiopathic curves of less than 25 degrees may sometimes improve and/or stabilize rapidly after only a few months of brace wear. In this event, night use of the brace alone may serve to maintain correction. Any progression of the curve calls for resumption of full-time brace wearing. Curves of 40 to 50 degrees require a minimum period of a year of full-time bracing, and it is seldom worthwhile to test for stability of correction earlier. If curves of this magnitude show significant increase while the brace is being worn, they should be considered surgical candidates (Fig. 6–21).

The testing for stability of correction should follow a definite pattern. A standing x-ray is taken in the brace, after which the brace is removed and the patient is asked to come back for another standing x-ray after a period of four hours. The films are then carefully compared. If there has been no loss or if the loss does not exceed five degrees, the patient is instructed to remove the brace daily for three hours. This period includes the usual one hour out of the brace that is routinely allowed for bathing and exercises. If the loss is greater than five degrees, the patient must continue full-time brace wearing (23 hours daily). In the event of such loss it is not

worthwhile to repeat the testing for at least six months. If the loss is minimal, the testing should be repeated in three months, this time for a six-hour period. In this way one can always be sure that the patient is properly weaned from the brace.

Stability may be occasionally achieved rather rapidly, even during juvenile years and in early adolescence. If the patient is growing rapidly, great care must be used in weaning. The patient must never be given promise of brace removal that might not be fulfilled.

Exercises alone will not correct a progressive curve, although bad posture may be improved. Exercises are a very important adjunct for patients using the brace.

We do not know the factors that contribute to a stable correction. There appears to be a great deal of variation among patients. It has been proposed that soft tissue maturation, including maturation of the discs, plays a major role. This may be true in many instances but does not apply to all patients.

## Nonoperative Treatment of Adolescent Idiopathic Scoliosis: The Milwaukee Brace

The important aspects of treatment in the adolescent are not to overtreat static small curves but to watch them carefully for evidence of progression and to institute proper treatment before they become severe.

Two recent follow-up studies of Milwaukee brace treatment have been made. Blount,[3] in a study of 47 patients who returned for a follow-up of 5 to 15 years after discontinuance of the brace, reported that there were no hard and fast rules of curve behavior during brace treatment and after brace removal. He found that the average curve returned to its original status after brace removal and that dramatic improvements were often offset by substantial losses. Skeletal maturation did not imply stability of correction, and no difference was found in variations in age, initial curve size, and curve pattern. He advised that unacceptable curves should be fused. Posture correction, compensation, and rib prominence were found to be as important as changes in the size of the curve. Improvement during use of the brace was noted in 42 out of 47, but after brace removal, 19 lost less than 5 degrees, 13 lost from 6 to 10 degrees and were considered

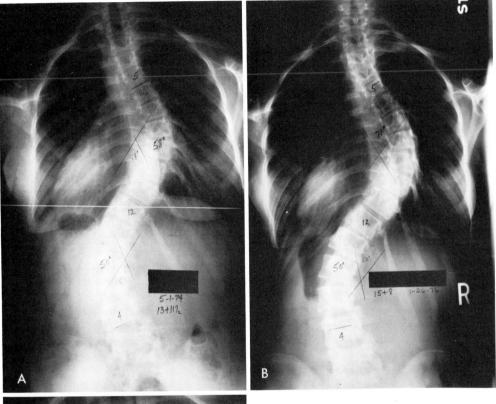

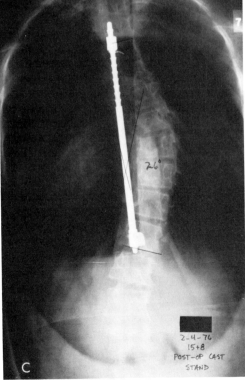

**Figure 6–21** *A,* S.D., 13+11½. This adolescent neglected curve—right thoracic major—measures 58 degrees. This 50 degree lumbar curve is minor and flexible. Use of the Milwaukee brace was instituted. *B,* S.D., 15+8. After two years in the Milwaukee brace, the right thoracic curve had increased. Surgical treatment was now advised. This should have been advised when the patient was first seen two years ago. Brace treatment in this patient was a useless expenditure of important adolescent years. *C,* S.D., 15+8. Surgical correction was satisfactory at 26 degrees.

acceptable, and 15 lost more than 11 degrees and were considered unacceptable.

Carr, Moe, and Winter[4] reviewed 75 patients who returned for personal inspection and evaluation after a minimum period of five years after brace removal. (These were patients from the 169 studied by Moe and Kettleson in 1970.[25]) In reanalyzing this group, they found that 36 had been uncooperative about wearing the brace and were removed from the study. Twenty-eight were treated surgically, and 30 were lost to follow-up. The conclusion reached from the follow-up study of the 75 patients was that the customary result was a return to the original curve. The most satisfactory results were in the curves of 45 degrees or less. The occasional patient maintained an excellent correction (see Fig. 6–33), but the main benefit of the brace was in the *prevention* of progression in curves of 20 to 45 degrees.

Curves measuring 40 degrees or less at spine maturation usually do not show later increase in magnitude, but larger curves often do. While there are no absolute guidelines, shorter multiple curves do not often increase a great deal. Short thoracic curves that have spontaneously fused in their central concavity will not increase, while long thoracic curves that extend into the upper lumbar spine will worsen. Usually, the greater the curve, the greater the likelihood and magnitude of the increase. Adolescent patients with curves beyond 50 degrees should not be treated with a Milwaukee brace. They require surgical treatment. Milwaukee brace treatment should be considered successful only if the results shown within a reasonably short time are satisfactory. The curve pattern is important, as is the maturity of the child. The double major thoracic pattern with a deforming high thoracic curve is not a good brace candidate. Small curves of this pattern (less than 25 degrees) should be observed for progression. If progression is noted, brace treatment should be tried. If a deforming state is reached, both curves should be corrected with Harrington instrumentation and fused without delay.

Curves in adolescence that worsen in spite of adequate brace wear become immediate surgical candidates. It is devastating to the morale of patient and parents to have an adolescent wear a Milwaukee brace for a curve or curves of 50 to 90 degrees through-

out her most emotionally important years and then be told by the doctor, "I'm sorry but we shall have to operate on your spine"; or, "I shall have to send you to a scoliosis center where they will probably advise surgical treatment." These wasted years will not return, and the child will not forget them. Sometimes this sad state occurs because the parents refused surgery, but most often it is due to ignorance about scoliosis by the attending physician.

Many questions remain unanswered at this moment. When the school screening program has had a great deal more time to obtain a computerized follow-up analysis of the child with a small curve, undoubtedly more light will be thrown on this enigma. Our former opinion that 80 per cent of adolescent idiopathic scoliosis occurs in girls has been questioned by the school screening program. The percentage of small curves in girls is closer to 50 per cent. Of patients surgically treated, a very high percentage are girls. All past writings on this subject indicated a great preponderance of girls over boys. Curves in adolescence tend to become more severe in girls than in boys.

It is of the utmost importance to diagnose adolescent scoliosis early. Since adolescent curves have their beginnings as small curves that are only slightly structural, our decisions about treatment must begin early. Flexibility plays a major role in decisions concerning small curves (less than 20 degrees). The term flexible curve is used to describe a spine that is shown to be completely flexible on supine voluntary side bending roentgenograms. The true idiopathic curve shown on the standing anteroposterior x-ray may exhibit variability in degree but is always present, and no clinical structural changes are apparent except that on the forward bending test such a curve usually shows a varying degree of rib prominence. Rotation is often absent on side bending views and is not more than that seen in the normal straight spine on side bending. Many curves remain small and flexible and are seen only in the standing position; such cases may persist into adult life. Some progress a little and then spontaneously cease progressing. How many of these temporarily progressive curves had unnecessary brace treatment? We will never know unless we observe them periodically without treatment. In how many cases is an increase of 5 to 10 degrees seen on anteroposterior x-ray because of a slight variation in torso rotation when the x-ray was taken? A fixation device[9] is needed in which the patient stands without change in body rotation. Our school screening program to date shows a 5 per cent incidence of curves less than 20 degrees, or 50 out of 1000. The incidence of curves greater than 20 degrees is 3 out of 1000.

Curves that have no known cause, that are persistently present in the standing position, and that show any evidence of a rib hump must be classified as idiopathic. As long as they are flexible on the side bending x-rays and measure 20 degrees or less they should only be watched. If they increase by 5 degrees and remain flexible, observation may demonstrate that the next x-ray shows no further loss. If so, brace treatment can be delayed. Posture and torso rotation when the x-ray is taken is of utmost importance. A lateral view should always be included in the initial evaluation.

If the curve not only increases by measurement but also shows increased cosmetic deformity and loss of flexibility, the decision for treatment becomes easier. Observation alone then may be hazardous to the patient, for in many instances progression may be rapid and often relentless. If the lateral x-ray demonstrates an abnormally flat thoracic spine, the decision for treatment is again made easier, for a flat thoracic spine may worsen in the Milwaukee brace. If there is progression beyond 35 to 50 degrees, surgical correction is the best answer. If the lateral view shows a normal dorsal rounding, the Milwaukee brace is the best answer. Careful watching is mandatory, for in the brace a normal lateral thoracic spine may rapidly become flat or even lordotic (see Fig. 6–24). Once begun, brace treatment should be continuous, accompanied by an accepted exercise program. No "weaning" from the brace should be permitted except for one to two hours of swimming until there is demonstrable proof that correction is stable, whereupon weaning can be gradually begun.

Curves that respond best to the Milwaukee brace are those of the moderate single thoracic pattern with a flexible lumbar curve. Also high in priority for brace treatment during early adolescence are the double major thoracic and lumbar pattern and the double major thoracic and thoracolumbar pattern of 40 degrees or less.

As pointed out by Blount,[3] the degree of correction obtained by Milwaukee brace treatment is not always the sole benefit that the brace may provide. The restoration of balance within the spine and good cosmetic improvement, may be accomplished through brace wearing and exercise, even without permanent correction of the curve.

We have had no experience with the Lyonnaise brace of Michel and Stagnara. The limitations on normal torso muscle activity in this brace, particularly in reference to respiratory excursion, are similar to those of a torso cast or jacket. Unlike the Milwaukee brace and the TLSO, there is little place for a systematic exercise program. It is true that Cotrel has, through use of large windows in the torso cast and a systematic and extremely well supervised exercise program, lessened this objection, but in the North American continent such a large scale of gymnastic procedures supervised by a large number of very enthusiastic and capable physical therapists will not be frequently found. Since the Milwaukee brace and the TLSO offer the most benefit in our service, we see little value in changing.

A review of books from Europe, with particular reference to Germany during the last century, shows the multitude of designs in torso bracing, nearly all of which have been discarded. The day has fortunately passed when idiopathic scoliosis patients were suspended and placed in an encompassing leather torso support such as that routinely prescribed in the 1930s in many areas including such hospitals as the Gillette Children's Hospital, St. Paul, Minnesota, where our scoliosis service was begun in 1947.

To be effective, a brace must be used with selected young growing children and must be carefully supervised and combined with exercises. Our experience to date indicates the superiority of a well-made Milwaukee brace for most curves. Braces that constrict the chest may show improvement of the curve radiographically but at the price of reduced pulmonary function—a price that the patient should not have to pay.

## THORACIC LORDOSIS AND OTHER COMPLICATIONS WITH THE MILWAUKEE BRACE

The creation of thoracic spine flattening or a thoracic lordosis by the Milwaukee brace has recently given rise to concern. In days past, the main thought in the minds of orthopedic surgeons using the brace treatment was the correction of the spine as viewed in the anteroposterior x-ray. In the study of the end results of the Milwaukee brace treatment by Moe and Kettleson,[25] it is of interest to note that only a few patients had adequate standing lateral x-rays taken prior to treatment and there were very few subsequent lateral views.

There is no doubt that a flat thoracic spine may be present before brace treatment. While the brace may not always cause this to worsen, it frequently does so, and one must watch carefully with lateral x-ray studies when such patients are placed in a Milwaukee brace. Under no circumstance should the thoracic pad exert pressure on the ribs close to the spine; instead it must lie more laterally. Patients with a flat thoracic spine should not do pelvic tilt exercises.

The brace often increases a high thoracic curve in the double thoracic pattern if only a right thoracic pad is used (see Fig. 6–9). Curves also progress in spite of brace treatment, especially when over 50 degrees (see Fig. 6–21).

When the curve in mid-adolescence is over 45 degrees and is deforming, surgical treatment is indicated without a trial of the brace. Even lesser curves should be fused if the rib deformity is great (see Fig. 6–22). Occasionally a juvenile curve of 60 degrees responds to the brace, but in the adolescent this is a surgical problem.

## INDICATIONS AND CONTRAINDICATIONS TO MILWAUKEE BRACE TREATMENT

All large curves in adolescence should be fused at once in the best correction. This includes thoracic curves, thoracic and lumbar curves, and double thoracic major curves. There is a "gray zone" in which curves in late adolescence of 50 degrees or less should be considered for correction and fusion. Double major thoracic and lumbar curves of 40 degrees may be so well balanced and show so little deformity that fusion is not indicated. The same is true of the double thoracic pattern (see Fig. 6–13). Single thoracic major curves of 50 degrees or more usually increase in adult life and should be fused in adolescence.

Indications and contraindications for the use of the Milwaukee brace vary according to the age and maturity of the patient and particularly according to the degree of the curve, its cosmetic deformity, and its flexibility. In early adolescence, as well as in juvenile years, minor nonstructural curves that are nondeforming and less than 25 degrees should not be given brace treatment but should be observed and standing x-rays taken at intervals of three to four months. If the curve demonstrates spontaneous improvement or no change, the intervals of observation may be increased. If definite signs of structural changes and progression are noted, the Milwaukee brace should be fitted and worn full-time for a period sufficient to establish control or improvement of the curve. Smaller curves will often require brace wear for only part of the day. In larger curves the brace should be worn full-time until stable correction has been shown to be present.

Occasionally one sees a patient with a small curve who would be a good brace candidate but whose rib deformity and decompensation contraindicates brace wear. We have seldom observed patients whose rib deformity was decreased by the brace, and in the presence of unacceptable deformity surgical treatment is often indicated even with curves of lesser magnitude.

It must always be kept in mind that the behavior of the curve with brace use is the determining factor in the length of time it must be worn each day. Stabilization of correction is necessary before the process of weaning the patient from the brace may begin.

Contraindications to Milwaukee brace treatment of adolescent idiopathic scoliosis include refusal by the patient, progression of the curve while the brace is being worn, a lordotic thoracic spine, large deforming rib elevations, maturity of growth, persistence of decompensation, and large curves of over 50 degrees. During growth, lumbar curves and thoracolumbar curves that are flexible and are less than 40 degrees respond to the TLSO.

## AGE OF THE PATIENT (BONE AGE)

***Age: 4 Months to 1 Year.*** The Milwaukee brace with plastic pelvic girdle is the best method to maintain or correct curvatures of 25 to 45 degrees. If effective, the brace should be continued into juvenile years. If the curve progresses, a cast may regain correction and should be followed in four to six months by the brace. If progression continues, the best correction should be obtained by the cast after fusion of the entire curve, and the Milwaukee brace should again be used. If progression after fusion occurs, an osteotomy should be performed and recorrection established, followed by further cast correction.

*Age: 4 Years to 8 Years.* This is often the crucial period in a curve's development. If the curve is now 60 degrees or less, the Milwaukee brace is worthy of a trial. When progression occurs in the brace, a trial of cast correction is indicated, which can again be maintained in the brace. Surgical fusion in the best possible correction is the only answer when progression occurs despite all attempts at external methods of correction.

In outline form, this age group should be treated as follows:

1) If the curve is less than 60 degrees, the Milwaukee brace.

2) If correction is maintained or improved, continue the brace.

3) If progressive in the brace, use a localizer cast as a trial.

4) All curves that progress in spite of external methods of correction should have maximal cast correction and surgical fusion with Harrington instrumentation.

5) Postoperative correction should be maintained in a cast for 8 to 12 months, followed by the brace.

6) If loss of correction occurs, osteotomize and recorrect.

*Age: 8 to 12 Years.* Curves of 50 degrees or less should have a trial in the Milwaukee brace. If progression occurs in the brace, surgery is indicated without delay. Never allow curves to progress beyond 60 degrees. Surgery is mandatory in large curvatures.

*Age: 13 to 15 Years.* All small curves less than 45 degrees should be given a trial in the brace.

a) If improved—continue brace.

b) If progressed—*surgery without delay.*

*Age: 15 and Older.* Curves less than 35 degrees should have a period of watching or bracing. Some do not progress without the brace. If responsive to brace, continue brace during remaining growth in spine. Unresponsive curves over 50 degrees should be fused. Larger curves over 60 degrees should not have brace trial. Fuse without delay.

*THINGS TO WATCH FOR*

1) Lordosis from brace. The brace with a right thoracic pad may be productive of a lordosis in the thoracic spine. An example is a girl, age 13, whose lateral x-ray measured +25 degrees and after one year in the brace was −20 degrees. The lateral curves did not improve but worsened from 30 to 40 degrees.

Immediate surgery is indicated in all curves that demonstrate progressive lordosis.

2) Never use a brace for severe curves in adolescence, whether single thoracic or multiple major thoracic and lumbar. These are surgical problems *at once.*

3) It must be remembered that a perfectly balanced (compensated) 40 degree thoracic and lumbar curve may be completely acceptable. In years past we often accepted compensated double curves of greater magnitude, but we now feel that they should be corrected, especially if the right thoracic is more major and the lumbar does not require fusion.

4) The lumbar or thoracolumbar curve:

a) Most respond in juvenile years to the TLSO and do not need a Milwaukee brace. The main requirement is flexibility to a considerable degree.

b) Always balance the pelvis so that the iliac crests are even. If the pelvis is low on the convexity of the lumbar curve, bracing will be less effective. Use a shoe lift to balance, and if the patient is growing, consider epiphysiodesis or stapling to equalize leg length.

**Operative Treatment: Preliminary Distraction and Casting**

This treatment may take the form of Cotrel halter and pelvic sling or halofemoral distraction. Nachemson and Nordwall[29] reported in 1976 on a trial of Cotrel dynamic traction carried out for three weeks preoperatively and found that subsequent implantation of the Harrington strut bar gave the same amount of correction as in operations performed without prior distraction. Our experience has been the same for curves under 80 to 90 degrees in adolescent and juvenile idiopathic scoliosis. We do not advocate preliminary distraction by either method in this group. For more severe curves halofemoral distraction often gives correction, which is advantageous and may lessen the risk of cord stretching and ischemia. Preoperative cast correction may likewise be advantageous because it allows greater and safer correction. The preoperative cast may also help in selection of the fusion area when there is a continuation of rotation in the lumbar spine beyond the thoracic curve.

In the past, cast correction prior to surgery was routine on our service for curves over 50 degrees. We no longer feel this is advisable except in larger curves of 85 to 100 degrees.

### OPERATIVE TREATMENT OF ADOLESCENT IDIOPATHIC SCOLIOSIS

The large deforming curve of 60 to 100 degrees in adolescence should have surgical treatment without waiting for maturity. Many smaller curves may be deforming, with decompensation, a dropped shoulder, and a large rib prominence. The Milwaukee brace will not change these except occasionally it will overcome decompensation. The result of surgical correction is much better. The flat or lordotic thoracic spine may be made worse by the brace, and in curves of 45 degrees or more, surgical treatment with a Harrington strut bar will give effective correction of both the curve and the lordosis.

When there are two moderate structural curves, the curves may balance each other so effectively that surgical correction in later adolescence is not indicated. In younger patients the brace may effectively prevent increase in curves that have been shown to be progressive. One must always bear in mind that curves of 25 to 30 degrees occasionally stop progressing even in mid-adolescence.

Pain in the curve area or at the junction of two curves may be an indication for fusion. In addition, the patient's or parents' desire for correction must not be disregarded.

**Harrington Contracting Assembly.** There is a disagreement among orthopedic surgeons about the indications for the contraction hook assembly in the Harrington instrumentation. Harrington and his followers use the contraction assembly routinely on the convexity of all curves. It is claimed that it adds stability and further correction to that obtained by the distraction strut bar on the concave side of the curve. When we first used the Harrington instrumentation in 1960 and during the fol-

lowing year we followed the same technique. It was during this period that we became aware of the thoracic lordosis of the spine so commonly found in idiopathic scoliosis and noted that such lordosis was worsened by the contraction assembly. It is well known that the bilateral insertion of the contraction assembly will flatten and improve a roundback deformity, and it therefore follows that a flat back will be worsened by its use. We discontinued the use of the contraction hook assembly in all scoliotic curves that did not demonstrate at least a normal kyphosis in the thoracic spine. We have found that the distraction bar when bent no more than 10 degrees will improve a flat or lordotic thoracic spine. The contraction assembly is always indicated in the presence of any abnormal kyphosis.

### CURVE PATTERNS IN SELECTION OF TREATMENT AND FUSION AREA

**Right Major Thoracic Pattern.** Indications for observation occur in patients with a curve of 30 degrees presenting in late adolescence with little evidence of remaining spinal growth. Even with evidence of loss of flexibility, such curves may show very little cosmetic deformity. Rib cage elevations, shoulder elevation, decompensation, and distortion of the torso are usually minimal or absent. Such curves seldom progress and do not require treatment, for they are scarcely ever deforming. The fact that they are still so small as spine growth terminates is evidence that they have progressed very little during the active growth period. Occasionally a 25 or 30 degree thoracic curve will show a marked rib elevation, and surgical treatment must be considered (Fig. 6–22). Brace treatment at the terminal period of growth is of little value, although occasionally it will rebalance the spine and improve some postural defects. If there is a sufficient cosmetic reason for correction in such small curves in late adolescence, surgical treatment is indicated.

Larger thoracic curves (above 50 degrees) at a period close to growth termination are nearly always deforming and do not respond to brace treatment. Surgical treatment is indicated. They often retain a considerable degree of flexibility, and a preoperative corrective cast does not change the amount of correction that can be obtained by Harrington

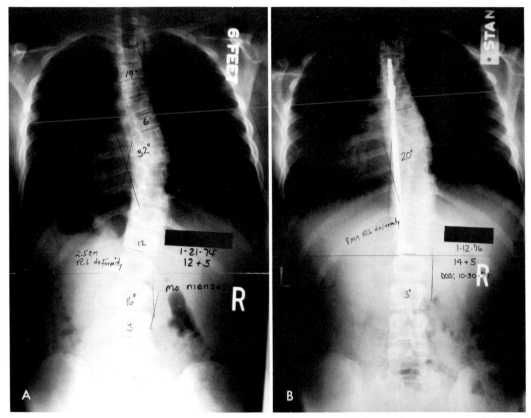

**Figure 6–22** *A,* L.P., 12+5. This young female adolescent had a 2.5 cm. rib deformity that gave cosmetic disfigurement. In spite of her immaturity and a thoracic curve of only 32 degrees, it was deemed inadvisable to use Milwaukee brace treatment because of the deformity. A brace was tried for 10 months. The rib deformity increased to over 3 cm. *B,* L.P., 14+5. Surgical correction of only 12 degrees resulted in an excellent reduction of the rib deformity to 8 mm. and a markedly improved cosmetic appearance.

instrument correction and is therefore not indicated. If the thoracic spine is flat on the lateral x-ray, a square-ended strut bar should be bowed toward the dorsal side and an extra vertebra should be added to the fusion area above and below, thus helping to bring the spine into a more normal dorsal rounding.

When vertebral rotation is neutral in the end vertebrae of the curve, only the vertebrae within the curve require correction and fusion. An extra vertebra added to the fusion length above and below does no harm and enhances security against the lengthening of the curve after the cast is removed. In larger curves with a thoracic displacement toward the convexity (overhang decompensation), the addition of one or two vertebrae beyond the neutral end vertebrae becomes mandatory (Fig. 6–23).

In the usual thoracic curve all vertebrae are rotated toward its convexity, except for the measured end vertebrae, which show no

rotation and are therefore considered neutral. Not infrequently, the lower end vertebra is still rotated toward the thoracic curve convexity, and this rotation continues in the same direction into the minor curve below. A curve with end vertebrae at T5 and T12 may have additional vertebrae L1, L2, or even L3 demonstrating continuation of the same rotation in the same direction, and the first neutral vertebra may even be L4. This situation must be recognized, for if the fusion area selected is T5–T12, there will be a lengthening of the curve and often a major or total loss of correction. One must fuse from neutral vertebra to neutral vertebra according to the rotation present. The fusion area must be lengthened accordingly. In the event of such continuing rotation, a preoperative corrective cast may be helpful in the selection of the fusion area, for such correction may eliminate the rotation in one or two lower vertebrae. If

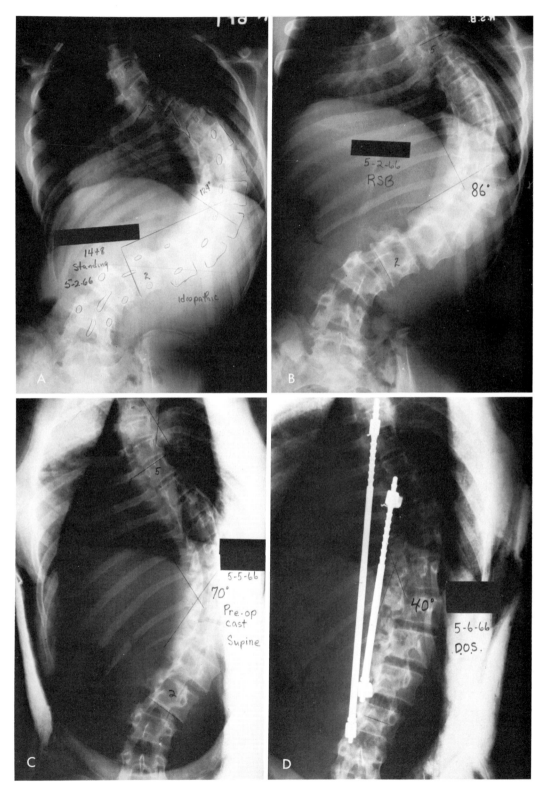

**Figure 6–23**  *A,* R.B., age 14+8. A 124 degree right thoracic curve, T5–L2. The upper thoracic left curve measured

*Legend and illustration continued on opposite page*

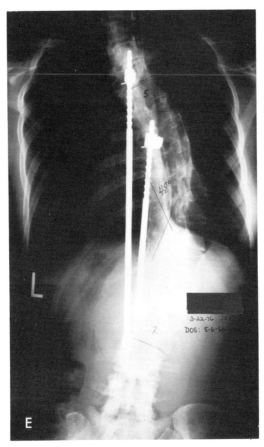

**Figure 6–23**  *Continued*
56 degrees. *B,* The right bending film showed a correction to only 86 degrees, indicating severe rigidity. *C,* 5/5/66. A preoperative Risser-Cotrel cast corrected the curve to 70 degrees. *D,* 5/6/66. Two Harrington distraction strut bars were inserted parallel; the fusion was performed from T4 to L3. Correction to 40 degrees was safely obtained. The operation was done the day following the cast application, operating through a large posterior window. *E,* R.B., 24+7. 3/22/76. Ten years after fusion, the correction was 48 degrees, and the cosmetic result was excellent. Loss of correction occurred during the early postoperative period.

so, it may be safe to shorten the fusion area by one vertebra, still fusing from neutral vertebra to neutral vertebra as shown in the corrective cast (Figs. 6–24 and 6–25).

We have never been convinced that thoracic curves should be treated by Dwyer anterior instrumentation, since the use of Harrington strut bars has proved entirely satisfactory. In severe and long curves, two bars placed parallel — one extending the entire length of the curve, the other spanning a shorter central portion — usually are of great help.

*Single Major Thoracolumbar Pattern.* During growing years this curve pattern responds very well to the TLSO worn full-time. In this pattern there is no higher curve requiring even night use of the Milwaukee brace, and correction in the TLSO is often satisfactory (Fig. 6–26).

After growth has ceased, the cosmetic result of continued decompensation must be given consideration. This pattern, even with a curve of 30 degrees, may produce a shift of the entire torso of several centimeters from the midpoint of the pelvis (Fig. 6–27). The response to posterior fusion of the curve with Harrington instrument correction is excellent. Fusion above or below the end vertebrae is best, extending the fusion to L4. There is never an indication for continuing to the sacrum in adolescents and young adults. The Dwyer instrumentation may be used, but only in patients with hyperlordosis, since it always increases kyphosis. The pseudarthrosis rate is higher for the Dwyer procedure than for

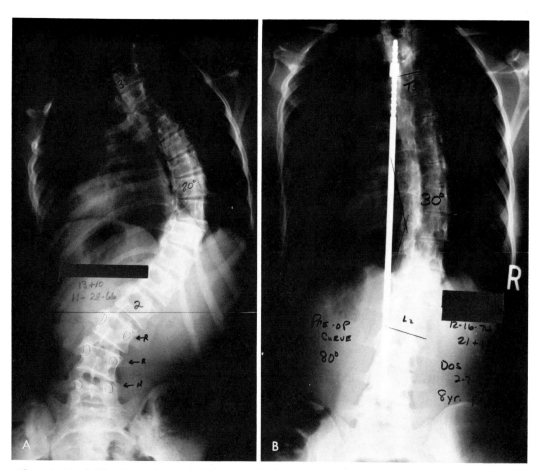

**Figure 6–24**   *A,* S.B., 13+10. A severely deforming right thoracic curve of 80 degrees. The curve is T5–L2, but vertebral rotation continues down to L5, which is the first neutral vertebra. L4 is very nearly neutral; therefore, the decision in selection of the fusion area was T4–L4. *B,* S.B., 21+1. Fusion T4–L4 gave excellent and permanent correction at 30 degrees. This x-ray was taken eight years postoperatively.

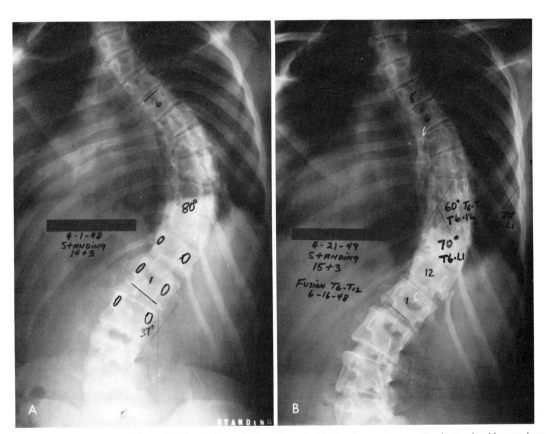

**Figure 6–25**   *A,* One of the early idiopathic scoliosis patients in 1948, when cast correction by turnbuckle was done. This 80 degree right thoracic curve was fused T6 to T12, disregarding the fact that L1 was rotated in the same direction as those vertebrae in the thoracic curve. Fusion to L3 was indicated. 4/1/48. *B,* Ten months after surgery the curve had lengthened and correction lost to 70 degrees. Note the widening of the convex interspace between T12 and L1. The fusion at T11–T12 does not appear to be very solid. No further loss of correction occurred, and no further treatment was carried out. 4/21/49.

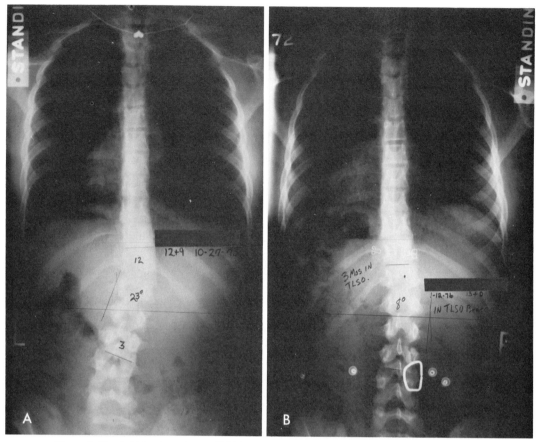

**Figure 6–26**  *A*, K.D., A 23 degree flexible lumbar curve. *B*, K.D., in TLSO brace three months.

Harrington instrumentation. In our experience the Harrington instrumentation alone is very satisfactory in adolescent idiopathic scoliosis.

*Major Lumbar Curve Pattern.* The major lumbar curve alone may not be deforming even at 45 degrees (Fig. 6–28), but most curves of this pattern distort the waistline and produce disfigurement (Fig. 6–29). This usually causes less concern in male patients than in females. Most curves of 40 degrees or less respond very well to the TLSO during growth (Fig. 6–26). In late adolescence, fusion is preferable in curves of 45 degrees or more. Curves of such magnitude will progress in later life and will cause disabling pain in a substantial percentage of patients. We do not agree with James[15] and Ponseti[31] that these are insignificant problems in adolescence from a cosmetic standpoint. Fusion need only encompass the curve itself. If the curve is excessively lordotic, the Dwyer procedure is most effective, although the posterior approach has given satisfactory results in our experience. One should avoid the production of a flat lumbar spine in fusing these curves by using a square-ended rod and lower hook, bending the bar to conform to the normal lordosis. A round rod will rotate if bent and will create a kyphosis rather than a lordosis.[27]

*Single Major High Thoracic Curve Pattern.* This rare pattern poses a problem that may be minimal or severe, both cosmetically and physiologically. High thoracic curves are usually accompanied by an elevation of the first ribs on the convexity, even in those with a thoracic opposite curve below. In double thoracic curves the rib elevation and its accompanying neck deformity is extremely variable, but in the single high thoracic curve, rib elevation and neck deformity are almost always present.

When the curve is small, there may be no

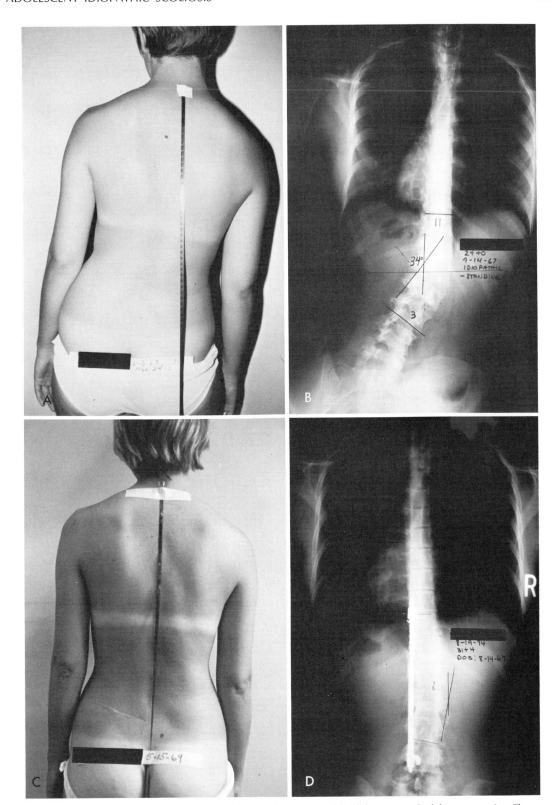

**Figure 6–27**   A and B, Idiopathic thoracolumbar curve in a 24 year old girl showing marked decompensation. The curve was T11–L3, + 34 degrees. C, After correction and fusion, T10–L4. D, Seven years postoperative. 8/19/74.

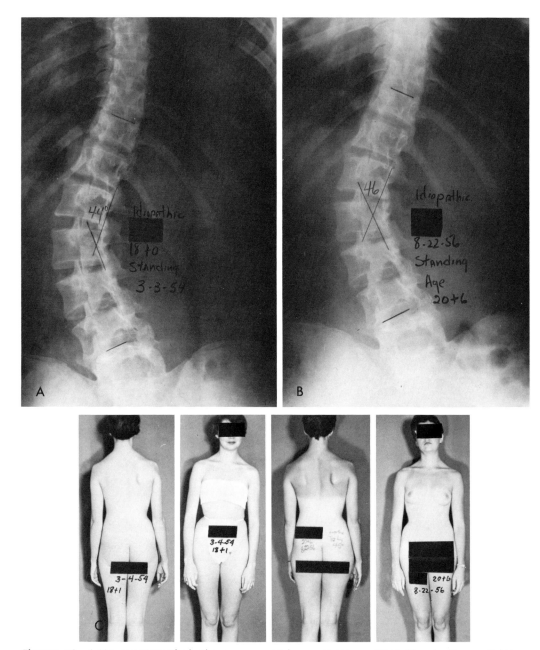

**Figure 6–28** *A*, N.J., age 18+0. The lumbar curve was 44 degrees. *B*, N.J., age 20+6. There had been a slight increase, to 46 degrees. There was still no cosmetic deformity. Our present experience indicates a strong probability of continued increase during adult years. 8/22/56. *C*, N.J., age 18+1. A lumbar curve in a late adolescent that gave no cosmetic deformity and was given no treatment. We do not know the outcome of this patient in later adult ages. Between 18+1 and 20+6, she increased from 44 degrees to 46 degrees. 3/4/54.

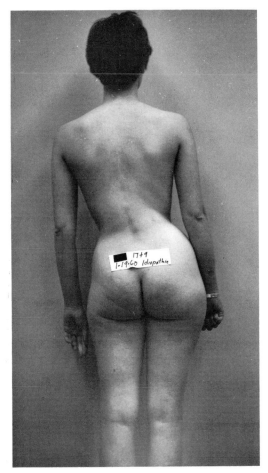

**Figure 6–29** K.C., 17+9. Although the curve was small, it created a great deal of cosmetic deformity. The patient was too old for a brace, and was a candidate for a fusion.

of treatment. Surgical correction and fusion are definitely warranted.

***Major Thoracic and Minor Lumbar Pattern.*** This situation offers opportunity for good judgment by the scoliosis surgeon. The thoracic curve must be corrected and fused. The judgment concerns the lumbar curve. What degree of flexibility is required to omit fusion of the lumbar curve? At what age is this judgment required?

Lumbar curves combined with thoracic curves in the standing anteroposterior x-ray often simulate in degree the thoracic curve, but side-bending x-rays differentiate the two. When the amount of structural fixation and degree of curvature in the lumbar curve are small, fusion is not required. When the degree of structural fixation is 20 degrees, the decision of whether to fuse is dependent on the amount of correction required in order for the spine to become completely or almost completely balanced (Figs. 6–30 and 6–31).

In young adolescents, the problem becomes more complicated because here a small amount of structural fixation in the lumbar curve may become greater after fusion of only the thoracic curve. The TLSO or the Milwaukee brace offers the best solution during most of the remaining growth period after the thoracic fusion is mature.

The older adolescent requires only the maintenance of balance. In the days when cast correction alone was used and corrections were less than at the present, we often achieved maximal cast correction of both curves, fused only the upper curve, and obtained good balance, even when there was a considerable amount of structural fixation of the lower curve.

***Double Major Thoracic and Lumbar Curve.*** When major curves develop simultaneously in the young adolescent, the Milwaukee brace should be prescribed unless there is a contraindication. Such double curve patterns may be well controlled with the brace during growth. Clarisse[5] has shown in an analysis of 100 patients that this curve pattern will usually worsen during juvenile and adolescent years.

When these curves become more severe and reach a balanced state at 50 degrees in late adolescence, one must judge their future progression and their present cosmetic balance and appearance. If growth is terminated, they will probably not worsen. If acceptable

cosmetic deformity or physiologic problem. When the curve is of greater magnitude there is a severe cosmetic deformity and often a pulmonary function depletion as well.

The high thoracic curve, when small and in the growing child, may be watched carefully for progression as well as for cosmetic neck deformity. A few do not progress and no treatment is required. The value of wearing a Milwaukee brace with a "trapezius pad" over the convex side is debatable but is probably worthy of trial in the juvenile or early adolescent.

The more severe curve with an obvious rib elevation, a marked neck asymmetry, and often a severe rib "hump" offers little choice

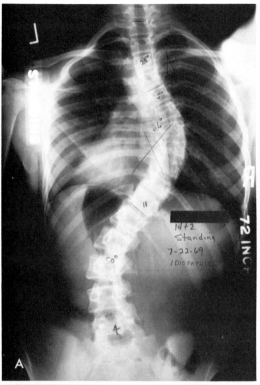

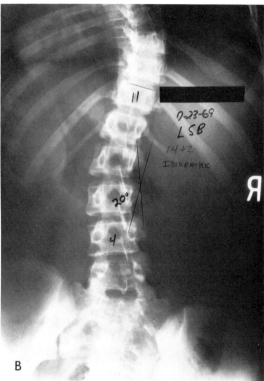

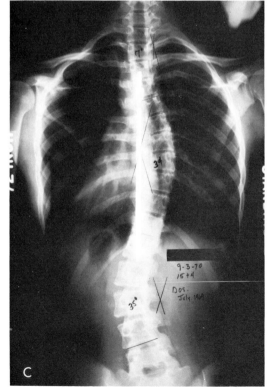

**Figure 6–30**  *A,* S.P., age 14+2. A right thoracic major curve with structural curves in high thoracic and lumbar. Right thoracic curve, 66 degrees; left lumbar curve, 50 degrees; high thoracic curve, 25 degrees standing. *B,* The left lumbar is 20 degrees on left bending. *C,* S.P., age 15+4. Only the right thoracic curve was corrected and fused, with a well-balanced, nondeforming spine resulting. Although the high thoracic curve was nearly 50 per cent structural, it was unnecessary to fuse it because of the major thoracic curve; the curves above and below were minor, although structural.

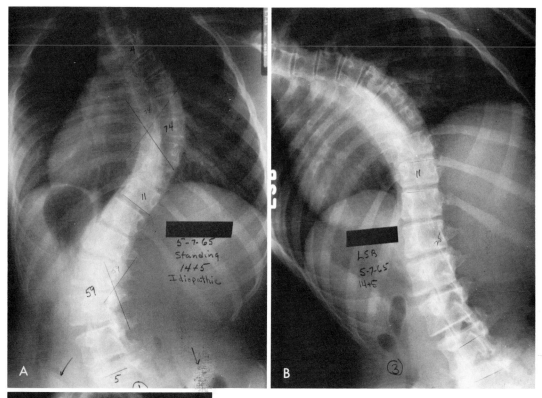

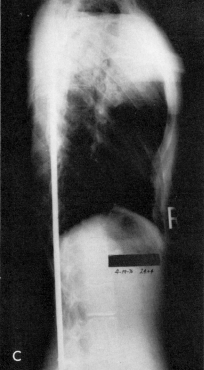

**Figure 6–31**  *A,* M.K., age 14+5. This patient first appeared for treatment at chronologic age 14+5. She presented a right thoracic curve, T4–T11, of 74 degrees and a left lumbar curve, T11–L5, of 59 degrees. Her iliac apophyses had almost completed their excursion. This might be interpreted as a right thoracic major and left lumbar minor. The side bending x-rays may tell the story. 5/7/65. *B,* The left bending film demonstrated a 25 degree structural component in the lumbar curve. The exact curve pattern was still questionable but favored a double major pattern. *C,* M.K., age 24+4. The use of the long straight round Harrington strut bar usually eliminates all thoracic kyphosis and lumbar lordosis. The loss of lumbar lordosis was compensated in this instance by an acute lumbosacral angulation. Loss of lumbar lordosis has created problems, especially in the adult, which will be discussed in the section on surgery in adults. 4/14/76.

cosmetically, they need not be given surgical treatment. This opinion is in agreement with Ponseti, James, and many others.

Curves of this pattern that have reached 60 or 70 degrees or more present a cosmetic problem although they may be well balanced, and they may appear more or less acceptable when the child is clothed. However, the torso is short, and the rotational disfigurement is very evident to the patient.

We recommend correction and fusion of both curves in this degree of progression. Progression in adult life often occurs. We have had experience with numerous adults with this pattern who have severely disabling pain and whose curves have progressed. These patients become surgical candidates. The pain is at the junction of the two curves or within the lumbar curve. The adolescent who has had these curves corrected and fused is generally very satisfied with the improvement and the cessation of progression. Fusion of both curves limits spine movement, but this does not become a serious problem. We have had practically no lumbosacral pain problems when fusing to L4 or L5. Lumbosacral fusion is not indicated (Fig. 6–31).

In correcting lumbar curves with Harrington strut bars, one must avoid elimination of lordosis by using a square-ended bar and bending it to fit the lordotic contour and often adding a short contracting hook assembly.

***Double Major Thoracolumbar and Thoracic Pattern.*** In this pattern the most major curve is usually the lower thoracolumbar, which is the larger and more deforming but also is usually the more flexible. If the thoracic curve is more than 25 degrees and is highly structural, both curves require correction and fusion. If the thoracic curve is small, only the lumbar should be fused.

In young adolescents, when the lower curve is less than 40 degrees, the Milwaukee brace can be expected to produce a satisfactory end result. If the thoracic curve is minimal during growing years, the TLSO may fulfill all requirements.

In surgical correction one sometimes inserts the lower Harrington hook in the lower end vertebra (L3), but usually it is inserted in L4, depending on the severity and flexibility of the curve. The upper hook is placed in the upper lumbar or lower thoracic end vertebra. If the thoracic curve requires correction it is best to use a separate distraction bar.

***Double Major Thoracic Curve Pattern.*** This pattern produces many contraindications. In some patients the high thoracic curve may not demonstrate an elevated rib on the convexity, and the shoulders may be level. There appears to be no need for inclusion of this high curve in the correction and fusion. It is recognized that in practically all mid-thoracic curves there is a high thoracic curve above that is often somewhat structural.

The operating surgeon is faced with the dilemma of whether to disregard this high curve or to correct and fuse both. While there is no inviolable rule, we have found that in structural high curves with first rib elevation and with cosmetic asymmetry of the neck both curves should generally be fused (Fig. 6–32).

Whether one or two corrective strut bars are to be used is an individual decision, but our own experience points to the single slightly bent "dollar sign" rod as the best way to instrument these curves. It is best to reverse the rod so that a small hook can be inserted into the T1–T2 or T2–T3 joint. The rod must be bent to conform with the existent kyphosis and to prevent upper hook displacement.

***Multiple Curve Patterns.*** These often do not constitute a problem, for most do not have a cosmetically unacceptable appearance. The greater the number of curves and the shorter the length of each, the less will be the total deformity. Nevertheless, not all behave in this benign manner, and one curve may worsen, creating a cosmetically unacceptable deformity that requires correction and fusion.

Multiple curve patterns are uncommon, especially patterns containing five or six curves. Four curves—two central major and two minor thoracic and lumbar—are more frequent. A true triple curve is less common, and likewise uncommon is the spine with complete balance in five or six small curves.

Most multiple curves do not require treatment, but there may be one curve that is major and requires surgical correction.

***Lumbosacral Area.*** There is no major lumbosacral curve that is productive of curves above it. The lumbosacral angulation is secondary to a lumbar curve above, and while it sometimes may require special consideration, it is seldom a problem in adolescent idiopathic scoliosis. Curves originating in the lumbosacral area are associated with congenital anomalies (see Chapter 7).

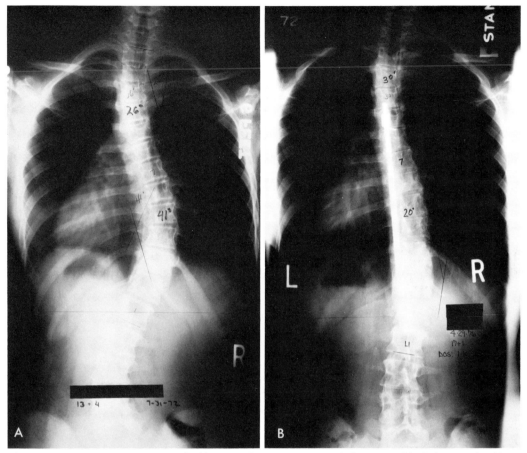

**Figure 6–32** *A,* K. F., age 13+4. A double major thoracic pattern. Both thoracic and high thoracic should require fusion. Note the high left first rib. This curve was 50 per cent structural. *B,* K. F., age 17+1. Only the right thoracic curve was fused, leaving the high thoracic now larger. The neck deformity worsened but was still not severely deforming; fusion of the high thoracic curve was not performed, although this was poor judgment.

## SUMMARY

As the foregoing text and references reveal, the enthusiasm for the Milwaukee brace in the treatment of the growing child with idiopathic scoliosis has diminished somewhat since the book by Blount and Moe[2] was published in 1973. This in no way lessens the value of this brace, for it remains the best orthosis for nonoperative treatment when used in properly selected patients. It will maintain or improve moderate juvenile or early adolescent curves of 30 to 50 degrees (see Figs. 6–13 and 6–33). Since the response to the brace has been shown to be variable and unpredictable, it must not be continued in patients whose curve or curves steadily worsen while wearing the brace. In a like manner, the brace must not be prescribed for large curves (over 50 degrees) in any period of adolescence.

There are rarely indications for the Dwyer anterior approach in adolescent idiopathic scoliosis, but its use is sometimes advisable in lumbar curves with hyperlordosis (Fig. 6–34). The production of thoracic lordosis by Milwaukee brace treatment is not uncommon and must be avoided. It must always be borne in mind that the thoracic spine in idiopathic scoliosis is often flat. This may constitute a contraindication to treatment with the brace.

Long-term wearing of the brace in adolescence should not be permitted in curves measuring over 50 degrees even when there is no great amount of progression. The adolescent is a sensitive individual. The Milwaukee brace, when worn throughout the most im-

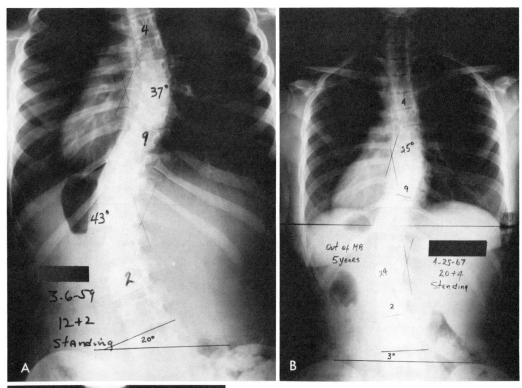

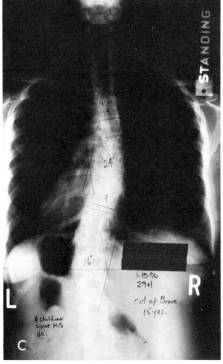

**Figure 6–33** *A,* A.R., age 12+2. A structural right thoracic and thoracolumbar curve. Note that there are 11 ribs and that the curve's apex is at T12. The patient was treated in a Milwaukee brace. Of interest is the fact that examination of the anterior chamber of the eye showed abnormalities of the pectinate lines characteristic of Marfan's syndrome. The patient was referred for surgical treatment because of this finding. *B,* A.R., age 20+4. The patient became pregnant at age 16 and delivered a child. The curves at age 20+4 were balanced at 25 degrees each. She had now been out of the brace five years. 4/25/67. *C,* A.(R.)N., age 29+1. After 15 years out of her brace, the curves were still balanced at 25 degrees each. It is of interest that she had four more pregnancies without change in the curve. 1/15/76.

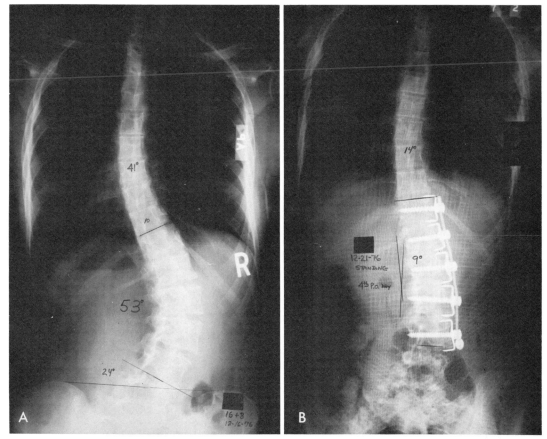

**Figure 6–34**   *A,* S.T., 16+8. A lumbar curve of 53 degrees; very deforming. She was hyperlordotic and was considered a satisfactory candidate for a Dwyer anterior procedure. An unusual lumbar curve, as most are to the left. 16/16/76. *B,* S.T., 12/21/76. It was felt that fusion should stop at L3 because she had a sacralized L5. This is an ideal candidate for the Dwyer in idiopathic major lumbar curves, since better correction can be obtained. Correction was to 9 degrees.

portant period of emotional maturation, may sometimes leave permanent emotional scars. Surgical correction, when indicated, should be done early. It is tragic to withhold surgery for several years when the brace is obviously not fulfilling its role of correcting a larger curve or maintaining a moderate curve. Worst of all is the common practice by the inexperienced orthopedic surgeon or physician of fitting a brace on an adolescent with a 70 or 80 degree curve. The excuse of fitting a brace because the doctor wishes to "do something" is completely unwarranted, for there are now many scoliosis centers available to which the patient can be referred for more expert advice.

Surgical treatment of idiopathic scoliosis in the adolescent is safe in good hands. The spectre of paralysis from surgery has been almost totally eliminated by the Stagnara

wake-up test (see Chapter 20) and clinical monitoring (both sensory and motor) of the lower extremities. This test, combined with adequate surgical skill and judgment, has made Harrington instrumentation a safe procedure.

## References

1. Brooks, H. L., Azen, S. P., Gerberg, E., Brooks, R., and Chan, L.: Scoliosis: A prospective epidemiological study. J. Bone Joint Surg., *57A*:968–972, 1975.
2. Blount, W. P., and Moe, J. H.: The Milwaukee Brace. Baltimore, Williams and Wilkins, 1973.
3. Blount, W. P.: Long term end results of Milwaukee brace. Clin. Orthop. *126*:47, 1977.
4. Carr, W. A., Moe, J. H., and Winter, R. B.: Long term end results of Milwaukee brace. In Publication.
5. Stagnara, P., and Phillips, C.: Reunion Come, Groupe d'Etude de la Scoliose. Presented at the Scoliosis

Research Society, Lyon, France, September, 1973.

6. Cobb, J.: Spine arthrodesis in treatment of scoliosis. Bull. Hosp. Joint Dis., *XIX*:187–209, 1958.

7. Cobb, J.: Instructional Course Lecture—Outline for Study of Scoliosis. J. W. Edwards, vol. V., 1948.

8. Collis, D. K., and Ponseti, I. V.: Long term follow-up in patients with idiopathic scoliosis not treated surgically. J. Bone Joint Surg., *51A*:425, 1969.

9. Dawson, E.: Personal communication.

10. De George, F. V., and Fisher, R. L.: Idiopathic scoliosis: genetic and environmental aspects. J. Med. Genet., *4*:251, 1957.

11. Fisk, J., Moe, J. H., and Winter, R. B.: Lumbosacral Joint in Idiopathic Scoliosis. Read at the Scoliosis Research Society, Guteberg, Sweden, 1974.

12. Harrenstein, R. J.: Die skoliose bei Sauglingen und ihre Behandling. Z. Orthop. Chir. L. *11*:1, 1929.

13. Harrenstein, R. J.: Sur la scoliose des nourressons et des jeunes enfants. Rev. Orthop., *23*:289, 1929.

14. James, J. I. P.: Two curve patterns in idiopathic structural scoliosis. J. Bone Joint Surg., *33B*:339–406, 1951.

15. James, J. I. P., Lloyd-Roberts, G. C., and Pilcher, M. E.: Patterns in idiopathic structural scoliosis. J. Bone Joint Surg., *41B*:719, 1959.

16. Langenskiold, A., and Michelsson, J. E.: The pathogenesis of experimental progressive scoliosis. Acta Orthop. Scand., Suppl. *59*:26, 1962.

17. Langenskiold, A., and Michelsson, J. E.: Experimental progressive scoliosis in rabbits. J. Bone Joint Surg., *43B*:116, 1961.

18. Lloyd-Roberts, C. G., and Pilcher, M. F.: Structural idiopathic scoliosis in infancy: A study of the natural history of 100 patients. J. Bone Joint Surg., *47B*:520–523, 1965.

19. MacEwen, D. G., and Cowell, H. R.: Familial incidence of idiopathic scoliosis and its implication in patient treatment. J. Bone Joint Surg., *52A*:405, 1970.

20. Mehta, M. H.: The rib-vertebral angle in the early diagnosis between resolving and progressive infantile scoliosis. J. Bone Joint Surg., *54B*:230–243, 1972.

21. Mehta, M. H.: Personal communication.

22. Moe, J. H.: Methods of correction and surgical techniques in scoliosis. Symposium on current pediatric problems. Clin. Orthop. North Am., *3*:17–48, 1972.

23. Moe, J. H.: Symposium on the Spine. St. Louis, C. V. Mosby, 1969.

24. Moe, J. H.: A critical analysis of methods of fusion for scoliosis. J. Bone Joint Surg., *40A*:529–554, 1958.

25. Moe, J. H., and Kettleson, D.: Idiopathic scoliosis: Analysis of curve patterns and preliminary results of Milwaukee brace treatment in 169 patients. J. Bone Joint Surg., *52A*:1509–1633, 1970.

26. Moe, J. H., Sundberg, B., and Gustilo, R.: A clinical study of spine fusions in the growing child. J. Bone Joint Surg., *46B*:784–785, 1964.

27. Moe, J. H.: Loss of lumbar lordosis. In publication.

28. Morel, G.: Personal communication from Yves Cotrel.

29. Nachemson, A., and Nordwall, A.: The Cotrel dynamics spine traction—an ineffective method for pre-operative correction of scoliosis. J. Bone Joint Surg., *58A*:158, 1976.

30. Nordwall, A.: Studies in idiopathic scoliosis. Acta Orthop. Scand., Suppl. 150. Copenhagen, Munksgaard, 1973.

31. Ponseti, I. V., and Friedman, B.: Prognosis in idiopathic scoliosis. J. Bone Joint Surg., *32A*:381–395, 1950.

32. Ponseti, I. V., and Separd, R. S.: Lesions of the skeleton and of other mesodermal tissues in rats fed sweet pea *(Lathyrus odoratus)* seeds. J. Bone Joint Surg., *36A*:1081, 1954.

33. Riseborough, T., and Wynne-Davies, R. A.: Genetic survey of idiopathic scoliosis in Boston, Mass. J. Bone Joint Surg., *56A*:974, 1973.

34. Risser, J. C.: Iliac apophysis, an invaluable sign in the management of scoliosis. Clin. Orthop., *11*:111–119, 1958.

35. Risser, J. C.: Important practical facts in the treatment of scoliosis. A.A.O.S. Instructional Course Lectures, *5*:248–260, 1948.

36. Risser, J. C.: Modern trends in scoliosis. Bull. Hosp. Joint Dis., *XIX-2*: 166–186, 1958.

37. Schulthess, W.: Die Pathologie and Therapie der Ruckgratsverkrummungen in Joachimsthal-Handbuch der Orthopadischen Chirurgie, Bd. 1 A. Pt. 2 Jena, Gustav Fischer, 1905–1907.

38. Scott, J. C., and Morgan, T. H.: The natural history and prognosis of infantile idiopathic scoliosis. J. Bone Joint Surg., *37B*:400–413, 1955.

39. Travaglini, F.: Multiple primary idiopathic scoliosis. Ital. J. Orthop. Traumat., *1*:67–80, 1975.

40. Walker, G. F.: An evaluation of an external splint for idiopathic structural scoliosis in infancy. J. Bone Joint Surg., *47B*:524–525, 1965.

41. Winter, R. B., Lovell, W. W., and Moe, J. H.: Excessive thoracic lordosis and loss of pulmonary function in patients with idiopathic scoliosis. J. Bone Joint Surg., *57A*:972–977, 1974.

42. Winter, R. B.: Scoliosis and growth. *In* Zorab, P. A. (ed.): Third Symposium Held at the Institute of Diseases of the Chest, Brompton Hospital, London, Nov. 13, 1970. Churchill, Livingstone, London, 1971.

43. Wynne-Davies, R.: Familial (idiopathic) scoliosis. A family survey. J. Bone Joint Surg., *50B*:24–30, 1968.

44. Wynne-Davies, R.: Genetic and other factors in the etiology of scoliosis. Ph.D. Thesis, University of Edinburgh.

45. Wynne-Davies, R.: Infantile idiopathic scoliosis—causative factors. J. Bone Joint Surg., *57B*:138–141, 1975.

# Chapter 7

# CONGENITAL SPINE DEFORMITY

## INTRODUCTION

Congenital spine deformities have had a tendency to be ignored in the past by most physicians and surgeons. Because they do not "look like" or "behave like" the more common idiopathic and paralytic curves, they were all too often passed by as being of "academic interest only." Actually, congenital spine deformities follow rather predictable patterns of behavior, these predictions being based primarily on an understanding of spinal embryology and spinal growth. For greater detail regarding spinal embryology and growth, the reader is referred to Chapter 5.

All children with congenital spine deformity are treatable. Some need no treatment, and some need extensive treatment. There may be considerable conflict between the goal of curve management and the goal of maximal vertebral growth. Should one fuse a two year old child with a congenital spine deformity? The answer varies. The authors hope the following material will help clear the confusion.

## CLASSIFICATION OF CONGENITAL SPINE DEFORMITY (Fig. 7–1)

A. Defects of Segmentation
  1. Anterior defect (failure of normal disc development)
    a. Complete failure of disc formation (block vertebra)
    b. Partial (anterior) failure of disc formation

    c. Incomplete disc development (apparent normal disc formation early, but later anterior "bars" form)
  2. Anterolateral defect producing kyphoscoliosis — very rare.
  3. Lateral defect. Unilateral unsegmented bar, both anterior and posterior. Produces a purely lateral scoliosis without kyphosis or lordosis.
  4. Posterolateral defect. Posterior unilateral unsegmented bar. This is the most common type of bar and produces lordoscoliosis.
  5. Posterior defect — bilateral. This produces a lordosis without or with minimal scoliosis. This is rare but may be severe.
  6. Total defect of segmentation. May be at single or multiple levels. This does not produce a curve, only shortening of the spine due to lack of vertical growth.
B. Defects of Formation
  1. Pure anterior defect (pure kyphosis)
    a. Partial absence of vertebral body
    b. Complete absence of vertebral body
    c. Absence of more than one vertebral body
  2. Anterolateral defect
    a. Absence of half of the anterior portion of one side of the vertebral body and complete absence of the other side. Produces kyphoscoliosis, is fairly common, and tends to produce a deformity progressive in both projections.
  3. Lateral defect (hemivertebra)
    Absence of the lateral aspect of the

**131**

vertebral body, both anteriorly and posteriorly. Scoliosis results.

   a. Single hemivertebra
1. nonsegmented, incarcerated
2. semisegmented, incarcerated
3. fully segmented, incarcerated
4. fully segmented, nonincarcerated

   b. Multiple hemivertebrae
1. unilateral, sequential
2. unilateral, nonsequential
3. balanced, adjacent
4. balanced, nonadjacent

   c. Associated with contralateral defect of segmentation

   d. Associated with myelomeningocele

C. Mixed
   1. Any of the above anomalies may be seen together, either in the same area of the spine or at another level. Single isolated anomalies are less common than multiple or mixed anomalies.

## GENETIC ASPECTS

When dealing with congenital anomalies of any type, one must always consider the genetic implications. Quite frequently the parents will ask, "If we have further children, will they also have this problem?" The mature patient will ask, "Will my children inherit this condition?"

Several papers dealing with this topic have been published. Because of the interest it stimulates, the positive family history is frequently reported. On the contrary, the

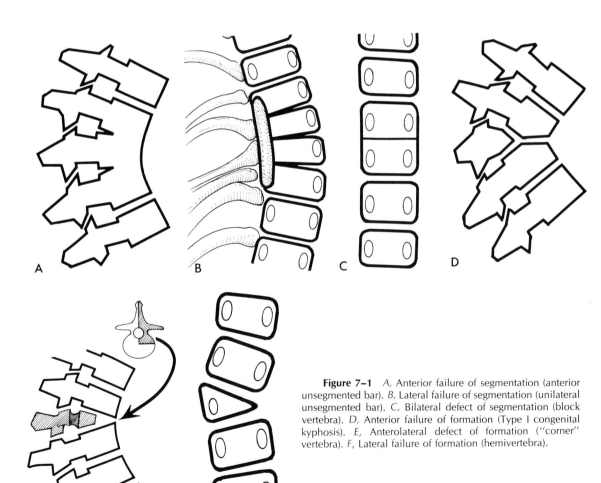

**Figure 7–1** *A,* Anterior failure of segmentation (anterior unsegmented bar). *B,* Lateral failure of segmentation (unilateral unsegmented bar). *C,* Bilateral defect of segmentation (block vertebra). *D,* Anterior failure of formation (Type I congenital kyphosis). *E,* Anterolateral defect of formation ("corner" vertebra). *F,* Lateral failure of formation (hemivertebra).

negative family history is not exciting, and so is not reported. Thus the medical literature tends to be filled with reports of positive family histories.

The only good overall view of this matter was published by Wynne-Davies,[93] who studied the families of 337 patients with congenital spinal anomalies. She found those with multiple anomalies without spina bifida cystica to have a definite hereditary tendency and "are also etiologically related to anencephaly and spina bifida cystica." Those with isolated single anomalies "are sporadic (non-familial) in nature, carrying no risk to subsequent sibs."

Rimoin et al.[67] reported on spondylocostal dysplasia with extensive areas of segmentation defects in both the spine and the ribs. Four members of four generations in one family had this condition. Bartsocas et al.,[3] Jarcho and Levin,[35] Langer and Moe,[42] and Lavy et al.[43] have reported positive family histories in consanguineous relationships.

Few extensive series of congenital spine deformities have been reported. Kuhns and Hormel[39] reported an analysis of 170 patients. There was no mention of family history.

Winter et al.[85] reported on 234 patients with congenital scoliosis. Family history was not reported. A very large number of patients with congenital spine deformity have subsequently been seen by the authors. Including those with either scoliosis or kyphosis, but excluding those with myelomeningocele, there are only 6 positive family histories in approximately 500 patient records. Of these 6, there were one instance of identical thoracic unilateral unsegmented bars in male and female siblings (the product of the marriage of first cousins), two instances of patients with lumbar congenital deformity whose sisters died of myelomeningocele, two instances of almost identical lumbar hemivertebrae in mothers and their daughters, and one instance of identical anterior defects of segmentation in a mother and son. Identical twins have been seen with only one twin having the anomaly.

Thus hereditary congenital spine deformity is rare. Complex lumbar anomalies are often hereditary and often associated with myelomeningocele. Multiple anomalies, especially with multiple rib synostoses, may be hereditary, especially in consanguineous families, but single anomalies are usually nonhereditary (Fig. 7–2).

## NATURAL HISTORY

### Defects of Segmentation

*LATERAL DEFECTS: SCOLIOSIS*

Asymmetric defects of segmentation may be purely anterior, purely posterior, purely lateral, or posterolateral. Since these anomalies have no growth potential in the nonsegmented area and may have normal or near-normal growth on the opposite side, deformity occcurs in direct proportion to growth. Normal spinal growth is characterized by rapid early growth, stable growth from age three to puberty, and accelerated growth during the adolescent growth spurt. It is thus no surprise that such anomalies are characterized by rapid increase in deformity during the first three years, steady increase during the years from age three to puberty, and accelerated increase during the adolescent growth spurt (Fig. 7–3).

The unilateral unsegmented bar is thus the "classic" example of absent growth on one side and virtually normal growth on the other. Such anomalies are certain to progress during growth. This has been amply demonstrated by MacEwen,[53] Blount,[8] and Winter.[86]

The authors have never observed a patient with a unilateral unsegmented bar in whom progression did not take place. Progression in these patients begins prior to birth, and continues throughout growth. The usual rate of progression has been 5 to 7 degrees per year. Thus, if a child has a 30 degree curve at age 3 years and has 12 more years of growth remaining, an increase of 60 degrees (12 years × 5 degrees/year) can be added to the existent 30 degrees, thus predicting at least a 90 degree curve by age 15. In fact, almost all the untreated patients seen by the authors have had curves above 100 degrees by age 15.

Unsegmented bars are more often in the thoracic spine and are usually posterolateral, thus producing some lordosis in addition to the severe scoliosis. This combination of deformities is very detrimental to lung function. These patients have usually presented to the authors with severe pulmonary deficits. We have, unfortunately, observed the deaths of several such patients who came to us too late to help (Fig. 7–4). An unsegmented bar in the lumbar spine will produce severe pelvic obliquity (Fig. 7–5).

*Text continued on page 139*

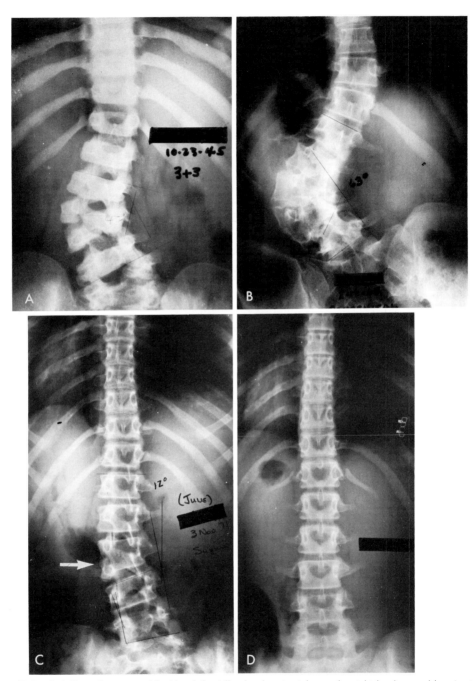

**Figure 7–2**  *A,* A.G., a three year old with a left midlumbar hemivertebra and a right lumbosacral hemivertebra. (An example of a hemimetameric shift). *B,* P.G., a first cousin, also demonstrates a midlumbar hemivertebra as well as asymmetric development of the upper sacrum. *C,* Julie M. This girl has a semisegmented hemivertebra in the midlumbar spine with a mild 12 degree curve. *D,* Jeanne M. Her identical twin sister, showing no congenital anomalies of the spine.

*Legend and illustration continued on opposite page*

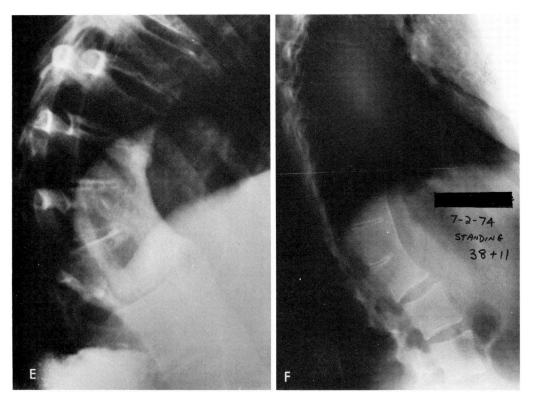

**Figure 7–2** *Continued*
    *E,* J.B., a male with an anterior defect of segmentation. *F,* His mother, showing the same anterior defect of segmentation but with less severe deformity.

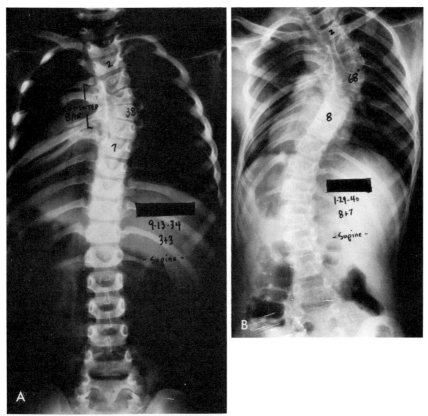

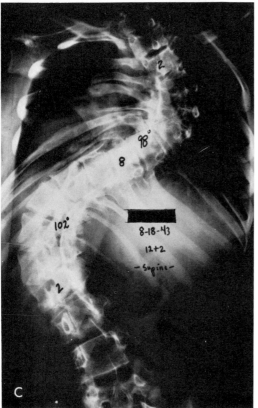

**Figure 7–3** *A,* Three year old child with a classic unilateral unsegmented bar involving four thoracic vertebrae with a 38° curve. Note the lack of any other significant curve, there being just a mild sweeping compensatory curve between T7 and L2. *B,* The same patient at age 8 years, 7 months. The curve due to the unsegmented bar has increased to 68 degrees, and the compensatory curve has also increased and is now developing rotation, a sign of structural change. *C,* The same patient at age 12 years, 2 months. The thoracic curve has now reached 98 degrees, and there is a highly structural 102 degrees left thoracolumbar curve. This lower curve, originally purely compensatory and nonstructural, has become severely structural and would require fusion at this time. This is an example of a condition where originally there was a single thoracic primary curve but on later follow-up the patient has a double major curve pattern.

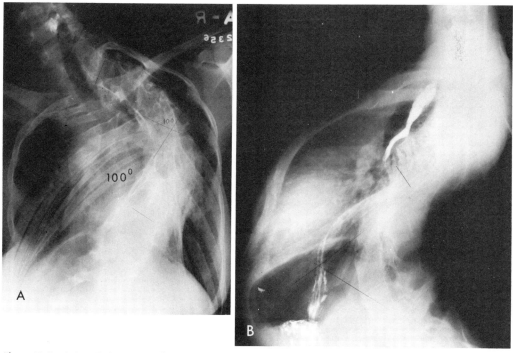

**Figure 7–4**  *A,* An AP chest x-ray of a patient with a 100 degree thoracic scoliosis due to congenital anomalies including unilateral unsegmented bar. She was 21 years of age at this time. *B,* Lateral x-ray of the same patient showing severe thoracolumbar lordosis. The patient expired at age 25 of cor pulmonale.

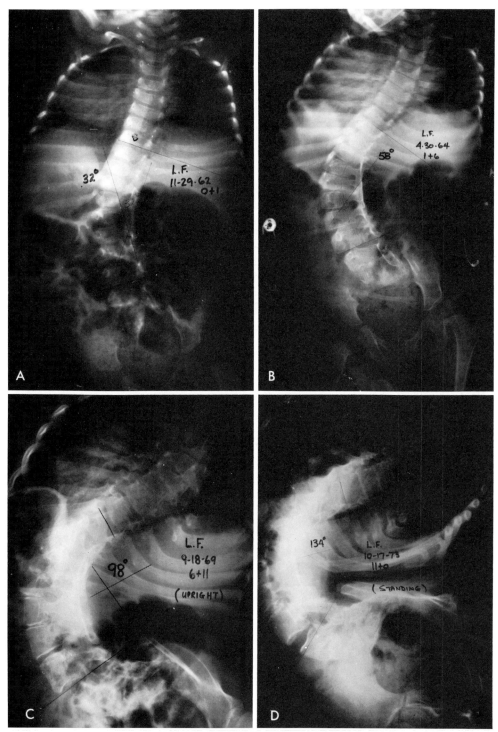

**Figure 7–5**   *A,* An AP x-ray of a one-month old child demonstrating 32 degrees curve. There is a unilateral unsegmented bar in the concave side of the lumbar curve, which does not show well on this x-ray. *B,* At age one year, six months, her curvature had already increased to 58 degrees. The bar can easily be seen at this time. *C,* By age six years, eleven months, the curve had increased to 98 degrees, and the pelvic obliquity had become quite noticeable. *D,* By age 11 the curvature had reached 134 degrees, the pelvic obliquity was extremely severe, and the pelvis was beginning to indent the rib cage.

*Legend and illustration continued on opposite page*

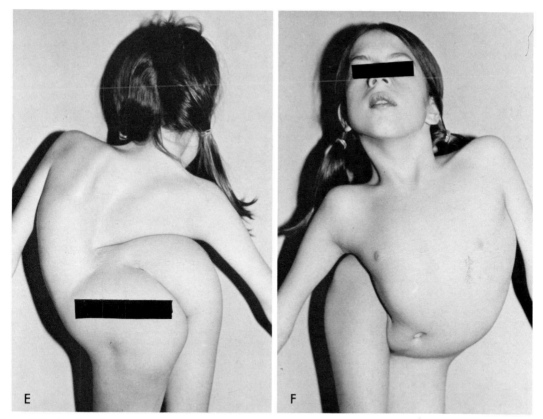

**Figure 7–5**  *Continued*
*E,* Posterior photograph of the patient at age 11 showing the severe pelvic obliquity and the impairment of the chest by the pelvis. *F,* An anterior view showing the extreme cosmetic deformity created by this bar.

## KYPHOSIS

Anterior defects of segmentation are much less common than lateral defects of segmentation. Such anterior defects, in the presence of posterior growth, will produce kyphosis. The severity of the kyphotic deformity will depend on the length of the area involved and the discrepancy of growth. A complete failure of disc formation from the anterior to the posterior part of the vertebral body has much less tendency to be "bent" by posterior growth than an incomplete failure of disc formation (posterior half of disc still present). The problem is further complicated by defects of segmentation that do not manifest themselves until later in growth. These have the appearance of normal or "near-normal" discs and end-plates for several years, yet can still develop severe deformity by the end of growth.[58]

The kyphotic deformities produced by defects of segmentation have seldom been as severe as those produced by anterior defects of formation. Paraplegia has not been reported (Fig. 7–6).

## LORDOSIS

Fortunately, this condition appears to be extremely rare. The authors have personally seen only three cases, two having severe deformity with significant respiratory compromise, one dying of respiratory failure at age 20 (Fig. 7–7).

## Defects of Formation

### ANTERIOR AND ANTEROLATERAL KYPHOSIS AND KYPHOSCOLIOSIS

Anterior failure of formation ranges from extremely mild to extremely severe. The mildest types show failure of development of

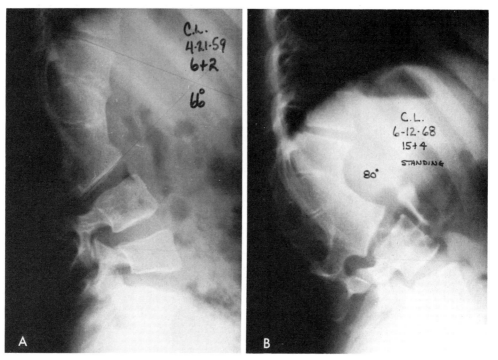

**Figure 7–6** *A,* Lateral x-ray of a six year old girl showing a 66 degree curve due to an anterior failure of segmentation. *B,* The same patient at age 15, showing an 80 degree curve.

the anterior 1/4 to 1/3 of a single vertebral body. The severe types have total absence of more than one vertebral body.

The anterior defect may be symmetrical, in which case a pure kyphotic deformity develops, or asymmetric, in which case kyphoscoliosis develops. There is a spectrum of deformity ranging from pure kyphosis to pure scoliosis with varying grades of kyphosis between.

The natural history of these deformities is generally poor. That is to say, most increase with growth, produce significant and often severe deformity, and quite often lead to paraplegia.

The most common cause of paraplegia due to spine deformity (other than tuberculosis) is congenital kyphosis. Kyphosis is most common at the thoracolumbar junction, secondly in the lower thoracic area, thirdly, upper thoracic, and finally, lumbar. Congenital cervical kyphosis has rarely been reported. Winter et al.[87] noted that of 30 patients watched without treatment during growth, all 30 progressed, the average progression being 44 degrees in six years, or an average of 7 degrees per year (Fig. 7–8).

Paralysis may have its onset at a wide variety of ages. Some children seem to be born with a neurologic problem which may be quite insidious. There may be subluxation at birth with a stenosis of the spinal canal due to the deformity. These children may have foot deformity at birth, or may appear neurologically normal, but do not develop bladder control.

In the review of congenital kyphosis by Winter et al.[87] 16 of the 130 patients developed cord compression due to the deformity. All had kyphosis (Type I) or kyphoscoliosis due to defects of formation. Paralysis was most likely to develop when the apex of the kyphosis was in the thoracic spine, especially when in the T3–T8 area. This anatomic area of the spine has the narrowest diameter of the spinal canal, and at this same level, the spinal cord has its most precarious blood supply (see Chapter 5). Furthermore, the cord at this level has the least elasticity. Paralysis has been noted with kyphoses as low as L2.

In summary, kyphotic or kyphoscoliotic deformities due to absence of all or parts of the vertebral bodies are not common but tend to produce progressive and severe deformities

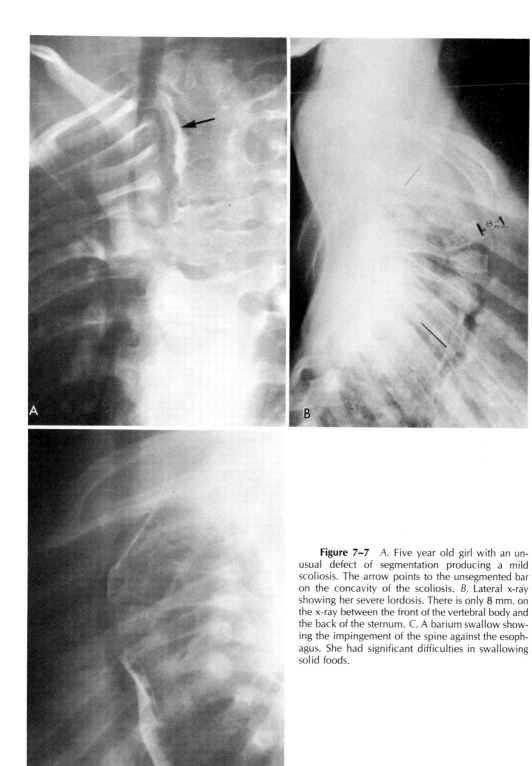

**Figure 7–7**   *A,* Five year old girl with an unusual defect of segmentation producing a mild scoliosis. The arrow points to the unsegmented bar on the concavity of the scoliosis. *B,* Lateral x-ray showing her severe lordosis. There is only 8 mm. on the x-ray between the front of the vertebral body and the back of the sternum. *C,* A barium swallow showing the impingement of the spine against the esophagus. She had significant difficulties in swallowing solid foods.

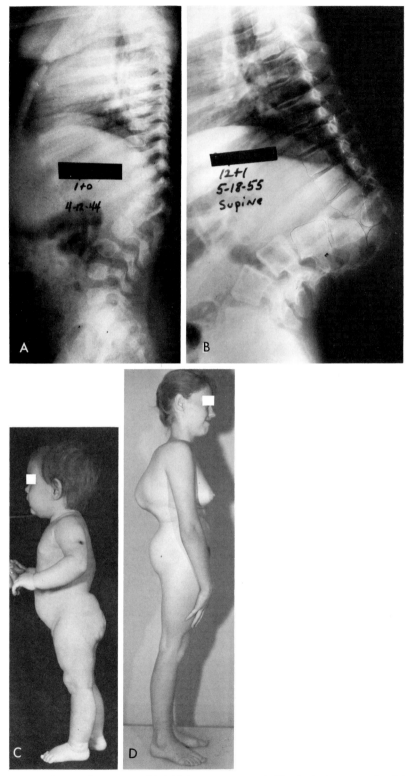

**Figure 7–8**   *A,* Lateral x-ray of a one year old child showing a congenital kyphosis due to anterior defects of formation. *B,* Same patient at age 12 showing the severe progression of her deformity without treatment. *C,* Lateral photograph of patient at age one. *D,* Lateral photograph of patient at age 15.

with an alarmingly high percentage of paraplegia. The most dangerous lesions are those in the upper thoracic spine (Fig. 7–9).

*LATERAL DEFECTS: HEMIVERTEBRA*

Probably the most common of all congenital spine anomalies is the hemivertebra, either singly or in association with other hemivertebrae or other anomalies. No other anomaly can cause such heated discussion concerning treatment: recommendations range from total excision to total neglect. In order to arrive at a rational program of treatment, it is necessary to have a complete understanding of the natural history of this anomaly. Unfortunately, not all hemivertebrae or all patients with a hemivertebra behave in the same manner.

As pointed out by Cotrel, Nasca et al.,[61] Tsou et al.,[77] and others, there are several recognizable types of hemivertebrae. These are classified as follows (Fig. 7–10):

a) Single hemivertebra (nonsegmented), incarcerated

b) Single hemivertebra (semisegmented), incarcerated

c) Single hemivertebra (fully segmented), incarcerated

d) Single hemivertebra (fully segmented), nonincarcerated

e) Multiple hemivertebrae (unilateral), sequential

f) Multiple hemivertebrae (unilateral), nonsequential

g) Balanced hemivertebrae (adjacent)

h) Balanced hemivertebrae (nonadjacent) (hemimetameric shift)

i) Posterolateral hemivertebra

Thus one can see that a multitude of anatomic possibilities exist, and thus a multi-

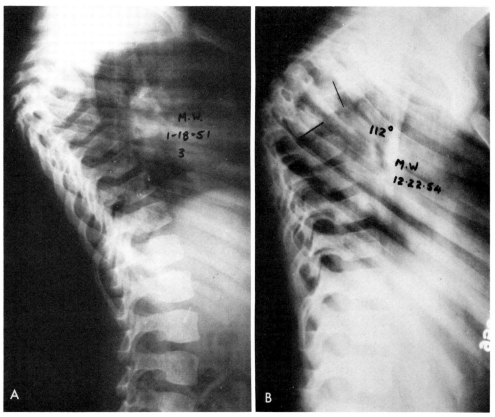

**Figure 7–9** *A,* Lateral x-ray of a 3 year old patient with kyphosis due to anterior failure of formation. He was neurologically normal at this time. The incorrect diagnosis of tuberculosis was made. *B,* The same patient three years later. At this time paraplegia had developed owing to the untreated kyphosis.

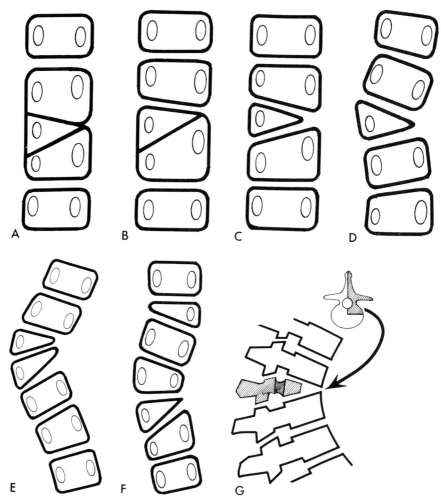

**Figure 7–10**  *A,* Single hemivertebra (nonsegmented, incarcerated). The hemivertebra is "tucked into" the spine and has no growth potential. Therefore, no curve is produced. *B,* A single hemivertebra (semisegmented, incarcerated). Because the hemivertebra is separated from the vertebra above but not the one below, it is "semisegmented." Because it is "tucked into" the spine without malalignment, it is "incarcerated." *C,* A single hemivertebra (fully segmented, incarcerated). *D,* A single hemivertebra (fully segmented, nonincarcerated). *E,* Multiple hemivertebrae (unilateral, sequential). *F,* Balanced double hemivertebrae. *G,* Posterolateral hemivertebra.

tude of natural histories may exist. It is therefore not surprising that confusion exists as to the true natural history of these problems. If one analyzes these variations carefully, one can see that it is the *potential for asymmetric growth* that makes the difference in prognosis.

In general, incarcerated hemivertebrae seldom cause problems, especially if nonsegmented from their adjacent vertebrae. Nonincarcerated hemivertebrae have a tendency to cause progressive curves, especially if there are multiple hemivertebrae on the same side. One can summarize the problem as follows: *Where asymmetric growth may exist, progression is probable. Where growth appears symmetric, progression of the curve is unlikely.* However, since the surgeon can only guess the growth potential, the ultimate answer is up to nature. No anomaly can be assumed to be benign. Time will give the answer, and thus the patient must be followed carefully.

There has been an unfortunate tendency

not to appreciate the progression of congenital spine deformities. This has been due to a combination of lack of knowledge, complacency on the part of the physician, lack of precise measurement of the curve, and failure to appreciate the slow but relentless progression of a curve due to the progress of only 5 to 6 degrees each year, an amount easy to attribute to "measurement error." All too often the physician looks only at the current x-ray plus the one taken six months earlier and the change is only two or three degrees — easy to ignore. The *initial* x-ray, the *most recent x-ray*, and the *current* x-ray must always be compared. Only then can true progression be appreciated (Figs. 7–11, 7–12, 7–13, and 7–14).

## OPERATIVE TREATMENT

### Defects of Segmentation

#### ANTERIOR DEFECTS: KYPHOSIS

The natural history is one of slow and steady increasing deformity throughout growth, with acceleration during the adolescent growth spurt.

Therefore, the ideal treatment is early recognition of the deformity and arthrodesis *before* significant deformity develops. A posterior arthrodesis stabilizes the curve and arrests posterior growth, thus preventing increasing deformity. Posterior arthrodesis under such circumstances will only prevent

*Text continued on page 150*

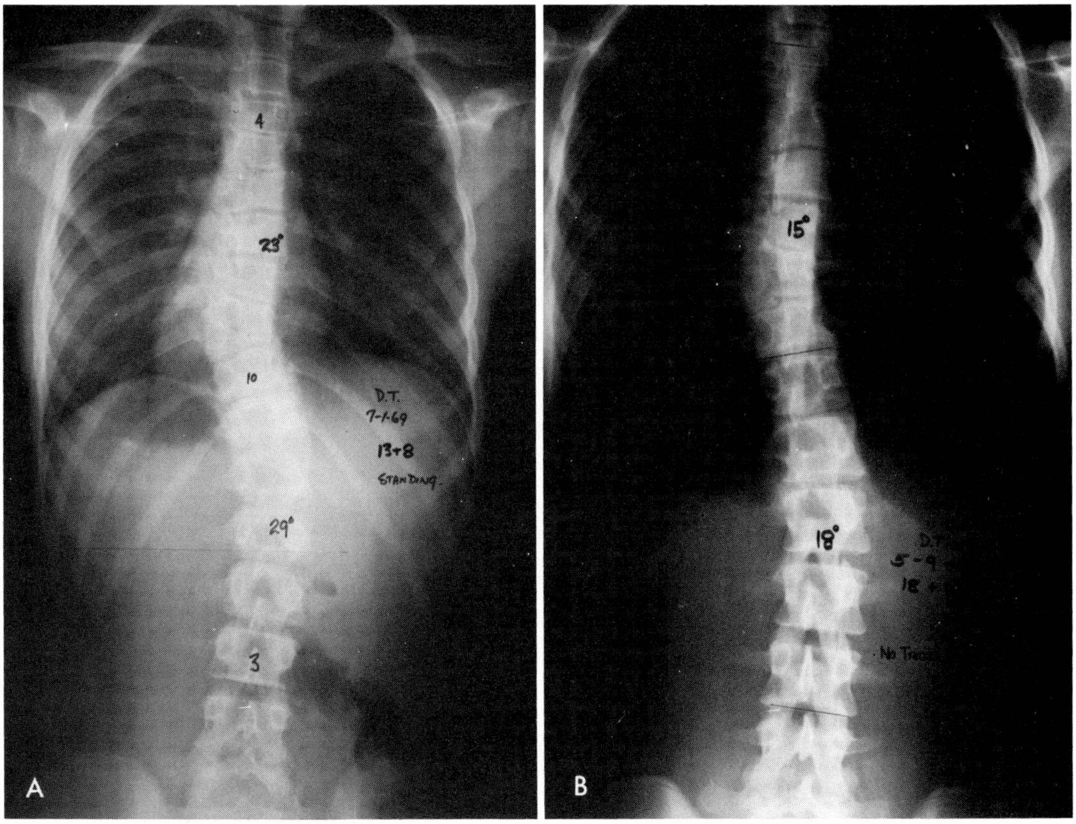

**Figure 7–11** *A,* Thirteen year old girl with congenital scoliosis. There are two hemivertebrae on the left side in the thoracic spine. The upper one, at T6, is incarcerated and nonsegmented. The lower one, at T9, is semisegmented and non-incarcerated. The T10–L3 curve appears to be a compensatory or secondary curve. *B,* The same patient at age 18, having had no treatment of any type whatsoever. There has been no increase in the curves. They actually measure better. If bracing or exercises had been given, it would have been easy to assume that the improvement or lack of progression was due to the treatment. Actually it was due only to the natural history of this particular patient.

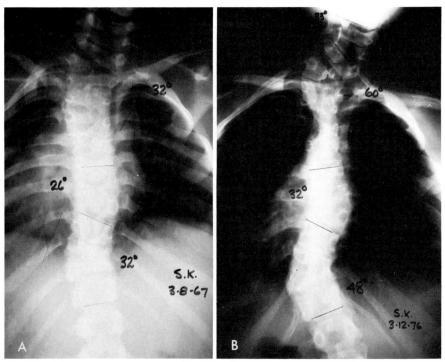

**Figure 7–12**   *A,* Five year old patient with a complex pattern of curvatures. In the lower cervical spine there is an 18 degree curve due to a unilateral unsegmented bar involving C5, C6, and C7. At the upper thoracic spine there is a hemivertebra at T1, which appears on this x-ray to be nonincarcerated and segmented. At T8–T9 on the right side there is another hemivertebra, which appears to be incarcerated and nonsegmented. At T11 on the left side there is another hemivertebra. This is segmented and nonincarcerated. *B,* The same patient nine years later without treatment. The cervical curve has increased from 18 degrees to 33 degrees, the high left thoracic curve has increased from 32 degrees to 60 degrees, the right mid-curve has increased from 26 degrees to 32 degrees, and the low left curve has increased from 32 degrees to 48 degrees. In this particular pat'ent all the curves increased. The predictability of the lower two curves was difficult, but the predictability of the two higher curves was not too difficult to establish.

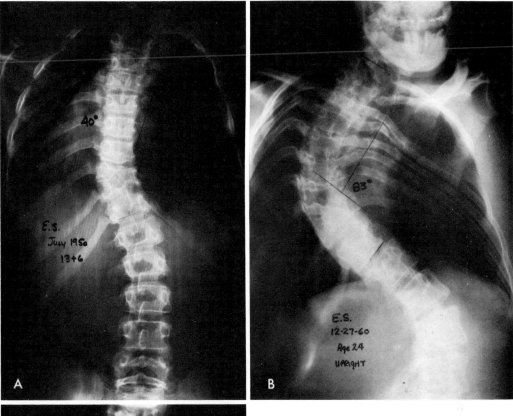

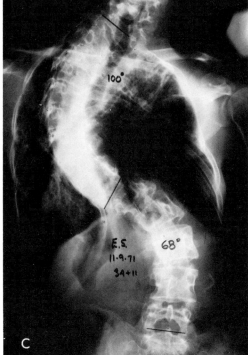

**Figure 7–13** *A,* This 13 year old girl presented to Gillette Children's Hospital with a 40 degree left thoracic curve due to a single hemivertebra on the left side at T10. This would be considered nonincarcerated and semisegmented. In the upper thoracic spine there are some vague anomalies, primarily bilateral defect of segmentation. There are some normal vertebrae in between, and the lumbar curve is compensatory. The patient was seen by Dr. Moe and surgical fusion recommended because of fear of progression. The family rejected this advice and did not return for follow-up as requested. *B,* The same patient at age 24, following admission to the hospital for delivery of a child. Following delivery she went into pulmonary edema requiring digitalization. The thoracic curve now measured 80 degrees. She had some thoracic lordosis. She disappeared from follow-up and was not seen again for several years. *C,* The same patient at age 35, when she appeared at the Twin Cities Scoliosis Center for treatment of cor pulmonale. She died three years later.

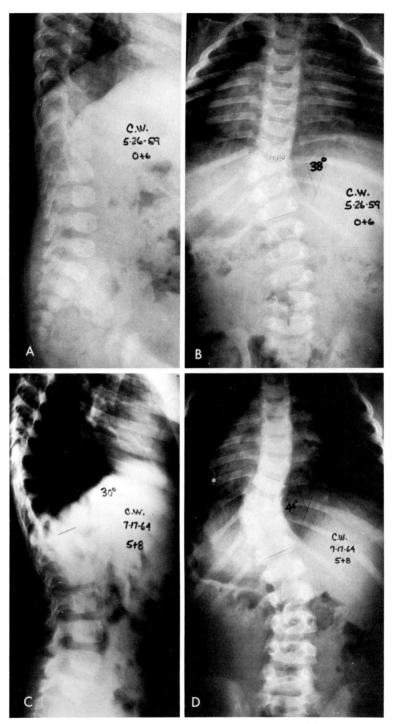

**Figure 7–14**    *A,* Lateral x-ray of a six month old child. No spine deformity is visible. *B,* AP x-ray taken at the same time showing a single nonincarcerated hemivertebra at T9. On the left there is a 38 degree scoliosis. *C,* At age five years, there is a 30 degree kyphosis. *D,* An AP x-ray at age five shows an increase in scoliosis to 44 degrees. This increase in both scoliosis and kyphosis was not appreciated, and no treatment was given.

*Illustration continued on the opposite page*

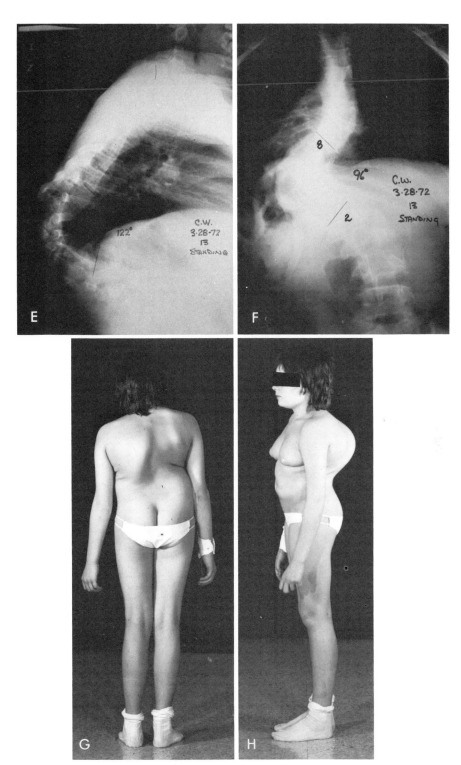

**Figure 7–14** *Continued*

*E,* Lateral standing x-ray at age 13 showing a 122 degree curve. *F,* AP x-ray at age 13 showing a 96 degree scoliosis. *G,* Posterior photographs showing a left scoliosis with prominent rib hump. *H,* Lateral view showing a severe kyphosis. This is a true kyphoscoliosis due to a posterolateral hemivertebra (corner hemivertebra).

increase of deformity but cannot improve the deformity, which is confined to the anomalous vertebrae.

However, it is possible to obtain some improvement if the arthrodesis includes one normal vertebra above and below the anomalous area. When fused early, the posterior element cannot grow, but the anterior portion of the normal vertebrae will grow, producing a trapezoidal vertebra and a compensatory lordosis just above and just below the kyphotic area. This will cause a pleasing cosmetic improvement. To accomplish these effects, the posterior arthrodesis must be done prior to age five (Fig. 7–15).

Not all patients are detected early, and many present to the surgeon with a significant and unsightly deformity. The surgeon must then choose between posterior arthrodesis alone to prevent increase (but not correct the existent deformity) or more extensive procedures to both *correct and stabilize* the spine. Prior to 1965, such corrective procedures were felt to be impossible, but pioneering efforts by Bickel[5] and Hodgson[28] led to the procedure of anterior osteotomy of the unsegmented bar. The exposure and techniques are almost identical to those used for the surgical treatment of severe Scheuermann's disease as outlined in Chapter 20.

Following anterior osteotomy (and filling of the osteotomy sites with cancellous bone chips), halofemoral or halo-Cotrel traction is applied in a hyperextension position for two weeks. A posterior fusion with Harrington compression instruments is then done over the entire area of kyphosis. The patient is ambulated in a hyperextension Risser cast. The total cast duration is six to nine months. In a small series reported by Mayfield et al.,[58] significant corrections were obtained with no complications (Fig. 7–16).

### LATERAL DEFECTS: UNILATERAL UNSEGMENTED BAR

Discussion of the treatment of this problem deserves special attention because of the extreme deformities that occur when it is not detected or treated early.

Early detection and aggressive treatment are the keys. Since the concavity of the curve is not growing and the convexity is growing, the curve should be fused early, *before* significant deformity occurs. No way is known to create growth in the concavity; therefore, balancing of the growth is done by *stopping growth on the convexity*. This is achieved with a good arthrodesis (Fig. 7–17).

It is frequently said that such early fusion is not indicated because it will "stunt the growth" of the child. This argument is without merit. The area of the anomalies cannot grow vertically because *nature did not provide growth potential*.

The two patients shown in Figures 7–18 and 7–19 illustrate clearly the contrast between procrastination and early prompt posterior fusion.

Another argument frequently heard is that "early posterior arthrodesis will cause progressive lordosis." This has not occurred in our experience. No such patient has developed an *increase* in lordosis following fusion, provided that the anomalous area was adequately fused. It is true that some patients finished growth with lordosis, but in such patients there was usually a pre-existent lordosis. Comparison of preoperative and end-of-growth lateral x-rays shows no increase of lordosis.

When the patient comes to the physician with an existent severe deformity, simple fusion can only halt progression; it cannot provide correction, since the unsegmented bar is unyielding to traction or bending. Correction of such severe curves can be accomplished only by osteotomy of the unsegmented bar. Fortunately, many of these bars are posterolateral and do not involve the vertebral bodies. Careful preoperative analysis by tomography can delineate whether the bar is posterior only or both anterior and posterior. If there is also lordosis, this is a sign that the bar is posterior.

Osteotomy of the bar is not difficult, if

*Text continued on page 158*

---

**Figure 7–15** *A,* Lateral x-ray at age 8 months, showing a congenital kyphosis. There is a defect of segmentation of two vertebral bodies at the apex of the curve. Just below this, there is an incomplete defect of segmentation and just above, a tendency for slipping forward of the upper vertebrae on the two nonsegmented vertebrae. *B,* Lateral x-ray at age two years and six months, one year after spine fusion. A pseudarthrosis is visible at the apex of the curve. Kyphosis measures 42 degrees. A pseudarthrosis repair was performed.

*Legend and illustration continued on the opposite page*

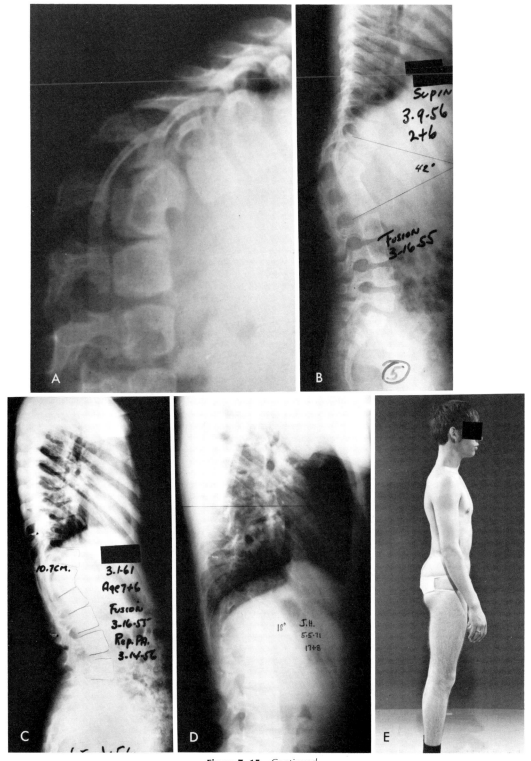

**Figure 7–15** *Continued*
*C*, At age 7, the kyphosis has decreased. *D*, At age 17, the kyphosis now measures only 18 degrees. There is normal torso alignment. *E*, Lateral standing photograph at age 17 shows totally normal body alignment. Note the relatively small amount of torso shortening considering the early age of the fusion. Note the totally normal lateral contour.

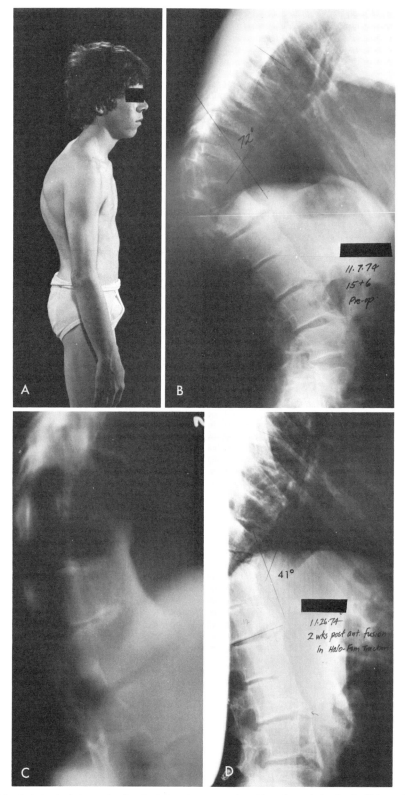

**Figure 7–16**  *A,* Lateral photograph of patient showing a prominent low thoracic kyphosis. This could easily be mistaken for Scheuermann's disease. *B,* A lateral standing x-ray taken at the same time shows a 72 degree kyphosis. There is a defect of segmentation anteriorly, particularly in the low thoracic area. *C,* A lateral laminogram shows the anterior defect in more detail. *D,* A lateral x-ray in halofemoral traction two weeks following anterior osteotomy of the unsegmented bar and division of the anterior longitudinal ligament with grafting of the disc spaces.

*Illustration continued on the opposite page*

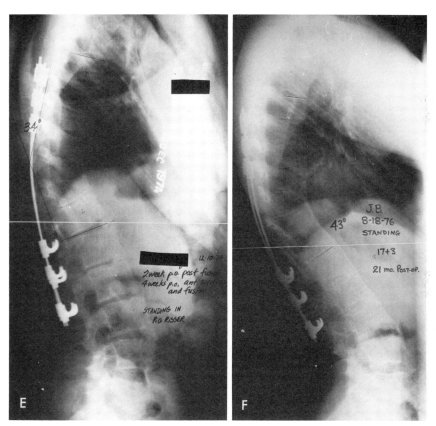

**Figure 7–16**  *Continued*
*E,* A lateral x-ray with the patient standing in a postoperative cast following posterior Harrington instrumentation using two parallel compression rod systems. The curve now measures 34 degrees. The patient was fully ambulatory, and the cast was removed at six months. *F,* At age 17, 21 months post fusion, his curve measured 43 degrees. There was some settling due to premature cast removal. The general result, however, was satisfactory.

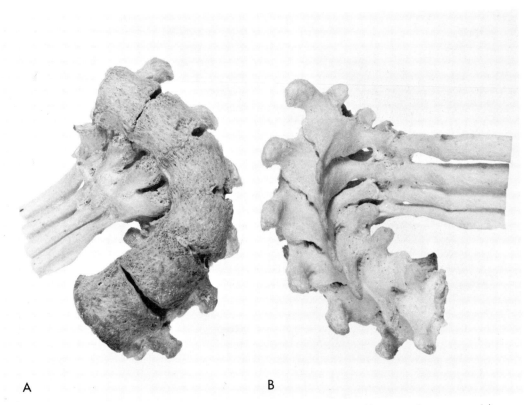

A                                                                    B

**Figure 7–17**  *A,* Anterior photograph of a specimen of a unilateral unsegmented bar. Note the presence of disc spaces on the convexity of the curve and the absence on the concavity. Note the defect of segmentation of the transverse processes and ribs. *B,* Posterior view of the same specimen showing the synostosis of ribs and transverse processes. The laminae are separated in the uppermost two vertebrae and have a defect of segmentation in the lower two. (Illustrations courtesy of Dr. G. D. MacEwen, DuPont Institute, Wilmington, Delaware, reproduced with his permission.)

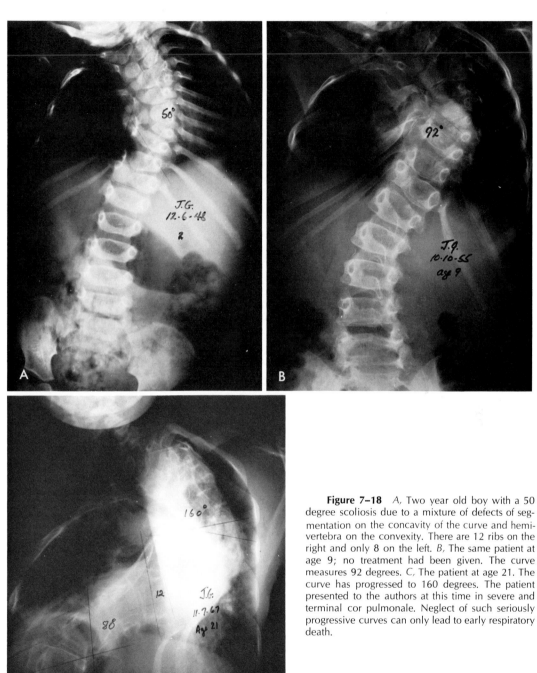

**Figure 7–18** *A,* Two year old boy with a 50 degree scoliosis due to a mixture of defects of segmentation on the concavity of the curve and hemivertebra on the convexity. There are 12 ribs on the right and only 8 on the left. *B,* The same patient at age 9; no treatment had been given. The curve measures 92 degrees. *C,* The patient at age 21. The curve has progressed to 160 degrees. The patient presented to the authors at this time in severe and terminal cor pulmonale. Neglect of such seriously progressive curves can only lead to early respiratory death.

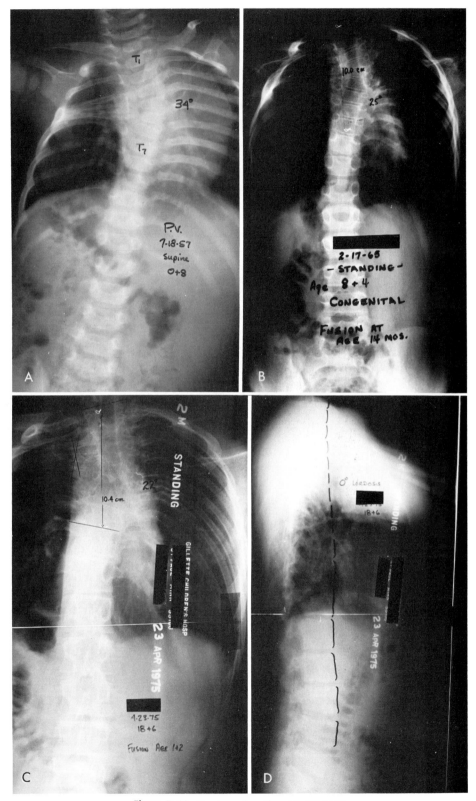

**Figure 7–19**  *See legend on the opposite page*

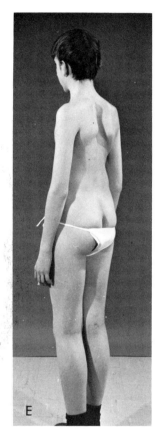

**Figure 7–19**  *Continued*   *A,* An eight month old boy with a 34 degree curve due to unilateral unsegmented bar. Note the similarity of this case with the untreated case shown in Figure 7–3. *B,* Patient at age 8, seven years after spine fusion from C7 to T9. The curve measures 25 degrees, and the distance from the imbedded markers at the top and bottom of the fusion areas is 10.0 cm. *C,* The same patient at age 18, 17 years after spine fusion. The curve measures 22 degrees. The distance between the two markers measures 10.4 cm. The patient's pulmonary function measured 80 per cent of normal. He had no respiratory symptoms. *D,* Lateral x-ray of the patient at age 18 showing a straight spine. This same condition existed prior to the fusion. *E,* Posterior oblique photograph to show the bodily contours and proportions. The torso is relatively shorter than that of a normal boy of this age. The hands, however, come only to mid-thigh.

care and delicacy of technique are used. The level of osteotomy must be carefully chosen preoperatively using tomography. There must be a normal or near-normal disc anteriorly at the level of osteotomy. Nothing is gained by a posterior osteotomy at an area with anterior nonsegmentation.

At the level of osteotomy, the ligamentum flavum on the convex side is identified and carefully removed, exposing the dura. With a Kerrison rongeur, the osteotomy is completed by working one's way toward the concavity, directing the osteotomy toward the foramen lying between two transverse processes. Any rib synostosis in this area should be excised at the same time. *A fusion of the entire curve is then performed* before closure.

Correction should be obtained by slow and gradual methods, with the patient awake and with careful neurologic monitoring. Correction with Harrington distraction rods alone is dangerous. The risks of paraplegia are high. Halofemoral traction has given the authors the best results. Good corrections have also been obtained with a halo-turnbuckle cast. Blount has obtained good correction using a Milwaukee brace postoperatively.[8] Figures 7–20 and 7–21 demonstrate osteotomy and correction of patients with curves due to unilateral unsegmented bars.

*POSTERIOR DEFECTS: CONGENITAL LORDOSIS*

The correction of severe deformity is virtually impossible. The answer lies in early detection and early *anterior* arthrodesis to prevent progressive deformity, respiratory failure, and early death.

**Defects of Formation**

*ANTERIOR DEFECTS: KYPHOSIS*

In this condition, as in all types of congenital defects, early detection and early fusion are the keys to treatment. Since the risk of paralysis is so high with congenital kyphosis, it is particularly important to fuse these early. This principle of early fusion was strongly recommended by James in 1955,[32] but his advice has been all too often forgotten.

What is the ideal age for fusion? The best results have been in patients fused prior to age 3, and prior to the development of a kyphosis of more than 50 degrees. Under these circumstances, a solid posterior arthrodesis can be obtained that not only stops progression but also usually results in gradual spontaneous correction because of continued anterior growth. Anterior fusion will destroy this anterior growth potential.

What is the earliest age at which fusion can be accomplished? Our youngest patient was six months at the time of fusion (using bank bone). Several cases fused at 12 to 24 months have also been successful. The most severe deformity solved by early posterior fusion was a 75 degree kyphosis in a three year old girl. Pseudarthrosis is frequent. If there is any question, reinforcement of the fusion at six months is strongly advised (Figs. 7–22, 7–23, and 7–24).

The more severe deformities and those in older children cannot be treated by posterior fusion alone. Kyphoses greater than 60 degrees and in children over age five rarely have been corrected by posterior arthrodesis alone, regardless of how many attempts at pseudarthrosis repair were done.

It was not until 1965, when Hodgson's anterior surgery for tuberculosis had proved so valuable, that anterior fusion for congenital kyphosis became utilized.[28] It rapidly proved to be the solution for this previously insurmountable problem. Like any other operative procedure, to be successful it must be properly performed. Our initial experience met with a few failures, always due to an inadequate arthrodesis. For example, we did a small, three segment fusion when we should have done a six or seven segment fusion. We put in one graft when we should have put in three (Fig. 7–25). For details of the operative technique, see Chapter 20.

Anterior fusion alone is seldom sufficient and should almost always be supplemented by posterior fusion, with or without Harrington instrumentation. Full Risser casts, a Milwaukee brace, or halocasts are needed for thoracic kyphoses. Underarm casts and braces are adequate for lumbar or thoracolumbar curves only. The cast should be worn for at least 10 months. We formerly felt that six months of bed rest was necessary, but recent experience

*Text continued on page 168*

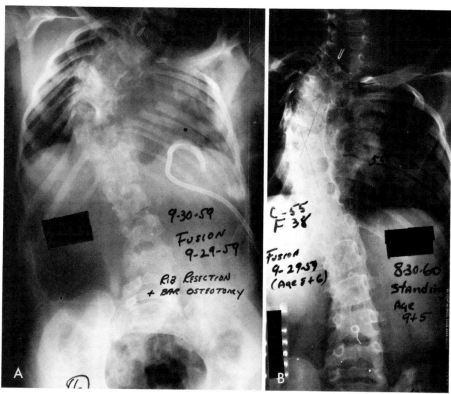

**Figure 7–20**   *A,* This 8 year old child had a 90 degree progressive curve due to unilateral unsegmented bar and defect of segmentation of the bases of the ribs. In a single operative procedure, the synostosis of the ribs was excised, the unilateral unsegmented bar was osteotomized, and a fusion of the entire thoracic spine was performed. Postoperative correction was performed by means of a turnbuckle cast. *B,* Same patient at age 9, one year following fusion. The curve has been corrected to 55 degrees. The fusion is solid.

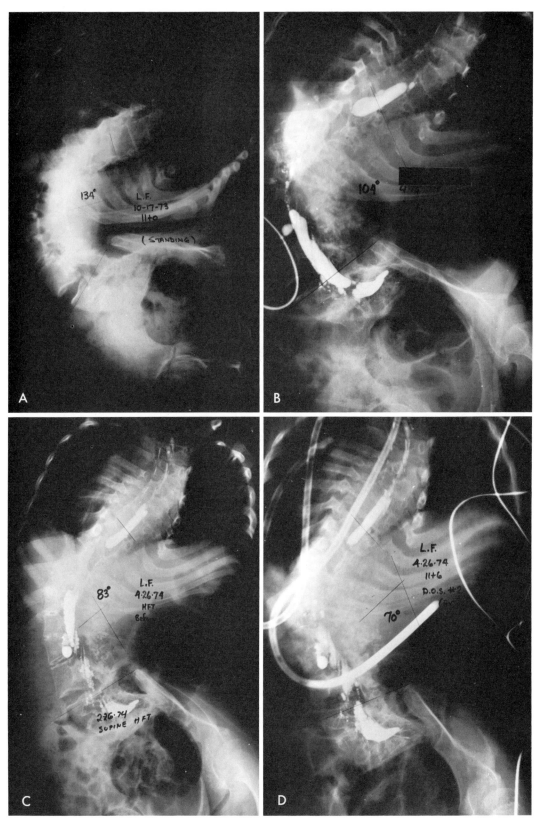

**Figure 7–21** *See legend on the opposite page*

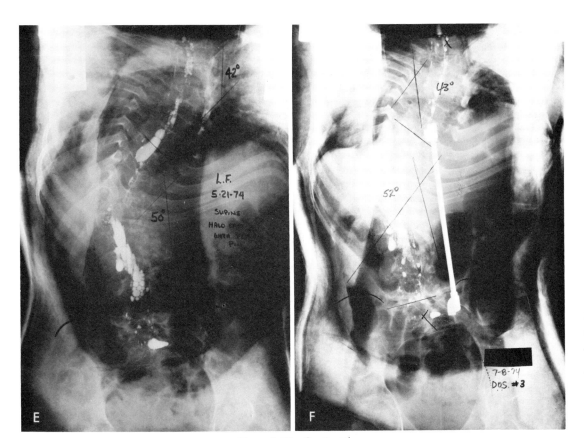

**Figure 7–21** *Continued*

*A,* This 11 year old girl presented with severe deformity due to a unilateral unsegmented bar involving the entire lumbar spine. (See Figure 7–5 for earlier films and the patient's clinical appearance.) *B,* The first operation consisted of a posterior excision of the entire unsegmented bar, which was situated posteriorly and did not involve the vertebral bodies. This resection extended from T10 to S1. A halo was applied and femoral pin inserted in the right distal femur. Traction was very slowly and cautiously begun. *C,* After two weeks, considerable correction had been obtained. *D,* She then had the second operation, which consisted of an anterior approach on the convex side excising all of the discs and wedges of bone from the end-plate from T10 to S1. No internal fixation was used. *E,* The postoperative traction with a halo and a single femoral pin was continued. Within four weeks, a level pelvis was obtained, and she was placed in a halo cast extending down one leg to include the right femoral pin. There was no cast on the left leg. She was sent home for a period of rest from the hospital. *F,* She was returned to the hospital two months later. The posterior operative area was re-exposed and a Harrington rod inserted as a strut bar to maintain the correction of the pelvis, permitting removal of the pin from the distal femur and the institution of hip motion on the right side. At the same time, a large amount of bone graft material was inserted throughout the lumbar fusion area, extending up to include the thoracic curvature. Unfortunately, the patient expired of pneumonia at home, three months later. Thus, no final follow-up is available on this patient.

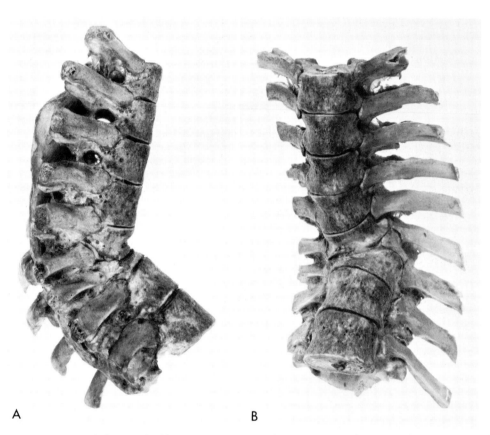

A                                                    B

**Figure 7–22**  *A,* Lateral photograph of the spine of a patient with a congenital kyphosis secondary to anterior failure of formation. A posterior fusion has been performed. The patient, unfortunately, succumbed to an automobile accident. *B,* An anterior view that shows particularly well the anterior failure formation of the vertebral body. There is a small triangular remnant of the missing body. The two vertebrae above and below the defect have then come together and made sufficient contact that they actually appear to be fused. (Illustrations through the courtesy of Dr. G. D. MacEwen and Dr. Albert Shands of the DuPont Institute of Wilmington, Delaware.)

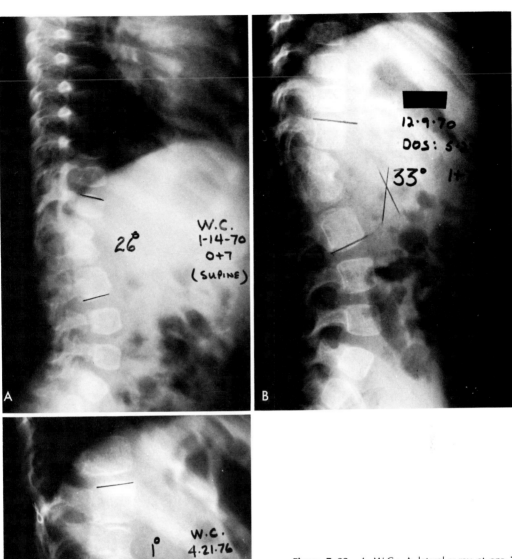

**Figure 7–23** *A,* W.C.: A lateral x-ray at age 7 months, showing a 26 degree congenital kyphosis. *B,* At age 1+ 7, a posterior fusion was performed of this area, which had shown a slight increase during the previous year. Only four segments were fused. *C,* The same patient five years later, at age 6 years and 9 months. There has been spontaneous correction to only a 1 degree kyphosis. It is anticipated that further correction into a normal lumbar lordosis will occur with time.

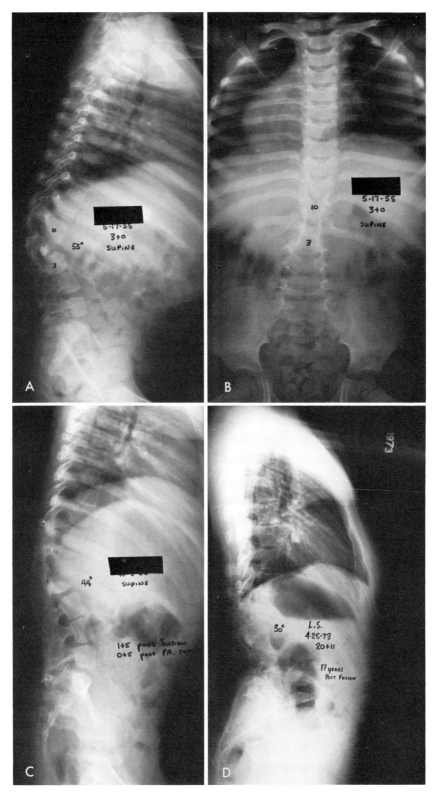

**Figure 7–24**   *See legend on the opposite page.*

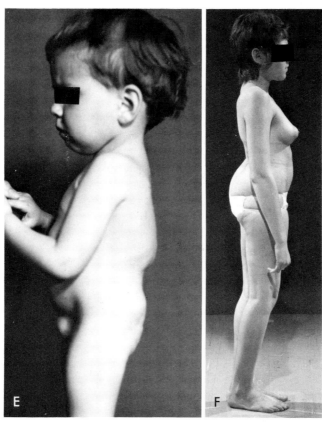

**Figure 7–24** *Continued.* *A,* Lateral supine x-ray at age 3 of a girl with congenital kyphosis due to anterior failure of vertebral body formation. There are actually several segments missing so that T10 and L3 are nearly approximated. There is a 55 degree curve, supine. The upright films showed a 75 degree curve. *B,* Anterior view taken at the same time shows the shortening of the lumbar spine due to the defect of formation of several vertebrae. There is a congenital spinal stenosis between T10 and L3. She had mild bladder symptomatology (enuresis only). *C,* She underwent posterior spine fusion at age 3. This x-ray was taken at age 4 years and 5 months, 1½ years after spine fusion and five months after a posterior pseudoarthrosis repair. Fusion was extended to the sacrum, which is probably an unnecessarily long area of posterior fusion in view of our present knowledge. Note the anterior defect at the apex of the curve. Correction was obtained by the use of plaster casts. *D,* Lateral x-ray at age 20 years and 11 months, 17 years after spine fusion. Her kyphosis has spontaneously improved to 30 degrees. The fusion is solid. *E,* Lateral photograph at age 3, showing the sharp kyphosis. *F,* Lateral photograph at age 20, showing lack of any kyphotic deformity. She has a short waist due to the combination of congenital absence of vertebrae plus the early arthrodesis.

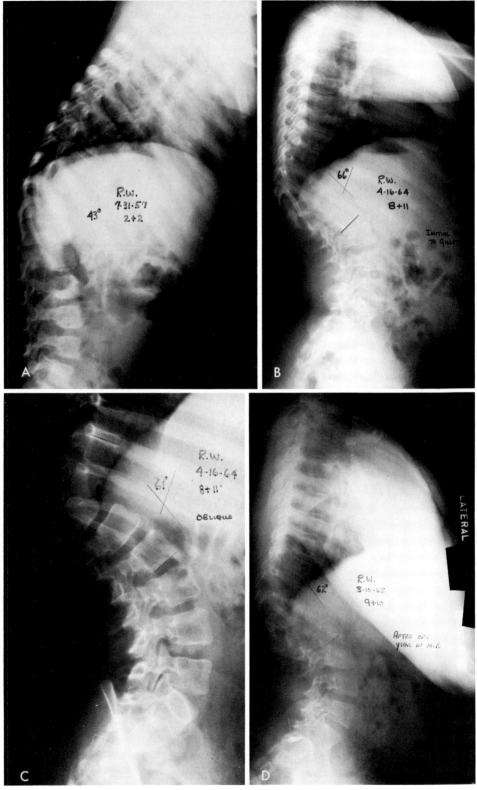

**Figure 7–25**  Legend appears on page 168.

*Illustration continued on the following page*

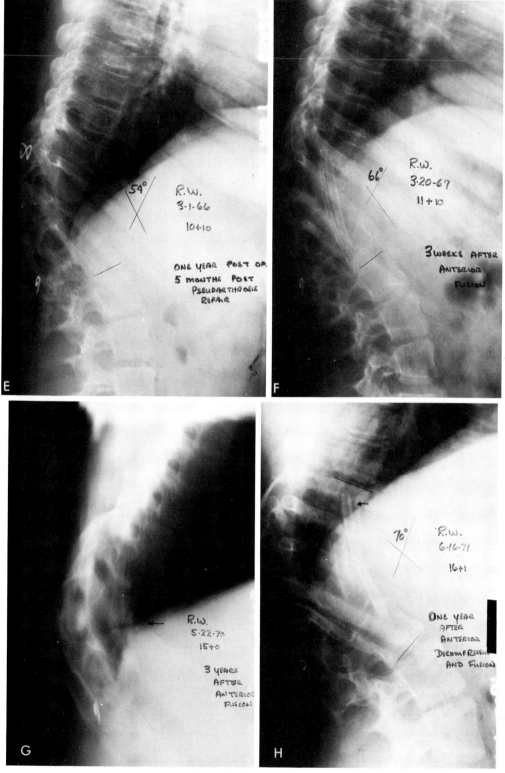

**Figure 7–25** *Continued*

*Illustration continued on the following page*

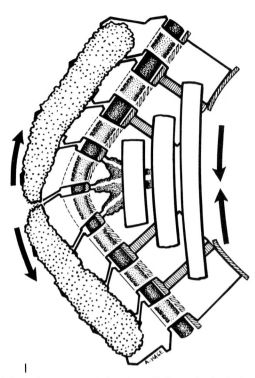

**Figure 7–25** *Continued*  *A,* Lateral x-ray at age 2 showing a 43 degree kyphosis due to the anterior failure of formation. The patient received no treatment at this time. *B,* When first seen by the authors at age 8 years and 11 months, the curvature had increased to 66 degrees. There were no neurologic symptoms. A Milwaukee brace was tried. *C,* An oblique x-ray at age 8 years and 11 months shows particularly well the posterior corner vertebra and the contact of the two vertebral bodies above and below the hemivertebra. *D,* On 3/10/65, after one year in a Milwaukee brace, the curve still measures 62 degrees. It was felt that further brace treatment was inappropriate and that surgery should be carried out. *E,* 3/1/66, one year after spine fusion, posteriorly, and five months after a posterior pseudarthrosis repair, the curve measures 54 degrees, and the pseudarthrosis is still quite visible. This is a classic example of the impossibility of obtaining a solid posterior arthrodesis in the face of an anterior defect of segmentation of this magnitude at this age. *F,* 3/20/67: An anterior fusion was performed using autogenous rib strut graft. The curve measures 66 degrees. The strut grafts are too far posteriorly and should have been longer and stronger. Harrington compression rods should have been used posteriorly in addition to the anterior fusion. *G,* 5/22/70: This x-ray, taken three years after the anterior fusion, shows a pseudarthrosis clearly evident straight through the anterior and posterior fusion masses. At this time, he was beginning to develop bladder paralysis and other evidence of long tract signs. *H,* 6/16/71: At age 16, one year after anterior spinal cord decompression and spine fusion, with new strut grafts, a solid fusion has been obtained and his neurologic condition has returned to normal. Subsequent follow-up to age 21 showed no further changes either in the x-ray or in the clinical condition. *I,* This diagrammatic representation of a congenital kyphosis shows that a posterior fusion mass is under distraction whereas an anterior strut grafting is under compression, thus providing optimal healing potential. The anterior strut must lie far in front of the apex of the curvature to obtain maximal effect.

has shown that early ambulation can be done with correction maintained if stable posterior fixation with Harrington rods has been accomplished. In cases of pure kyphosis, compression rods only should be used. In kyphoscoliosis, a compression assembly should be inserted first on the convex side, followed by a slightly bent distraction rod on the concave side. Posteriorly, one must fuse at least one vertebra above and one below the kyphotic area. The anterior fusion must include all vertebrae in the *structural* portion of the kyphosis (Fig. 7–26).

Recently, we have been very pleased with an anterior distracting device developed by Pinto and Avanzi of Sao Paulo, Brazil (see Chapter 21). This distractor fits into the two "limbs" of an angular kyphosis and can be gradually elongated by a reverse "turnbuckle" mechanism. Once adequate distraction has been accomplished, the strut graft or grafts are inserted, and the distractor is removed. It is *not* an implant. There is no tendency for stretching of the spinal cord, since the cord is relaxed as the kyphosis is corrected in this manner.

Traction is a two-edged sword in the treatment of congenital kyphosis. Contrary to neurofibromatosis kyphosis, which is usually fairly flexible, congenital kyphosis is usually rigid, and traction may not cause change of spinal alignment. It may only stretch the spinal cord, resulting in a tension lesion where the cord is pulled against the apex of the kyphosis. Hyperextension x-rays are quite valuable in distinguishing rigid from nonrigid deformities. *Paraplegia has been reported several times in the traction treatment of congenital kyphosis.* Paraplegia is most likely to develop a) in cases of pure kyphosis, b) where the apex is T4–T8, c) when the kyphosis is severe and rigid, and d) when the cord is tethered distally by a diastematomyelia or other type of dysraphism.

For flexible curves, particularly when there is a significant amount of scoliosis and when the apex is at the thoracolumbar junction, traction may be helpful. As always, careful twice-daily neurologic checks are mandatory for all patients in skeletal traction. Patients being considered for skeletal traction should have myelography to rule out a tethering lesion.

Figures 7–27 and 7–28 illustrate the combined anteroposterior approach for patients with severe congenital kyphoscoliosis or kyphosis.

***Paralysis with Congenital Kyphosis.*** This constitutes one of the greatest challenges to the spine surgeon. Not only does the paralysis need to be relieved but also the curvature must be stabilized so that paralysis will not recur. Each case must be fully analyzed, a plan developed, and the surgery done with great care.

Preoperatively, myelography is essential. Either a high-volume technique or low-volume with the needle removed and the patient supine is critical. The conventional prone myelogram with 10 to 15 ml. of dye is useless. (See Chapter 3 for details regarding this technique.)

Precise neurologic evaluation and documentation are essential. Only with a good baseline evaluation can one appreciate subtle changes postoperatively. When there is significant cord compression, and when the cause of cord compression is a prominence of bone (and/or disc) anterior to the cord, this prominence must be removed *by an anterior approach.* Cord decompression can be done

via a costotransversectomy approach (the Capener technique), but this approach does not give adequate exposure for anterior fusion.

The authors prefer the anterior transthoracic approach of Hodgson in order to *both* decompress the cord and simultaneously perform an anterior fusion. The technique is described in Chapter 20. In addition to the anterior decompression and fusion, posterior fusion with or without Harrington rods is recommended. In the classic paper on spinal cord compression and its treatment, Lonstein et al.[49] reported the results of such surgery.

In the past, laminectomy has often been attempted for the relief of cord compression due to kyphosis. The results, as noted by Lonstein, have been poor, with a high tendency for worsening of the paralysis rather than relief. Since the cause of the compression is anterior to the cord, the removal of laminae cannot alter the compression but can only add the problems of postlaminectomy kyphosis to the already existent congenital kyphosis. If one attempts to retract the cord to remove the offending bony prominence, irreversible cord damage may result.

For cord compression due to congenital kyphoscoliosis rather than pure kyphosis, one must decide whether to approach the cord from the convex or the concave side of the scoliosis. The goal is to allow the cord to take a more normal course; i.e., the cord must be allowed to move both forward and toward the midline of the body, or toward the concavity of the scoliosis. Thus the surgical approach should generally be on the concavity of the scoliosis, *not* the convexity.

This approach makes the exposure more difficult, since the spine is farther from the chest wall and rotated away from the surgeon. Nevertheless, this disadvantage must be accepted in order to achieve truly adequate cord decompression. If there is considerable rotation of the apical vertebrae, the approach can be through the convex thorax, even though the concave side of the curve is decompressed.

It is very important to place anterior strut grafts in the mid-axial body line, or line of gravity-loading. Except when there is severe rotation, it is difficult to achieve this from the convex side, and therefore, to achieve adequate anterior fusion, the concave side is usually preferred (Fig. 7–29).

Not all patients with cord compression

*Text continued on page 178*

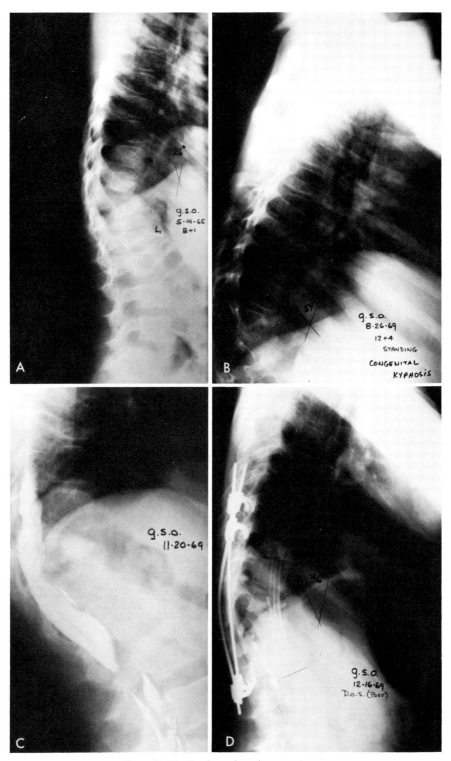

**Figure 7–26**   *See legend on the opposite page.*

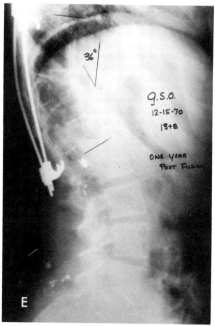

**Figure 7–26** *Continued*   A, Lateral x-ray of an 8 year old boy with a 26 degree kyphosis due to anterior failure of formation. No treatment was given. B, The same patient at age 12 shows a 57 degree rapidly progressive kyphosis with pain at the apex of the curvature. C, A myelogram shows the indentation of the dye column by disc material protruding at the apex of the curve. Despite this myelographic appearance, the neurologic examination was completely normal. It was therefore felt that decompression was not indicated. D, 12/16/69: Patient had anterior fusion with autogenous rib strut grafting followed two weeks later by posterior fusion and Harrington compression instrumentation with correction of the curve to 36 degrees. No neurologic difficulties were encountered in the performance of the surgery. E, 12/15/70: A lateral standing x-ray, one year following combined anterior and posterior fusion, shows full maintenance of the curvature at 36 degrees. The patient was neurologically normal.

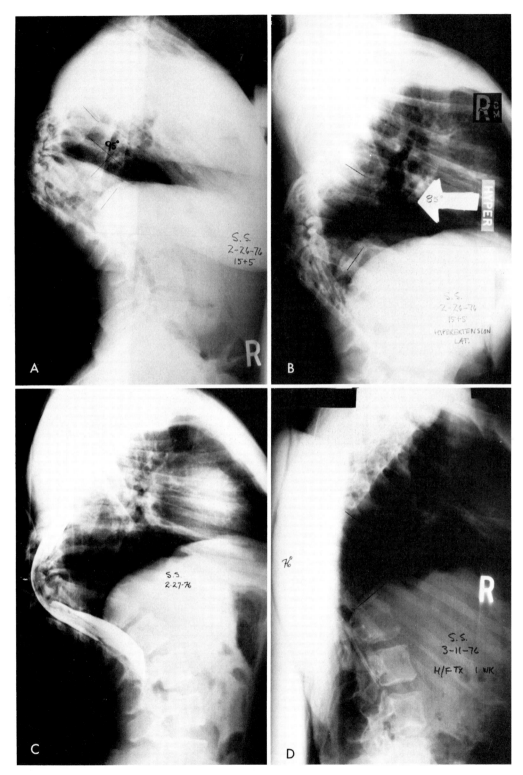

**Figure 7–27**  *See legend on the opposite page.*

*Legend and illustration continued on the opposite page*

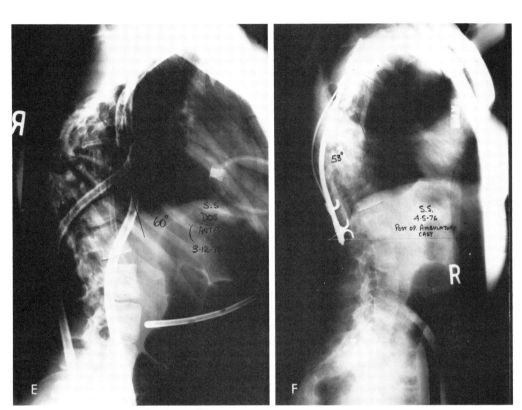

**Figure 7–27** *Continued* A, Lateral standing x-ray of a 15 year old girl shows a 95 degree congenital kyphosis due to anterior failure of segmentation. She had a slight scoliosis in conjunction with this. She was neurologically normal. B, Hyperextension lateral x-ray shows the curve to be quite rigid, correcting only to 85 degrees. C, Lateral high volume myelogram shows marked indentation of the dye column by the apex of the curvature. Despite this x-ray, the patient was neurologically normal. No attempt was thus made to visualize or "decompress" the spinal cord because of this normal neurologic condition. D, 3/11/76: The patient was placed in very carefully monitored halofemoral traction. The curvature improved to 76 degrees, only 9 degrees better than the hyperextension x-ray, but there was considerable improvement above and below the central rigid area. E, The patient underwent transthoracic spine fusion using the anterior distractors to obtain further correction of the kyphosis without stretching the spinal cord. Six anterior strut grafts were utilized to gain maximal stability and bone grafting of this kyphosis. The patient had no neurologic difficulties from the surgery, and the curve was further corrected to 60 degrees. F, Two weeks after the anterior surgery, a posterior spine fusion with Harrington instrumentation was performed. Owing to the slight scoliosis, it was possible to insert a bent distraction rod in addition to the customary contraction rod. One year later, three months after cast removal, her kyphosis measured 55 degrees, only a two degree loss.

*Legend and illustration continued on the following page*

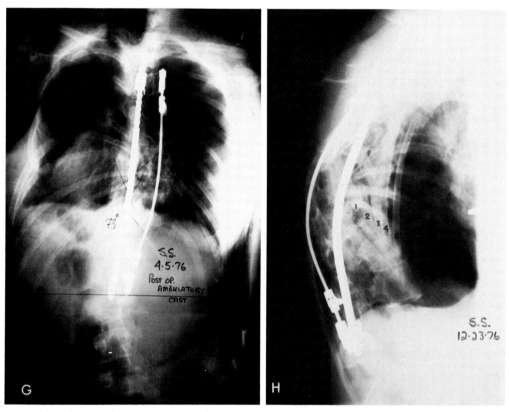

**Figure 7–27** *Continued* *G,* An AP x-ray shows the scoliosis with the convex compression rod and the concave distraction rod. The patient was managed postoperatively in a Risser cast, fully ambulatory. *H,* An oblique x-ray nine months postoperatively, showing five of the anterior strut grafts.

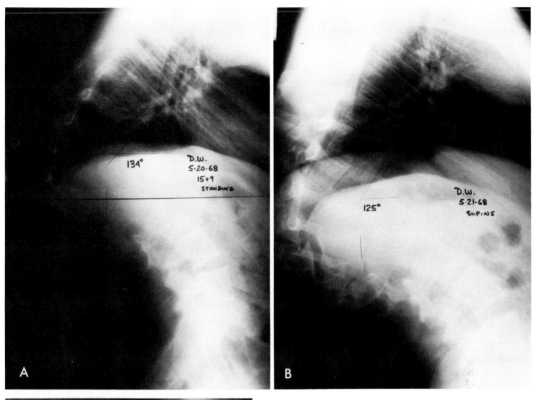

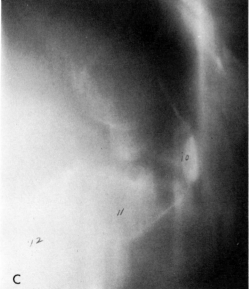

**Figure 7–28** *A,* D.W.: Lateral standing x-ray at age 15+ 9 shows a 134 degree congenital kyphosis. He had been followed by an orthopedic surgeon who was waiting for the completion of growth before attempting surgery. Such neglectful waiting cannot be condoned. *B,* The same patient. The supine x-ray shows a much better detail of the deformity. *C,* A lateral laminogram shows nearly total absence of the body at T10 plus wedge shape deformity of the body at T11.

*Legend and illustration continued on the following page*

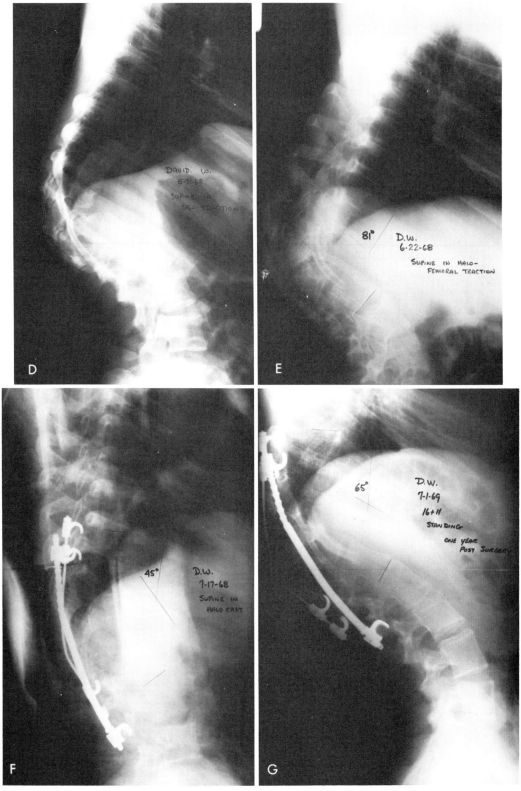

Figure 7–28   *Continued*

*See legend on the opposite page*

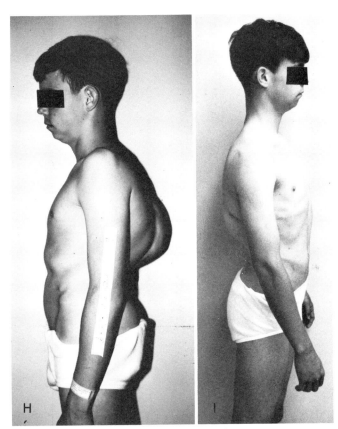

**Figure 7–28** *Continued*

*D,* The patient was placed first in skin traction to test the effectiveness of traction. There were no neurologic difficulties so he was subsequently changed to halofemoral traction. *E,* An anterior spine fusion was performed with an anterior strut graft. Under present conditions this would be considered as far too meager a grafting procedure. *F,* Lateral x-ray following posterior fusion with Harrington compression and distraction instrumentation. Once again, use of the distraction rod was possible owing to a slight scoliosis. Correction to 45 degrees was obtained by this program. *G,* Lateral standing x-ray one year following surgery shows the final curve at 65 degrees. He had no neurologic problems related to the surgery. His only complication was the pressure sore from the cast. *H,* Lateral photograph prior to treatment, showing the severe kyphotic deformity. *I,* Lateral photography one year later showing a very significant correction of his deformity.

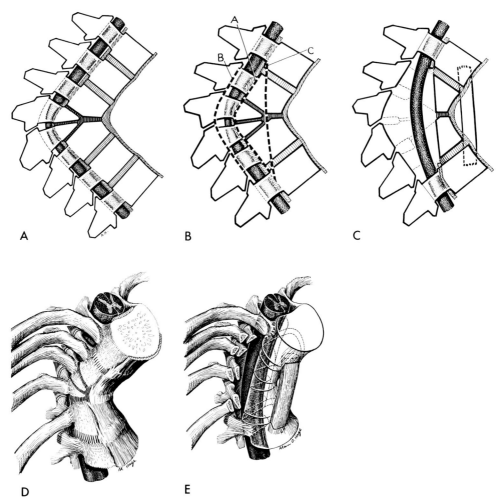

**Figure 7–29**   *A,* Lateral diagram of a congenital kyphosis with defect of formation of two vertebral bodies. The spinal cord is noted to be brought forward tightly against the back of the vertebral bodies, and the cord is thinned in this area. *B,* When planning an anterior spinal cord decompression and fusion, the triangular area of bone outlined by lines A and C must be removed. If there is a concomitant scoliosis, the concave pedicles must also be removed along line B. *C,* Diagrammatic representation of the release of pressure from the spinal cord. It moves forward after resection of the apical vertebral bodies, and then anterior strut grafting is also performed. Laminae are not removed, thus maintaining normal posterior stability. Posterior fusion should also be done. *D,* An oblique drawing to show the usual view confronting the surgeon. *E,* Diagrammatic oblique view showing the forward transposition of the spinal cord and the anterior strut grafting.

require an operation exposing the cord. It is important to realize that the spinal cord can be decompressed by reducing the severity of the spine deformity. The European literature has emphasized this "orthopaedic" treatment of cord compression. When is such an approach indicated rather than direct cord decompression? The authors recommend such an approach when a) there is a relatively minor quantity of cord compression, as in spasticity, hyperactive reflexes, and positive Babinskis,

but no major motor deficit, sensory deficit, or sphincter loss, and b) the kyphosis has flexibility as demonstrated by hyperextension x-rays. Totally rigid kyphoses cannot be alleviated by this technique.

Correction of the curve should be done by hyperextension casts or direct anterior surgery, with correction of the kyphosis and then both anterior and posterior fusion in the corrected position. *Traction should be avoided.*

## LATERAL DEFECTS: HEMIVERTEBRA

The treatment of scoliosis related to a hemivertebra has been highly controversial. Seldom should such controversy exist. Ideally, curvatures caused by hemivertebrae should be detected early and watched carefully, and if no progression occurs, no treatment is necessary. If progression is noted, early fusion will stop the progression before significant deformity occurs. Brace treatment is of virtually no value for hemivertebra problems. If all hemivertebrae could be detected early, progression noted early, and fusion performed early, there would be little trouble with curvatures due to hemivertebrae. Since they are not all detected early, the progression is not always appreciated, and worst of all, the progressive curve has often not been adequately treated.

Figures 7–12, 7–13, and 7–14 give adequate testimony to the ill effects of neglectful observation. What then should be done? The answer is easy—*fuse the curve!* Figure 7–30 illustrates the problem well. Arthrodesis salvaged the problem but should have been done much sooner.

A more ideal example is the patient shown in Figure 7–31, whose progressive curve was recognized early and fused early, and an ideal end result was obtained.

The major objection to early fusion has been stunting of growth. It is true that the fused area does not grow, but the anomalous area does not grow vertically either, and thus *the surgical procedure will not cause loss of trunk height. The anomalous development is what causes shortening of the trunk height.*

The other problems associated with early fusion are elongation ("adding on") of the original curve, bending of the fusion area, and development of structural changes in portions of the spine that originally were purely compensatory curves in normal, nonanomalous vertebrae.

All of these problems must be of concern to the physician. However, they should never deter an early fusion when this is the procedure of choice. The answer to these problems is not easy—but one answer is the Milwaukee brace. Not all patients fused early require a Milwaukee brace postoperatively, once the fusion is solid. However, when the fusion mass is in a curved position (i.e., a residual curve exists of 40 to 50 degrees or more), a Milwaukee brace should be used during growth. An already bent fusion mass is more likely to bend than a straight one (Fig. 7–32).

The problem of development of structural and progressive changes in areas of the spine that were originally nonanomalous, nonstructural, and purely compensatory demands perseverance. One of the best answers to this is to fuse the primary congenital curve as early as possible and as straight as possible. In addition, one should use the Milwaukee brace to control these troublesome secondary curves. These can usually be managed well until the adolescent growth spurt, but then they may need to be fused.

***Hemivertebra Excision.*** The reader must obviously ask, is excision of the hemivertebra of value? The answer, as usual, is variable. In general, hemivertebrae need *not* be excised, but in specific circumstances, they should be removed. Hemivertebra excision has been reported many times in the past (Fig. 7–33).[11, 41, 44, 69, 81, 84, 91]

Patients with curvatures *in compensation* (head centered over pelvis) do not need hemivertebra excision. Those in whom a compensated alignment cannot be obtained by cast correction or traction, especially when the hemivertebra is low in the lumbar spine, should be considered for hemivertebra resection (Fig. 7–34).

In performing such excisions, the two-stage technique of Leatherman[44] is strongly recommended (Fig. 7–35). Single stage anterior and posterior resection is not recommended, owing to the high percentage of paralysis reported from such procedures.[91]

It must always be remembered that hemivertebra removal is merely a wedge excision of the apex of a structural scoliosis. *The entire curve must always be fused!* The authors prefer to do the anterior wedge excision first and the posterior excision and curve fusion during the second stage. Harrington compression instruments have proved useful in closing and stabilizing the wedge excision. Others have reversed the procedure, doing the posterior wedge excision and fusion first, and the anterior second, using the Dwyer apparatus to close the gap. *Kyphosis must be avoided in using such an approach.*

In children too small to use either Harrington rods or Dwyer instruments, closure of the gap and correction of the curve can be done best by turnbuckle casts, of either the Risser or the halo-cast type (Fig. 7–36).

*Text continued on page 193*

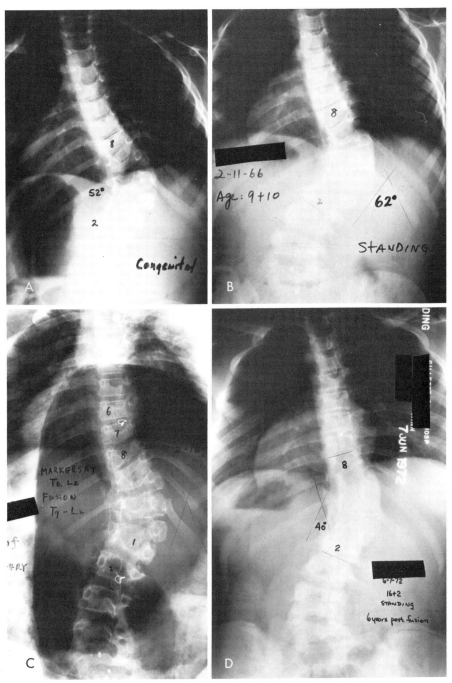

**Figure 7–30**   *A,* Five year old girl with a 52 degree congenital scoliosis due to hemivertebra at the thoracolumbar junction. There are actually two hemivertebrae, one just above the apical vertebra and one just below. Brace treatment was attempted. *B,* The same patient at age 9, showing a 62 degree curve. The brace was a failure. *C,* The patient was treated by correction in a Risser localizer cast with correction of the curve to 41 degrees and fusion from T6 to L2. The anatomic details of the hemivertebrae can be best seen on this x-ray. *D,* The same patient is seen six years following spine fusion. The x-ray shows the curve to measure 40 degrees, solidly fused with no loss of correction whatsoever. This is a good example of the progressive type of hemivertebra situation successfully managed by simple posterior spine fusion. Hemivertebra excision in such cases is not necessary. Note the normal body alignment, with the torso vertically oriented directly above the center of the pelvis.

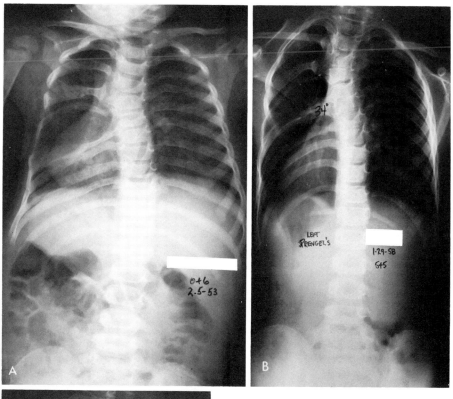

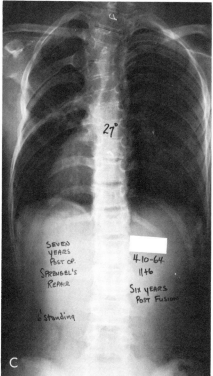

**Figure 7–31** *A,* This six month old patient presented with Sprengel's deformity and a congenital scoliosis due to a midthoracic hemivertebra on the left. She also has obvious defects in rib development on the left. No treatment was given at this time. *B,* The same patient, age five, showing an increasing 34 degree curve and the Sprengel's deformity. *C,* The same patient at age 11, six years following a posterior spine fusion and seven years following the repair of the Sprengel's deformity. Her progressive curve has been arrested and her spine returned to normal alignment.

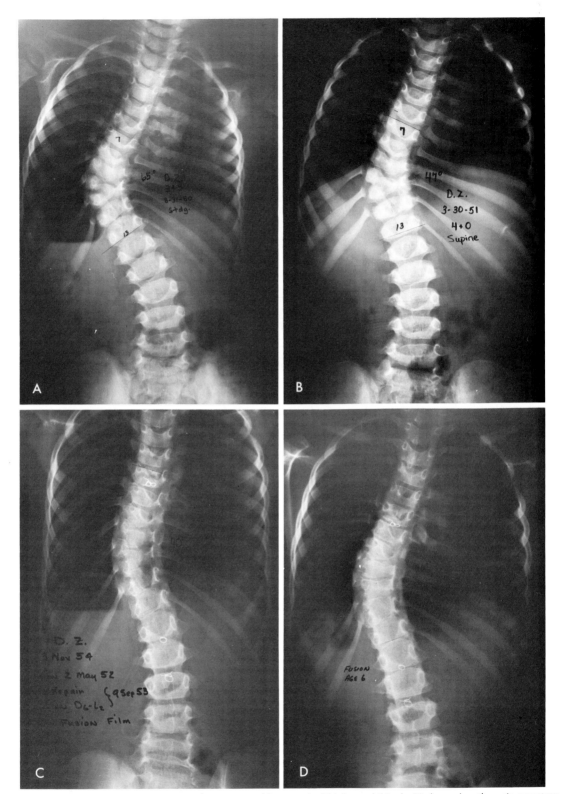

**Figure 7–32** *A*, D.Z. An x-ray at age three years and five months. This boy exhibited a 65 degree low thoracic curvature due to a single hemivertebra on the left side at T10. This is an excellent example of a nonincarcerated and fully segmented hemivertebra producing a very significant curve. Such a curve can always be expected to progress. *B*, Supine x-ray at age four shows better detail. Note the compensatory curves above T7 and below T13. *C*, This AP standing x-ray was taken one year following posterior spine fusion from T6 to L2. The wire markers indicate the top and bottom of the fusion area. The curve has been corrected to 40 degrees. *D*, Five years later, at age 12, the measured curve is still 40 degrees, but the patient's general condition has deteriorated in terms of body alignment. L3 is now becoming part of the original curve, and proximally T5 is showing evidence of becoming part of the curve. The fusion is solid with no evidence of pseudarthrosis. These subtle changes were not appreciated at that time, and no treatment was given.

*Legend continued on the opposite page*

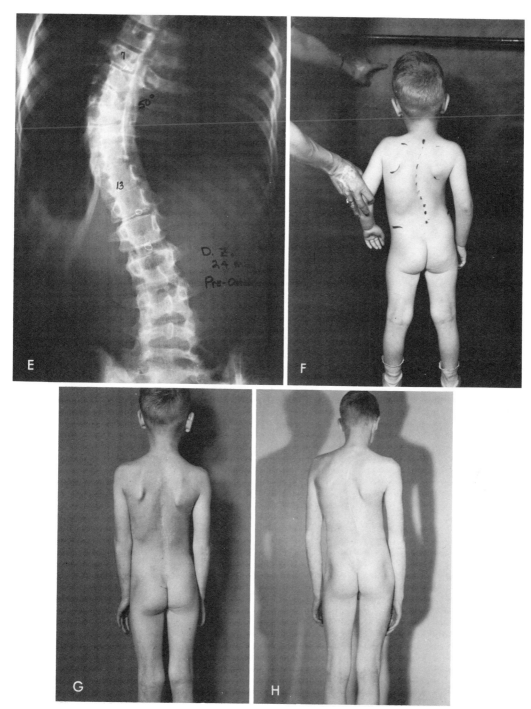

**Figure 7–32** *Continued*   *E,* AP standing x-ray at age 14 shows the significant lengthening of the curve both above and below the fusion area. The fusion area now measures 50 degrees, indicating that there has been some bending of the fusion in addition to extension. T5 and T6 are now fully incorporated into the major curve, as is L3. This is an excellent example both of the bending of a fusion mass and of lengthening of a curve. The patient did not wear a Milwaukee brace during his growing years. The fusion was explored at age 14, and there was no evidence of pseudarthrosis. *F,* Posterior photograph of the patient at age 3, prior to treatment. *G,* Posterior photograph of the patient at age 7, with the curve corrected to 40 degrees. Notice the level shoulders, level hips, and well-balanced torso. *H,* final posterior photograph at age 14. Notice the loss of body alignment, elevation of the left shoulder, tipping upward of the left scapula, and so forth.

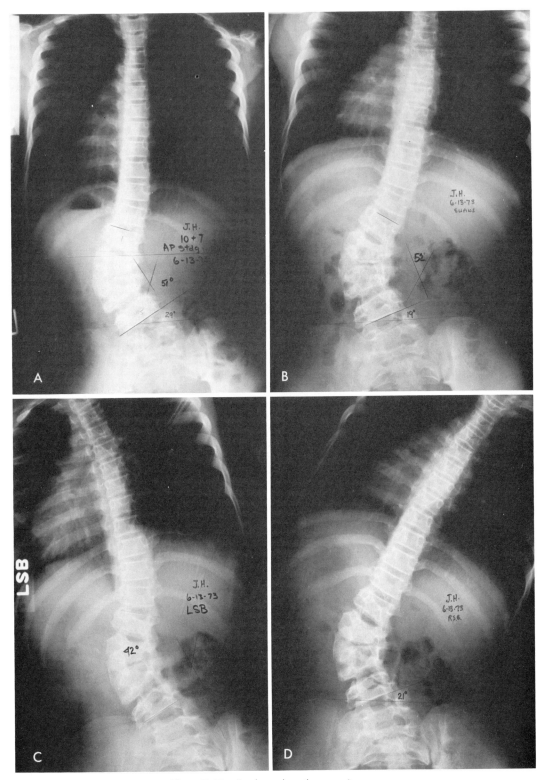

**Figure 7–33**   *See legend on the opposite page.*

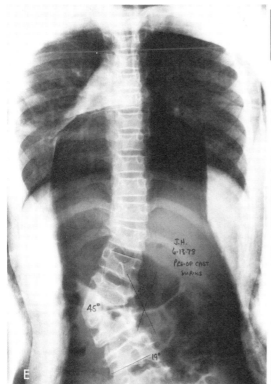

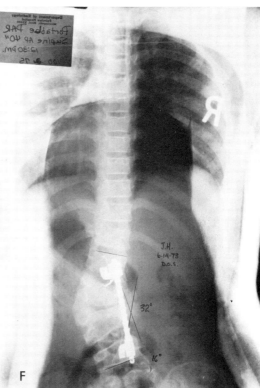

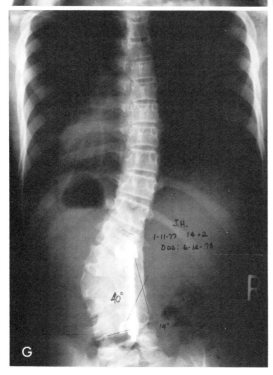

**Figure 7–33** *Continued   A,* J.H.: An AP standing x-ray of this 10 year old boy shows a 51 degree, L1–L5 left lumbar scoliosis due to a single hemivertebra at L3. This is a fully segmented nonincarcerated hemivertebra. There is a 29 degree right lumbosacral curve. The plumb line is off to the left and is deviated to the left 3 cm. Should such a patient have a hemivertebra excision? The answer is a resounding NO. Excision of the L3 hemivertebra would result in a far greater degree of misplacement of the torso to the left. Careful analysis of x-rays will help to determine this situation. *B,* Supine x-ray of the same patient shows a 52 degree curve, no change from the upright film, but the patient's torso is now well centered over the pelvis, owing to improvement of the lumbosacral curve to 19 degrees. *C,* Supine left side bending film shows correction of the major curve to 42 degrees. *D,* Right side bending film shows correction of the lumbosacral curve to only 21 degrees. However, T12 is noted to lie directly over the center of the sacrum. This lack of ability to correct L5 fully over the sacrum indicates that excision of the L3 hemivertebra would be absolutely contraindicated. *E,* The patient was placed in a preoperative cast with correction of the major curve to 45 degrees. *F,* Fusion was performed from L1 to L5 with a short Harrington distraction bar. The curve measures 32 degrees. The "wakeup" test was performed, and there was normal ability to move the legs. *G,* 3½ years later, there are a solid fusion and excellent maintenance of the curvature at 40 degrees. The pelvis is level, and the torso is perfectly centered over the pelvis. This is an excellent example of where correction and fusion of the primary lumbar curve *are* indicated, but hemivertebra excision is contraindicated.

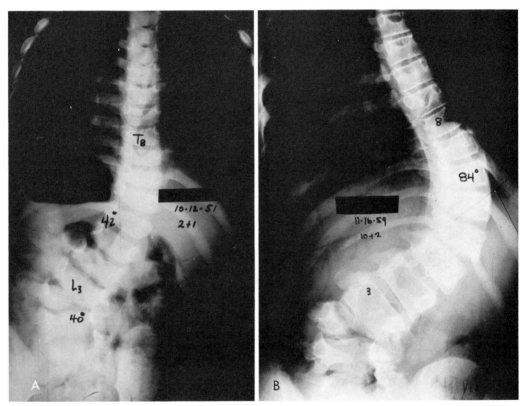

**Figure 7–34** *A,* This two year old girl has a hemivertebra between L3 and L5. Her torso is markedly deviated to the right. There is no compensatory curve below the hemivertebra. This type of hemivertebra *should* be excised. There is a 42 degree secondary curve proximal to the hemivertebra. No treatment was given. *B,* The same patient at age 10+2 shows increase of the secondary curve to 84 degrees with development of rotation and other structural changes. At this age, one must correct and fuse both curves to the greatest degree possible, and the golden opportunity for hemivertebra excision has been lost.

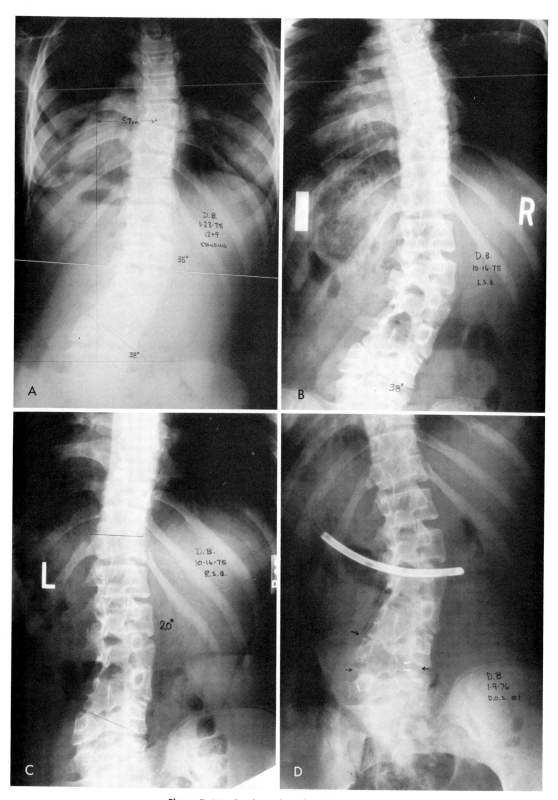

**Figure 7–35** *See legend on the following page.*

*Illustration continued on the following page*

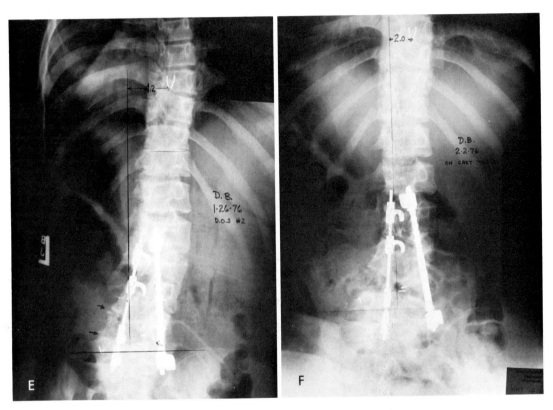

**Figure 7–35** *Continued A,* This 12+9 year old girl presented with torso deviation of a progressive nature, unresponsive to two years of Milwaukee brace treatment. She has a 38 degree structural lumbosacral curve due to a hemivertebra at L4. There is a 35 degree right curve. The upper lumbar spine also contains congenital anomalies, as does the lower thoracic spine. A line erected vertically from the midpoint of the sacrum is 5.7 cm. to the left of the spinous process of T9. This is a good measurement technique for evaluating the quantity of torso displacement. *B,* A bending film to the left shows a very rigid lumbosacral curve due to the hemivertebra. T12 does not come directly above the sacrum, and the entire spine remains deviated to the right. *C,* Supine right side bending shows correction of the upper lumbar curve to 20 degrees. A hemivertebra can be noticed at the apex of the curve. It is a nonsegmented incarcerated hemivertebra, however. *D,* An anterior hemivertebra excision was performed as a first stage. The three arrows mark the triangle of bone removed. *E,* Two weeks later, a posterior wedge of the same magnitude was removed and a Harrington compression rod placed on the convex side and a distraction rod on the concave side. The correction was not satisfactory, since there was still a 4.2 cm. displacement of the spinous process in the midthoracic spine. *F,* The patient was taken to the plaster room, where a cast was applied incorporating both thighs and extended to the axilla level. Great care was taken on the table to maintain the pelvis level and then to push the torso toward the midline. The patient was kept on full bed rest for five months to allow consolidation in this position. Ambulation is not possible for such problems of torso deviation. The fusion extended from T9 to the sacrum.

*Legend continued on the opposite page*

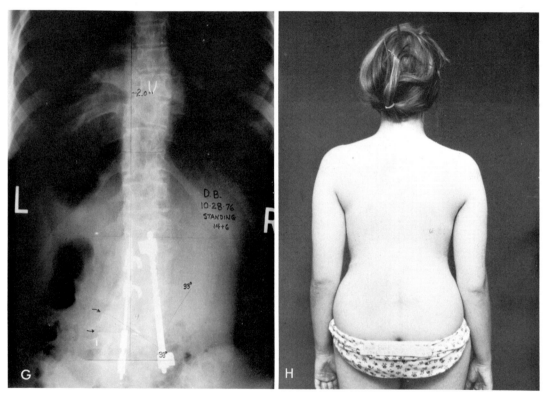

**Figure 7–35** *Continued* G, A standing x-ray one year postoperatively, showing maintenance of good torso alignment. A plumb line from the head fell directly in the midline. H, A posterior photograph of the patient at one year following spine fusion, showing totally normal body alignment.

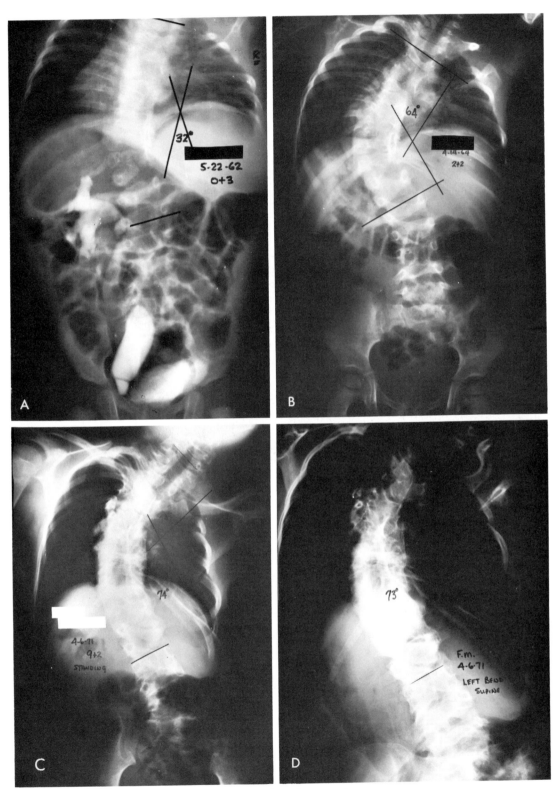

**Figure 7–36**  *See legend on opposite page.*

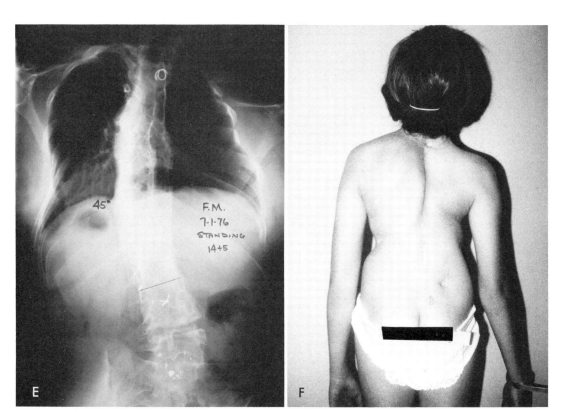

**Figure 7-36** *Continued* A, Three month old child had an intravenous pyelogram performed because of urinary infection problems. She was noted to have a solitary left kidney with severe hydronephrosis and hydroureter due to a distal ureteral vesicle obstruction. Her life was saved by appropriate urologic surgery. No treatment was rendered to the congenital scoliosis due to the unilateral unsegmented bar. B, At age 2, her curve had already doubled to 64 degrees. This rapid increase in curve in young children is due to their rapid growth at this time. Since one side of the spine grows and the other does not grow, it is not unusual to have this rapid increase. No treatment was given. C, When first seen by the authors at age 9, she had a 74 degree curve extending from the lower cervical spine to the midlumbar spine. A localized posterior fusion from T5 to T12 had been performed at age 5. This did not halt the advance of her deformity. D, A supine left side bending film showed the curve to be totally rigid. It was thus felt that traction, casting, or bracing would not provide any correction whatsoever and that to obtain correction, spinal osteotomy was necessary. She underwent a double anterior wedge osteotomy performed through a left thoracotomy, with the higher wedge at T5 and the lower wedge at T12. Two weeks later, she had an osteotomy of the posterior fusion mass in four places, two of them overlying the anterior osteotomies. Correction was performed by a halo-turnbuckle cast. There were no neurologic deficits. E, An x-ray at age 14+5, five years following surgery, shows a completely solid spine fusion and marked improvement of alignment. F, Photograph showing the patient's condition following surgery.

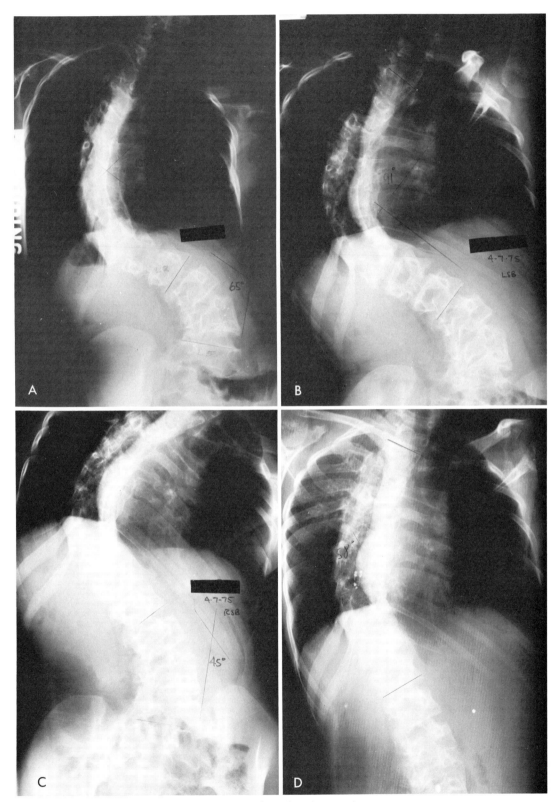

**Figure 7–37**   *See legend on the opposite page.*

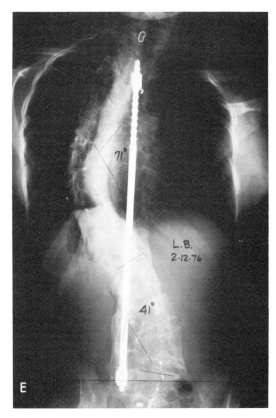

**Figure 7–37** *Continued* *A,* Standing x-ray of a 9 year old girl with a 103 degree left thoracic congenital scoliosis previously fused elsewhere from T5 to T12. She also has a structural right lumbar scoliosis of 65 degrees due to a wedged vertebra at L4. Note the severe torso malalignment. *B,* A left side bending film shows better detail of the thoracic spine including the area of previous fusion. There is improvement only to 91 degrees. *C,* Right side bending shows the structural nature of the lumbar curve with correction to 45 degrees. Following analysis of these bending films, it was felt necessary to osteotomize the previous thoracic fusion to obtain correction of this curve and to include the lumbar curve in the total correction and fusion program. *D,* This x-ray was taken two weeks following osteotomy of the old fusion with correction over a two week period by halo-femoral traction. There was improvement to 58 degrees. *E,* The patient was treated postoperatively in a halo cast. One year following spine fusion, the patient shows good general balance. There is slight elevation of the left shoulder. The thoracic curve has been corrected to 71 degrees and the lumbar curve to 41 degrees.

## COMPLEX CONGENITAL SPINE DEFORMITIES

The previous discussions have assumed a single well-defined congenital anomaly. Unfortunately, the problems are often more complex (Fig. 7–37). Multiple anomalies frequently are present. However, the basic principles remain the same. Short rigid progressive curves must be fused regardless of the specific anomaly. Nonprogressive curves, regardless of the anomaly, can safely be watched.

### Scoliosis with Diastematomyelia

Diastematomyelia and other types of neurospinal dysraphism (see Chapter 3) may be seen in conjunction with deformities of the spine. In the authors' experience, about five per cent of patients with congenital scoliosis have been found to have diastematomyelia,[88] and another five per cent have some other type of neurospinal dysraphism.

The problem is how best to manage the patient who presents with spinal deformity plus a diastematomyelia. The concern is, of course, that the techniques used to correct the spinal deformity do not cause a paralysis or increase an already existent neurologic defect.

In our experience, routine myelography has not been performed in all patients with congenital spine deformity. Myelography is indicated whenever there is a possibility of a dysraphic condition. Our indications for myelography are: 1) Any evidence of localized widening of the interpediculate distance, 2) any hair patch, hemangioma, or nevus over the spine, 3) any neurologic deficit in the bladder or lower extremities, 4) any foot deformity, e.g., club foot or vertical talus, and 5) any patient in whom we contemplate correction of a curvature by traction or in whom a Harrington rod will be used. We do not perform myelography when none of the above conditions exists, even though we may do a fusion.

Whenever a diastematomyelia is found during growth, we believe it should be removed, *regardless of whether or not the patient has a neurologic deficit*. It has been our experience that when a neurologic problem develops in a patient with diastematomyelia, removal of the spur seldom results in correction of that neurologic deficit but only prevents further deficits. We therefore agree

with Guthkelch,[20] who strongly urges removal of such lesions *before* neurologic damage occurs. It is possible to have more than one diastematomyelia (Fig. 7–38).

When treating a patient with diastematomyelia and scoliosis, the diastematomyelia must be removed first, before the curve is treated. Following removal of the spur, scoliosis treatment can be carried out more safely. In our experience, most neurosurgeons would prefer not to have a spine fusion performed simultaneously with spur removal. We usually do the spine fusion 10 to 14 days after the laminectomy. There have been no problems from this approach, provided that the neurosurgeon does a limited laminectomy (Fig. 7–39).

When traction is necessary for correction of the scoliosis prior to spine fusion, the spur is first removed and traction begun a week later. After two to three weeks of traction, the fusion is performed. Harrington rods should *not* be used in patients with spinal dysraphism, since their spinal cords have very limited capacity to resist stretching. Catastrophes have been reported in patients with dysraphism subjected to Harrington distraction instrumentation (Fig. 7–40).[89]

### Harrington Instrumentation in Congenital Spine Deformity

Their use in congenital scoliosis carries a higher risk than for idiopathic scoliosis. It is preferable to obtain correction by traction and/or casting and to insert the rods for stabilization only, and not for correction. We have in the past used (and continue to use occasionally) rods to correct the curve, providing there is no dysraphic lesion and providing an immediate "wake-up" test is performed.

## NONOPERATIVE TREATMENT OF CONGENITAL SPINE DEFORMITY

### Defects of Segmentation

Patients with defects of segmentation, whether anterior, lateral, or posterior, do *not* respond to bracing of any type. One may accomplish the development of compensatory curves above and below the area of nonsegmentation, but one cannot stop the progression of the primary curve.

Furthermore, the development of com-

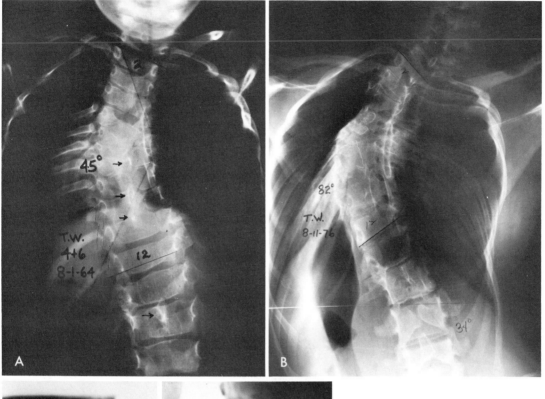

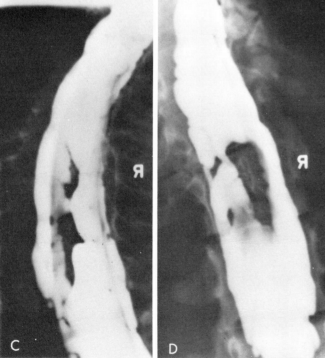

**Figure 7–38** *A*, An AP x-ray at age 4 years and 6 months shows a congenital thoracic scoliosis of 45 degrees due to a unilateral unsegmented bar extending from T4 to T10. There is widening of the interpediculate space from T5 through L3. Midline bony prominences can be noted in several areas. (See arrows.) *B*, An AP x-ray at age 18 shows increase of the curvature to 82 degrees. No treatment had been given. Owing to the rotation of the spine from the curvature, the increased interpediculate space and the midline bony prominences are not as obvious at this time. *C* and *D*, A large volume myelogram revealed three separate spurs, two in the lower thoracic spine and one in the upper lumbar spine.

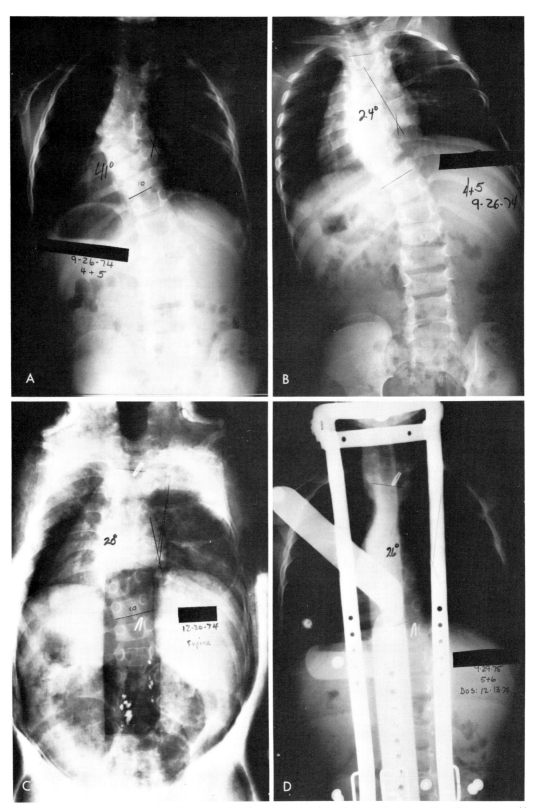

**Figure 7–39** *A,* This 4+5 year old girl presented with a progressive thoracic curve due to a unilateral unsegmented bar. She was also noted to have widening of the interpediculate distance at L1, L2, and L3. *B,* A supine left side bending film shows correction of the thoracic curve to 24 degrees. A midline bony spur at L1 is readily seen on these films.

*Legend continued on the opposite page*

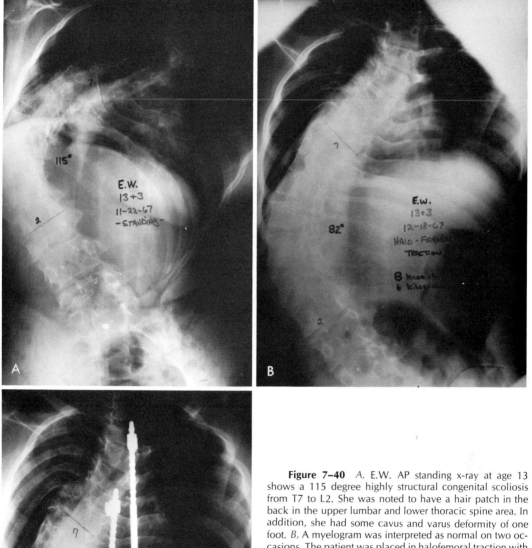

**Figure 7–40** *A,* E.W. AP standing x-ray at age 13 shows a 115 degree highly structural congenital scoliosis from T7 to L2. She was noted to have a hair patch in the back in the upper lumbar and lower thoracic spine area. In addition, she had some cavus and varus deformity of one foot. *B,* A myelogram was interpreted as normal on two occasions. The patient was placed in halofemoral traction with correction of the curve to 82 degrees. Weights above 8 kg. on the head and 6 kg. on each leg produced bladder paralysis. No further weights were therefore added. *C,* On the day of surgery, two Harrington rods were inserted and additional correction attempted. The Stagnara wake-up test was not being performed at that time. She awoke from surgery completely paraplegic. The rods were removed and she subsequently regained about 50 per cent of the function of her lower extremities. This is a classic example of the paralysis secondary to excessive elongation of the spine in the presence of a tethered spinal cord.

**Figure 7–39** *Continued   C,* The patient was referred for appropriate neurosurgical consultation, and excision of the hemivertebra was performed. Ten days later, a posterior spine fusion of the thoracic curve was done. Correction is shown here, supine, in a Risser cast. The patient was then ambulated, and an upright film showed no loss of correction so ambulation was felt to be safe and it was continued throughout her convalescent period. *D,* This x-ray, nine months following surgery, shows a solid fusion at 26 degrees without loss of correction. She is now wearing a Milwaukee brace. She had no neurologic problems as a result of the surgery.

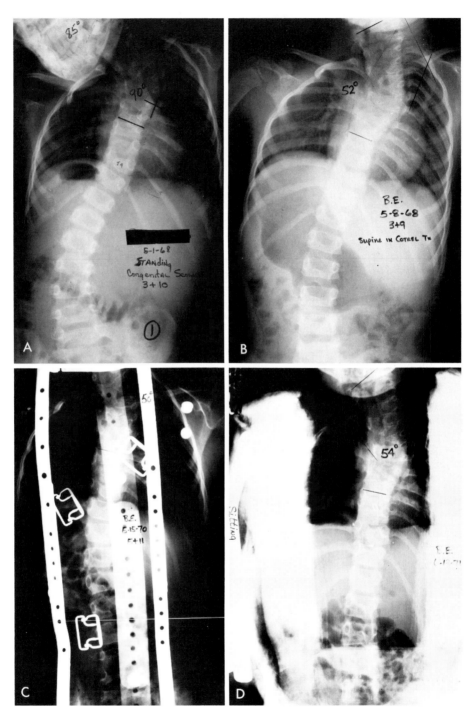

**Figure 7–41**  *A,* B.E. AP standing x-ray of this 3 year old girl shows a 90 degree very severe high cervicothoracic scoliosis with severe head tilt. *B,* The patient was placed in Cotrel traction and showed an unexpected and pleasing correction of her curve to 52 degrees. It was therefore elected to place her in a Milwaukee brace. *C,* After two years in a Milwaukee brace, her curve was still being maintained at 50 degrees. Thus, in this particular patient, the brace did an excellent job of preventing increase in deformity and maintained the deformity at a much improved degree. Whether fusion should have been performed or not at age 3 is a difficult question to answer. *D,* At age 6, she was placed in a halo cast and a posterior fusion performed from C5 to T8. Correction to 54 degrees was accomplished in the halo cast.

*Legend continued on the opposite page*

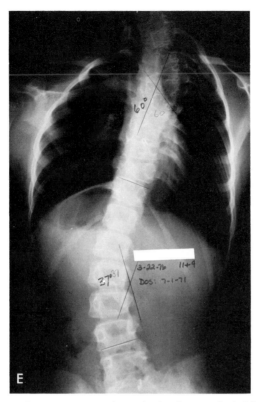

**Figure 7–41** *Continued   E,* A follow-up at age 11 shows the fused area to be holding at 60 degrees. There is a compensatory 37 degree lumbar curve.

pensatory curves may be hazardous. As pointed out by Mayfield et al.,[58] the compensatory hyperlordotic areas created by bracing of a congenital kyphosis may prove more harmful than the primary curve. The best way to minimize the problems of the secondary curve is to provide maximal correction and early fusion of the primary curve.

## Defects of Formation

Patients with defects of formation are more amenable to brace treatment, provided that the curvature has flexibility. Patients with short rigid curves (e.g., multiple sequential hemivertebra on the same side) are not responsive to bracing and should be fused early. Patients with congenital kyphosis due to defects of formation have not responded at all to bracing and should be fused early. This has been well documented by Winter et al.[87]

When is bracing of value in the nonoperative treatment of congenital scoliosis? In the only review of such patients, Winter et al.[90] noted that good results were found in two groups: 1) those with long but flexible curves in which the anomalous area constituted only a small percentage of the total curve, and 2) those with cervicothoracic curves in which there was significant head tilt. The Milwaukee brace was highly effective in restoring normal head alignment and shoulder level. Braces other than the Milwaukee brace have never been shown to be of benefit for such curvatures.

Brace treatment is almost never sufficient for total curve management. The brace usually keeps the curve under control until a more optimal time for fusion is reached. This is particularly true of long flexible curves, in which early fusion will indeed cause some stunting of total trunk height. (For a more detailed discussion of trunk growth and early fusion see Chapter 5.) Figure 7–41 illustrates a good combination of early brace treatment and later fusion. Figure 7–42 demonstrates the use of the brace in a long but flexible curve pattern resulting from scattered anomalies.

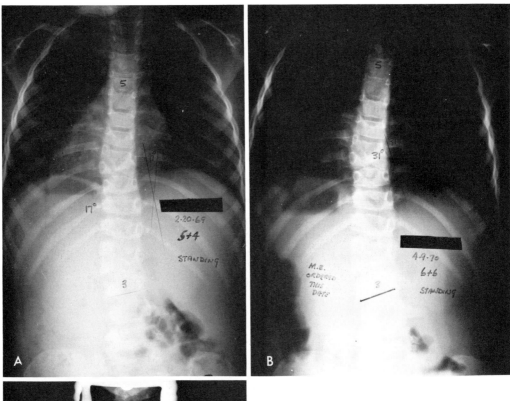

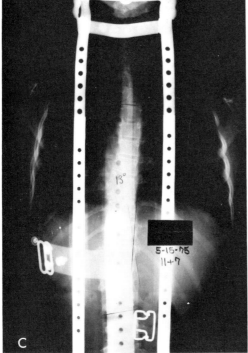

**Figure 7–42** *A,* M.C. A five year old girl had a 17 degree left long T5–L3 scoliosis due to a hemivertebra on the left at T9 and a second one on the left at L2. Both hemivertebrae are nonsegmented and incarcerated. The patient had been followed since age 2, and there had been no increase in the curve until this time. *B,* At age 6+6, the curve was noted to increase suddenly to 31 degrees, and a Milwaukee brace was prescribed at this time. *C,* The patient in her Milwaukee brace at age 11+7, after five years of the Milwaukee brace use. The curve is 13 degrees, and adequate growth of the spine has occurred. To fuse such a lengthy curve at a young age would have produced significant stunting of the spine, which can be prevented by the use of the Milwaukee brace. This case is an excellent example of the use of the Milwaukee brace for a long but flexible congenital curve having scattered areas of anomalies.

# References

1. Athanassow, P.: Uber congenitale Skoliose. Arch. Orthop. Mechanother., *1*:353, 1903.
2. Bartolozzi, P., and Frontino, G.: The surgical treatment of congenital kyphoscoliosis due to posterolateral hemivertebra in the dorsal spine. Arch. Putti Chir. Organi. Mov., *26*:221–226, 1971.
3. Bartsocas, C. S., Kiossoglou, K. A., Papas, C. V., Xanthou-Tsingoglou, M., Anagnostakis, D. E., and Daskalopoulou, H. D.: Costovertebral dysplasia. Birth Defects, *10*:221–226, 1974.
4. Bauer, H.: Uber angeborenen Wirbelsaulenmissbildungen In besondere angeborenen Kyphosen. Z. Orthop., *58*:354–381, 1933.
5. Bickel, W.: Personal communication.
6. Billing, E. L.: Congenital scoliosis: An analytical study of its natural history. Proceedings of the Western Orthopaedic Association. J. Bone Joint Surg., *37A*:404–405, 1955.
7. Bingold, A. C.: Congenital kyphosis. J. Bone Joint Surg., *35B*:579–583, 1953.
8. Blount, W. P.: Congenital scoliosis. Huitieme Congres de la Société Internationale de Chirurgie Orthopedique et de Traumatologie. Brussels, Imprimerie des Sciences, 1961, pp. 748–762.
9. Bowen, D. I., Collum, M. T., and Rees, D. O.: Clinical aspects of oculo-auricular-vertebral dysplasia. Br. J. Ophthalmol., *55*:154, 1971.
10. Bremer, F. W.: Klinische Untersuchungen und Aetiologie der Syringomyelie der Status dysraphicus. Deutsch. Z. Nervenheilkd, *95*:1, 1926.
11. Compere, E. L.: Excision of hemivertebrae for correction of congenital scoliosis. Report of two cases. J. Bone Joint Surg., *14*:555–562, 1932.
12. Cramer, K.: Beitrag zur Kasiustik der angeborenen Skoliosen. Arch. Orthop. Mechanotherap. Unfall Chir., *5*:341–349, 1907.
13. DePalma, A. F., and McKeen, W. B.: Congenital kyphoscoliosis with paraplegia. Clin. Orthop., *39*:190–196, 1965.
14. DeWald, R., and Ray, R.: Congenital kyphosis with successful treatment. J. Bone Joint Surg., *53A*:587–590, 1971.
15. Fischer, F. J., and Vandemark, R. E.: Sagittal cleft (butterfly) vertebra. J. Bone Joint Surg., *27*:695–698, 1945.
16. Giannini, M. J., Borrelli, F. S., and Greenberg, W. B.: Agenesis of the vertebral bodies, a cause of dwarfism. Am. J. Roentgenol., *59*:705–711, 1948.
17. Gillespie, R., Faithful, D., Hall, J. E., and Roth, A.: Intraspinal anomalies associated with congenital scoliosis. Clin. Orthop., *93*:103, 1973.
18. Gjorup, P. A.: Dorsal hemivertebra. Acta Orthop. Scand., *35*:117–125, 1964.
19. Grieg, D. M.: Congenital kyphosis. Edinburgh Med. J., *16*:93–99, 1916.
20. Guthkelch, A. N.: Diastematomyelia with median septum. Brain, *97*:729–742, 1974.
21. Gold, L. H. A., Kieffer, S. A., and Peterson, H. O.: Lipomatous invasion of the spinal cord associated with spinal dysraphism: Myelographic evaluation. Am. J. Roentgenol., *107*:479–485, 1969.
22. Hansen, R.: Some anomalies, deformities and diseased conditions of the vertebrae during their different stages of development, elucidated by anatomical and radiological findings. Acta Chir. Scand., *60*:309, 1926.
23. Harrenstein, R. J.: Angeborenen Kyphose mit Gibbus Infolge Wirbel Missbildungen. Z. Orthop. Chir., *52*:332–339, 1930.
24. Hendrick, E. B.: On diastematomyelia. Progr. Neurol. Surg. (Basel), *4*:277–288, 1971.
25. Herbert, J. J.: Ostéotomie vertébrate pour cyphose congénitale. Rev. Chir. Orthop., *37*:506–508, 1951.
26. Hilal, S. K., Marton, D., and Pollack, E.: Diastematomyelia in children, a radiographic study of 34 cases. Neuroradiol., *112*:609–622, 1974.
27. Hirschberger, A. K.: Beitrage zur Lehre der angeborenen Skoliose. Z. Orthop. Chir., *7*:129, 1900.
28. Hodgson, A. R.: Correction of fixed spinal curves. A preliminary communication. J. Bone Joint Surg., *47A*:1221–1227, 1965.
29. James, C. C., and Lassman, L. P.: Diastematomyelia. Arch. Dis. Child., *33*:536, 1958.
30. James, C. C. M., and Lassman, L. P.: Spinal dysraphism. J. Bone Joint Surg., *44B*:828–840, 1962.
31. James, C. C. M., and Lassman, L. P.: Spinal Dysraphism, Spina Bifida Occulta. London, Butterworth & Co., 1972.
32. James, J. I. P.: Kyphoscoliosis. J. Bone Joint Surg., *37B*:414–426, 1955.
33. James, J. I. P.: The management of infants with scoliosis. J. Bone Joint Surg., *57B*:422–429, 1975.
34. James, J. I. P.: Paraplegia in congenital kyphoscoliosis. J. Bone Joint Surg., *57B*:261, 1975.
35. Jarcho, S., and Levin, P. M.: Hereditary malformations of the vertebral bodies. Bull. Johns Hopkins Hosp., *62*:216, 1968.
36. Johnson, J. T. H., and Robinson, R. A.: Anterior strut grafts for severe kyphosis. Clin. Orthop., *56*:25–36, 1968.
37. Jordan, C. E., Dorst, J. P., Fischer, K. C., Mell, C., and White, R. I.: The scoliosis of congenital heart disease. Am. Heart J., *84*:463, 1972.
38. Keim, H. A., and Greene, A. F.: Diastematomyelia and scoliosis. J. Bone Joint Surg., *55A*:1425–1435, 1973.
39. Kuhns, J. G., and Hormel, R. S.: Management of congenital scoliosis. Review of 170 cases. Arch. Surg., *65*:250–263, 1952.
40. Lance, M.: Deux cas de cyphose avec gibbosité par anomalies osseuses congénitales. Rev. Orthop., *10*:55–60, 1923.
41. Langenskiold, A.: Correction of congenital scoliosis by excision of one-half of a cleft vertebra. Acta Orthop. Scand., 38:291–300, 1967.
42. Langer, L. O., and Moe, J. H.: A recessive form of congenital scoliosis different from spondylothoracic dysplasia. Birth Defects, *11*:83–86, 1975.
43. Lavy, N. W., Palmer, C. G., and Merritt, A. D.: A syndrome of bizarre vertebral anomalies. J. Pediatr., *69*:1121, 1966.
44. Leatherman, K. C.: The management of rigid spinal curves. Clin. Orthop., *93*:215, 1973.
45. Lichtenstein, B. W.: Spinal dysraphism, spina bifida, and myelodysplasia. Arch. Neurol. Psychiatr., *44*:792–809, 1940.
46. Lichtenstein, B. W.: Distant neuroanatomic complications of spina bifida (spinal dysraphism). Arch. Neurol. Psychiatr., *47*:195, 1942.
47. Lindeman, K.: Zur Kasiustik der angeborenen Kyphosen. Arch. Orthop. Unfallchir., *30*:27–33, 1931.
48. Lombard, P., and Legenissel: Cyphoses congénitales. Rev. Orthop., *25*:532–550, 1938.
49. Lonstein, J., Moe, J., Winter, R., Chou, S., and Pinto,

W.: Spinal deformity and cord compression. J. Bone Joint Surg., *56A*:1304, 1974.

50. Love, J. G., Daly, D. D., and Harris, L. E.: Tight filum terminale. Report of condition in 3 sibs. JAMA, *176*:115, 1961.

51. Luke, M. D., and McDonnell, E. J.: Congenital heart disease and scoliosis. J. Pediatr., *73*:725, 1968.

52. MacEwen, G. D.: Acute neurologic complications in the treatment of scoliosis. (A report of the Scoliosis Research Society.) J. Bone Joint Surg., *57A*:404–408, 1975.

53. MacEwen, G. D.: Congenital scoliosis with a unilateral bar. Radiology, *90*:711–715, 1968.

54. MacEwen, G. D., Hardy, J. H., and Winter, R. B.: Evaluation of kidney anomalies in congenital scoliosis. J. Bone Joint Surg., *54A*:1451–1455, 1972.

55. Marsh, H., Gould, A. P., Chitton, H. H., and Parker, R. W.: Transactions of the Clinical Society, London, 1885.

56. Matthaus, H.: Ein Beitrag zur Behandlung der angeborenen Lumbalkyphose. Z. Orthop., *112*:1312–1314, 1974.

57. Mayer, L.: Treatment of congenital scoliosis due to hemivertebrae. J. Bone Joint Surg., *17*:671–674, 1935.

58. Mayfield, J., Winter, R. B., Moe, J. H., and Bradford, D. S.: Congenital kyphosis due to defects in vertebral body segmentation. (Submitted for publication.)

59. Mensink, H. J. A., and Rogge, C. W. L.: Congenital scoliosis. Arch. Chir. Neerl., *26*:109–129, 1974.

60. Muller, W.: Die angeborene Gibbusbildung mit Wirbelkorperspaltung anderunterren brust Wirbelsaule. Arch. Orthop. Unfallchir., *30*:319–330, 1931.

61. Nasca, R. J., Stelling, F. H., and Steel, H. H.: Progression of congenital scoliosis due to hemivertebrae and hemivertebrae with bars. J. Bone Joint Surg., *57A*:456–466, 1975.

62. Perret, G.: Diagnosis and treatment of diastematomyelia. Surg. Gynecol. Obstet., *105*:69, 1957.

63. Perret, G.: Symptoms and signs of diastematomyelia. Neurol., *10*:51, 1960.

64. Peterson, H. A., and Peterson, F. F. A.: Hemivertebrae in identical twins with dissimilar spinal columns. J. Bone Joint Surg., *48A*:938, 1967.

65. Putti, V.: Die angeborenen Deformitaten der Wirbelsaule. Fortschr. Roentgenstr., *15*:65–92, 1910.

66. Reckles, L. N., Peterson, H. A., Bianco, A. J., and Weidman, W. H.: The association of scoliosis and congenital heart defects. J. Bone Joint Surg., *57A*:449–455, 1975.

67. Rimoin, D. L., Fletcher, B. D., and McKusick, V. A.: Spondylocostal dysplasia—a dominantly inherited form of short-trunked dwarfism. Am. J. Med., *45*:948–953, 1968.

68. Roth, A., Hall, J. E., Mizel, M., and Rosenthal, A.: Scoliosis and congenital heart disease. Clin. Orthop., *93*:95, 1973.

69. Royle, N. D.: The operative removal of an accessory vertebra. Med. J. Aust., *1*:467, 1928.

70. Şarpyener, M. A.: Congenital stricture of spinal canal. J. Bone Joint Surg., *27*:70, 1945.

71. Shands, A. R., Jr., and Bundens, W. D.: Congenital deformities of the spine. An analysis of the roentgenograms of 700 children. Bull. Hosp. Joint Dis., *17*:110–133, 1956.

72. Shaw, J. F.: Diastematomyelia. (Editorial.) Dev. Med. Child Neurol., *17*:361–364, 1975.

73. Simmons, E. H.: Congenital kyphosis. J. Bone Joint Surg., *55B*:233, 1973.

74. Simmons, E. H.: Observations on the technique and indications for wedge resection of the spine. J. Bone Joint Surg., *50A*:847–848, 1968.

75. Stanislavjevic, S., and St. John, E. G.: Congenital fusion of three lumbar vertebral bodies. Radiology, *71*:425, 1958.

76. Till, K.: Spinal dysraphism—A study of congenital malformations of the lower back. J. Bone Joint Surg., *51B*:415–422, 1969.

77. Tsou, P. M., Yau, A. C. M. C., and Hodgson, A. R.: Congenital spinal deformities: Natural history, classification, and the role of anterior surgery in management. Paper read at the annual meeting of the Scoliosis Research Society, 1974. J. Bone Joint Surg., *56A*:1767, 1974.

78. Ullrich, H. F.: Experiences with congenital scoliosis. Clin. Orthop., *7*:163–170, 1956.

79. Van Assen, J.: Angeborene Kyphose. Acta Chir. Scand., *67*:14–33, 1930.

80. Vitko, R. J., Cass, A. S., and Winter, R. B.: Anomalies of the genitourinary tract associated with congenital scoliosis and congenital kyphosis. J. Urol., *108*:655–659, 1972.

81. VonLackum, H. L., and Smith, A.: Removal of vertebral bodies in the treatment of scoliosis. Surg. Gynecol. Obstet., *57*:250–256, 1933.

82. Von Rokitansky, C.: Handbuch der Pathologischen Anatomie. Vol. II. Wien, Braumuller und Seidel, 1844.

83. Wakeley, C. P. G.: A case of congenital scoliosis due to suppression of half a vertebra. J. Anat., *57*:147, 1923.

84. Wiles, P.: Resection of dorsal vertebrae in congenital scoliosis. J. Bone Joint Surg., *33A*:151–154, 1923.

85. Winter, R. B., Moe, J. H., and Eilers, V. E.: Congenital scoliosis. J. Bone Joint Surg., *50A*:1–47, 1968.

86. Winter, R. B.: Congenital spine deformity: Natural history and treatment. Isr. J. Med. Sci., *9*:719–727, 1973.

87. Winter, R. B., Moe, J. H., and Wang, J. F.: Congenital kyphosis. J. Bone Joint Surg., *55A*:223–256, 1973.

88. Winter, R. B., Haven, J., Moe, J. H., and Lagaard, S.: Diastematomyelia and congenital spine deformities. J. Bone Joint Surg., *56A*:27–39, 1974.

89. Winter, R. B.: Spinal deformity in neurological and muscular disorders. *In* Hardy, J. (ed.): *Congenital Spinal Deformities*. St. Louis, C. V. Mosby Co., 1974.

90. Winter, R. B., Moe, J. H., MacEwen, G. D., and Peon-Vidales, H.: The Milwaukee brace in the non-operative treatment of congenital scoliosis. Spine, *1*:33–49, 1976.

91. Winter, R. B.: Congenital kyphoscoliosis with paralysis following hemivertebra excision. Clin. Orthop., *119*:116–125, 1976.

92. Winter, R. B.: The effects of early fusion on spine growth. *In* Zorab, P. A. (ed.): *Scoliosis and Growth*. Edinburgh & London, Churchill & Livingston, 1971.

93. Wynne-Davies, R.: Congenital vertebral anomalies: Aetiology and relationship to spina bifida cystica. J. Med. Genet., *12*:280–288, 1975.

# Chapter 8

# NEUROMUSCULAR DEFORMITIES

## INTRODUCTION

There is a large spectrum of neuromuscular disorders that may affect the growing child. All may cause a progressive spinal deformity. Sometimes the deformity is due to asymmetric paralysis and sometimes to symmetric paralysis of such a degree that the spine "collapses." The neurologic condition may be stable or progressive. The curvature can be progressive even though the neurologic condition is not. There may be breathing difficulty due to the paralysis or the curve or both. Sensation may be present or absent. Mental function may be normal or subnormal.

Thus, in many ways, neuromuscular spine deformities are different from idiopathic scoliosis. Many serious errors of treatment have resulted from the application of concepts appropriate for idiopathic scoliosis to the more complex neuromuscular scoliosis.

## CLASSIFICATION

The reader is referred to Chapter 2 for the comprehensive classification of scoliosis. The neuromuscular section is repeated here:

A. Neuropathic
  1. Upper motor neuron
    a. Cerebral palsy
    b. Spinocerebellar degeneration
      i. Friedreich's ataxia
      ii. Charcot-Marie-Tooth
      iii. Roussy-Levy
    c. Syringomyelia
    d. Spinal cord tumor
    e. Spinal cord trauma
  2. Lower motor neuron
    a. Poliomyelitis
    b. Other viral myelitides
    c. Traumatic
    d. Spinal muscular atrophy
      i. Werdnig-Hoffmann
      ii. Kugelberg-Welander
    e. Dysautonomia (Riley-Day)
B. Myopathic
  1. Arthrogryposis
  2. Muscular dystrophy
    a. Duchenne (pseudohypertrophic)
    b. Limb-girdle
    c. Facioscapulohumeral
  3. Fiber type disproportion
  4. Congenital hypotonia
  5. Myotonia dystrophica

## GENERAL PRINCIPLES

What distinguishes the patient with neuromuscular scoliosis from the patient with idiopathic scoliosis? Why is one so different from the other when the end result—a crooked spine—seems the same?

In idiopathic scoliosis we do not know the etiology. We do know, however, that certain curve patterns exist and are amazingly constant. If there is any defect in pulmonary function, it is due to the curve and not to any underlying process. If we halt the progress of the curve before breathing is affected, we know the patient can expect a lifetime free from pulmonary function deficit. This is not true in the paralytic. Intercostal paralysis may cause a significant deficit of pulmonary function in the absence of a curvature. A small curve, however, may "tip the scales," causing a case with borderline breathing capacity to become a real catastrophe.

The patient with idiopathic scoliosis does not have a curve that extends to the pelvis. There is no need for fusion of an idiopathic curve to the pelvis. In the neuromuscular curves, fusion to the pelvis is quite often necessary.

Generally speaking, the patient with a neuromuscular curve requires a longer fusion than does the idiopathic patient. The paralytic patient may need a fusion up into the cervical spine or, on rare occasions, to the occiput. The idiopathic patient never requires fusion above T1.

The paralytic patient has thinner, more osteoporotic bone. The iliac crests are quite often atrophic and a meager source of bone graft. Because of the small amount of bone, a solid fusion is more difficult to obtain. Pseudarthrosis repair is more likely to be necessary. The fusion mass does not heal as rapidly, so postoperative immobilization must be of longer duration. Because of the soft bone, hook dislodgement is more frequent.

Because the bone is more osteoporotic, the venous channels in the bone are larger, and therefore the blood loss at surgery is higher. Because of the smaller muscle bulk, the circulating blood volume is smaller. Thus, the paralytic patient not only loses more blood but also tolerates the loss less well.

Because of weak cough, postoperative respiratory complications are more frequent in the paralytic. Special attention must be directed to the neuromuscular patient in the postoperative period to prevent atelectasis and pneumonia. Tracheotomy or nasotracheal intubation with positive ventilatory support may be needed. This is not true of the idiopathic patient, except in the most severe cases.

In the idiopathic patient, one never worries about pelvic obliquity, sitting balance, or the presence of contractures about the hip. In the paralytic, these must be constantly kept in mind.

Because of his normal skin sensation, the idiopathic patient seldom has problems with pressure sores. But how does one manage the patient who needs surgery for a spine deformity but who has no sensation about the hips?

The list can go on and on, but the message should be clear by now. The paralytic patient is not the same as the idiopathic. There are a large number of factors that must be taken into consideration, and management of the paralytic patient is far more complicated than care of the patient with idiopathic scoliosis.

## PHYSICAL EXAMINATION

Physical examination of the scoliosis patient has been discussed fully in Chapter 3. A few points are worth repeating, and a few others need adding.

In examining the spine, one should note the pattern of the curve. Is it thoracic only? lumbar only? thoracolumbar? cervicothoracic? Is the pelvis level while sitting, standing, and lying? Is it a "collapsing" spine, i.e., is it very deformed while sitting, but much improved with traction? Or is it a very structural curve, with little change from sitting to supine and with or without traction? Is it a pure scoliosis, a kyphoscoliosis, or a lordoscoliosis?

Next, one should examine the hips and pelvis. Is the pelvis level? If not, why not? Is the pelvic obliquity due to the spine only? Is the pelvic deformity due to contractures of the iliotibial bands? Are there hip flexion contractures? Unilateral contracture of the iliotibial band produces pelvic obliquity.[26] Contracture of the hip flexors produces lumbar lordosis. Contracture of both the hip flexors and an iliotibial band produces both lumbar lordosis and pelvic obliquity. Hip extensor contracture (seen usually in cerebral palsy) produces anteflexion of the pelvis and a lumbar kyphosis (Figs. 8-1 and 8-2).

Pulmonary function and breathing capacity must be carefully evaluated. Clinical examination is most important. One can accurately see whether the chest expands well or not. The quality of the cough is of utmost importance, actually of far more importance than laboratory tests of pulmonary function. Can the patient blow out a match 12 cm. from the mouth? Functional capacity, including sitting stability, should be determined. Does the patient need the use of hands for torso support? Is sitting impossible without the external support of others or a brace? Is the patient ambulatory? How ambulatory? Can the patient transfer from wheelchair to bed?

In summary, the physician wishes to determine the severity and pattern of the

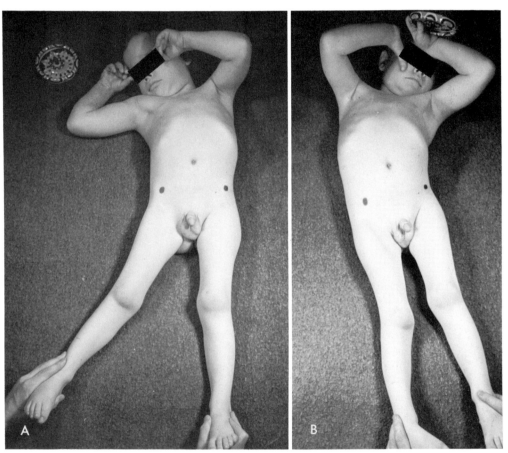

**Figure 8–1**   *A,* A patient with residuals of poliomyelitis. The pelvis is level with the right hip abducted. *B,* When the right leg is brought into neutral alignment, the pelvis become oblique. Such a patient requires surgical release of the contracted iliotibial band.

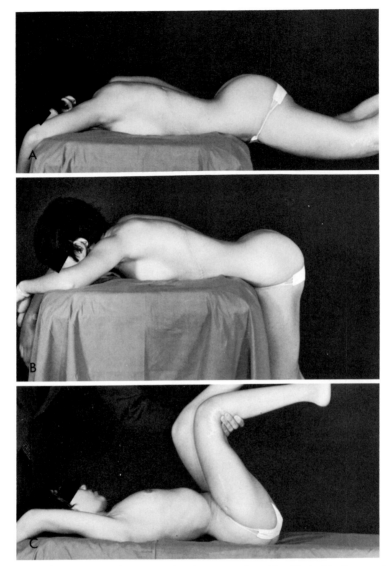

**Figure 8–2**    *A,* Physical examination of a patient placed prone on the table with the hips in extension shows a significant increase of lumbar lordosis. Is this lordosis due to contractures of the hip flexors, or is this a lordosis which is fixed in the spine? *B,* Flexion of the hips to 90 degrees reveals improvement but not total elimination of the lumbar lordosis. This examination shows this particular patient has a lordosis that is a combination of structural lordosis within the spine, plus aggravation by hip flexion contractures. Hip flexion contracture release alone would not correct her lordosis. She underwent both hip flexor release and surgical correction and fusion of her lumbar lordoscoliosis.

curve, the presence or absence of pelvic obliquity, the status of muscles about the hips, sitting stability, transferability, pulmonary capacity, and cough strength. In addition, mental capacity, motor strength, and general functional ability need careful assessment, especially the existent or potential effect of the deformity on functional ability.

## RADIOLOGIC EVALUATION

Many of the features noted in the physical examination can be refined and documented in the radiologic examination. Once again, the reader is referred to Chapter 3 for more information regarding radiologic examination of the scoliosis patient.

Certain special views aid considerably in evaluation of the neuromuscular patient. Standing films are appropriate for those able to stand, but often sitting films are more valuable, showing the spine with the effect of gravity but eliminating the suspension effect of crutches and the effect of hip flexion and iliotibial band contractures on pelvic obliquity. Crutch-dependent patients show a greater curve on sitting films than on standing films.

Bending films (voluntary) are of little value in the paralyzed patient. Passive bend films or traction ("stretch") films provide far better information about the correctability or rigidity of a curve. Hyperextension films are of great value for kyphosis, and hyperflexion films are useful for lordosis.

## UPPER MOTOR NEURON LESIONS

### Cerebral Palsy: Incidence and Natural History

There are four major studies of the prevalence of scoliosis in children with cerebral palsy. Robson[52] examined 152 adolescents and young adults. He noted that "fixed" or structural scoliosis was present in 23 (15.2 per cent). Fixed scoliosis was defined as a curve that persisted in the prone position and demonstrated rotation on forward bending. Curves disappearing in the prone position and without rotation on forward bending were defined as postural curves. Fifty patients (32.8 per cent) had postural curves. Structural curves were equally prevalent in males and females but were not found in patients below age 15. The study group was composed mostly of diplegics and athetoids. Only six curves were felt to be "moderately severe" (approaching 60 degrees on clinical examination). X-rays were not taken.

Rosenthal et al.[53] examined 50 adolescents from a cerebral palsy clinic population of 500. All patients between 14 and 19 were examined. All patients had x-rays. There was an equal number of males and females. Of the 50 adolescents, 19 were found to have scoliosis (38 per cent). The curves ranged from 10 to 146 degrees. Of the 19 curves, 18 were less than 40 degrees. Two patients had pain.

Balmer and MacEwen[2] reviewed 100 children in a cerebral palsy clinic. There were 21 with scoliosis of 10 degrees or more. Fourteen children had curves under 30 degrees, 4 had curves between 30 and 60 degrees, and 2 had curves between 60 and 95 degrees.

Samilson and Bechard[54] reviewed the spines of 906 institutionalized, severely involved patients. Of this group, 232 (25 per cent) had scoliosis, and 193 of these were spastic quadriplegics. Of the 232 with scoliosis, 135 (58 per cent) had fixed pelvic obliquity, and 199 had hip contracture, subluxation, or dislocation. The most severe curves were thoracolumbar. Of these patients, 84 per cent had pelvic obliquity, 82 per cent had hip contractures, and 70 per cent had hip subluxation or dislocation.

In an unpublished review of patients at Gillette Children's Hospital, the authors have found approximately 25 per cent of the patients in a large cerebral palsy clinic to have structural scoliosis of 10 degrees or more, most curves being under 25 degrees. However, as a large referral center for scoliosis treatment, the authors have also seen a relatively large number of very severe curvatures (90 to 180 degrees) in patients with cerebral palsy. Most of the patients with very severe curves are spastic quadriplegics or diplegics with fairly severe involvement and who are usually nonambulatory.

Postural deformity, especially kyphosis, is very common, particularly early in the child's development. This appears to be due to delayed development of the trunk extensors with relative overactivity of the trunk flexors. There is delay in establishment of the normal truncal reflex activity necessary to maintain an erect posture.

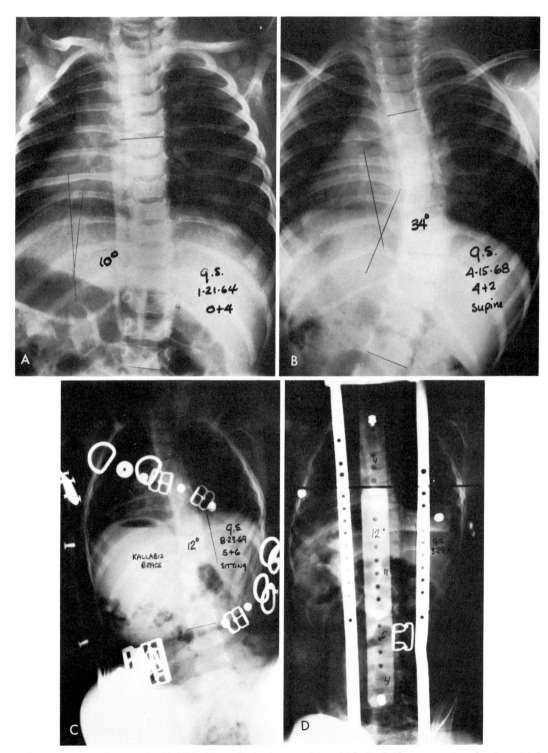

**Figure 8–3** *A,* A four month old child with cerebral palsy, spastic quadriplegia. *B,* The same patient showing a 34 degree curve on a supine x-ray at age four. *C,* Brace treatment was started at age four using a three point kalibis brace with excellent improvement even in the upright position. *D,* The same patient three years later, at the age of eight, having been changed to a Milwaukee brace to permit better respiratory function. The curve measures 12 degrees in the brace.

*Legend continued on opposite page*

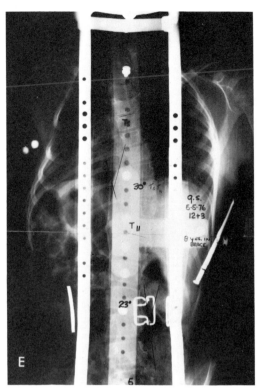

**Figure 8–3** *Continued.* *E,* The same patient at age 12 years and 3 months. After eight years of bracing, her curve is still well controlled at 30 degrees.

## NONOPERATIVE TREATMENT

There has been a tendency to ignore nonoperative treatment of the child with cerebral palsy. This has largely been due to general discouragement about the child with cerebral palsy, coupled with poor experiences in use of the Milwaukee brace. Recent advances in orthotics and more enthusiasm for the child with cerebral palsy have led to much improved nonoperative treatment.[32]

Like all paralytic spine deformities, one cannot begin orthotic treatment after the patient has developed a major structural curve. Early structural curves must be detected and braced promptly. The purpose of bracing structural curves is to delay fusion until age 12 to 14, when more adequate spine length will have developed. If the child is already age 13 and has a 60-degree structural curve, prompt surgical fusion is the procedure of choice, not bracing.

For thoracic curves, the Milwaukee brace is still the orthosis of choice. Underarm level braces are not effective for thoracic curvatures. For thoracolumbar and lumbar curves (the more common patterns in cerebral palsy) molded plastic underarm body jackets are preferable. The conventional TLSO used in lumbar idiopathic scoliosis (see pp. 379–383) is *not* recommended for paralytic curves.

Bracing should continue until a better age for fusion is reached, or until the curve becomes worse in the brace, at which time fusion should be done regardless of age. There is no need to wait until the end of growth (Figs. 8–3 and 8–4).

## SURGICAL TREATMENT

There are two main problems in the surgical treatment of spine deformity in cerebral palsy — the actual technique and the indications. Prior to the development of efficient internal fixation devices, surgical treatment of these patients was so unrewarding and so frought with complications that the surgical approach was virtually abandoned. Advances in surgical technique, including halofemoral traction, Dwyer instrumentation, Harrington instrumentation, and lumbar transverse process fusion, have now essentially solved the technical problems.

The indications, however, remain controversial. When is spine surgery indicated in a child with mental retardation? Should such a child be offered all the medical expertise available to children of normal mentality? Is early death due to respiratory compromise a fate that should be prevented or a blessing with which we should not interfere? If a child is nonambulatory, is it of benefit to correct the scoliosis and pelvic obliquity, or is it a waste of precious health care money?

These are difficult and sometimes unanswerable questions. The authors feel that *the child with cerebral palsy should not be ignored and forgotten. When it will benefit the child, surgery should be done.* The benefits may be the freedom from back pain, the freedom from a painful dislocated hip, the ability to sit all day without fatigue, the ability to sit without using the hands for trunk support, the ability to breathe easily, and the opportunity to sit tall and straight rather than twisted and grotesque when there is the mentality to appreciate the difference. We do not feel that surgical correction should be done in those circumstances where no benefit would be obtained.

The indications for surgical correction and fusion are therefore many:
1. A curve interfering with respiration
2. A curve with pain
3. A curve interfering with sitting balance
4. A curve associated with pelvic obliquity and a painful subluxation of the hip
5. Curves obviously progressing to one or more of the above.

The number of degrees of curvature is of less importance than the malfunctions noted above.

Little has been published about the surgical treatment of cerebral palsy scoliosis. Haas[20] described the correction of a 45-degree lumbar curve in a 13 year old girl by extensive muscle releases and transfers. MacEwen[33] reported on the operative treatment of 16 patients with posterior fusion and Harrington instrumentation. Three had preliminary halofemoral traction. The average curve was 72 degrees. The average correction was 36

degrees (50 per cent), with 26 degree maintenance (35 per cent). There was an average 10 degree (14 per cent) loss of correction. Two patients had poor results, one with total loss of correction, the other with persistent pseudarthrosis.

Bonnett, Brown, and Brooks[4] reported 13 patients operated by the Dwyer technique. The average curve was 80 degrees. Posterior fusion with Harrington rods was also done in four patients. Rapid resumption of upright activity in molded plastic body jackets was permitted. Bonnett et al.[6] also reported an extensive series of patients with paralytic curves of various etiologies, predominantly poliomyelitis. A few were cerebral palsy patients. These authors emphasized the importance of long fusions, secure internal fixation with Harrington rods, the use of large alar hooks, and broad transverse process fusion, especially in the lumbar spine.

O'Brien et al.[43] described the surgical treatment of scoliosis with pelvic obliquity. These were all poliomyelitis patients, but the principles demonstrated are quite applicable to cerebral palsy. They emphasized the great benefit to correction of the pelvis by combined Dwyer *and* Harrington instrumentation and fusion. In the 39 patients reviewed, the average correction of pelvic obliquity was 78 per cent.

The surgical techniques vary depending on the location and magnitude of the curve. A few patients have purely thoracic curves. These may be only idiopathic curvatures in patients with cerebral palsy. In such cases, posterior fusion of the curve with Harrington instrumentation is all that is necessary. The management is essentially the same as with idiopathic scoliosis (Fig. 8–4).

Lumbar curves and especially thoracolumbar curves are the most likely to be considered for arthrodesis. There is a high prevalence of pelvic obliquity and subluxated or dislocated hips on the "high" side. For mild curves, posterior fusion with Harrington instrumentation, coupled with a wide transverse process fusion of the lumbar spine, is the procedure of choice.

The more major lumbar and thoracolumbar curves require a more extensive approach. The patient is first placed in halofemoral traction for two to three weeks, with unequal weights on the lower extremities if there is pelvic obliquity. The second stage is an anterior correction and fusion by the Dwyer technique, usually at about T10 to L4 or L5.

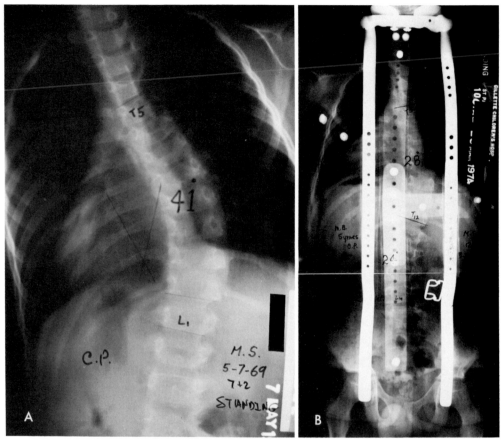

**Figure 8–4** *A,* A 7 + 2 year old male with cerebral palsy, mild spastic diplegia. A 41 degree right thoracic curve is present on a standing x-ray. A Milwaukee brace was prescribed. *B,* The same patient at age 12, after five years in the Milwaukee brace; this curve is well controlled at 28 degrees. He later required surgical fusion.

Halofemoral traction is continued for two more weeks. The third stage is a posterior fusion with Harrington instrumentation, *from the upper thoracic spine to the sacrum.*[1] It is tempting to "stop short" and fuse only up to T8–T9, based on the anteroposterior x-ray before treatment. However, experience has shown that the scoliosis will progress in the thoracic spine, and, even more importantly, a progressive thoracic kyphosis will take place above the upper end of the fusion. For this and other reasons (better internal fixation, better control of pelvic obliquity, and fewer pseudarthroses) the authors feel strongly that *both* are needed, and *never* the Dwyer alone.

Postoperative management has caused many problems in the past, especially with pressure sores. This has been, for the most part, eliminated in our hospitals by a combination of rigid internal fixation, better plaster technique, better padding under the casts,

early return to the upright position, and better nursing care.

Depending on the level of the curve and degree of internal fixation, we use halo casts, Risser casts, underarm casts, or bivalve polypropylene body jackets postoperatively. The casts do *not* extend down onto the legs. The patients are returned to the upright position within two weeks of final surgery. Prolonged bedrest is no longer necessary.

Athetoid and combative patients may require six to eight halo pins rather than the customary four in order to give superior fixation. Halofemoral traction is used liberally, even for some of the milder curves. Uncooperative patients need a general anesthetic for cast application. When doing posterior fusion with Harrington instrumentation but without halofemoral traction, it is advisable to apply the Risser cast while the patient is still under the same anesthetic as for

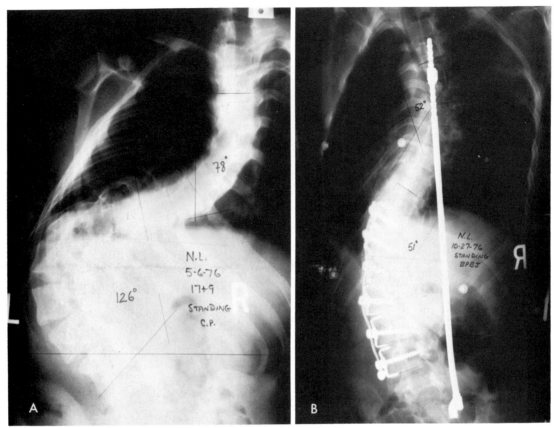

**Figure 8–5**  *A,* A 17 + 9 year old boy with cerebral palsy and spastic quadriplegia. He exhibits a 126 degree T10–L4 left lumbar curve and a 78 degree T4–T10 right thoracic curve. His pelvis is level. The torso is deviated to the right. There is no pelvic obliquity. He was developing considerable pain in the lumbar spine. This curve was also progressive. Curves of this magnitude cannot be treated by bracing. *B,* The same patient nine days following posterior fusion and three weeks following the Dwyer procedure, standing in a bivalve polypropylene body jacket. There is excellent maintenance of curve correction with the thoracic curve measuring 52 degrees and the lumbar curve 51 degrees and the torso well centered over the pelvis.

surgery. This will prevent hook dislocation due to uncontrolled activity by the patient.

For extremely severe curves, preliminary fasciotomy and tenotomy may be beneficial. While the patient is under the same anesthetic as for the application of the halo and femoral pins, the concavity of the curve is exposed as for a fusion. The muscle attachments around the facets *and* transverse processes are released, the sacrospinalis is released from the sacrum and iliac crest, and the lumbodorsal

fascia is released from the iliac crest. Hip flexion and adduction contractures can be released at the same time.

We have not found the halopelvic device to be beneficial in patients with cerebral palsy. Most of these patients require fusion to the sacrum, and this cannot be done adequately with the halopelvic device in place. Obtaining an adequate autogenous iliac bone graft is also compromised by the pelvic pins (Figs. 8–5 and 8–6).

**Figure 8–6**  *A,* A 9 year, 11 month old boy with spastic quadriplegia, nonambulatory. He has a T9–L4 left thoraco-lumbar curve measuring 100 degrees. Because of mental retardation, treatment was not recommended. *B,* The same patient at age 18. He now has a curve of 185 degrees from T7 to L4. Note the lengthening of the curve proximally. Previously he had been able to sit, but with the steady increase in curvature, he had totally lost all sitting stability and has become a bed-ridden patient. This greatly increased the difficulty of management of the patient, and therefore, surgical treatment was elected, despite his retardation. *C,* Halofemoral traction corrected the curve to 120 degrees, and the Dwyer added further improvement of the curve to 70 degrees. *D,* The patient is seen here upright in a halo cast two weeks following posterior fusion with rods. His curve was maintained at 59 degrees, only a 5 degree change from the supine x-ray on the day of the final surgery. The hips were not immobilized. A halo cast was used to avoid excessive forces on the upper hook. A regular Risser cast was not possible, owing to a drooling problem.

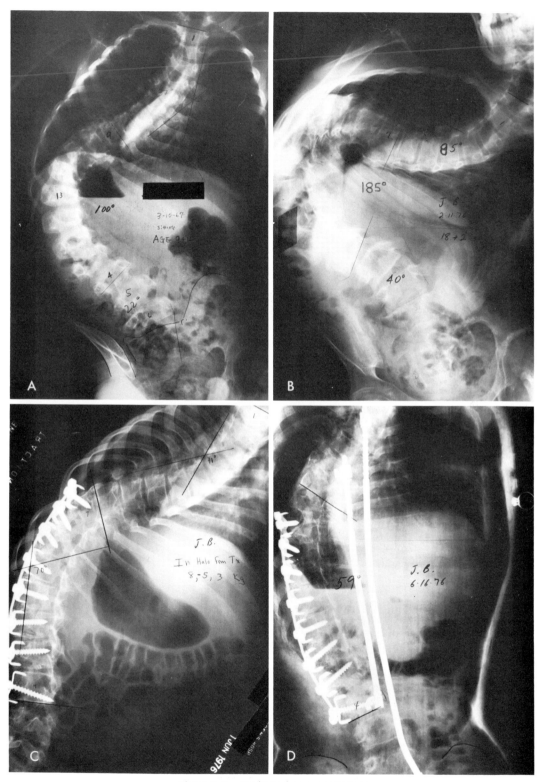

**Figure 8–6** *See legend on opposite page.*

## Spinocerebellar Degenerative Diseases

These conditions are usually familial, have a chronic course, progress slowly over several decades, cause degeneration of one or more neurologic tracts, and frequently result in orthopedic deformities and frequent cardiomyopathy.[15, 23] The most common of these conditions are Friedreich's ataxia, Charcot-Marie-Tooth disease, and Dejerine-Sottas disease. Of those, scoliosis is most likely to occur in Friedreich's ataxia.

Nonoperative treatment has not been rewarding in Friedreich's ataxia. Owing to the patient's generalized neurologic condition, braces are poorly tolerated, and the curves seem to progress relentlessly. Progressive curves should usually be stabilized surgically, unless the patient is terminal or has significant cardiomyopathy (Fig. 8–7).

## Syringomyelia

### NATURAL HISTORY AND REVIEW OF LITERATURE

Syringomyelia existing in the growing child will commonly produce a scoliosis; reports in the literature of the frequency range from 25 to 88 per cent. There are some unusual aspects to this type of scoliosis. Unlike most neuromuscular problems, the

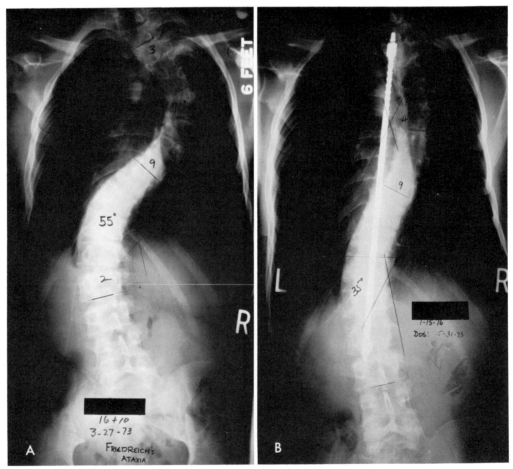

**Figure 8–7** *A,* A 16 + 10 year old male presented to the authors with a 70 degree right thoracic and a 55 degree left thoracolumbar curve secondary to Friedreich's ataxia. *B,* Posterior instrumentation and fusion were done from T3 to L2. In retrospect, the fusion should have extended to at least L3 or even L4.

curves produced are not long and sweeping, but more closely resemble idiopathic scoliosis. This similarity of curve pattern, coupled with the very subtle neurologic changes early in syringomyelia, leads to frequent misdiagnosis of these curves as idiopathic.

Simmons and Weber[57] reviewed 50 patients with syringomyelia; 20 of them had scoliosis (12 males and 8 females). A single structural curve was present in 17, and 3 had double curves. Of these curves, 15 were thoracic, 4 thoracolumbar, and 4 lumbar. There was a close correlation between the neurologic level and the level of the curve.

Huebert and MacKinnon[25] reviewed 43 patients with syringomyelia. Of these, 27 had scoliosis; 15 had curvatures of less than 25 degrees, 5 had curves of 25 to 50 degrees, and 7 had curves over 50 degrees.

## NONOPERATIVE TREATMENT

Experience with nonoperative treatment has been quite limited. The author's single case treated in a Milwaukee brace had progression of the scoliosis despite brace treatment, and fusion was required to control the scoliosis. A progressive cervical hyperlordosis that developed in the area of the laminectomy in this same patient was corrected and controlled by the brace.

## SURGICAL TREATMENT

Progressive scoliosis should be treated, and if greater than 40 degrees, it should be fused. The length of the fusion should follow the rules set down for idiopathic scoliosis (see page 114).

One should never hesitate to treat the patient with scoliosis and syringomyelia. Most patients with this condition live many years, sometimes having a normal life span. One of Simmons and Weber's patients with scoliosis was 73 years old.

Many if not most patients with syringomyelia have a laminectomy for the diagnosis and/or treatment of the lesion. The laminectomy may considerably compound the spine deformity problem, particularly if it is thoracic. Anterior fusion may be necessary in the patient with thoracic kyphoscoliosis due to a mixture of syringomyelia, scoliosis, and post-laminectomy kyphosis (Fig. 8–8).

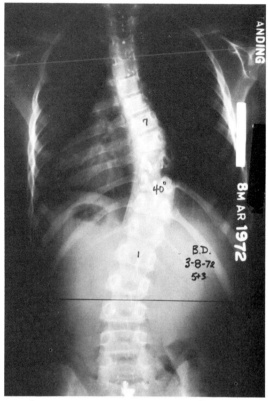

**Figure 8–8** A 5 year old girl with a T7–L1 right thoracic curve that totally resembles an idiopathic curve radiologically and clinically. Weakness in her hands had led to the diagnosis of syringomyelia. This curve was treated with a Milwaukee brace, but progression occurred despite the brace, and fusion was done at age 9.

## Spinal Cord Tumor

Although uncommon, one of the causes of spinal deformity is the neurologic condition resulting from a spinal cord tumor. These are most often either astrocytomas or ependymomas. Both tumors are notoriously unpredictable in regard to disability and life expectancy.[60]

All too often, the patient presents with a scoliosis of a peculiar nature, and a detailed neurologic examination reveals pathologic signs such as abnormal reflexes. A myelogram is performed, a tumor diagnosed, and a laminectomy performed. If an astrocytoma is found, a biopsy is performed (the tumor is unresectable) and irradiation given. The patient is then presumed to be terminal, although this is not always the case. Several such

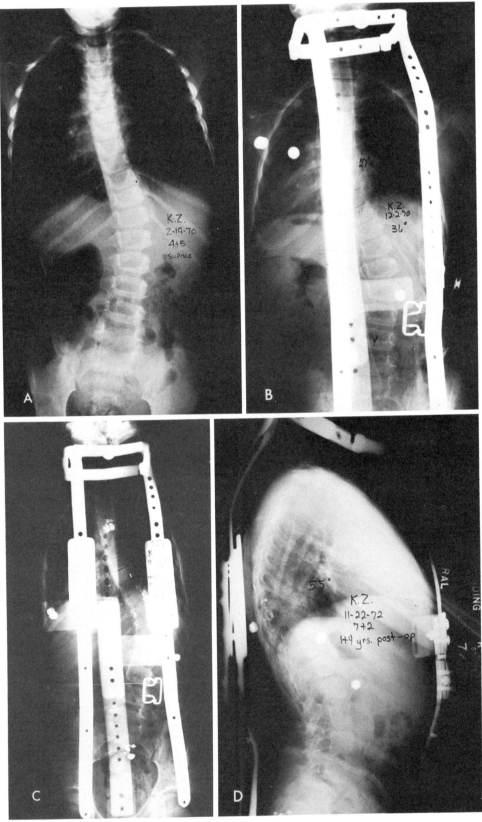

**Figure 8–9**   *See legend on opposite page.*

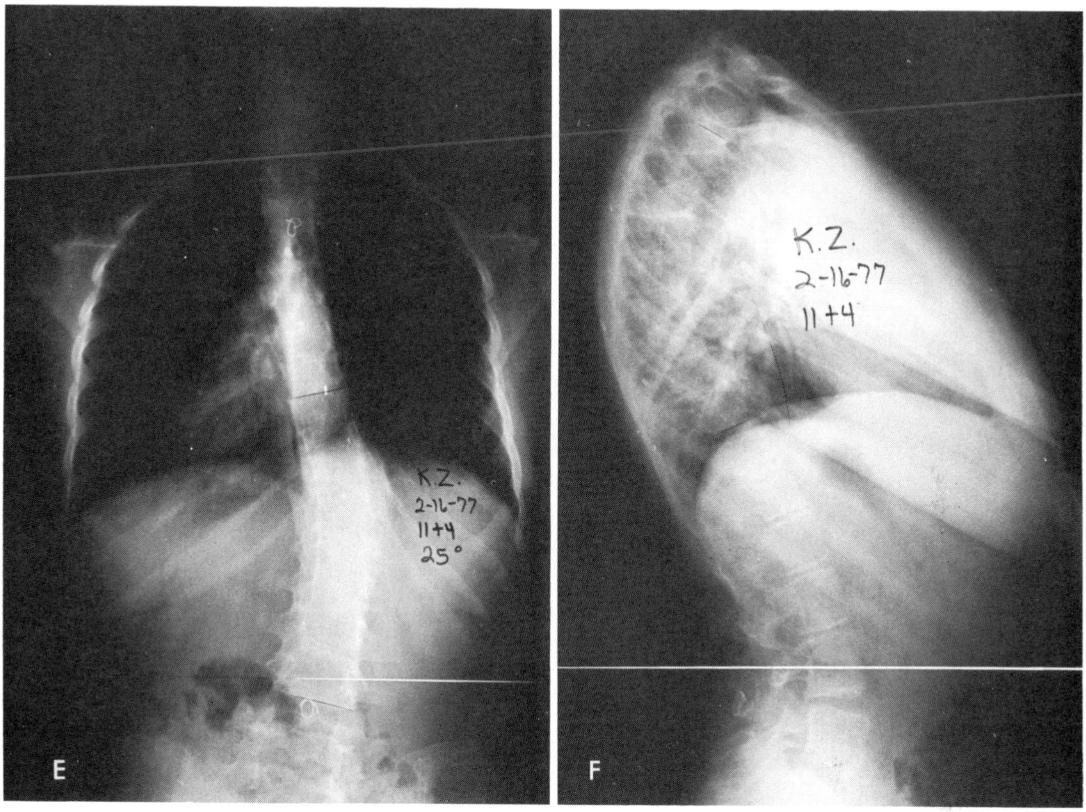

**Figure 8–9** *A,* This 4 year old girl presented with a right thoracolumbar curve that was mistakenly diagnosed as an idiopathic scoliosis. The pelvic obliquity on this supine film should have alerted us to the possibility of other than idiopathic scoliosis. *B,* She was placed in a Milwaukee brace, but the curve responded poorly. Complaints of a burning, itching pain across the right abdomen finally led to the correct diagnosis—astrocytoma of the thoracic cord. A laminectomy and biopsy were done and the tumor irradiated. *C,* One and a half years later, her scoliosis was showing an increase of curvature despite constant use of a Milwaukee brace. *D,* A lateral view showing a thoracic kyphosis of 55 degrees. She has had a T5–T11 laminectomy and was showing a progressive postlaminectomy thoracic kyphosis as well as the progressive paralytic scoliosis. Posterior fusion from T3 to L4 was done in combination with an anterior fusion of T3 to T10 (area of the laminectomy). *E,* At age eleven years, she shows a solid fusion. The scoliosis measures 25 degrees. She is neurologically normal except for residual hyperactive deep tendon reflexes. Bowel and bladder function are normal. She is fully ambulatory and attends regular school. This is four years following spine fusion and 5½ years following her laminectomy. *F,* A lateral view at age 11 + 4. The spinal contours are normal.

patients have presented to the authors with curvature problems several years after tumor treatment. Whether or not the tumor is still present is rather an academic question. The patient is alive and functioning well, but has a progressive curve. The curve may be due to paralysis from the tumor; it may be kyphosis caused by the laminectomy; it may be an irradiation-induced curve; or it may be some combination of these. Regardless of the etiology of the curve, treatment is appropriate.

Paralytic curves require surgical stabilization if the patient is of adequate age (10 +). Under this age, brace treatment should be attempted. Fusion should extend to the sacrum if there is pelvic obliquity or a flail, collapsing spine. In the area of the laminectomy, posterior fusion is seldom adequate, and anterior fusion should be done (Fig. 8–9).

## Spinal Cord Trauma

### REVIEW OF THE LITERATURE

The child with a cord injury has a compound problem. There is the paralysis, itself a severe problem, and also a secondary paralytic spine deformity.[37, 59]

Kilfoyle et al.[29] analyzed 104 children with paraplegia. There were 73 congenital paralyses (myelomeningocele), and 31 were acquired. Of the 104 children, 97 developed spine and pelvic deformity, with lordosis most common, scoliosis second, and kyphosis least common. All deformities tended to become worse during growth unless surgically stabilized. These authors emphasized the concept of spines "balanced," "partially balanced," or "off balance." (See Chapter 9.) It was felt by these authors that "early intervention is now considered an expression of conservatism."

Bonnett et al.[5] analyzed 123 patients under the age of 18 with acquired spinal cord injury. Of these, 57 had significant deformity, and 66 did not. The average age at injury of the 57 with deformity was 6.8 years and for the 66 without deformity, 16 years. Thus, progressive curvatures are seen in children with growth remaining, not in the late adolescent with growth complete or nearly so. All 57 patients had scoliosis (average, 72 degrees, usually flexible and "collapsing"), and 12 of the 57 had lordosis (average, 88 degrees). Thirty of the 57 were treated nonoperatively. Corsets were found to be more effective than Milwaukee braces for most patients. Twelve patients remained the same in the brace, nine worsened, and nine improved. The authors emphasized that brace treatment should begin *before* structural curves developed.

Surgery was performed on 22 patients. Pelvic obliquity was a strong indication for surgery. Bonnett[7] emphasized the total care needs of the cord-injured child. The patient with cervical injury and quadriplegia requires varying amounts of external supportive devices, depending on the level of paralysis. The Milwaukee brace was found best for spinal support of injuries above T10. For injuries below T10, bivalve plastic body jackets were recommended. The orthoses are worn only when the patient is upright. Surgery was indicated for spinal stabilization. This permitted stable sitting, prevented respiratory compromise, freed the hands for useful activity rather than trunk support, and provided significant improvement of self-image. Most patients required spinal fusion at the beginning of the growth spurt.

Wedge and Gillespie[62] reported on spine surgery in 20 paraplegic children. They emphasized the need for a long fusion—midthorax to sacrum. Pelvic obliquity should be fully corrected, and the combination of Dwyer and Harrington procedures was quite helpful in selected cases (Figs. 8–10, 8–11, and 8–12).

## NONOPERATIVE TREATMENT

The experience of the authors confirms the published data. Nearly all children rendered paraplegic or quadriplegic prior to the growth spurt develop significant spine deformity that is sufficient to require bracing during early growth and fusion at the time of the growth spurt (or earlier if refractory to bracing). A Milwaukee brace is necessary for cervical and high thoracic lesions and bivalve polypropylene or similar plastic underarm braces for low thoracic and thoracolumbar lesions. The brace should be lined with cushioning (but nonabsorbent) material. The braces should not be worn at night or while recumbent. They must be worn whenever the patient is upright, either sitting or standing. In order to preserve lung function, the thorax must not be tightly constricted. Bracing should be started as soon as the upright position is assumed following the injury. The brace is to *prevent* deformity, not to correct a structural curve.[9]

## SURGICAL TREATMENT

Surgical stabilization will be needed in virtually all children rendered quadriplegic or paraplegic prior to the growth spurt, and in most children paralyzed before the end of growth.[34, 41, 48] The indications for surgery are the existence of such a paralysis, the existence of a structural curve, the development of pelvic obliquity, and progression of a deformity while under brace treatment. The goals of surgery are: sitting stability, freedom of the hands for useful activity rather than trunk support, preservation of respiratory function, and prevention of pressure sores (e.g., those due to fixed pelvic obliquity).

Internal fixation is quite important, since the anesthetic skin prevents the use of corrective casts. The authors have obtained the best results by internal fixation with one or two Harrington distraction rods, wide transverse process fusion throughout the lumbar spine, fusion to at least two levels above the

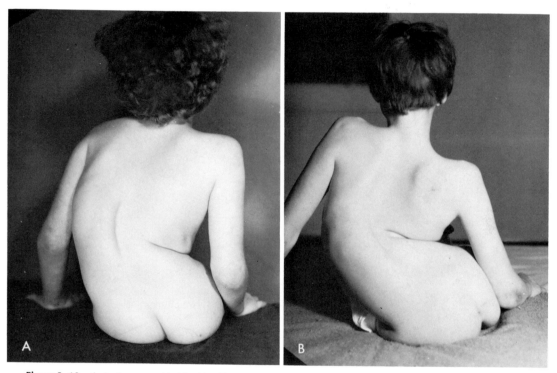

**Figure 8–10**  *A,* A nine year old girl with a T6 traumatic paraplegia from a car accident at age 3. Note the need for hand support to maintain sitting balance. This curve has already progressed beyond the point where brace treatment would help. *B,* The same patient four years later without treatment. She now has problems with recurrent left ischial pressure sores. Such neglectful "treatment" cannot be justified.

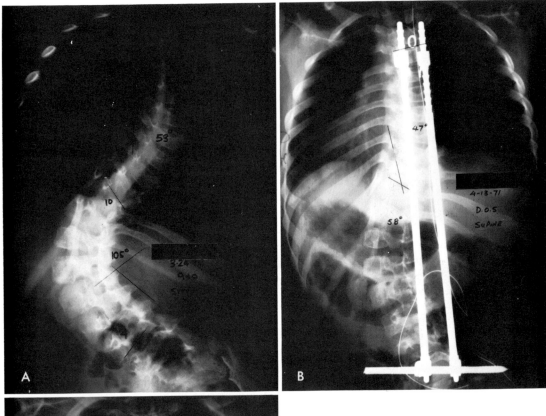

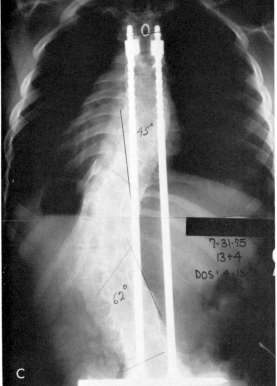

**Figure 8–11**  *A,* A sitting film of a nine year old boy who suffered paraplegia from an exchange transfusion at the time of birth. He exhibits a 105 degree left thoraco-lumbar curve, T9–L4, and a 53 degree upper thoracic curve. There is a significant pelvic obliquity. *B,* An AP x-ray taken on the day of surgery for the scoliosis. In this particular case, a transverse sacral bar and two long distraction rods were utilized. The entire surgery was accomplished in one stage. Despite the residual 58 degree left lumbar curve, the pelvis is level, and the torso is vertical and well centered over the level pelvis, thus accomplishing the goals of treatment. *C,* The patient at age 13 + 4, four years after the spine fusion. Note the solid fusion and the maintenance of the proper torso-pelvic relationship. This patient did have a pseudarthrosis at L2–L3 requiring a pseudarthrosis repair six months after the original fusion. (See Chapter 16, page 415, section on Complications of Surgery.) This boy's postoperative care consisted of a standard but well-padded Risser cast without immobilization of the hips. Upright activities were permitted throughout the entire healing.

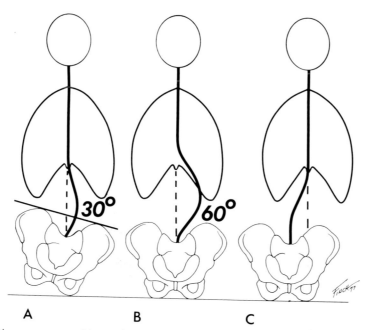

**Figure 8–12** In the management of the paralytic patient, it is of the utmost importance to obtain a vertical torso centered over a level pelvis. *A,* The curve is small, but pelvic obliquity persists. This is *not* a satisfactory situation. *B,* The torso is well centered over a level pelvis. Even though the curve is 60 degrees, this is preferable to *A. C,* The torso is vertical and the pelvis is level, but the torso is not centered over the sacrum. This is called "lateral translation." This is not a good situation either, since the line of gravity falls over one ischium. Pressure sores can be expected.

neurologic lesion, and postoperative immobilization in a well-padded halo-cast for cervical level lesions and in a bivalve polypropylene body jacket for lower thoracic and thoracolumbar lesions. The hips are *not* immobilized, and the patient is returned to the upright position within two weeks of surgery. Combined Dwyer and Harrington procedures are ideal for severe structural pelvic obliquity. Postoperative immobilization is required for 10 to 12 months.

## LOWER MOTOR NEURON LESIONS

### Poliomyelitis

All major spine treatment centers developed their skills in the treatment of neuromuscular spine problems during the era of the great poliomyelitis epidemics.[10] Despite the eradication of poliomyelitis from most advanced countries by the Salk and Sabin vaccines, many less developed areas of the world still suffer from endemic poliomyelitis.[28] Even in the United States and Canada, there are many adults with untreated poliomyelitis curvatures. Many such curves are seen yearly by the authors. Most of these should have

been treated years ago by proper correction and fusion.

Curvatures due to poliomyelitis take one of two forms; either asymmetric paralysis and secondary curvature or a collapsing spine due to extensive symmetrical paralysis.[17, 21] The differentiation is quite important, since the collapsing spine always requires fusion to the sacrum.[16, 17] Asymmetric paralysis with curvature quite often can be managed by a shorter fusion that does not extend to the sacrum.

The most severe curvatures seen at our center have been those due to poliomyelitis. The worst was a 200 degree curve in a 36 year old woman who presented with cor pulmonale due to the curve (Fig. 8–13).

Poliomyelitis curves may affect any part of the spine, including the neck. Some curves are short and limited and may resemble an idiopathic curve. Most are long and sweeping and may extend up into the neck or down to the pelvis. The most grotesque curves are the long "C" curves extending from neck to pelvis. The higher the curve, the more severe will be the pulmonary function deficit.[27] This is caused by both the thoracic deformity and the intercostal paralysis.

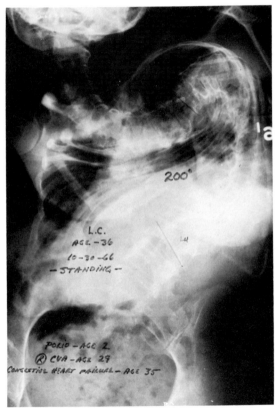

**Figure 8–13**   A 200 degree post-poliomyelitis scoliosis. The patient had polio at age 2, and presented to the authors at age 36 with severe cor pulmonale.

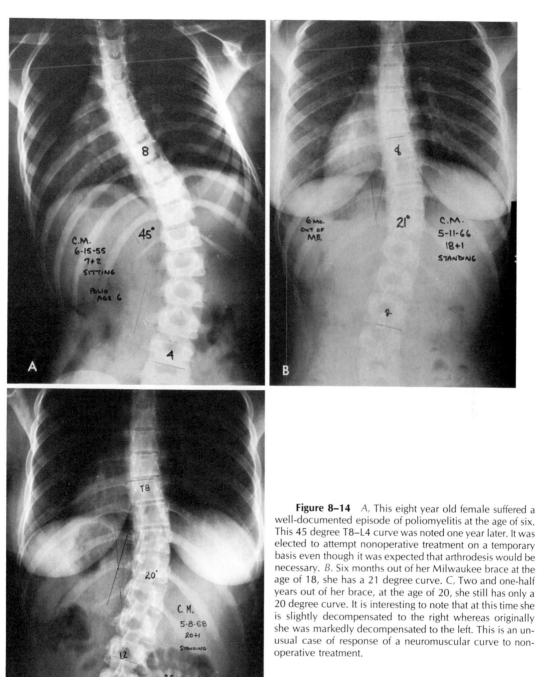

**Figure 8–14** *A,* This eight year old female suffered a well-documented episode of poliomyelitis at the age of six. This 45 degree T8–L4 curve was noted one year later. It was elected to attempt nonoperative treatment on a temporary basis even though it was expected that arthrodesis would be necessary. *B,* Six months out of her Milwaukee brace at the age of 18, she has a 21 degree curve. *C,* Two and one-half years out of her brace, at the age of 20, she still has only a 20 degree curve. It is interesting to note that at this time she is slightly decompensated to the right whereas originally she was markedly decompensated to the left. This is an unusual case of response of a neuromuscular curve to nonoperative treatment.

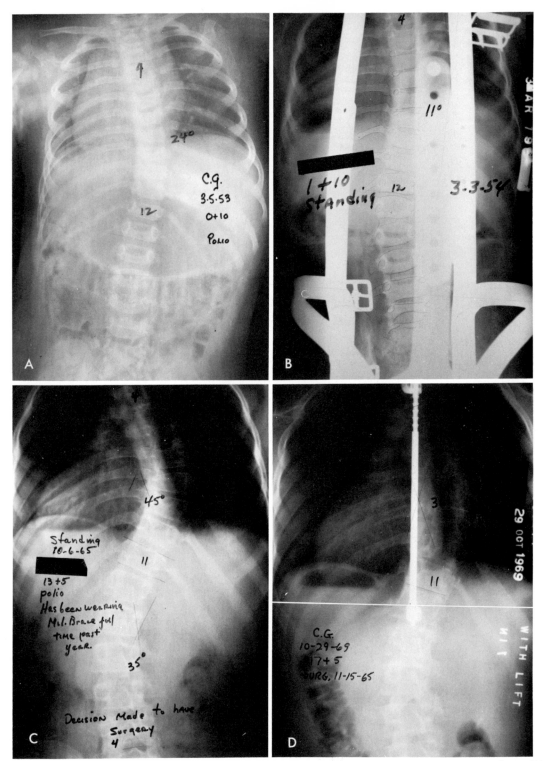

**Figure 8–15** *A,* This 10 month old boy exhibits a 24 degree T4–L1 right thoracic scoliosis secondary to poliomyelitis, which he suffered at the age of two months. *B,* The child was placed in a Milwaukee brace at the age of 1 year. This x-ray at the age of 1 year and 10 months shows correction of the curve to 11 degrees with excellent vertical position of the torso over the pelvis. *C,* He continued to be kept under 40 degrees until the age of 13 at which time his curve started to show deterioration, coinciding with the adolescent growth spurt. The thoracic curve now measures 45 degrees. There is a compensatory nonstructural 35 degree left lumbar curve. There is no pelvic obliquity, and the structural curve is limited to the thoracic spine. *D,* This x-ray, four years after Harrington instrumentation and spine fusion from T3 to T12, shows correction and stabilization of the curve at 36 degrees. It was not necessary to fuse the lumbar curve. There is a level pelvis and only a minor lumbar compensatory curve.

High cervicothoracic curves produce extremely unsightly deformities even though the angle of measurement may be relatively small. Pelvic obliquity due to a lumbar curve can produce marked gait disturbance or sitting balance malfunction. Thus one must pay attention not only to the severity of the curve but also to its functional defects.[30]

## NONOPERATIVE TREATMENT

Although on rare occasions a polio curve can be permanently treated by bracing, the prime purpose of nonoperative treatment is to delay fusion to a more optimal age (age 10 years in girls and age 12 in boys). Good results have been obtained in many patients, provided the bracing was begun before any structural curve developed and provided the bracing was continuous.[14] Exercises and other forms of nonoperative treatment are *not* of any value for polio curves. For lumbar curves, the modern molded plastic braces are quite useful. For thoracic curves, a Milwaukee brace is best. Under no circumstances should the chest cage be compressed. This is one great advantage of the Milwaukee brace. Releases of contractures about the hip (e.g., flexors and iliotibial bands) may be useful in conjunction with bracing. For details of bracing, see Chapter 15 (Figs. 8–14 and 8–15).

To be effective, bracing must be applied early in the development of the curve. The basic purpose of the brace is to *prevent* the development of a serious curvature. In essence, any curve of 20 degrees or greater on an erect film should be braced.

## SURGICAL TREATMENT

The surgical technique for these curves is no different than for other types of curves; i.e., a careful subperiosteal exposure, meticulous facet excision and grafting, thorough decortication, instrumentation, and the addition of autogenous bone graft. These techniques are well covered in Chapter 21 and need not be repeated here. However, the timing of surgery, the selection of the fusion area, whether or not to use traction, whether or not to do anterior surgery in addition to posterior, and what type of immobilization to use are all topics needing discussion.

***Timing of Surgery.*** Surgery should not be done either too early or too late. Since the area fused will no longer grow, and since the poliomyelitis patient usually requires a long fusion, an early arthrodesis will significantly stunt the growth of the spine. Nevertheless, it may still be necessary to do early fusion when the curve is too severe to brace or the brace is not controlling the curve. The alternative is that the child will be even shorter, because of the progressive curve, plus the obvious disadvantages of the curve itself. Generally speaking, one would like to fuse the spine just before the adolescent growth spurt, since it is at this moment that curve progression accelerates and bracing tends to fail.

Since individuals vary considerably as to when the growth spurt occurs, it is best to observe the child for the early signs of puberty (e.g., pubic hair development) and do the fusion at that time. From a practical point of view, as long as the brace is controlling the curve (maintaining a curve of 40 degrees or less), nonoperative treatment can continue. Whenever the brace loses its ability to control the curve, fusion should be done, regardless of the age. Under no circumstances should fusion be delayed until the end of growth (Figs. 8–15 and 8–16).

***Selection of Fusion Area.*** The most common error we see in patients coming to us after fusion elsewhere is too short a fusion. The paralytic patient needs a long fusion. How does one select exactly the proper length? The decision is based on both clinical and radiographic criteria. The goal of surgery is to stabilize the spine in an optimal position. That optimal position is a level pelvis, a vertical torso centered over the level pelvis, and the head centered over the thorax and pelvis. Does the patient have only scoliosis, or is there kyphosis or lordosis also? Is it a collapsing spine, or does the patient have some muscle control of the spine? Does the patient have head and neck control? Is the head tilted to one side by a curve extending up into the neck? These clinical features are of utmost importance.

Radiologically, one needs long films showing the entire area from the head to the pelvis. The films of most value for the selection of the fusion area are the sitting AP and the lateral fims. The absolute minimum fusion area is the measured curve area. One should *never* fuse less than this. For polio patients, more length is required. All rotated vertebrae must be fused, and the fusion should

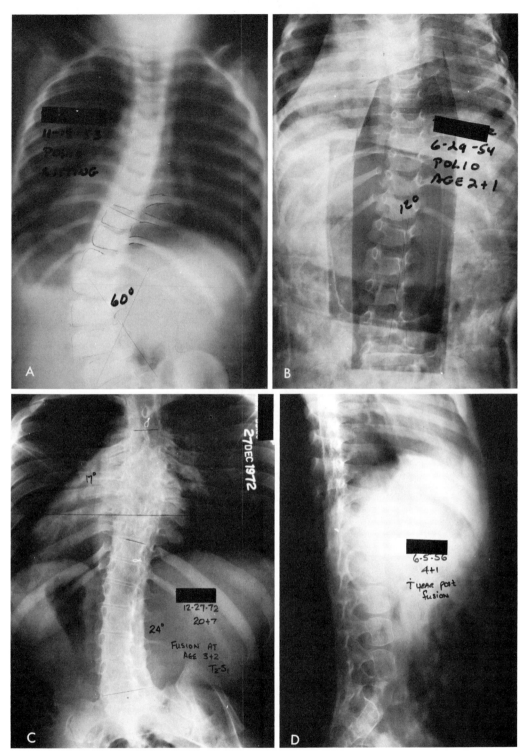

**Figure 8–16**  *A,* This one year and six month old boy suffered poliomyelitis at the age of three months. He presented to the authors at this age with a 60 degree lumbar curve and marked pelvic obliquity in the sitting position. *B,* The patient was placed in a Risser cast to test the ability to control this curve nonoperatively. It was possible to maintain the curve at 12 degrees in the cast. Nonoperative treatment should have continued until early adolescence or until such time as the curve went out of control in the brace. *C,* The patient underwent fusion from T3 to the sacrum at the age of three years and two months. This x-ray was taken at the age of 20 years and 7 months, 17 years and 4 months after the fusion. A solid fusion is noted. There is some mild residual pelvic obliquity. There are no sclerotic changes about the sacroiliac joints, a frequently voiced fear of long fusions to the sacrum. Metallic markers were imbedded in the fusion at the time of surgery and measured at yearly intervals thereafter. There was only 3 mm. of lengthening of the fusion mass in the 17 years following the fusion. Young fusions do not grow. *D,* This lateral x-ray was taken one year following the spine fusion. The spine is straight without either lordosis or kyphosis.

**226**

*Legend continued on opposite page*

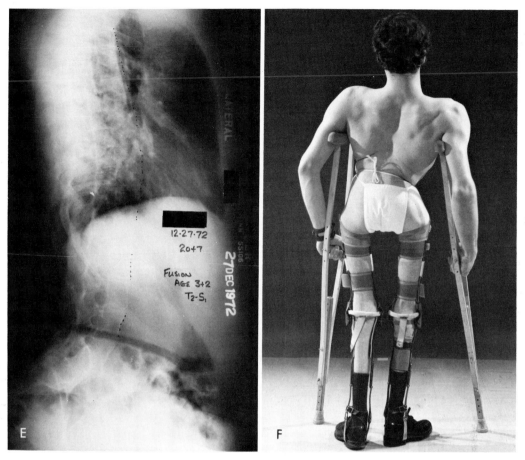

**Figure 8–16** *Continued.* *E*, A lateral x-ray 16 years later shows some increase of lordosis, particularly in the lower thoracic area. This indicates that there has been a slight bit of anterior growth with bending of the fusion posteriorly. In this particular case, the amount of lordosis is minimal. More severe lordosis has been reported by others. The thicker the posterior fusion mass, the less likely it is that lordosis will occur, owing to anterior growth. *F*, A posterior photograph of the patient at age 20. Note the relatively normal torso-leg proportion. Although the torso is quite short owing to the early fusion, the legs are short owing to the extensive bilateral paralysis. His total body height is in the third percentile.

extend to the first nonrotated vertebra. In addition, the top and bottom of the fusion area should lie in a line directly above the center of the sacrum. This provides balance of the fusion mass and prevents curve lengthening.

Collapsing spines require fusion from the upper thorax to the sacrum.[51] Fusion to the sacrum is always necessary for the collapsing type of spinal deformity. It is *not* always necessary for the noncollapsing type of polio curve. Purely thoracic structural curves with good lumbar musculature and no pelvic obliquity do not require fusion to the sacrum. Do all patients with pelvic obliquity require fusion to the sacrum? No, not if the pelvic obliquity is caused by iliotibial band contractures that can be released. When the sacrum

behaves like a segment of the curve, it must be included in the fusion. When there is obvious asymmetry of the lumbar and abdominal wall muscles, the fusion should extend to the sacrum (Fig. 8–17).

***Preoperative Traction.*** If at all possible, traction should be avoided. The 13 year old child with a 60 degree curve does not need traction. At this age, there is sufficient "slack" in the curve to allow a decent correction, which can be obtained readily on the operating table. For this reason, we have found the preoperative bending and/or stretch films to be of considerable value in patient evaluation. If on the bending or distraction film, an acceptable correction is noted, preoperative traction is unnecessary. Not only is it unnecessary, but

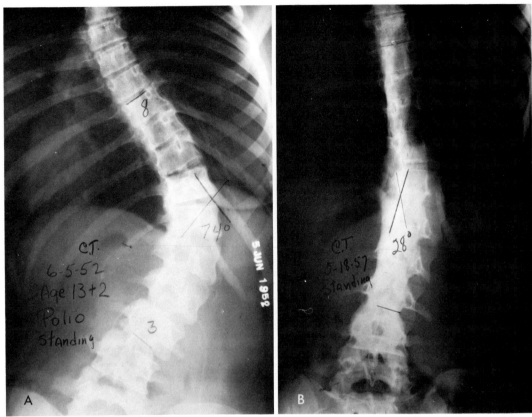

**Figure 8–17** *A,* This 13 year old girl has a curvature due to poliomyelitis. There is a 74 degree T8–L3 right thoracolumbar curve. Note that above T8 and below L3 there is an immediate development of compensatory curves and the pelvis is level. This is an example of the type of poliomyelitis curve that does *not* require fusion to the sacrum. Note that T7 is rotated in the same direction as T8, and the apex of the curve, and T6 is neutral in rotation. T6 is also centralized above the sacrum. Note that L3 is significantly rotated but L4 is not. The fusion area should be T6 to L4. *B,* This x-ray, five years later, shows a solid fusion. This case demonstrates well that metallic fixation is not absolutely necessary for scoliosis correction. Good corrections can be obtained by good cast techniques. Correction was maintained by a good arthrodesis.

also it is time consuming, expensive, and psychologically unpleasant, and it may result in complications in and of itself. The paralytic patient is already osteoporotic; why make him more so? (See Fig. 8–23.)

Traction has proved beneficial for curves of large magnitude, especially when soft tissue contractures have made the curve "tight." It is especially valuable for patients with limited vital capacity due to the curve. Placing the patient in traction for two or three weeks may significantly improve the vital capacity, thus making the patient a better operative risk. If the patient presents with cor pulmonale, six to eight weeks of traction may be needed to reverse the cardiac decompensation and create an operable patient.

For patients presenting with pelvic obliquity that does not fully correct on the bend or stretch film, traction with a single femoral pin on the "high" side of the pelvis will gradually correct the pelvic obliquity. At surgery, one then has a much easier task, since the correction has already been accomplished and only stabilization is required (Figs. 8–18 and 8–19).

***Anterior Surgery.*** When, if ever, is anterior surgery necessary for poliomyelitis curvatures? Generally speaking, one should never have to do anterior surgery, provided that the patients all came with mild to moderate deformities and were still in the growing years. Poliomyelitis curves were treated quite successfully long before anterior surgery was devised.

At the present time, the main indication for anterior surgery is in the lumbar or thoracolumbar "C" curve with the severe pelvic obliquity. Traditional methods of traction and posterior fusion with instrumentation often failed to fully correct the pelvic obliquity. The advent of the Dwyer procedure has markedly improved our ability to correct and stabilize this type of curve. O'Brien and Yau[42] reported three patients treated by both the Dwyer and the Harrington procedures. One patient was corrected from 72 degrees to zero, the second from 85 degrees to 12 degrees, and the third from 70 degrees to 18 degrees. A more extensive paper on this subject was subsequently published by O'Brien et al.[43] Not only is there excellent correction of the pelvic obliquity but also there is rigid internal fixation both front and back, and an interbody fusion is obtained in addition to the posterior fusion. Pseudarthrosis is most unlikely. The Dwyer procedure alone is *never* sufficient for the paralytic poliomyelitis patient. In our opinion, the C curve is the only real indication for anterior fusion in the polio patient (Fig. 8–20).

***Harrington Rods.*** Harrington instruments were originally designed for the poliomyelitis patient. Paul Harrington recognized that the traditional methods of cast correction, especially the turnbuckle cast, had serious deleterious effects on pulmonary function. Although the patient's spine looked straighter on the x-ray after fusion, his lungs didn't work as well.[18, 47, 57] A method of internal correction was needed, and Dr. Harrington successfully met that need.

This original purpose of the Harrington rods still holds true today. Internal fixation is very useful in most curves, and particularly so in severe curves, patients with decreased pulmonary function, and patients with pelvic obliquity.[19, 44]

The use of Harrington rods in poliomyelitis curves is more complex than in the idiopathic patient. When fusing to the sacrum, a long rod should be used, contouring as necessary for thoracic kyphosis and lumbar lordosis. Against the sacrum, we use an alar hook placed on the ala just lateral to the articular facet of S1. If the rod has been bent for lumbar lordosis, a square-ended rod and a square-holed hook should be used to prevent rotation. When fusing the lumbar spine, a bilateral transverse process fusion should be done. Bonnett et al. from Rancho Los Amigos have reported an extensive series of paralytic patients.[6] This article is strongly recommended to the reader.

Harrington rods should not be placed into the cervical spine. When a curve needs fusion up to the neck, a halo cast is mandatory for postoperative immobilization. Rods can be inserted as high as T1, and the fusion can be extended. For extensive neck paralysis, with the ability to hold up the head, fusion to the occiput can be done. This will markedly improve the patient's functional capacity.[46]

***Postoperative Immobilization.*** No single type of postoperative immobilization is best. Several modalities must be available, depending upon the patient's curve area, curve severity, pulmonary function, patient reliability, and patient age. The Milwaukee brace was originally invented for the postoperative support of the poliomyelitis patient.[3] At that time, the patient was kept recumbent for six to eight months and then gradually ambulated. This was because there was no internal fixation, and curve correction could not be maintained when upright. With secure internal fixation by Harrington rods, the Milwaukee brace gives good external immobilization, is lighter in weight than a cast, permits full chest expansion, is "air-conditioned," and can be opened for skin inspection and bed baths. The main disadvantages are the need for a skilled orthotist and its "removability" by the unreliable patient.

For the patient with minimal pulmonary function deficit and good leg strength, a standard Risser-Cotrel cast has been used at this center with excellent results.

For the patient with a fusion extending high into the cervical spine, a halo cast or halo-Milwaukee brace is essential. Halo casts have also been found useful for patients with large thoracic curves, soft bone, and poor pulmonary function. The halo cast permits prompt ambulation, prevents hook dislocation by decreasing the forces on the Harrington hooks, and allows large windows to be cut, thus permitting full chest expansion. Pressure on the chest wall is not necessary for curve protection. The halo hoop may be useful on rare occasions to obtain correction but should never be used for long-term immobilization.

For the patient with a lumbar or thoracolumbar curve, halo casts or Risser casts are not necessary, provided adequate internal fixation is present. In these patients, an underarm body cast is sufficient. Recently we have switched to lightweight casts made of fiber glass or lightweight plastic body jackets

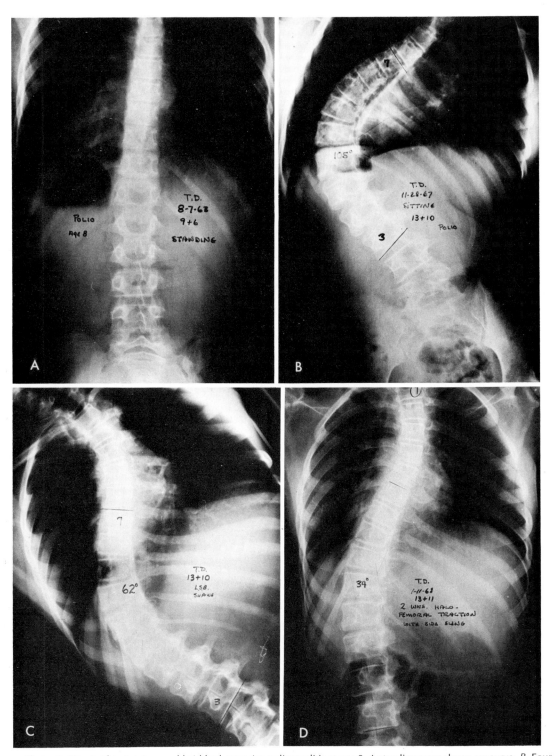

**Figure 8–18**   *A,* This 9 + 6 year old girl had extensive poliomyelitis at age 8. A standing x-ray shows no curve. *B,* Four years later, at age 13, she presented to the authors with a 105 degree curve in the sitting position. She had been under constant care by "rehabilitation experts" the entire four years. They had totally ignored her spine. *C,* On passive supine left bending, the curve measures 62 degrees, documenting its structural nature. *D,* After two weeks of halofemoral traction, the curve was 34 degrees.

*Legend continued on opposite page*

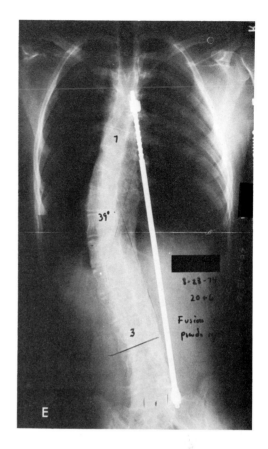

**Figure 8–18** *Continued.* *E,* Six years later (5½ years after pseudarthrosis repair) her curve is solidly fused at 39 degrees.

(the bivalved polypropylene body jacket) similar to those used for patients with myelomeningocele. The light weight of the plastic supports usually increases the patient's functional capacity considerably.

What if the fusion extends to the sacrum? Should one or both thighs be included in the cast? Is bed rest mandatory? Formerly we felt that both a longer cast plus six months of bed rest were necessary. *This is no longer true.* Even when the fusion extends to the sacrum, the cast or brace does *not* immobilize the hips, and the patients are back to upright activities within two weeks of surgery. Although not completely avoided, pseudarthroses have been less frequent with this program than formerly.

## MANAGEMENT OF THE PATIENT WITH LIMITED PULMONARY FUNCTION

Poliomyelitis patients are often limited in their breathing capacity, owing to intercostal and abdominal muscle paralysis. Careful evaluation of pulmonary function should be done of all patients for whom surgery is planned. If the patient has 40 per cent or better of normal vital capacity and has an effective cough, complications are relatively unlikely. Surgery can proceed without need for tracheotomy, nasotracheal intubation, or positive ventilatory support.[35, 40]

The patient with an ineffective cough needs either a nasotracheal tube or a tracheotomy in order that secretions can be adequately removed in the immediate postoperative period. Once the patient is no longer receiving narcotics and is in the upright position, he is back to his preoperative status and no longer needs the tube or positive ventilatory support.[39]

The Rancho group still prefers preoperative tracheotomy for high-risk patients. At the Twin Cities Scoliosis Center, we have abandoned preoperative tracheotomy and prefer to use postoperative nasotracheal intubation with positive ventilatory support for the first few days after surgery. Once the surgical pain is gone, the patient is weaned off the respirator, and then the tube is removed. We have not done a tracheotomy in the past five years.

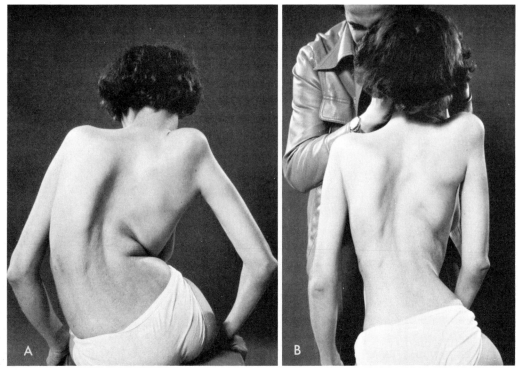

**Figure 8–19**   *A,* This 28 year old poliomyelitis victim has a 118 degree scoliosis in the sitting position. *B,* Simple suspension of the patient shows marked correction of her curve (to 42 degrees). This is an example of a "collapsing" curve, and traction prior to surgery is not necessary for such curves.

Most nasotracheal tubes have been removed in four to five days, the longest being in for nine days (Fig. 8–21).

### Spinal Muscle Atrophy

*NATURAL HISTORY AND REVIEW OF LITERATURE*

This entity has had many other names — Werdnig-Hoffmann disease, Kugelberg-Welander Disease, amyotonia congenita, etc. At the present time, a wide spectrum of clinical manifestations are gathered under the single title of spinal muscle atrophy. This is a disorder of the anterior horn cells and is thus actually a lower motor neuron disorder and not a muscle disease. In the earlier onset type (Werdnig-Hoffmann) the infants are very "floppy," and many of them die by the age of six, usually of respiratory failure. In a few of these patients, the disease ceases to progress and they live a full life span, usually with severe paralysis.[55, 61]

A later onset type (Kugelberg-Welander) makes itself apparent in midchildhood. This type is slower to progress, most children remaining ambulatory until age 13 to 15.[45]

Hardy[22] reviewed 88 children, dividing them into two groups, those dying early and those surviving beyond age 7. Scoliosis was present in only 19 per cent of those under age 5, in 58 per cent between 6 and 11, and in 84 per cent of those age 12 or older. The Milwaukee brace was helpful in some. Spine fusion was considered necessary in progressive curves. Owing to the respiratory compromise in these children, special attention to the lungs was strongly recommended.

Dorr et al.[11] reviewed 34 patients who were treated surgically. The curves were long and nonresponsive to bracing, and the average fusion was 18 levels. Postoperative respiratory assistance by positive pressure was frequently needed. The average period of postoperative support was 17 months. Internal fixation with Harrington rods was important. The Dwyer procedure was quite helpful for lumbar lordoscoliosis.

*NONOPERATIVE TREATMENT*

Like all collapsing-spine problems, bracing must begin early, before the development

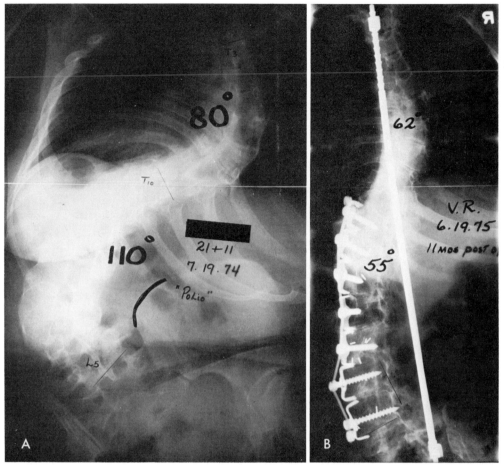

**Figure 8–20** *A,* This 21 year old female has a post-poliomyelitis scoliosis with an 80 degree right thoracic curve and a 110 degree left lumbar curve plus severe pelvic obliquity. The goal of treatment here is to obtain a level pelvis and two balanced curves above. A halo plus a single femoral pin on the right were used for two weeks, followed by a Dwyer procedure and, two weeks later, a posterior spine fusion with Harrington instrumentation. *B,* Eleven months following combined anterior and posterior instrumentation and fusion.

of structural deformity. Milwaukee braces are not well tolerated by these patients, and bivalved polypropylene body jackets seem to work best. The brace will be necessary as long as there is growth, or until the curve shows progression despite the brace.

### SURGICAL TREATMENT

The indications for surgery are similar to those stated previously for the collapsing spine in poliomyelitis or spinal cord injury. Since these children already have respiratory compromise due to their muscle weakness, the physician must not allow the curve to progress to the point of further respiratory compromise. In surgical management, particular attention must be directed toward pulmonary function, which must be tested preoperatively.

Those with *severe* limitation should have preoperative tracheostomy and positive respiratory support. Those with borderline moderate to severe limitation may require tracheostomy but usually do well with nasotracheal intubation and positive support for three to seven days postoperatively until pain has decreased and narcotic support is no longer needed. With a vital capacity of 40 per cent or greater, supported respiration is rarely needed.

Internal fixation with Harrington rods is virtually essential. Usually two rods are preferable in order to distribute the fixation forces over four purchase points rather than two.

Fusion from the upper thoracic spine to the sacrum is always necessary. One should use either the large alar hooks or a transsacral

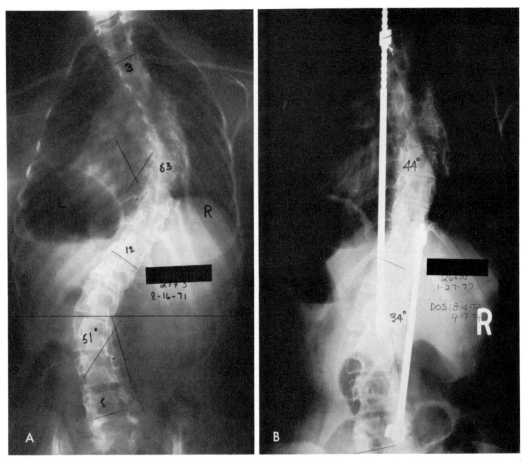

**Figure 8–21**   *A,* A post-poliomyelitis patient with respiratory function so severely involved that she must use a rocking bed at night and can breathe only upright during the day using accessory muscles of respiration. *B,* She was fused in 1972 with a preoperative tracheostomy and positive ventilation for 10 days postoperatively. She was ambulated in a halo cast, and the tracheostomy was found unnecessary and was removed. A pseudarthrosis required further surgery in 1973, at which time a nasotracheal tube was used rather than a tracheostomy. She required the nasal tube for only three days.

bar. Little bone is obtained from the iliac crest, and homogenous bank bone or parental bone should be added.

Postoperative immobilization is best done with a bivalved polypropylene body jacket or some other type of very lightweight but rigid support, well molded to the patient's new contour. The hips should not be immobilized, and the patient should be returned to the upright position as soon as possible. Immobilization time is prolonged, at least 15 to 18 months (Fig. 8–22).

## DYSAUTONOMIA (RILEY-DAY SYNDROME)

This is a rare autosomal recessive disorder found exclusively in children of Ashkenazi Jewish origin and was first described in 1949.[31] There are profound disturbances of autonomic nervous system functions with decreased or absent tears, unstable tempera-

ture regulation, unstable blood pressure, and excessive perspiration. Many have a disturbed swallowing reflex, leading to frequent aspiration. Scoliosis is frequent, occurring in 90 per cent of those age 10 years. The patterns "look" idiopathic rather than paralytic, but there is a high frequency of kyphoscoliosis rather than lordoscoliosis.[31]

Spine fusion has been performed in a few patients, but the risks are high. Bracing is frought with many problems, especially pressure sores due to poor skin sensation.[64]

## MYOPATHIC DISORDERS

### Duchenne Muscular Dystrophy

Spine deformity is common in patients with this condition. Lordosis is often the presenting complaint at the time of the first diagnosis of muscle disease. This lordosis is caused by weakness of the hip extensors,

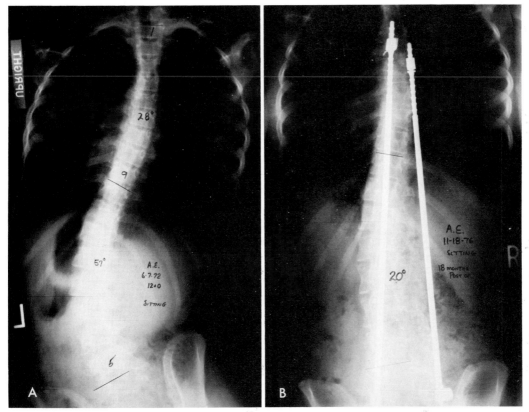

**Figure 8–22** *A,* A 12 year old girl with spinal muscle atrophy and a progressive collapsing scoliosis problem. *B,* Fusion from T5 to the sacrum was performed utilizing two long distraction rods and a broad transverse process fusion. Both iliac crests were used for bone graft. This x-ray is 18 months following fusion. Brace treatment had been attempted from 1972 to 1975.

which are the first muscles around the pelvis to become involved, and active extension of the trunk by the patient in order to maintain the center of gravity over the feet.[58] Later, lordosis is accentuated by hip flexion contractures. Scoliosis seldom occurs in the child who is still ambulatory. Bunch[8] describes two patterns of scoliosis onset, one occurring before cessation of walking (rare), and the second after one to three years of wheelchair existence (common).

Siegel[56] stated that "almost all" patients with Duchenne dystrophy develop scoliosis after going to the wheelchair. Robin and Brief[49] analyzed 27 patients with various types of childhood muscular dystrophy. Of these, 24 had spine deformity, 23 with scoliosis, the other with severe lordosis. The curves were typically long, thoracolumbar, and with pelvic obliquity. Eleven curves progressed rapidly (15 degrees to 30 degrees per year) during later growth. The curves were characteristic of the collapsing spine.

Dubowitz,[12, 13] in a review of 63 children

with Duchenne dystrophy, noted no scoliosis in those still ambulatory or in a wheelchair for one year or less. Of the 50 children who had been off their feet one year or more, 32 had scoliosis. Dubowitz recommended the routine use of a well-molded plastic body jacket as soon as the child lost ambulation.

Wilkins and Gibson[63] analyzed 62 patients in the later stages of Duchenne dystrophy, all having ceased ambulation. Several observations were made from the x-rays, including kyphotic index, sacral angle, lateral curvature, vertebral rotation, and pelvic rotation. Five patterns of deformity were noted: Group I consisted of patients with early straight spines (9 patients); Group II, kyphotic spines (16 patients) with minimal scoliosis but conversion of the normal lumbar lordosis to lumbar kyphosis with a vertical sacrum; Group III, kyphoscoliotic spines (9 patients) with severe scoliosis, pelvic obliquity and lumbar kyphosis; Group IV (14 patients), scoliosis without kyphosis, this group having the most severe deformities; and Group V (14

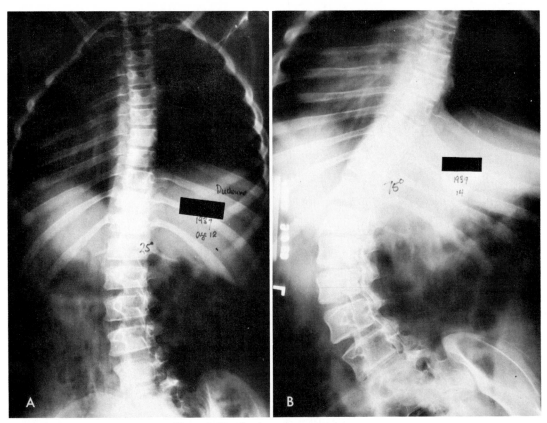

**Figure 8–23** *See legend on opposite page*

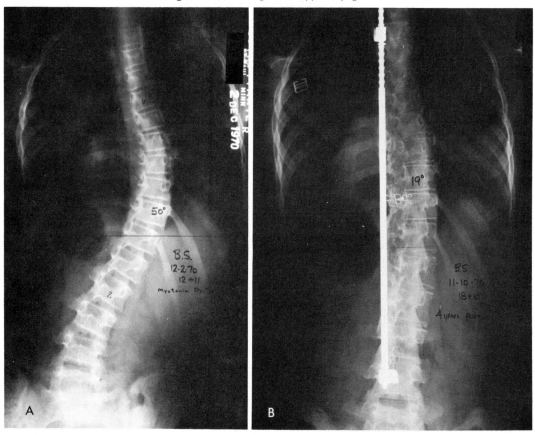

**Figure 8–24** *See legend on opposite page*

patients), "extended" spines. Group V had little deformity, and the spine was stiff in this position. These authors suggested that treatment should be directed toward developing this extended spine position and in this way perhaps avoiding the other more disabling deformities.

Nonoperative treatment is usually preferable, since most patients do not develop significant scoliosis until about age 12 and usually die by age 18, thus making surgery of doubtful benefit. Milwaukee braces are not well tolerated, and the orthosis of choice is either a well molded bivalved firm plastic body jacket or a specially molded plastic wheelchair insert. These should be started as soon as a curve of 20 degrees or more is noted in the sitting position. Routine sitting x-rays every six months are recommended. Bracing is not necessary while the patient is recumbent (Fig. 8–23).

## Limb-Girdle Dystrophy, Facioscapulohumeral Dystrophy, and Dystrophia Myotonica

These dystrophies are less common than Duchenne dystrophy but have a much better prognosis. Siegel[56] states, "The childhood form of facioscapulohumeral dystrophy is often complicated by scoliosis, which can be treated with traditional methods of corrective plaster, spinal surgery, and orthoses, such as the Milwaukee brace. Patients with dystrophia myotonica or limb-girdle dystrophy seldom develop structural scoliosis."

Our experience with these conditions is limited. We have seen three patients with scoliosis due to dystrophia myotonica, one of whom required spine fusion. One patient has been seen with scoliosis due to limb-girdle dystrophy. This was, however, a severe 105 degree thoracic curve with significant respiratory compromise (Fig. 8–24).

## References

1. Akbarnia, B., Winter, R. B., Moe, J. H., Bradford, D. S., and Lonstein, J. E.: Surgical treatment of spine deformity in cerebral palsy. Scoliosis Research Society, Ottawa, 1976.

2. Balmer, G. A., and MacEwen, G. D.: The incidence and treatment of scoliosis in cerebral palsy. J. Bone Joint Surg., 52B:134–137, 1970.
3. Blount, W. P., Schmidt, A. C., Kevver, D., and Leonard, E. L.: The Milwaukee brace in the operative treatment of scoliosis. J. Bone Joint Surg., 40A:511, 1958.
4. Bonnett, C., Brown, J., and Brooks, H. L.: Anterior spine fusion with Dwyer instrumentation for lumbar scoliosis in cerebral palsy. J. Bone Joint Surg., 55A:425, 1973.
5. Bonnett, C. Perry, J., and Brown, J.: Cord injury and spine deformity in children. Presented at the Scoliosis Research Society, 1972.
6. Bonnett, C., Brown, J., Perry, J., Nickel, V., Walinski, T., Brooks, H. L., Hoffer, M., Stiles, C., and Brooks, R.: The evolution of treatment of paralytic scoliosis at Rancho Los Amigos Hospital. J. Bone Joint Surg., 57A:206–215, 1975.
7. Bonnett, C. A.: The cord injured child. In Lovell, W. W., and Winter, R. B. (eds.): Children's Orthopaedics. Philadelphia, J. B. Lippincott, 1978.
8. Bunch, W. H.: Muscular dystrophy. In Hardy, J. H. (ed.): Spinal Deformity in Neurological and Muscular Disorders. St. Louis, C. V. Mosby Co., 1974.
9. Campbell, J., and Bonnett, C.: Spinal cord injury in children. Clin. Orthop.,112:112–114, 1975.
10. Colonna, P. C., and Vom Saal, F.: A study of paralytic scoliosis based on 500 cases of poliomyelitis. J. Bone Joint Surg., 23:335, 1941.
11. Dorr, J., Brown, J., and Perry, J.: Results of posterior spine fusion in patients with spinal muscle atrophy — A review of 34 cases. Presented at the Scoliosis Research Society, 1972.
12. Dubowitz, V.: Progressive muscular dystrophy: Prevention of deformities. Clin. Pediatr., 3:323–328, 1964.
13. Dubowitz, V.: Some clinical observations on childhood muscular dystrophy., Br. J. Clin. Pract., 17: 283–288, 1963.
14. Duval-Beaupere, G., Poiffaut, A., Bovier, C. L., Garibol, J. C., and Assicot, J.: Plexidur jackets for correction of paralytic scoliosis. Results after seven years. Acta. Orthop. Belg., 41:652, 1975.
15. Forgan, L., and Munsat, T. L.: Spinocerebellar degenerative diseases. In Hardy, J. H. (ed.): Spinal Deformity in Neurological and Muscular Disorders. C. V. Mosby Co., St. Louis, 1974.
16. Garrett, A. L., Perry, J., and Nickel, V. L.: Paralytic scoliosis. Clin. Orthop., 21:117, 1961.
17. Garrett, A. L., Perry, J., and Nickel, V. L.: Stabilization of the collapsing spine. J. Bone Joint Surg., 43A: 474, 1961.
18. Gucker, T.: Experience in poliomyelitic scoliosis after correction and fusion. J. Bone Joint Surg., 38A: 1281, 1956.
19. Gui, L., Savini, R., Vicenzi, G., and Ponzo, L.: Surgical treatment of poliomyelitic scoliosis. Ital. J. Orthop. Traumat., 2:191–205, 1976.
20. Haas, S. L.: Spastic scoliosis and obliquity of the pelvis. J. Bone Joint Surg., 24:774–780, 1942.

**Figure 8–23**   A, An AP supine x-ray of a 12 year old boy with Duchenne hypertrophic muscular dystrophy. There is a 25 degree curve with rotation and early pelvic obliquity. B, The same patient just two years later, showing a 75 degree curve and severe pelvic obliquity. This pattern of curvature is typical of the patient with Duchenne dystrophy.

**Figure 8–24**   A, A 12 year old girl with scoliosis due to myotonic dystrophy. For curves with this lateral displacement of the thorax, the fusion must extend to L4. B, Four years following spine fusion from T4 to L4. The patient is still ambulatory. Her neurologic condition is stable.

21. Hamel, A., and Moe, J. H.: The collapsing spine. Surgery, 56:364, 1964.

22. Hardy, J.: Neuromuscular scoliosis. J. Bone Joint Surg., 52A:407–408, 1970.

23. Hensinger, R. N., and MacEwen, G. D.: Spinal deformity associated with heritable neurological conditions: Spinal muscle atrophy, Friedreich's ataxia, familial dysautonomia, and Charot-Marie-Tooth disease. J. Bone Joint Surg., 58A:13–24, 1976.

24. Hipps, H. E.: Changes in the growing spine produced by anterior poliomyelitis. Clin. Orthop., 21:96–105, 1961.

25. Huebert, H. T., and MacKinnon, W. B.: Syringomyelia and scoliosis. J. Bone Joint Surg., 51B:338–343, 1969.

26. Irwin, C. E.: The iliotibial band: Its role in producing deformity in poliomyelitis. J. Bone Joint Surg., 31A:141–146, 1949.

27. James, J. I. P.: Paralytic scoliosis. J. Bone Joint Surg., 38B:660, 1956.

28. James, J. I. P.: Scoliosis. Edinburgh, London, and New York, Churchill-Livingstone, 1967.

29. Kilfoyle, R. M., Foley, J. J., and Norton, P. L.: Spine and pelvic deformity in childhood and adolescent paraplegia—A study of 104 cases. J. Bone Joint Surg., 47A:659–682, 1965.

30. Levine, D. B.: Poliomyelitis. In Hardy, J. H. (ed.): Spinal Deformity in Neurological and Muscular Disorders. St. Louis, C. V. Mosby, 1974.

31. Levine, D. B.: Orthopaedic aspects of familial dysautonomia. In Zorab, P. A. (ed.): Scoliosis and Muscle. Philadelphia, J. B. Lippincott, 1974. (Spastics International Medical Publications.)

32. MacEwen, G. D.: Cerebral palsy and scoliosis. In Hardy, J. H. (ed.): Spinal Deformity in Neurological and Muscular Disorders. St. Louis, C. V. Mosby, 1974.

33. MacEwen, G. D.: Operative treatment of scoliosis in cerebral palsy. Reconstr. Surg. Traumatol., 13:58–67, 1972.

34. Makin, M.: Spinal problems of childhood paraplegia. Isr. J. Med. Sci., 9:732, 1973.

35. Makley, J., Herndon, C., Inkley, S., Dvershuk, C., Matthews, L., Post, R., and Littell, A. S.: Pulmonary function in paralytic and non-paralytic scoliosis, before and after treatment: A study of 63 cases. J. Bone Joint Surg., 50A:1379–1390, 1968.

36. Mayer, L.: Further studies of fixed paralytic pelvic obliquity. J. Bone Joint Surg., 18:87–100, 1936.

37. McSweeny, T.: Spinal deformity after spinal cord injury. Paraplegia, 6:212, 1969.

38. Moe, J. H.: The management of paralytic scoliosis. South. Med. J., 50:67, 1957.

39. Nickel, V., Perry, J., Affeldt, J., and Dail, C.: Elective surgery on patients with respiratory paralysis. J. Bone Joint Surg., 39A:989, 1957.

40. Nickel, V., and Perry, J.: Respiratory evaluation of patients for major surgery. In The American Academy of Orthopaedic Surgeons Instructional Course Lectures, vol. 18. St. Louis, C. V. Mosby, 1961.

41. Norton, P. L., and Foley, J. J.: Paraplegia in children. J. Bone Joint Surg., 41A:1291–1309, 1959.

42. O'Brien, J. P., and Yau, A. C.: Anterior and posterior correction and fusion for paralytic scoliosis. Clin. Orthop., 86:151–153, 1972.

43. O'Brien, J. P., Dwyer, A. P., and Hodgson, A. R.: Paralytic pelvic obliquity—Its prognosis and management and the development of a technique for full correction of the deformity. J. Bone Joint Surg., 57A:626–631, 1975.

44. Pavon, S. J., and Manning, C.: Posterior spine fusion for scoliosis due to anterior poliomyelitis. J. Bone Joint Surg., 52A:420–431, 1970.

45. Pearn, J. H.: Scoliosis in the spinal muscle atrophies of childhood. In Zorab, P. A. (ed.): Scoliosis and Muscle. Philadelphia, J. B. Lippincott, 1974. (Spastics International Medical Publications.)

46. Perry, J., and Nickel, V. L.: Total cervical spine fusion for neck paralysis. J. Bone Joint Surg., 41A:37, 1959.

47. Roaf, R.: Paralytic scoliosis. J. Bone Joint Surg., 38B:640, 1956.

48. Roaf, R.: Scoliosis secondary to paraplegia. Paraplegia, 8:42–47, 1970.

49. Robin, G. C., and Brief, L. P.: Scoliosis in childhood muscular dystrophy. J. Bone Joint Surg., 53A:466–476, 1971.

50. Robin, G. C.: Surgical treatment of paralytic scoliosis. Isr. J. Med. Sci., 9:813, 1973.

51. Robin, G. C.: Treatment of the paralytic collapsing spine. S. Afr. J. Surg., 9:173–182, 1971.

52. Robson, P.: The prevalence of scoliosis in adolescents and yount adults with cerebral palsy. Dev. Med. Child Neurol., 10:447–452, 1968.

53. Rosenthal, R. K., Levine, D. B., and McCarver, C. L.: The occurrence of scoliosis in cerebral palsy. Dev. Med. Child Neurol., 16:664–667, 1974.

54. Samilson, R., and Bechard, R.: Scoliosis in cerebral palsy: Incidence, distribution of curve patterns, natural history, and thoughts on etiology. Curr. Pract. Orthop. Surg., 5:183–205, 1973.

55. Schwentker, E. P., and Gibson, D. A.: The orthopaedic aspects of spinal muscular atrophy. J. Bone Joint Surg., 58A:32–38, 1976.

56. Siegel, I. M.: Scoliosis in muscular dystrophy. Clin. Orthop., 93:235–238, 1973.

57. Simmons, E., and Weber, F. A.: The associations of syringomyelia and scoliosis. J. Bone Joint Surg., 56B:589, 1974.

58. Spencer, G. E., Jr.: Orthopaedic Considerations in the Management of Muscular Dystrophy. Curr. Pract. Orthop. Surg., 5:279–293, 1973.

59. Stauffer, E. S.: Trauma. In Hardy, J. H. (ed.): Spinal Deformity in Neurological and Muscular Disorders. St. Louis, C. V. Mosby, 1974.

60. Tachdjian, M., and Matson, D. D.: Orthopaedic aspects of intra-spinal tumors in infants and children. J. Bone Joint Surg., 47A:223–248, 1965.

61. Tsairis, P.: Motor unit disorders. In Hardy, J. H. (ed.): Spinal Deformity in Neurological and Muscular Disorders. St. Louis, C. V. Mosby Co., 1974.

62. Wedge, J. H., and Gillespie, R.: The problems of scoliosis surgery in paraplegic children. J. Bone Joint Surg., 57B:536, 1975.

63. Wilkins, K. E., and Gibson, D. A.: The patterns of spinal deformity in Duchenne muscular dystrophy. J. Bone Joint Surg., 58A:24–32, 1976.

64. Yoslow, W., Beeker, M. H., Bartels, J., and Thompson, W.: Orthopaedic defects in familial dysautonomia: A review of 65 cases. J. Bone Joint Surg., 53A:1541–1550, 1971.

# Chapter 9

# MYELOMENINGOCELE

## INTRODUCTION

Of all the causes of spine deformity, myelomeningocele is the most severe and most difficult to treat. The advances in neurosurgery with early sac closure and effective shunting procedures for hydrocephalus, coupled with the advances in urology with management of the paralytic bladder, have led to an increased survival rate for these children. When they become older, spine deformity becomes an increasingly prominent problem. All too often the spinal deformity becomes so severe and creates such a disability that all previous rehabilitative efforts are destroyed.

The treatment of these spinal deformities has advanced remarkably in the past ten years. Problems once thought difficult are now routine, and problems once thought impossible are being conquered. We now have the capability to manage any spine deformity in myelomeningocele. The challenge is how to do it with the most safety, efficiency, and reliability.

A word of caution is worthwhile. These children are best managed in centers accustomed to and competent in the general care of the child with myelomeningocele. Their spine deformity cannot be treated in isolation from their other problems. A team effort is essential.

A second word of caution also seems necessary. The orthopedic surgeon caring for the spine problem must be highly experienced in scoliosis treatment. The person must *first* have mastered the treatment of idiopathic scoliosis and *second* must have mastered the

treatment of other neuromuscular spine deformities. Only then should that person proceed with the myelodysplastic child. A sound foundation in the principles of scoliosis is essential.

## NATURAL HISTORY

### Classification

- I. Developmental (paralytic)
  - A. Scoliosis
  - B. Lordosis
  - C. Kyphosis
  - D. Lordoscoliosis
  - E. Kyphoscoliosis
- II. Congenital
  - A. Scoliosis
  - B. Lordosis
  - C. Kyphosis
- III. Mixed

### REVIEW OF THE LITERATURE

Raycroft and Curtis[35] reviewed the natural history of myelomeningocele spine deformity in 130 consecutive admissions at Newington Children's Hospital. They distinguished two basic types, developmental (paralytic) and congenital (with anomalous vertebral development in addition to the spina bifida). Each group was subdivided into scoliosis, lordosis, and kyphosis.

Of the 103 patients without congenital anomalies other than the spina bifida, 53 (52 per cent) had spine deformity. Of these 53, 41 had scoliosis, 30 had lordosis, and 12 had

**239**

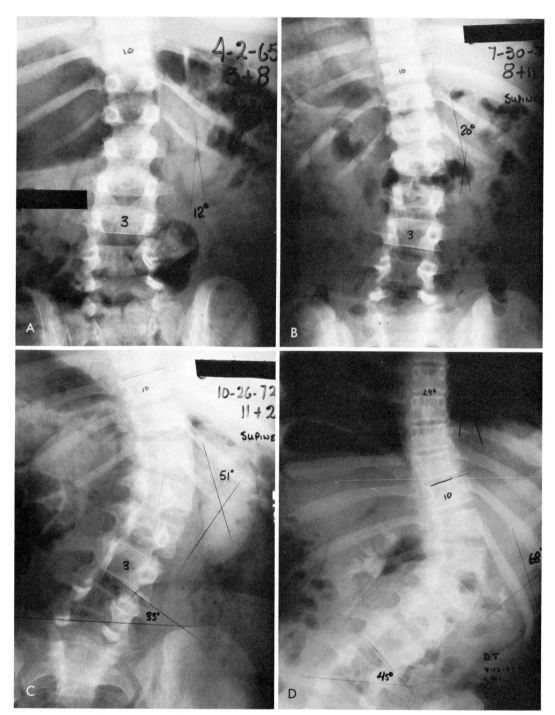

**Figure 9–1**  *A,* This 3 + 8 year old girl demonstrated a 12 degree, T10–L3 paralytic curve on this supine film. *B,* The same patient at age 8 years, 11 months, showing a 20 degree curve on supine x-ray. *C,* The patient at age 11 years and 2 months, showing a rather rapid development of structural curves at the start of the growth spurt. A supine x-ray shows the T10–L3 curve to have reached 51 degrees, and significant rotation has developed within this curve. In addition, there is a 33 degree fractional curve between L3 and the sacrum. From this x-ray, one does not know whether this fractional curve is purely compensatory or structural. *D,* A sitting x-ray at age 11 years and 9 months shows a 68 degree, T10–L3 curve with marked decompensation of the torso to the right. This decompensation would hint that there is structural character to the fractional lumbosacral scoliosis.

*Legend continued on opposite page*

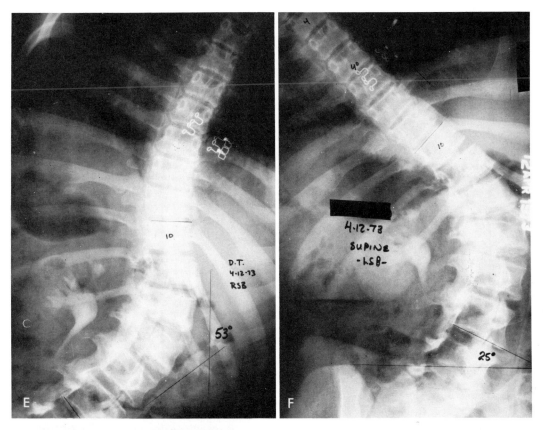

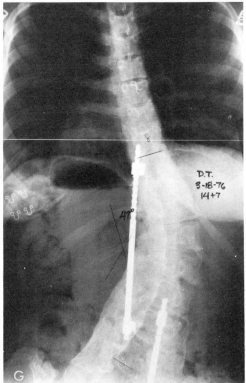

**Figure 9–1** *Continued.* *E,* Supine right side bending film shows the highly structural character of the T10–L3 curve correcting only to 53 degrees. *F,* A supine maximal left side bending film also shows the structural character of the L3 to sacrum fractional curve. This fixed lumbosacral curve adds very considerably to the complexity of surgical management of this patient. *G,* An AP sitting x-ray obtained three years after surgical correction and fusion. Two distraction rods were used, one to correct each curve, thus obtaining a balanced situation with the torso well centered over a horizontal sacrum. The fusion extends up to T6 and down to the sacrum. Note the extremely wide transverse process fusion in the lumbar spine. She did have a pseudarthrosis at L1, requiring pseudarthrosis repair six months after the initial fusion. Failure to appreciate the structural lumbosacral curve in this patient might have led to disastrous decompensation if a rod had been inserted only on the left side.

kyphosis, with most patients having a mixed deformity, Twenty-seven patients (100 per cent of those with vertebral body anomalies) had congenital spine deformity, 21 with scoliosis and 8 with kyphosis (2 having a mixed deformity). In total, 80 of the 130 patients (62 per cent) had spine deformity, one-third with the congenital type and two-thirds with the developmental type. Of the 50 children without curves, many had significant growth remaining, so further curves could be expected.

The congenital types usually had some curvature at birth whereas the developmental did not. The age at curve onset in the developmental type was noted: 0–5 years, 33 patients; 6–10 years, 18 patients; and 11–15 years, 2 patients. Of the patients with developmental scoliosis, 70 per cent also had dislocation of one or both hips. Of those with hip dislocation, 83 per cent had pelvic obliquity. The authors felt that there was a relationship between hip dislocation and pelvic obliquity but not necessarily a cause and effect relationship, since the same muscle imbalance may cause both problems. It was also noted that the higher the level of paralysis, the greater was the likelihood of spine deformity.

Hall and Martin,[18] in an unpublished report, analyzed a group of 130 myelomeningocele patients, all of whom had finished growth (all were age 20 or older). There were 101 (78 per cent) with obvious (clinically apparent) spine deformity.

Mackel and Lindseth[26] reported 82 patients who were at least 10 years old at the time of analysis. Of these, 54 (66 per cent) had spine deformity, 42 developmental and 12 congenital. All of the patients paralyzed at the level of T12 or higher had a curve. Of those with an L4 level paralysis, 70 per cent had spine deformity. By age 10, 83 per cent of the congenital group and 36 per cent of the developmental group had developed a scoliosis of 45 degrees or more. All curves appeared by age 10 and, once they had appeared, progressed relentlessly.

Roth[37] reviewed the x-rays of 149 patients with myelomeningocele. Twenty-six per cent had congenital spine deformity. Of the 149 patients, 29 had scoliosis, 32 had kyphosis, and 13 had lordosis. Of the total group, 47 had T12 or higher and 62 per cent of these had deformity, kyphosis predominating. Of the seven who had L1 or L2 lesions, 43 per cent

had deformity; of the 49 with lesions at the level of L3 or L4, 24 per cent had deformity; and of the 26 with L5 lesions, 23 per cent had deformity. Twenty patients had lesions at the S1 level, and none of these had spine deformity.

Banta et al.[2] studied 268 patients followed for at least four years. Of those with T12 or higher lesions, 58 per cent had lordosis by age 4, and 100 per cent had lordosis by age 15. Of those with L3 lesions, lordosis was present in 60 per cent by age 4, and 80 per cent by age 15. Of those with S1 lesions, 20 per cent had lordosis by age 4, and 40 per cent had lordosis by age 15. In reference to scoliosis, Banta noted that of the total group, 16 per cent had scoliosis by age 4, 35 per cent by age 9, and 52 per cent by age 15. In the nonfunctional ambulators, at least 80 per cent had scoliosis. For lesions at T12 or higher, there was a 100 per cent incidence of scoliosis.

Shurtleff et al.[41] analyzed a large group of patients as to the level of the lesion and the age of development of "significant" scoliosis and kyphosis. Scoliosis of greater than 30 degrees was considered significant. At age one, only 3 per cent had scoliosis. By age 4, 17 per cent of those with thoracic lesions, 14 per cent of those with L3–L5 lesions, and only 3 per cent of those with S1 lesions had scoliosis. By age 10, 33 per cent of the T12 levels, 22 per cent of the L1–L2 levels, 18 per cent of the L3–L5 levels, and 3 per cent of the S1 levels had scoliosis. By age 13, the figures for these groups were 55 per cent, 44 per cent, 23 per cent, and 3 per cent, respectively. At the end of growth, the percentages were as follows: 88 per cent (thoracic), 63 per cent (L1–L2), 23 per cent (L3–L5), and 9 per cent (S1). Kyphosis rarely occurred except in patients with the high-level lesions. Kyphosis of greater than 35 degrees in the lumbar spine or greater than 65 degrees for the whole spine was noted in 30 per cent of patients with high lesions by age 3, 36 per cent by age 12, and 62 per cent by age 20. Those with L1–L2 level lesions had only 12 per cent kyphosis by age 20; the L3–L5 lesions, 2 per cent; and the S1 lesions, 9 per cent.

It is the experience of the authors that these observations are reliable, accurate portrayals of the spine deformity incidence in myelomeningocele. The higher the level of paralysis, the more likely is the occurrence of deformity. Generally speaking, one can anticipate a 100 per cent incidence of curvature in

T12 level paraplegia or above, 90 per cent at L1, 80 per cent at L2, 70 per cent at L3, 60 per cent at L4, 25 per cent at L5, and 5 per cent at S1. Those without congenital vertebral anomalies (except spina bifida) do not have a curve at birth but gradually develop a curve, usually beginning before age 10 and then progressing until the end of growth or beyond. There is a rapid increase in the curve during the adolescent growth spurt.

## NATURAL HISTORY

The developmental curvatures (Fig. 9–1) are customarily long, sweeping "C" curves, extending from midthorax to sacrum and frequently producing pelvic obliquity. This obliquity becomes fixed and may result in loss of sitting stability and cause unilateral ischial decubiti (on the low side of the pelvic obliquity). These curvatures are most often a lordoscoliotic pattern.

Lordosis and kyphosis may also be of the developmental (paralytic) type. Most patients develop lordoscoliosis, but some develop pure lordosis. This may be caused by paralysis with collapse; may be aggravated by hip flexion contractures; or may be due to contractures posteriorly in the spine caused by scarring in the region of the myelomeningocele. This last problem seems to be less common in those who have had early closure and good skin coverage.

Developmental kyphosis usually progresses slowly, but is not present at birth. It is a paralytic kyphosis, aggravated by lack of laminar and intraspinous ligament stability.

The natural history of patients with congenital scoliosis is similar to that seen with congenital scoliosis without spina bifida. They are born with a curvature that usually progresses even in early childhood. They commonly have lumbar hemivertebrae, which may cause or aggravate the pelvic obliquity. Con-

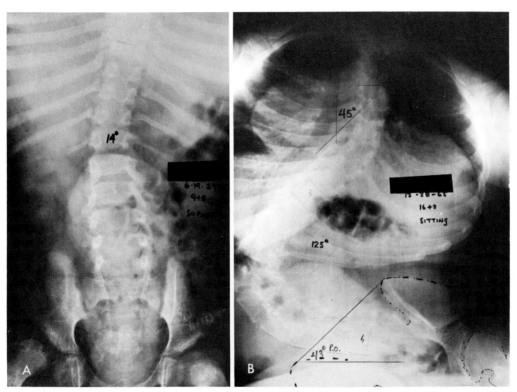

**Figure 9–2**  *A,* J.N.: This 9 + 8 year old girl is seen here with a 14 degree, T8-to-pelvis curve on a supine film. Her sac had never been excised. She has an L1 level paraplegia. *B,* Without treatment, this curve progressed to a highly structural 125 degree curve with 43 degrees of pelvic obliquity by age 16. This is a classic example of the severe progression that can occur during the adolescent growth spurt. It is easy to assume that the existence of only a 14 degree curve at age 9 means that the patient will not have a bad curvature problem. This patient had totally lost all sitting stability and had recurrent difficulties with pressure ulcers on the left ischium and trochanter. Reconstructive surgery at this time is most difficult, and curvatures should never be allowed to deteriorate to this severity.

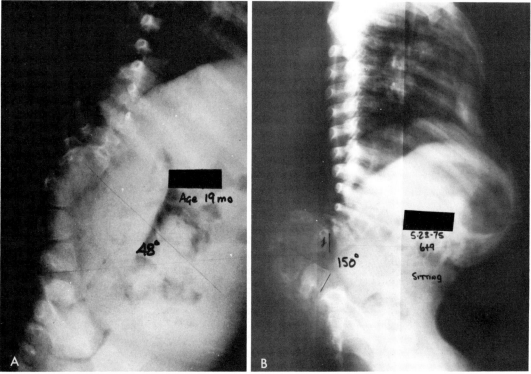

**Figure 9–3** *A,* A.B.: A lateral supine x-ray at age 19 months, showing a 48 degree congenital type kyphosis of the lumbar spine. No treatment was given. *B,* Same patient at age 6 years and 9 months. A sitting x-ray shows a 150 degree lumbar kyphosis.

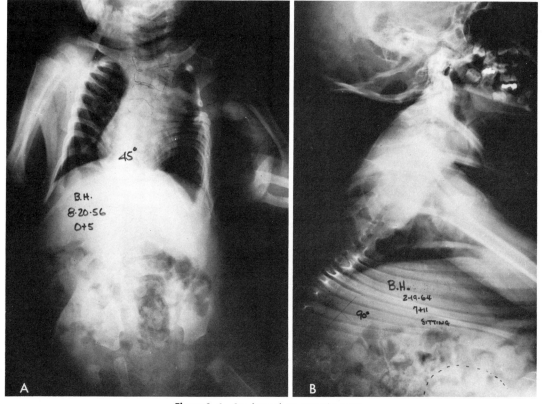

**Figure 9–4** *See legend on opposite page.*

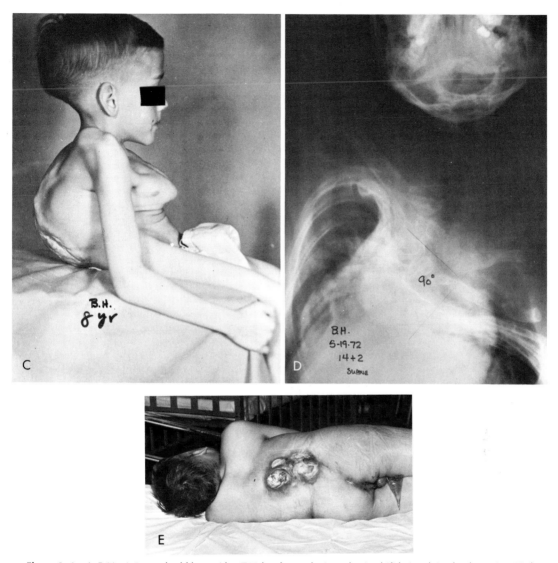

**Figure 9–4**  A, B.H.: A 5 month old boy with a T12 level paraplegia and spina bifida involving lumbar spine. He has a congenital type of kyphoscoliosis not well seen on this radiograph. There was a 45 degree scoliosis at the age of 5 months. B, A lateral sitting x-ray at the age of 7 years and 11 months showing a 90 degree kyphosis centered at the thoracolumbar junction. C, Clinical photo of patient at age 8. D, At age 14 + 2, a supine x-ray shows a severe 90 degree thoracic scoliosis. The more significant findings on this film are the markedly diminished chest space, the markedly enlarged heart, and the bilateral pneumonia. The patient was in terminal cor pulmonale when he presented to us at this time. E, The patient at age 14 years and 2 months, just prior to his death. He had osteomyelitis of the exposed spinous processes.

trary to the developmental curve, which is flexible until late, the congenital curve is quite rigid. Most such patients have a mixture of congenital and paralytic (developmental) spine deformity.

The single most difficult problem is the myelomeningocele patient with congenital kyphosis (Figs. 9–3 and 9–4). These children are born with a kyphosis usually 80° or more at

birth and have a T12 level total paraplegia. Skin closure at birth may be difficult. The kyphosis is rigid, progressing during infancy and commonly reaching 120 degrees by age 3. The average rate of progression is 8 degrees per year.[3] The severe kyphosis causes several problems, including ulceration of the skin over the spine, loss of sitting balance, and an excessively short abdominal wall, which may make ileal diversion difficult or even impossible.[5, 39] The ultimate poor functional level of these patients despite maximal treatment has led Lorber[24] to recommend "non-salvage" of these infants at birth.

## PATIENT EVALUATION

### History

The physician should first ask several questions regarding the general condition of the patient, followed by questions regarding the spine itself.

In terms of general condition, one needs to know about the child's mental capacity, the presence or absence of hydrocephalus, history of shunting procedures, the presence or absence of urinary tract infection, what urologic procedures have been performed, the current state of bladder function, the child's functional level in school, home, and social activities, and whether or not the child is using ambulatory aids for the lower extremities.

In regard to the spine, one needs to know the following: Is the deformity progressive? Is it causing functional problems such as lack of sitting stability, need for the use of the hands to support the torso, decreased ambulatory ability, or decreased wheelchair sitting tolerance? Have there been decubiti on one ischium as a result of pelvic obliquity? Have there been sores over a prominence of the back? Is there pain? Is there shortness of breath? Is there deterioration of neurologic function?

### Physical Examination

The physical examination must be complete, paying attention to the whole child. The head must be examined for hydrocephalus, the presence of a shunt, abnormal eye motion, blindness, and the quality of cerebral function. The chest should be examined for deformity, pneumonia, and an increased breathing rate. The abdomen should be examined for an ileal diversion, ileostomy, colostomy, and any sores or irritation of the skin from braces or stomal collecting devices. The hips should be examined for dislocation and contractures, particularly in the flexors, extensors, abductors, and iliotibial bands. Are there scars from previous surgical procedures performed about the hip? The knees should be examined for

contractures and for range of motion. The feet should be examined for sores and deformities. The buttocks should be examined for current or previous ulceration. The upper extremities should be examined for subtle paralysis, as hydromyelia may extend up into the cervical cord, even with a lumbar myelomeningocele.

The spine should be examined for scoliosis, lordosis, and kyphosis. A statement should be made as to which combination of deformities is present. The skin over the spine is of utmost importance. It should be noted whether there are pressure sores, open areas, paper-thin skin, sensitive areas, and the presence of or lack of bony elements. With careful physical examination in myelodysplastic patients, the exact level of the laminar defect can be palpated, and the presence of the bony ridges along each side of the sac can be easily felt. The skin must be examined for the absence of sensation. This may be critically important around the hip area when dealing with the need for braces or casts. The child's functional level of performance should be noted. Is he a walker, an assisted walker, a sitter, or a bed care patient?

### Radiologic Examination

Many of the customary x-rays taken for the patient with idiopathic scoliosis are not applicable to the patient with myelomeningocele spine deformity. Thus special views are recommended. The baseline films should be anteroposterior and lateral upright films if the child is old enough to sit independently. There should also be anteroposterior and lateral supine x-rays. The supine x-rays should be taken with the hips flexed at least 45 degrees and abducted 30 degrees. This will eliminate the forces of any muscle contractures about the hips that may pull on the pelvis and thereby distort the true picture of the spine deformity.

To test the rigidity or flexibility of an idiopathic curve, one usually obtains voluntary bending films. The myelodysplastic patient cannot bend voluntarily, and it is better to obtain films in correction using either longitudinal traction or passive bending. If there is a kyphosis, a supine hyperextension film should be obtained. If there is a lordosis, a hyperflexion film should be obtained. The x-ray in the knee-chest position is particularly valuable for determining the quantity of fixed lumbar lordosis in the patient who has a mixture of intrinsic spinal lordosis and lordosis secondary to hip flexion contractures. See Chapter 3 for technical details regarding x-ray evaluation.

## Other Evaluations

Other evaluations are concerned with the general state of health of the child. One would not wish to proceed with spinal surgery until maximum knowledge was available concerning the health of the child. Intravenous pyelography should be obtained at least once and sometimes twice a year. The urinary tract must be free of any obstructive problems and, if possible, free of infection prior to spinal surgery. Quite often a child will present with a significant spine problem, but surgery of the spine must be delayed until adequate management of the urinary tract has been accomplished. The exact status of the child's cerebral function is important to know. Spinal surgery can occasionally precipitate hydrocephalus in a child who has never had hydrocephalus or has had an arrested hydrocephalus.

## GENERAL PRINCIPLES AND GOALS

In dealing with neuromuscular problems in general, the physician should strive toward certain goals. These include preservation of respiratory function, maintenance of sitting stability, a level pelvis, and maximal torso length without unsightly prominences prone to decubiti. Although cosmetic aspects are secondary, it must be remembered that paralytic patients, even with myelomeningocele, have concepts of self-image. Solely in terms of self-image, it is far better to be sitting straight in a wheelchair than to be withered and deformed while sitting in the same wheelchair.

Hip subluxation and dislocation are frequent in all paralytic problems, and especially in children with myelomeningocele. It is critically important to hip stability to maintain a level pelvis. The more oblique the pelvis, the more likely is hip dislocation on the "high" side. Hip reconstruction is useless if there is pelvic obliquity.

The goal is to maintain good alignment until an adequate amount of growth has taken place, then stabilize the spine, striving always to obtain an *erect torso over a level pelvis.*

Congenital curves, whether scoliotic or kyphotic, become rigid early in life. Normal vertical growth *cannot* occur in the anomalous area. Early intervention for the anomalous area is necessary. The goal is to convert the situation to a paralytic pattern and treat accordingly.

## NONOPERATIVE TREATMENT

Nonoperative treatment has been mentioned by various authors, but there has been little published data concerning results of such treatment. Nonoperative treatment *can* be done and has been for many patients. It is never easy in patients with paralysis, especially with absent sensation.

There is a great need for nonoperative treatment in many of these patients, particularly those with purely paralytic deformities. Since they have long sweeping curves extending to the sacrum, a great deal of stunting of growth of the spine will occur if fusion is done at a very young age. It is preferable to brace the curve for several years and then fuse at a later time. *Under no circumstances should fusion be delayed until after the growth spurt,* as irretrievable progression will have occurred. The ideal age for fusion treatment is about age 10 in girls and age 12 in boys. Fusion should be performed earlier if the curve cannot be controlled with braces.

## Casts

Casts are difficult to use for nonoperative treatment and are not recommended. They are heavy, hindering the child's function, and it is difficult for the mother to check the skin for sores.

## Braces

### MILWAUKEE BRACE

The Milwaukee brace has been used fairly extensively in the treatment of myelomeningocele patients, particularly those with thoracic scoliosis. The Milwaukee brace may require some modification, including a different pelvic girdle to accommodate an ileal diversion. Sometimes the pelvic section is modified to contour around the lower rib cage to give some support to the torso.[7] The pelvic girdle should be lined with nonabsorbent cushioning material to distribute forces and lessen the likelihood of pressure sores. The brace should be removed by the mother several times a day and the skin carefully checked. Sometimes the child can sleep without the brace since the curve is a collapsing type and less likely to increase during the night. This is quite contrary to the management of idiopathic scoliosis. If the child can sleep with the brace, this is preferable. The lateral holding pad should be large, carefully contoured, and lined with cushioning material. The skin beneath the pad must be checked frequently (Figs. 9–5 and 9–6).

## OTHER BRACES

Underarm braces have been extensively used in children with myelomeningocele, as they tend to tolerate the Milwaukee brace poorly. These lumbar braces are effective for flexible lumbar and thoracolumbar curves.

They should be made from a strong but lightweight plastic material and from a cast of the patient taken in the corrected position. To obtain an adequate cast, the patient should be placed in a Risser frame and traction applied with a head halter and hip bandages or bilateral Buck's traction. Leg traction is preferable if there is any pelvic obliquity, since the obliquity can best be corrected by asymmetric leg traction. Drennan[12] recommends partial suspension of the child in the brace by attaching the brace to the wheelchair with a special swivel bracket (Figs. 9–7 and 9–8).

## GENERAL PRINCIPLES OF BRACE TREATMENT

There are three components to brace treatment, regardless of type of brace or curve problem. The first is the selection of brace treatment. Which curves can be braced? At

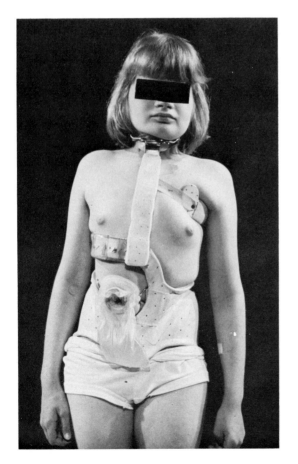

**Figure 9–5**  A Milwaukee brace, showing the special design of the abdominal section to accommodate an ilial stoma. The pelvic section is made of orthoplast with metal reinforcement around the stoma hole.

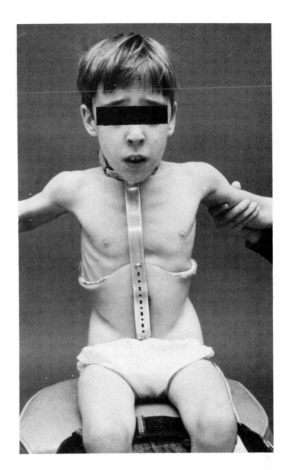

**Figure 9–6** A Milwaukee brace designed with a special pelvic section carried high underneath the torso for support via the chest cage. This will diminish the forces on the crest area.

what age can brace treatment be started? At what curve magnitude should brace treatment be started? Are there any contraindications to brace treatment?

The second component is the actual treatment itself—the technique of brace manufacture, details of application and daily management, and recognition of problems.

The third component is the termination of brace treatment. In myelomeningocele, a curve is virtually never controlled by brace treatment alone until the end of growth without spine arthrodesis. Thus the desired goal of brace treatment is to delay fusion until an optimal age. The physician must recognize when the brace is failing or when the optimal time for fusion has arrived.

## SELECTION OF PATIENT

Patients with developmental deformity, whether pure scoliosis, lordoscoliosis, or kyphoscoliosis, are the best candidates for brace treatment. The indications for treatment are deformities of 20 degrees or more, as viewed on upright films. It is dangerous to procrastinate beyond this point, as the optimal chance to achieve adequate correction is past.

Most certainly any *progressive* deformity should be treated. It is important to start treatment *before* fixed deformity develops, because braces are of little value in treatment of fixed deformity, especially pelvic obliquity. To procrastinate is to invite disaster. Most of these patients have collapsing deformities, and the brace is a passive holding device. Exercises for the spine are of no value. In fact, the brace is used to develop fixation of the spine in the optimal position. Any attempt to increase spinal mobility is contrary to the goals of treatment.

When should bracing be stopped? Obviously, if the patient has a curve that is relentlessly progressing despite adequate brace treatment, further bracing is futile, and fusion should be performed promptly. A second indication for cessation of brace treatment is inability of the patient to tolerate bracing. Despite the best attempts of physician and orthotist, recurrent pressure areas

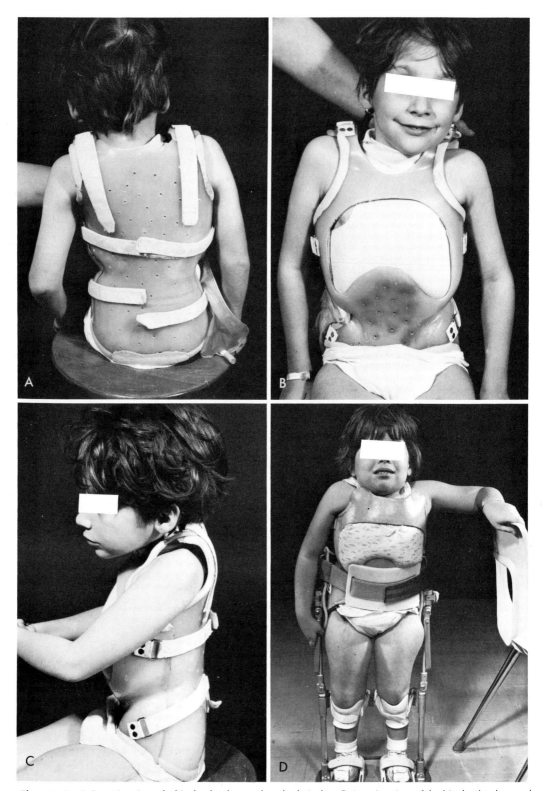

**Figure 9–7**   *A,* Posterior view of a bivalved polypropylene body jacket. *B,* Anterior view of the bivalved polypropylene body jacket. *C,* Lateral view of the bivalved polypropylene body jacket. The sides overlap in the midaxillary line and are held together with Velcro straps. The plastic extensions over the shoulders are optional depending upon the individual case. *D,* A different patient showing the same body jacket without the shoulder straps and showing her standing in a parapodium.

*Legend continued on opposite page*

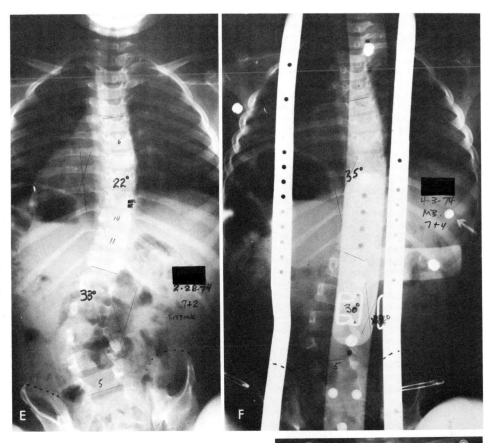

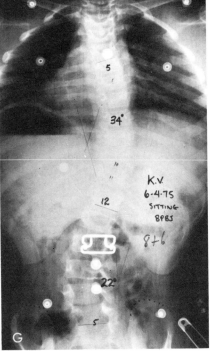

**Figure 9–7** *Continued.* *E,* A patient with a 22 degree right thoracic T5–T12 scoliosis and a 33 degree left lumbar curve with pelvic obliquity. *F,* The patient was fitted with a Milwaukee brace, which gave some correction of the lumbar curve to 30 degrees, but the thoracic curve was worse at 35 degrees. *G,* One year later she was switched to a bi-valved polypropylene body jacket, which significantly improved her functional capabilities and gave better correction of the lumbar curve and at least as good a correction of the thoracic curve. Note the excellent maintenance of a level pelvis.

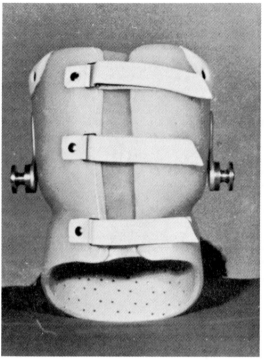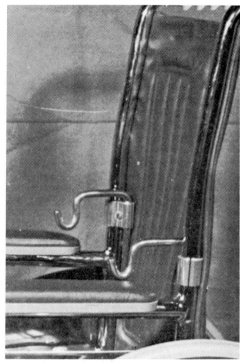

**Figure 9–8**   The plastic body jacket as used at Newington Hospital. The brace is an anterior opening brace with lateral swivel supports that fit on special brackets on the wheelchair to give some semisuspension effect. The swivel brackets allow forward and backward tilting of the body for wheelchair function. (Figure reproduced with permission of the author.)

may defeat a brace program. If this happens, fusion should be carried out promptly.

Finally, a patient may be wearing a brace without difficulty, but has reached 10 to 12 years of age. Since fusion is inevitable, one should not procrastinate longer. Adequate spine length will already have been achieved. Under no circumstances should fusion be delayed until the end of growth. From a practical point of view, braces usually cease to be effective when the adolescent growth spurt has been reached. The curve usually begins to worsen despite the brace, and the need for fusion becomes obvious (Figs. 9–9 and 9–10).

Congenital deformities are much less responsive to brace treatment than are developmental curves. Only if the curve has significant flexibility will the brace be successful.

In our experience, congenital kyphosis has been totally nonresponsive to brace treatment, and we do not feel there is any reason to use a brace for such patients (Fig. 9–11).

## SURGICAL TREATMENT

### Preoperative Evaluation

Preoperative evaluation has been covered to a large extent earlier in this chapter. The physical examination must include careful observation as to the nature and pattern of spine deformity, the functional problem it creates, the quality of the skin of the back and abdomen, and the extent of the area of spina bifida.

General examination must determine that the child is in the best possible general health. Any hydrocephalus problem must be stabilized, the lungs must be clear, and special attention must be directed to the urinary tract. Any obstructive uropathy must be corrected, and urine that is as sterile as possible must be obtained. Obviously, a sterile urine is not always possible, but active infection, especially with bacteremia, is a contraindication to spinal surgery. One should routinely obtain both blood and urine cultures prior to spine surgery. The genitourinary tract should be declared free of any acute problems by a competent urologist.

## Selection of Fusion Area

As in any spine deformity, the area requiring spine fusion must be carefully determined prior to the procedure itself. The determination of the extent of fusion is made on criteria developed years ago in the treatment of neuromuscular spine problems such as poliomyelitis. These fundamental rules do not change because a patient has myelodysplasia. *The most common error* (outside of failure to fuse) *is the selection of an inadequate fusion area.*

In patients with developmental (paralytic) spine deformity, the entire area involved in the paralysis must be fused. Fusion to the sacrum is necessary in all collapsing spines. One must fuse at least one vertebra and preferably two vertebrae above the uppermost vertebra on the curve as measured on the *upright* x-ray. Thus, if the patient has a T6–S1 curve, the fusion must extend from T4 to the sacrum. *Whether one operates from front or back, or whether or not one uses Harrington rods, Dwyer cables, or both, the extent of the fusion does not change.* This rule applies whether the problem is scoliosis, kyphosis, lordosis, or a combination thereof.

Congenital spine deformities must also have fusion of the entire extent of the curve. One of the major problems in dealing with congenital kyphosis has been the tendency to do osteotomy and fusion of the apex of the kyphosis but failure to fuse the entire length of the kyphotic deformity. This is intellectually comparable to the surgeon who resects a hemivertebra for congenital scoliosis but fails to fuse the entire curve of which the hemivertebra was only the apical segment. In patients with mixed congenital and developmental curves, the longer fusion area demanded by the developmental curve should apply.

## Operative Technique for Developmental Curves

Having decided that surgical stabilization is necessary and having selected the area requiring fusion, the operative program must now be planned. What is the best surgical technique? There is no single "best" technique. Each patient must be regarded individually.

The main problems are two: 1) obtaining a solid fusion to the sacrum and 2) obtaining a solid fusion of the area of spina bifida. The area proximal to the spina bifida, where the laminae are intact, seldom presents a problem.

For the patient with lumbar scoliosis and lordosis (but never with kyphosis) and who has bones large and strong enough to accept the Dwyer apparatus (age 10 or older), a combined approach with anterior fusion *to the sacrum* and posterior fusion of the entire curve, also to the sacrum, must be done. Harrington rods should be used posteriorly if at all possible. Dwyer instrumentation should be done anteriorly, if possible.

In the sac area, avoid entering the scarred, potentially infected midline. There are no useful laminae there. One posterior incision can follow the concave facet joint area extending into the thoracic spine. A second parallel posterior incision can be made over the convex facet area in the lumbar spine in order to obtain bilateral transverse process fusion throughout the lumbar spine and down to the alae of the sacrum. The Harrington rod should extend from the uppermost fused vertebra to the ala of the sacrum on the high side of the pelvic obliquity. When using this parallel incision technique, the intervening tissues must not be undermined or dissected in any way (Fig. 9–12). If the posterior skin is good, a single incision is preferable.

If there is some residual fixed lumbar lordosis after the anterior procedure, a straight Harrington rod will not lie against the transverse processes but will "bowstring" above the muscle area and make closure difficult and erosion of the rod through the skin quite likely. In such cases, the rod should be bent to conform to the residual lordosis. Unfortunately, an ordinary rod bent into lordosis will usually rotate to another alignment, even 180 degrees the opposite. To prevent this, the surgeon must use the hook with a square hole and a square-ended Harrington rod (see Chapter 20.

Dwyer instrumentation to the sacrum is not easy. It requires dissection beneath the iliac artery and vein and attachment of the distal screw to the sacrum. A screw head must never protrude beneath the artery or vein, as vascular erosion has been reported. If satis-

*Text continued on page 261*

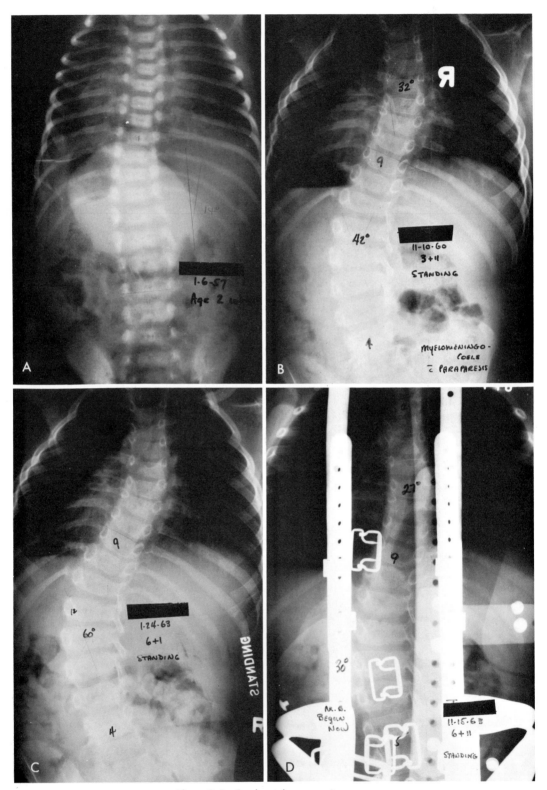

**Figure 9–9** *See legend on opposite page.*

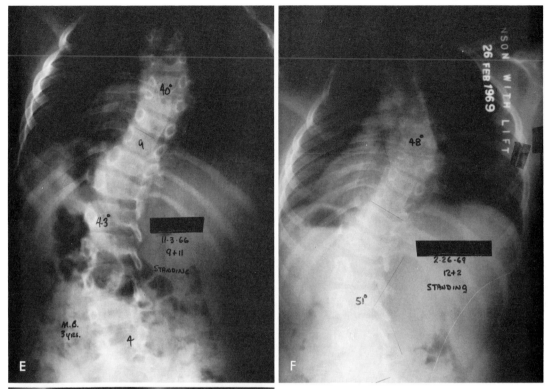

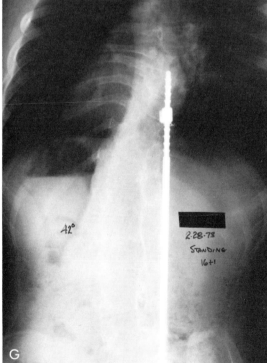

**Figure 9–9**  *A,* This 2 week old child had a large upper lumbar myelomeningocele. The sac was excised and closed at this age. The lesion, although high, was incomplete. *B,* The same patient at 3 years and 11 months, shown standing. There is a 32 degree right thoracic curve, a 42 degree left lumbar curve and quite significant pelvic obliquity already developing at this age. The patient is ambulatory with crutches and two short leg braces. *C,* At age 6, the curvature had increased to 60 degrees although the pelvic obliquity had not worsened. Because of the progressive nature of his curve, it was elected to attempt treatment nonoperatively with a Milwaukee brace. *D,* At age 6 years and 11 months, a standing x-ray shows the right thoracic curve at 27 degrees and the left lumbar curve at 30 degrees, a 50 per cent improvement in the Milwaukee brace. He was able, with gradual weaning into the brace, to develop the ability to wear the brace full time. *E,* After three years in a Milwaukee brace, a standing film out of the brace shows the thoracic curve at 40 degrees and the lumbar at 43 degrees, thus indicating some improvement of the curve in addition to preventing deterioration. Brace treatment was successfully continued for three more years. *F,* The patient at age 12 showed a 48 degree thoracic curve and a 51 degree lumbar curve, with minimal pelvic obliquity. At this time, he was becoming somewhat refractory to wearing his brace full time plus it was obvious that the curves were beginning to deteriorate in the brace. By this time, sufficient torso growth had occurred so that fusion could be done. *G,* A final x-ray of the patient at age 16. He underwent surgical correction and fusion at age 12. The fusion extended from T3 to the sacrum with instrumentation from T9 to the sacrum. A bilateral transverse process fusion was performed throughout the spina bifida area. No anterior fusion was performed. Note the level pelvis and the vertical torso well centered. Instrumentation of the upper (thoracic) curve would have resulted in decompensation of the torso and head to the right.

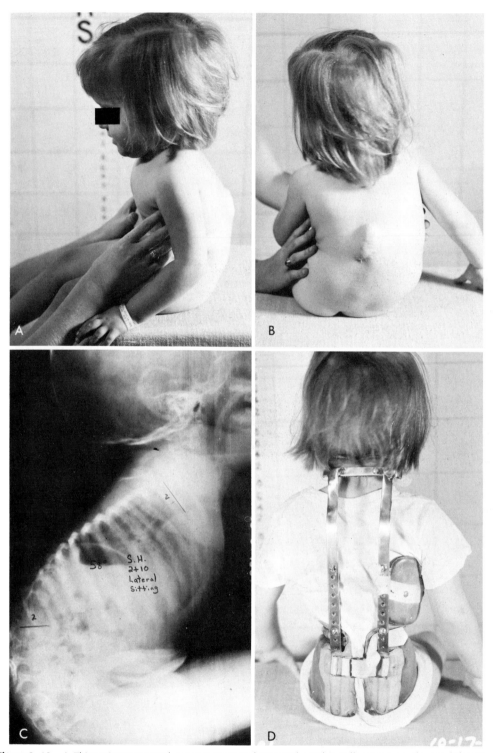

**Figure 9–10**   *A,* This patient presented at age 2 years and 10 months with a collapsing type of spine deformity, a mixture of kyphosis and scoliosis. *B,* Clinical photo of patient at age 2 years 10 months. *C,* A lateral x-ray at age 2 years and 10 months shows a long sweeping collapsing type of kyphosis extending from the upper thoracic spine to the sacrum. *D,* The patient was fitted with a Milwaukee brace, which adequately corrected both the kyphosis and the scoliosis.

*Legend continued on opposite page*

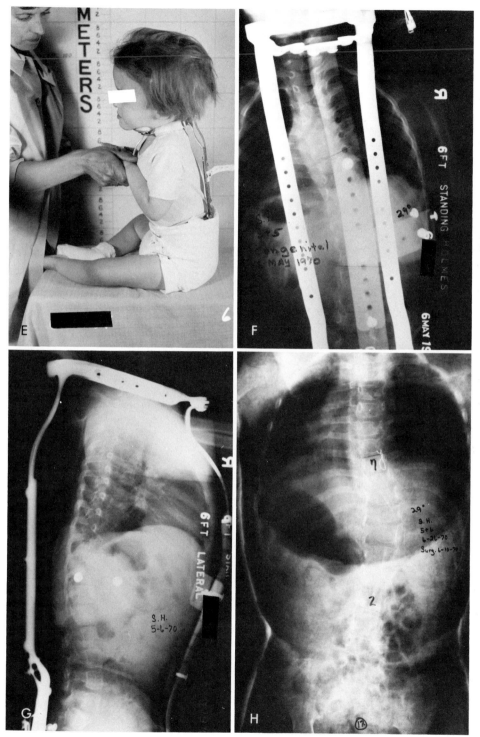

**Figure 9–10** *Continued.*   *E,* The brace considerably improved her sitting stability. *F,* A standing x-ray at age 5, showing a 29 degree scoliosis. *G,* A lateral standing x-ray at age 5 showing correction of a long sweeping kyphosis but persistence of a localized kyphosis in the upper lumbar spine in the region of her myelomeningocele. In this particular case, the kyphosis seemed to be predominantly due to lack of posterior stabilizing elements. *H,* The patient was fused from T6 to L4 using a bilateral transverse process posterior fusion leaving the sac intact, since she had good function distally. A Risser cast was used for correction.

*Legend continued on following page*

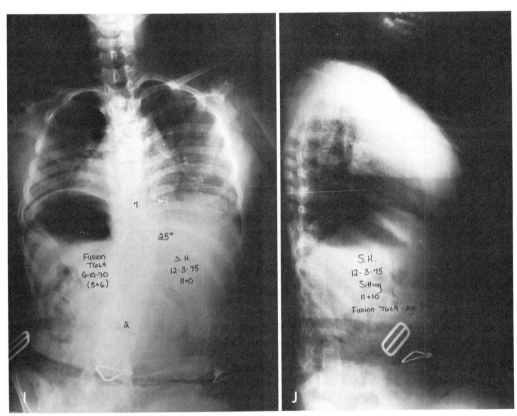

**Figure 9–10** *Continued.* *I,* An AP sitting x-ray at age 11, five years after spinal fusion, shows no loss of correction of scoliosis. It still measures 25 degrees. *J,* A lateral sitting x-ray at age 11, five years after fusion, shows full maintenance of normal lateral alignment. Only a posterior fusion had been done.

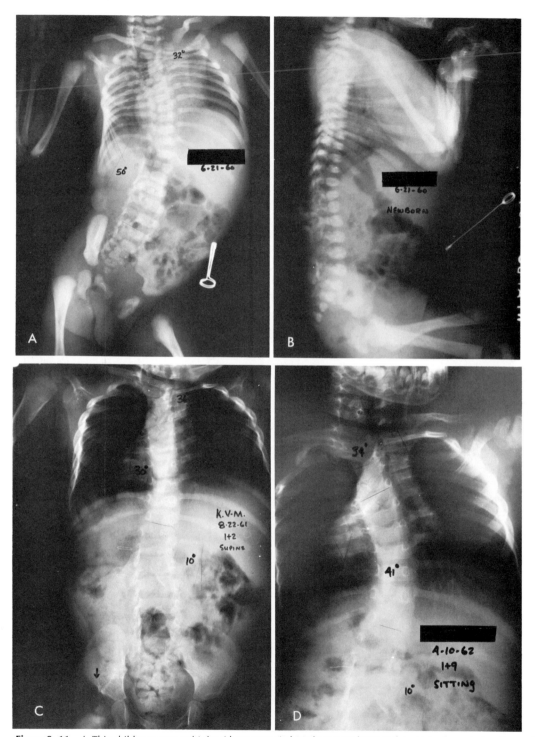

**Figure 9–11** *A,* This child was seen at birth with a congenital 32 degree scoliosis at the cervicothoracic junction and a 50 degree long curve extending down to the pelvis. She had a myelomeningocele in the lumbar spine and a meningocele at the cervicothoracic junction. She had no paralysis of the upper extremities and an incomplete paralysis of the lower extremities. *B,* A lateral x-ray of the same patient at birth, showing the bizarre development of the posterior elements in the lumbar spine. *C,* A supine x-ray at the age of 1 year and 2 months. The upper thoracic congenital scoliosis now demonstrates a unilateral unsegmented bar. This curve measures 36 degrees. The congenitally anomalous lumbar area shows only a 10 degree left curve. The intervening area between the two anomalous areas shows a right thoracic curve of 30 degrees. A dysplastic hip on the left side was treated by abduction splinting. *D,* A sitting x-ray at age 1 year and 9 months shows the two structural congenital areas to be unchanged, but there is a collapsing tendency of the intervening nonanomalous area.

*Legend continued on following page*

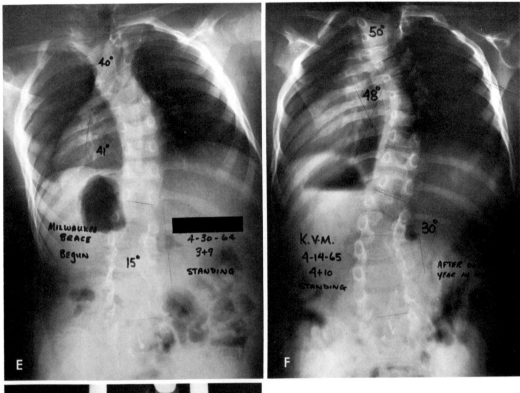

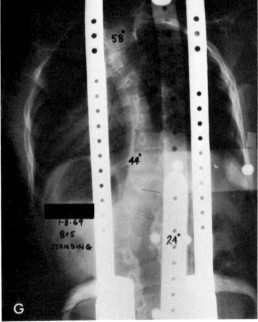

**Figure 9–11** *Continued. E*, A standing x-ray at the age of 3 years and 9 months shows increasing torso deformity, particularly in the thoracic curve, with tilting of the torso to the left. The congenital unsegmented bar area in the upper thoracic spine has increased to 40 degrees. There has been very little increase of the lumbar curve. An unsegmented bar is now obvious here also. A Milwaukee brace was begun at this time. *F*, At the age of 4 years and 10 months, this standing film shows further increase of all curves. Both the congenital curves, lumbar and upper thoracic, have increased, and the mid curve has increased to 48 degrees to balance the others, but the general torso alignment is much improved. Thus the brace accomplished compensation but not a curve correction. *G*, At the age of 8, the high thoracic curve had now reached 58 degrees, and it was very obvious that it was behaving in a fashion typical to all unilateral unsegmented bars, i.e., relentless progression throughout growth. Braces cannot be expected to accomplish anything for such a curve. The lumbar curve was being reasonably maintained at 24 degrees. The intervening thoracic curve at 44 degrees was really necessary to balance the high thoracic curve. It was elected to proceed with the surgery at this time. The brace has successfully managed general alignment of the spine, has kept the nonanomalous right thoracic curve within acceptable limits, and has permitted spine growth. (See Fig. 9–18 for surgical results of this case.)

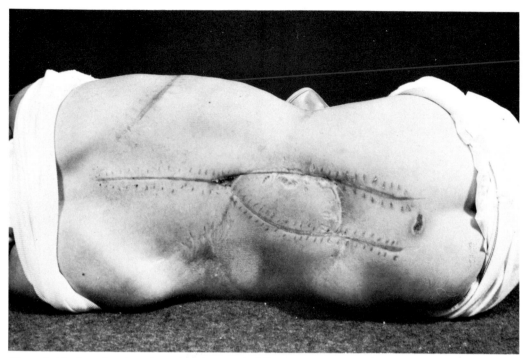

**Figure 9–12** Posterior view of a patient three weeks following posterior spine fusion from T3 to the sacrum utilizing two transverse process incisions in the lumbar spine, brought together as a single midline incision. This was all done in one stage. The anterior fusion via a right thoracotomy had been done two weeks prior to that. There is a small pressure sore over the sacrum due to poor fitting of the plastic brace on the first attempt. This was revised with success.

factory fusion and instrumentation to the sacrum posteriorly are possible, the Dwyer instrumentation can extend to L4 or L5 and not S1. Nevertheless, the anterior fusion should go to S1. If the posterior route is impossible owing to bad skin or previous infection, one should attempt to obtain a fusion and instrumentation to the sacrum. Never use the Dwyer in a patient with kyphosis; it will increase the kyphosis.

In patients with developmental curves requiring fusion but with bones too small for Dwyer instruments, the same procedures are performed, but without instrumentation.

Traction prior to surgery has *not* been found helpful. It leads to disuse osteoporosis, pressure sores, and problems with shunts.

The basic operative technique is that used for any spine fusion. The reader is referred to Chapter 20 for detail. The chief difference in the myelomeningocele child is the region of the spina bifida. Here the surgeon must identify the lateral bony ridges and dissect these and lateral to these to include the vestigial transverse processes bilaterally. The hypoplastic facet joints are excised with a rongeur. Large amounts of bone graft are laid in this trough along the transverse processes, especially between L4 and the alae. The fusion must extend to the alae of the sacrum bilaterally. Excision of the contents of the spinal canal is *not* indicated in developmental curves. Interbody fusion is better done by an anterior approach.

**Postoperative Management**

At the present time, the authors have completely abandoned the use of plaster casts in the myelomeningocele child. The standard postoperative support is a bivalved polypropylene body jacket made from a plaster model of the patient taken on a Risser frame *after* surgical correction of the deformity. This is a "total contact" orthosis. The brace is worn until the fusion is solid, usually one year. The hips are *not* immobilized, even though the fusion extends to the sacrum. The patient returns to normal upright activities as soon as the brace fits well, usually within 10 days of surgery. The brace is frequently removed for skin checks but is worn 24 hours a day. While the patient is horizontal, one of the halves of the brace can be left off for treatment of skin problems if necessary (Figs. 9–13, 9–15, and 9–16).

*Text continued on page 270*

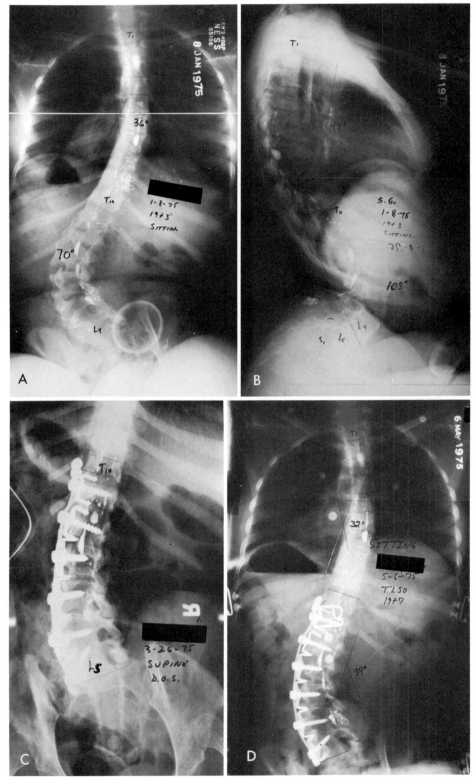

**Figure 9–13**  *See legend on opposite page.*

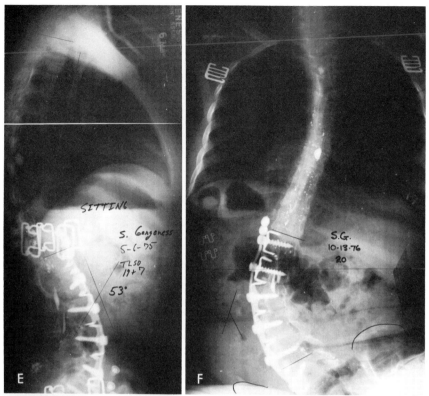

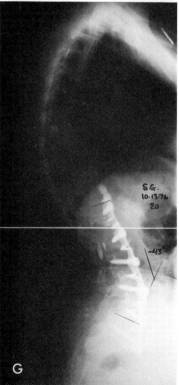

**Figure 9–13** *A,* An AP sitting view of a 19 year old girl with a lumbar myelomeningocele. She has an L1 paralysis to the customary examination but has bilateral intrinsic palsy of both hands. Her curve was progressive even though she was past the end of growth. *B,* A lateral x-ray shows her major problem, that is, a severe lumbar lordosis. Her sac had not been excised and produced a very dense scar posteriorly. Because of her progressive curve and her progressive loss of sitting balance, it was felt necessary to proceed with correction and fusion. Because of the very poor skin posteriorly, an attempt was made to solve her problem by anterior surgery only, using a Dwyer procedure. *C,* On the day of surgery she had excellent correction of the scoliosis to 35 degrees, and the pelvis is now level. Extension distally of the Dwyer procedure was quite difficult but was successfully accomplished to L5. *D,* A sitting view in her bivalved polypropylene body jacket two months after surgery shows maintenance of the curve at 39 degrees, only a 4 degree loss by resumption of the sitting position. The pelvis shows only slight pelvic obliquity. *E,* A lateral x-ray at the same time shows the excellent improvement of the lordosis to 53 degrees. Note the anteroposterior direction of the lowermost Dwyer screw. She was kept in the body jacket full time for 15 months following the surgery. *F,* This AP x-ray sitting at the age of 20 shows deterioration of the curve. There is no evidence of fraying of the Dwyer cable except at the junction of the uppermost and second screws. One can see an increasing distance between the two staples plus thinning of the cable. This, however, is not the major cause of the increased deformity but rather is the extension of the curve upward due to the more extensive paralytic disease. She has now had a cosmetic excision of her sac and providing of good skin. Extension of her fusion upward will be necessary. Note the marked increase in pelvic obliquity. *G,* Lateral x-ray at the age of 20 shows continued maintenance of excellent correction of the lumbar lordosis.

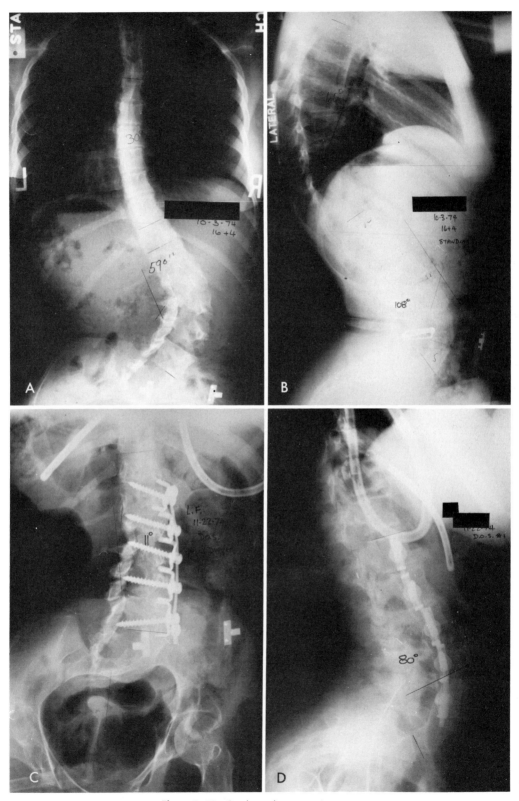

**Figure 9–14**  *See legend on opposite page.*

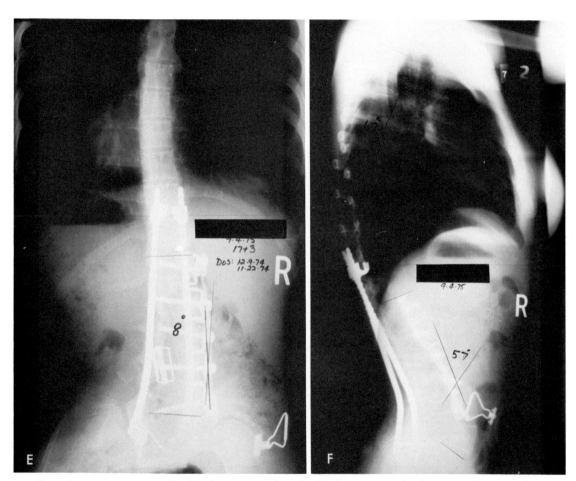

**Figure 9–14** *A,* A 16 year old girl with an L4 neurologic level and a progressive lumbar lordoscoliosis. *B,* A lateral x-ray of the same patient. Her lordosis was also progressive. *C,* Patient is shown on the day of surgery following a short, five-segment Dwyer procedure. The scoliosis has been corrected to 11 degrees. The pelvis is nearly level. *D,* A lateral x-ray on the same date shows correction of the lordosis to 80 degrees. Note the excellent correction of lordosis in the area where the Dwyer has been inserted but also the sharp persistence of lordosis between L4 and the sacrum below the lower end of the Dwyer procedure. *E,* An AP standing x-ray of the patient nine months following combined Dwyer and Harrington instrumentation. Note the perfectly level pelvis, the 8 degree residual scoliosis, and the vertical torso without scoliosis. *F,* A lateral standing x-ray, nine months following fusion, showing residual 57 degrees of lumbar lordosis. Note the contoured Harrington rods. These are square-ended rods in square-holed alar hooks. This patient was managed entirely with underarm support without extension to the legs, with the rapid resumption of upright activity and total avoidance of prolonged bed rest.

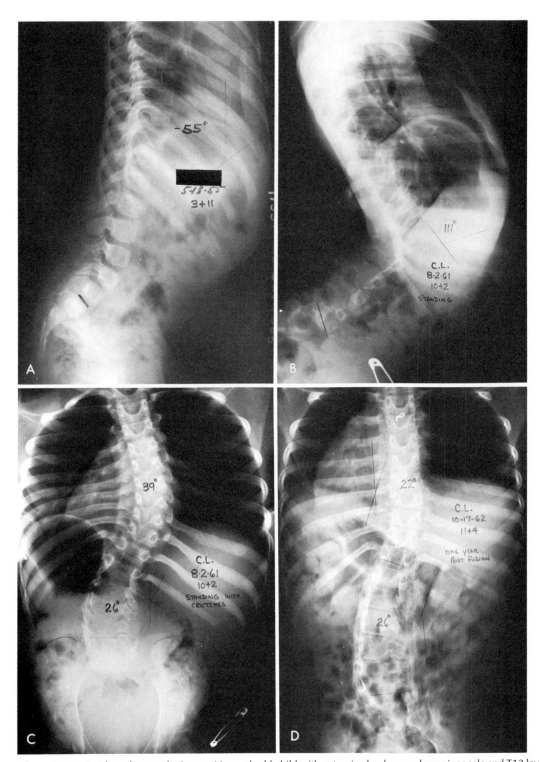

**Figure 9–15** *A,* A lateral x-ray of a 3 year, 11 month old child with extensive lumbar myelomeningocele and T12 level total paralysis. Note the thoracic lordosis of minus 55 degrees. *B,* When first seen by the authors at age 10 years and 2 months, in 1961, she demonstrated a marked increase in her lordosis, now measuring 111 degrees. Part of this was due to structural changes within the spine and part due to hip flexion contractures. Part also was due to a frail collapsing type of spinal deformity. *C,* An AP standing x-ray with crutches (therefore in partial suspension) shows a 39 degree right thoracic scoliosis with a 26 degree left lumbar curve and the extensive spina bifida extending from T11 to the sacrum. She had never had hydrocephalus or shunting and had a normal I.Q. Because of her progressive deformity, particularly the lordosis, she was treated by Dr. Moe with correction in a Risser cast and fusion from T3 to the sacrum in three stages, a single midline posterior fusion from T3 to T10 and transverse process fusion done one month apart. She was treated by extensive bed rest and plaster immobilization for one year. Bank bone as well as autogenous iliac bone was used for the fusion.

*Legend continued on opposite page*

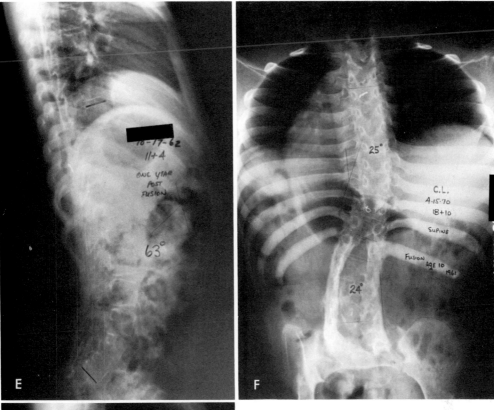

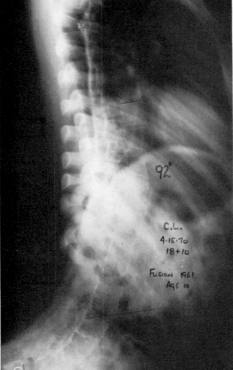

**Figure 9–15** *Continued.*

*D,* One year post fusion, her curves were 22 degrees in the thoracic area and 26 degrees in the lumbar area. The pelvis was level. *E,* A lateral x-ray one year following fusion shows excellent correction from the severe 111 degree lordosis to a 63 degree lordosis. The fusion was solid. No pseudarthroses occurred. *F,* An AP spine x-ray at age 18, eight years following fusion, shows the very solid arthrodesis from T3 to the sacrum with complete preservation of her correction. Note the hypertrophy of the fusion mass with time. There have been some radiological changes around the sacroiliac joint but there have been no clinical problems related to this. *G,* A lateral x-ray eight years following the fusion shows a solid arthrodesis; there has been some increase of lordosis but not to the severity that it was prior to surgery. She has no difficulties with breathing. Note the excellent AP chest diameter. This case demonstrates that even prior to the availability of internal fixation devices, a satisfactory correction and fusion could be obtained.

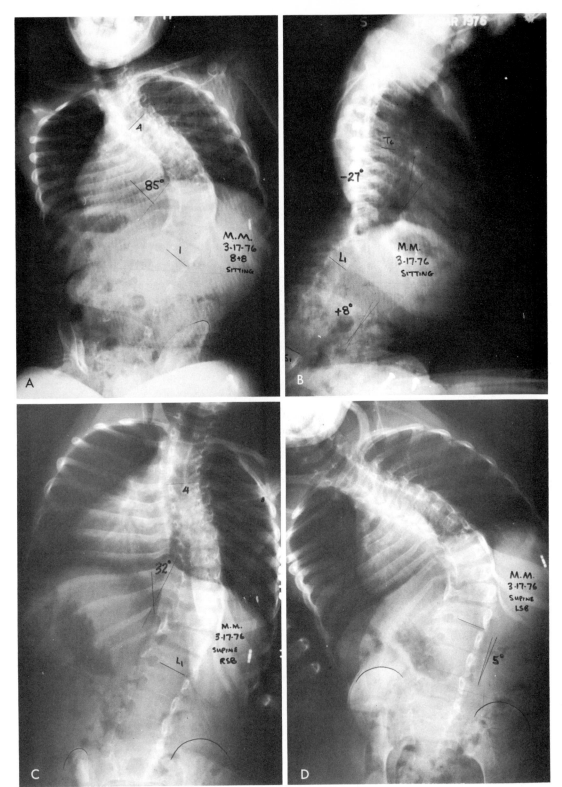

**Figure 9–16** *A,* An 8 year old boy presented to the authors with an 85 degree T4–L1 curve. His spina bifida extended from T12 to the sacrum. There was no pelvic obliquity. He has a T12 level paralysis. *B,* A lateral sitting x-ray shows a minus 27 degree thoracolumbar lordosis. *C,* A supine right side bending film shows correction of the major curve to 32 degrees. This indicates that adequate correctability exists and that traction is not necessary prior to surgery. *D,* A supine left side bending film shows structural characteristics in the lumbar spine. The lumbar spine lacks normal flexibility, but L1 does center over the sacrum.

*Legend continued on opposite page*

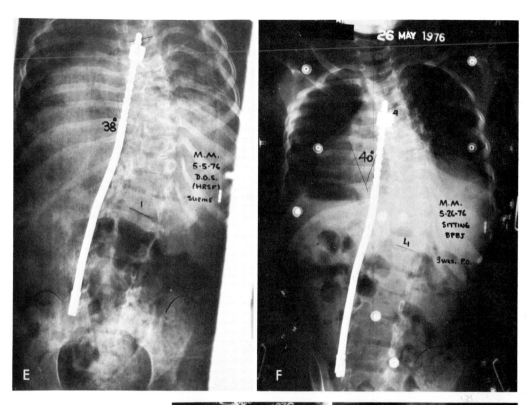

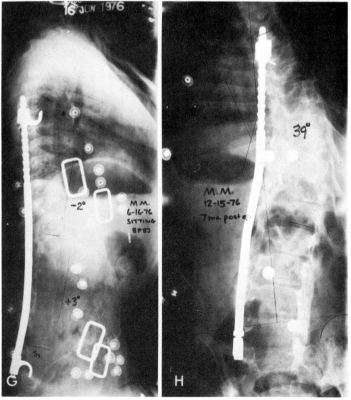

**Figure 9–16** *Continued.* *E,* A supine x-ray taken on the day of surgery shows correction of the curve to 38 degrees. The fusion extends from T3 to the sacrum. He also had an extensive anterior fusion (See Fig. 9–12 for the incision view.) *F,* An AP sitting x-ray three weeks postoperatively in a bi-valved polypropylene body jacket. This x-ray demonstrates that normal torso alignment, a level pelvis, and only a 2 degree loss of correction has occurred by the use of this brace. *G,* Lateral x-ray three weeks following surgery sitting in the bi-valved polypropylene body jacket. Note the correction of the abnormal lordosis existing prior to surgery and the bent rod to maintain a normal lumbar lordosis. This is a square-ended rod and a square-holed hook placed in the ala of the sacrum. *H,* An AP x-ray seven months following surgery showing full maintenance of correction and a fusion mass that is incorporating well although not fully solid yet.

## Congenital Scoliosis

Patients with congenital scoliosis and myelomeningocele usually require fusion at a much younger age than those with developmental curves. The typical patient has a lumbar scoliosis with pelvic obliquity and one or two hemivertebrae on the side of the convexity of the lumbar curve. The curves are customarily rather rigid and tend to be progressive despite external bracing. Our best results have been from a combination of anterior fusion (convex side) and bilateral transverse process fusion without instrumentation. Fusion is commonly necessary at about age 4 or 5, and the bones are too small or soft to accept any type of metallic fixation.

Hemivertebra excision is not recommended except in severe and rigid lumbar curves where the pelvic obliquity cannot be corrected by any other means. If such wedge osteotomy is done, one must remember also to fuse the entire length of the curve.

Some congenital patients have two areas of anomalies, one in the lumbar spine associated with the spina bifida and a second area in the upper thoracic spine. These two anomalous areas are separated by several normal vertebrae. If the interval area has good muscle control, one can fuse the two areas separately. Brace treatment may be necessary to control the noncongenital component of the curve. After adequate growth has been obtained, correction of the two fused areas by another fusion may be necessary (Figs. 9–17, 9–18, and 9–19).

## Congenital Kyphosis

Hoppenfeld[20] dissected 10 autopsy specimens of this condition. He noted the pedicles to be widely spread and that the rudimentary laminae were everted so that the inner laminar surface, which should face ventrally (in the normal spine) or medially (in nonkyphotic myelomeningocele), was actually facing posteriorly. The dorsal surfaces of the laminae were actually facing forward. The anterior longitudinal ligament was short and thick. Resection of both the anterior longitudinal ligament and the annulus fibrosus did allow some correction. The paraspinal muscles were present but were displaced far anterolaterally.

Drennan[11] also did anatomic dissections in 12 cases, paying particular attention to the muscle pattern, and analyzed the x-rays of 35 cases. The average kyphosis was 80 degrees in the newborn. The erector spinae muscles, instead of being posterior to the spine, were lateral, with portions even anterior to the axis of flexion. The quadratus lumborum was similarly displaced so that a majority of its fibers were anterior to the axis of flexion.

The psoas was particularly far anterior to the kyphosis. When innervated, it had a capability of producing marked kyphosis. The lower fibers of insertion of the diaphragm were also noted to aggravate the kyphosis.

Donaldson[10] noted that congenital kyphosis was a very severe problem and that he had never seen one that did not increase. He noted that the great vessels did not follow the kyphosis and thus created a significant problem in treatment. He also noted the fixed lordosis just above the kyphosis. Excessive correction of the kyphosis resulted in a hyperlordotic spine.

Park and Watt[32] did aortograms on seven children with congenital kyphosis averaging 88 degrees. The aorta was short and "bowstringed" across the kyphosis.

Sharrard pioneered resection of the kyphosis, particularly in the newborn in order to gain skin closure. Other children were done at older ages (average, 7.5 years) for progressive deformity. Similar procedures were reported by Eyring and Wankin[16] and Eckstein and Vora.[14] The patients had a good short-term correction of kyphosis, but no follow-up was reported by any of these authors.

It has been the experience of the authors that corrections by such osteotomies tend to last only a short time. Even though the level of the osteotomy may fuse, the deformity recurs owing to lack of surgical stabilization of the whole curvature.

Poitras and Hall[34] stated the problem well: "Correction can be accomplished *only* by excision of bony elements of the kyphosis, but *maintenance of correction* can be obtained only by solid interbody and posterior fusion of the entire length of the deformity." They reported six cases operated by a posterior approach with excision of the sac, excision of the bony elements to reduce the spine to satisfactory alignment, and fixation of the osteotomy with compression rods, achieving an interbody and posterior fusion all in a single procedure. The recommended age was 3 to 8 years.

In 1975, McKay[25] reported the development of a special anterior plate for the correction of kyphosis in myelomeningocele. This was, however, designed for correction and stabilization of the more flexible developmental kyphosis and *not* for the rigid congenital type with a short aorta.

The problem can be summarized: The child is born with severe lumbar kyphosis, usually about 80 degrees. Considerable difficulty will have been encountered in skin closure as a newborn. The skin over the back is precarious and frequently ulcerated. The child has a high level paralysis at birth. The deformity progresses with growth, even within the first two or three years of life. Braces are totally ineffective for control of the curve.

If the child presents to the surgeon before age 3 and has a rapidly progressive curve, direct anterior fusion with excision of the anterior longitudinal ligament, annulus, and discs and strut graft fusion will give modest correction and good stabilization (Fig. 9–20). If the patient presents at 5 to 10 years of age, the Hall single stage surgical procedure is performed. A long vertical posterior incision is used, the exact nature of which depends upon the local skin condition. The exposure continues past the lateral bony ridges from the sacrum upward to the upper level of the fixed lordosis above the kyphosis. Three or four levels with intact laminae are exposed.

The surgeon then must remove the entire sac. This is done only in children with complete, flaccid paraplegia. First, the surgeon dissects down the *inside* of the laminae until the foramina are exposed along each side. Within each foramen there will be a nerve root, an artery, and a vein. The nerve is transected sharply, and the artery and vein coagulated. This must be carefully done at each level on both sides, from normal laminae above (usually about T12) to the sacrum. The sac is then sharply transected with a scalpel *at the apex of the kyphosis,* where it is thin and quite scarred. If not so scarred, it is best to begin the sac excision at one end or the other and proceed either proximally or distally.

The caudal portion is then slowly and carefully removed, proceeding from the apex distally. Large, open fragile venous channels connect the sac to the posterior vertebral bodies. These vessels are located just lateral to the posterior longitudinal ligament in the midportion of the vertebral bodies. The bleeding from the hole in the vertebra is controlled with bone wax, and from the sac by cautery.

Once the distal half of the sac is removed, the proximal part is resected up to the level of good dura, which is transected and closed by pursestring suture. The cord may be absent or hypoplastic. The cord should not be sutured shut, but transected and left open so that spinal fluid can escape from the central canal of the cord to the arachnoid space. Deaths have been reported due to the resultant acute hydrocephalus.

Once the sac has been removed, the dissection continues subperiosteally around the vertebral bodies. The anterior longitudinal ligament is dissected away from the vertebral bodies over the entire length of the kyphosis. The anterior longitudinal ligament must be preserved, as it is the stabilizing hinge upon which correction depends. Sufficient vertebrae are then removed in order to realign the spine. These are *not* the most posteriorly displaced vertebrae, but rather those vertebrae *between the apex of the lordosis and the apex of the kyphosis.* This allows realignment of the lower lumbar spine with the thoracic spine.

Once these vertebrae are removed, the spine is aligned and held in position by Harrington compression rods, the upper hooks being in the laminae of the lower thoracic vertebrae and the lower hooks in the vertebral bodies and/or pedicles of L5 and S1. The bones removed (vertebral bodies, pedicles, and everted laminae) are cut up into the small fragments and placed anteriorly between the anterior longitudinal ligament and the vertebral bodies and some on the posterior aspect, especially in the lower thoracic spine. All lumbar discs are removed prior to instrumentation.

The wound is then irrigated and closed over suction drains. Antibiotics are given intravenously during the procedure and for several days postoperatively.

About one week after surgery a plaster model is taken for a bivalved plastic body jacket. This is ready within a few days and as soon as it is applied, the patient is started on tilt-table and sitting. The hips are *not* immobilized. Rapid return to the postoperative functional level is critical in order to prevent

*Text continued on page 286*

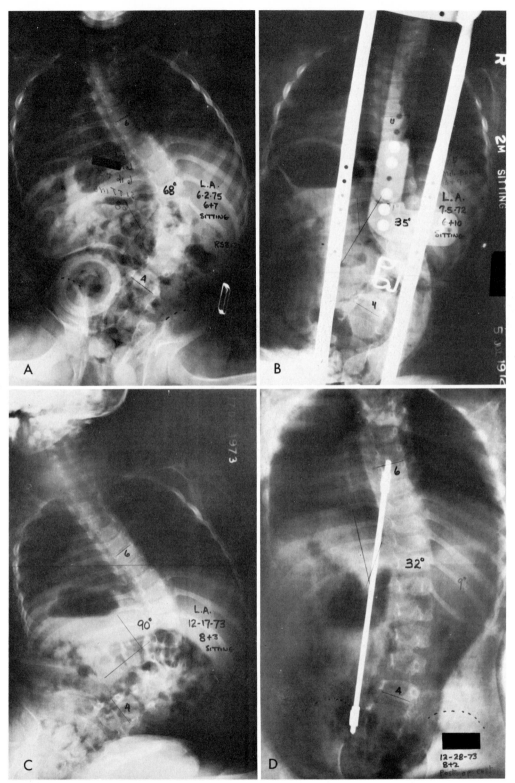

**Figure 9–17**  *A,* L.A. is a 6 year, 7 month old boy with a 68 degree curve and early pelvic obliquity on sitting film. A right side passive bending film showed correction to 27 degrees. Because of his young age and the extensive area that would require arthrodesis, it was elected to attempt brace treatment. This curve, however, has progressed to a great degree and has considerable structural qualities, thus making brace treatment difficult. Brace treatment must be started earlier than this if it is to be successful. *B,* An AP sitting x-ray of the patient shortly after brace application. There has been correction of the curve to 35 degrees. Bracing was, however, fraught with many difficulties, including recurrent pressure sores and poor parental cooperation. *C,* An AP sitting x-ray two years later, at the age of 8. His curve has deteriorated to 90 degrees. Surgical treatment is now absolutely necessary.

*Legend continued on opposite page*

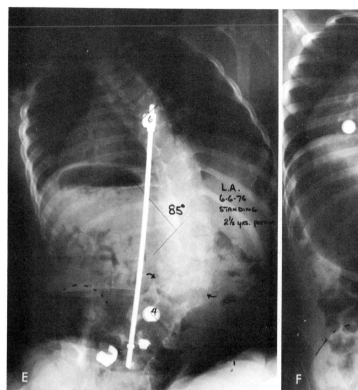

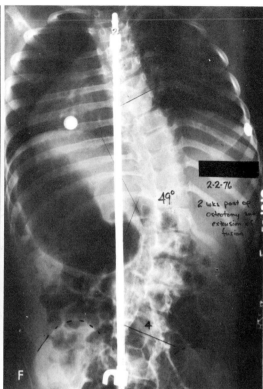

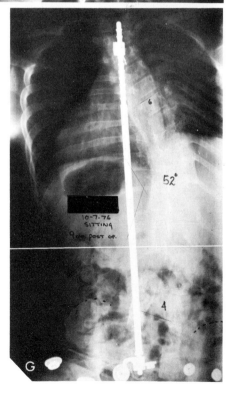

**Figure 9–17** *Continued.* *D,* This supine x-ray taken on the day of surgery shows Harrington instrumentation from T6 to the sacrum with fusion of the same area posteriorly. Correction to 32 degrees was obtained. Pelvic obliquity was greatly but not completely corrected. Note also that the arthrodesis should have extended upward to T4. The lowermost hook is on the ala of the sacrum. *E,* This patient's surgical procedure was fraught with many complications. As seen here, 2½ years later, the curve has increased to 85 degrees, it has lengthened approximately to T3, pelvic obliquity has recurred, the lower hook has dislocated, and there is a large pseudarthrosis at the L2–L3 level. Extensive revision was felt necessary. *F,* This x-ray taken on the day of surgical revision shows considerable improvement of the curve to 49 degrees and considerable although not full correction of the pelvic obliquity. Pseudarthrosis was extensively cleaned out, thus rendering the spine quite correctable again. A new Harrington rod was inserted, this time from T2 to the sacrum. The peculiar location of the lower hook is intentional. The previous hook had eroded downward in the sacrum and then stabilized in a relatively bony pocket which was utilized for the newer rod insertion. An anterior fusion was also performed in the area of pseudarthrosis. *G,* His operative course management was in a bivalved polypropylene body jacket. Nine months later he has a solid fusion with really no loss of correction. Thus, a deteriorating situation has been reasonably well salvaged.

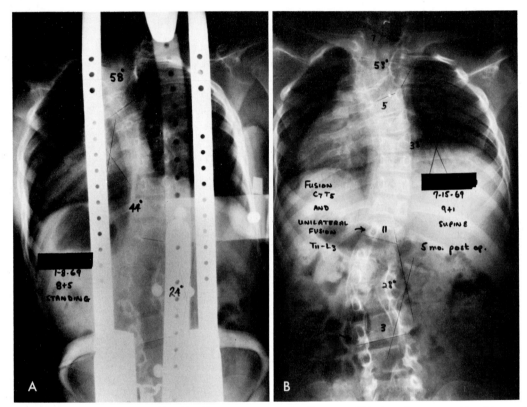

**Figure 9–18**  *A,* This 18 year old girl had been seen previously (Fig. 7–11). This time she was considered for surgical management. Because of the two progressive congenital areas, it was absolutely necessary to fuse these. The question remained as to whether the fusion had to include the central right thoracic curve, which did not contain anomalous vertebrae and in which there appeared to be good spinal musculature. It was therefore elected to attempt fusion of the two congenital areas and to continue brace treatment of the center area. *B,* This x-ray, taken five months following surgery, shows the procedures performed from C6 to T5. She underwent a conventional bilateral posterior spine fusion to arrest and stabilize the congenital curve due to the unilateral unsegmented bar. From T11 to L3 she underwent a unilateral fusion on the left side. There was a short unilateral unsegmented bar at the T12–L1–L2 area, and the fusion went one above and one below this to try to get compensatory correction in this curve. Postoperative management was with the Milwaukee brace. She was kept supine for five months and then ambulated in the brace.

*Legend continued on opposite page*

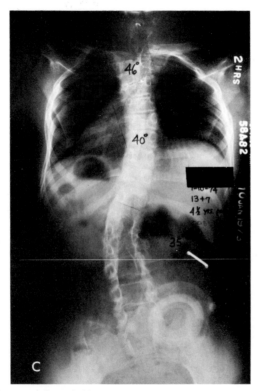

**Figure 9–18** *Continued.*    C, Four and one-half years postfusion and with continued bracing, we note continued successful management of her curve problem without fusion of the intervening curve area. The torso is well centered over a nearly level pelvis, and the high curve has been successfully stabilized and has not progressed further. The lumbar curve is stabilized at 35 degrees, and the mid curve is holding well at 40 degrees. We are continuing nonoperative treatment of this center curve, hoping that she may never require fusion of this area.

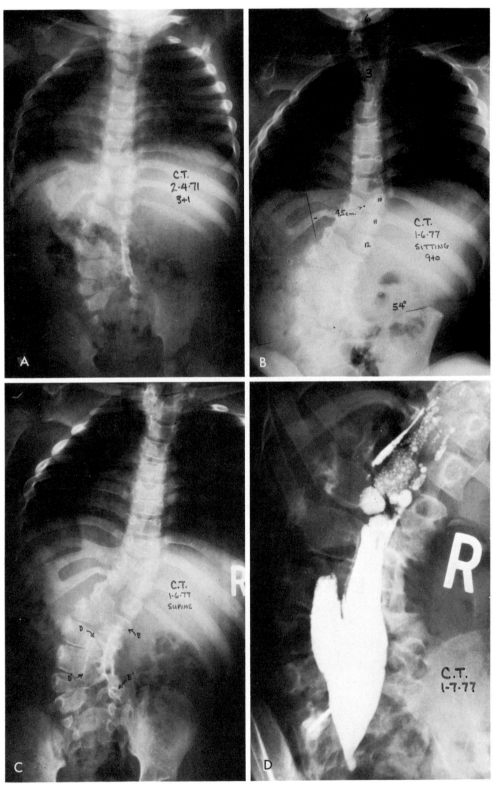

**Figure 9–19**  *See legend on opposite page.*

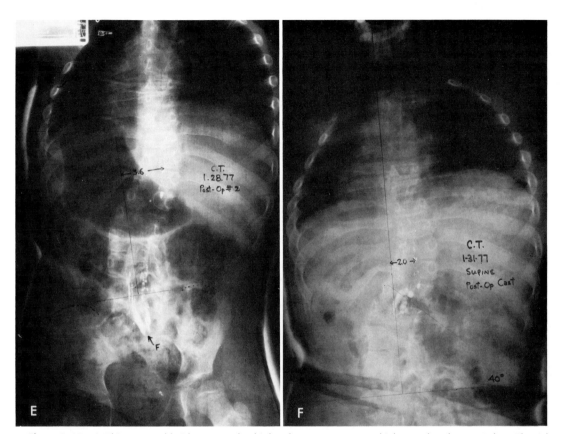

**Figure 9–19** *A,* This 3 year old girl was noted at birth to have an open sac, which was closed at age 2 days. The right leg was neurologically normal, the left completely paralyzed. Note the unilateral unsegmented bar in the convexity of the lumbar curve. No treatment was given to the scoliosis. *B,* When presented to the authors at age 9, the neurologic picture was unchanged, but the deformity was increasing. She also has a small right cervicothoracic curve associated with a Sprengel's deformity of the left shoulder. *C,* The supine film shows the anatomic details with better clarity. B–B¹ delineates the unilateral unsegmented bar. D–D¹ denotes the midline bony spur of a diastematomyelia. Note the persistent decompensation of the thorax relative to the pelvis. *D,* A myelogram shows more clearly the diastematomyelia. The heavy thick dye column obscures neurologic detail below the spur. *E,* The patient was treated by: a) removal of the diastematomyelia spur, b) resection of a posterior wedge of bone at L5, c) osteotomy of the unsegmented bar at L5–S1, d) posterior fusion of T11 to S1, and e) anterior hemivertebra excision of L5 on the left. A pin was inserted in the right distal femur and correction obtained by bending the patient to the left. In this x-ray, the correction is inadequate. Note the low-lying conus and thick filum terminale (F). *F,* The cast was wedged to give further correction. Her head is now centered over the sacrum. The thorax is slightly to the right (2.0 cm.), but the high congenital curve must also be taken into consideration. There were no neurologic complications. Attempting to treat such a curve by distraction would be catastrophic.

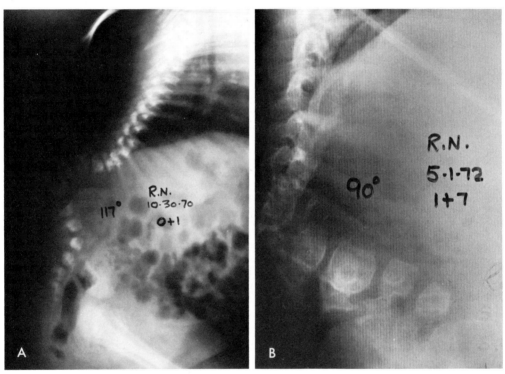

**Figure 9–20** *A,* A 1 month old child with myelomeningocele, a T12 level paraplegia, and a severe, 117 degree kyphosis of the lumbar spine. *B,* At age 1, she underwent a Sharrard apical wedge osteotomy. By age 1 + 7, she was progressing again.

*Legend continued on opposite page*

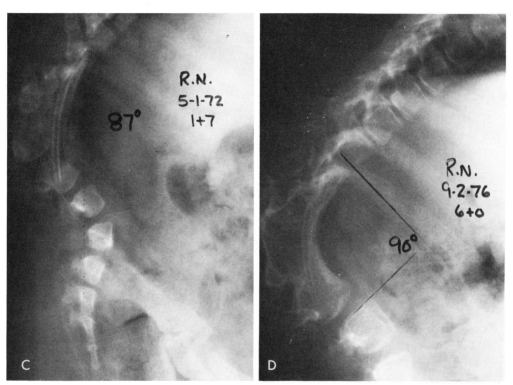

**Figure 9–20** *Continued.* *C,* At age 1 + 7, an anterior strut grafting procedure from ⌈11 to L4 was done in an effort to stabilize the kyphosis. *D,* At age 6, 4½ years later, the kyphosis is 90 degrees, showing only a 3 degree loss. She now has a kyphosis extending up into the thoracic spine. This is being braced in order to permit more growth before extending the fusion.

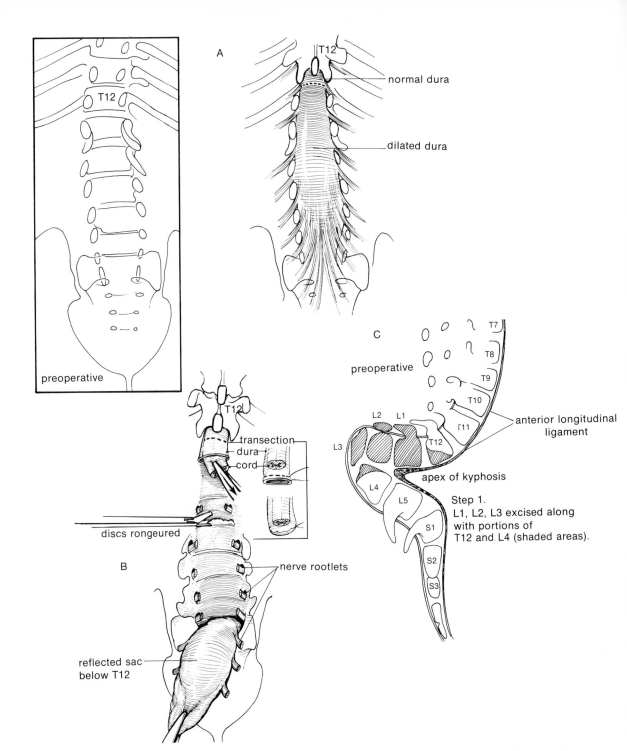

**Figure 9–21**  *A,* A posterior drawing showing the extensive spina bifida from T11 to the sacrum. The dotted line indicates the line of resection of the sac at the level of normal dura. *B,* The sac has been divided proximally and gradually reflected distally. The nerve routes are sectioned at each foramen and the highly vascular artery and vein in each foramen electrocoagulated. Extensive venous connections between the sac and the posterior aspect of the vertebral body (not pictured here) are coagulated at the sac and bone waxed at the bone. Following sac removal, the discs are removed by curette and rongeur. The cord is transected at a higher level than the dura, and the dura is closed, but the end of the sac is left open. This will prevent acute hydrocephalus. *C,* (An actual tracing of the patient.) The striped areas denote the actual bone removed in this particular case in order to obtain proper alignment. It is most important that the vertebrae contained in the upper horizontal segment of the curve be removed, not the most apical vertebra. The amount of bone removed depends on the individual case. Only that amount of bone should be removed which will allow satisfactory alignment of the distal segment with the proximal segment without tension.

**280**

*Legend continued on opposite page*

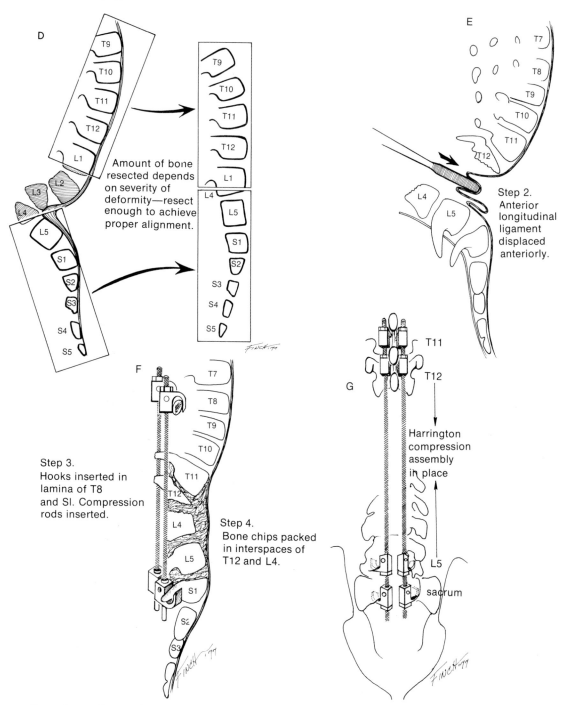

**Figure 9–21** *Continued.* *D,* A diagrammatic representation of the pathologic relationship existing. The thoracic segment in this particular case is tipped forward, and the L4–L5 sacrum unit is anteflexed. This is very common. These two segments must be placed in a straight alignment and that amount of bone should be removed which will permit this proper alignment. *E,* After resection of the bone, the anterior longitudinal ligament, which is carefully preserved, is pushed forward, thus allowing the two segments of the spine to be placed in proper alignment. *F,* Once proper alignment can be achieved, the spine is held in the proper alignment by Harrington compression apparatus. The lowermost hooks are placed in the foramina of L5 and S1. In this diagram, the lower hooks are placed in the foramina of S1. The upper hooks are placed over the laminae of normal vertebrae above the spina bifida. In this diagram, there are one set of hooks proximally and one set distally. *G,* An AP diagram showing the proper positioning of the Harrington rods. The upper hooks are placed directly over the laminae here, showing two pairs of hooks. The transverse processes are too thin and flimsy in these children to provide adequate fixation. The lowermost hooks are in the foramina, which is the only bone strong enough to give adequate support. These hooks will always lie in this semirotated position, owing to the oblique angle of the pedicle in the myelomeningocele patient.

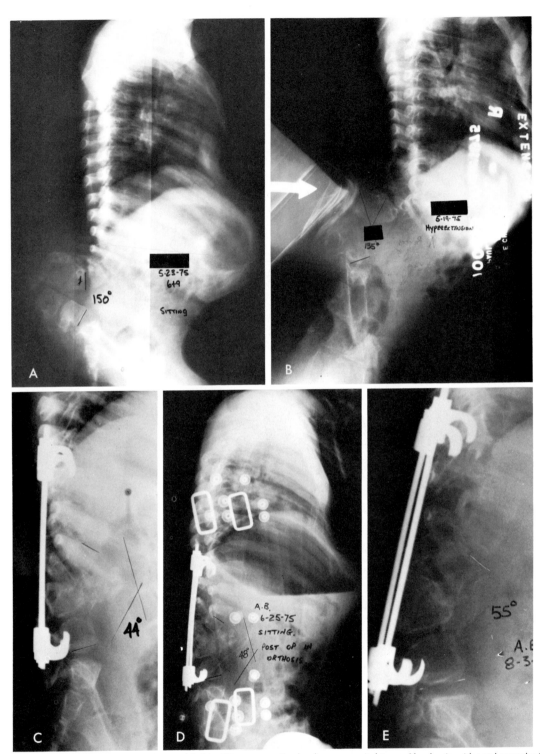

**Figure 9–22**   *A,* A.B.: A 6 + 9 year old girl with a progressive lumbar congenital type of kyphosis with total paraplegia at the T12 level. She has developed a chronic ulceration over the apex of the kyphosis and a very short anterior abdominal wall, which was significantly complicating her ilial stoma. *B,* A hyperextension x-ray demonstrates the very rigid curve correcting only to 135 degrees. *C,* A lateral x-ray following radical kyphosis resection and interbody and posterior fusion from T10 to L5. This is on the day of surgery. Fusion and instrumentation should have extended to S1. *D,* A sitting x-ray in her postoperative bivalved polypropylene body jacket showing maintenance of correction with only a 4 degree change. *E,* A sitting x-ray one year and three months following the surgery, showing maintenance of correction at 55 degrees.

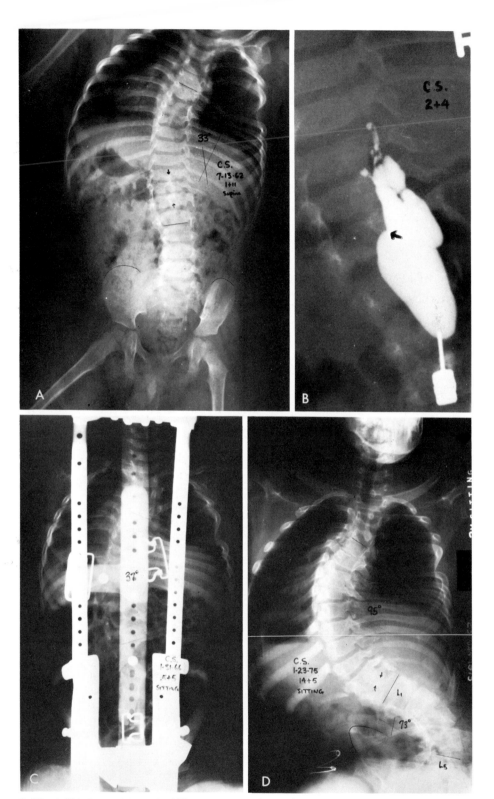

**Figure 9–23**  *A,* This 1 year, 11 month old boy was seen with a 33 degree curve containing both paralytic and congenital elements. The arrow points to a diastematomyelia at T11–L1. *B,* The myelogram demonstrates the diastematomyelia. This was removed. *C,* At age 5, an x-ray in Milwaukee brace shows satisfactory alignment of the curve at 37 degrees. Unfortunately, he disappeared from our care at this time. *D,* The patient reappeared at age 14 with this severe spinal deformity. He had almost totally lost his sitting balance. He has severe translation of the thorax to the left. There is a 95 degree thoracic curve and a 73 degree lumbar curve that is highly structural. There are no pedicles or laminae on the concavity of the curve from T6 to T12.

*Legend continued on following page*

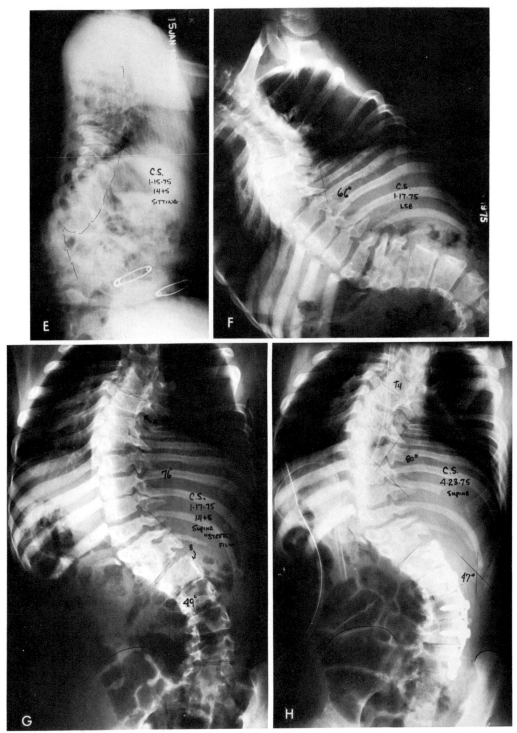

**Figure 9–23** *Continued. E,* A lateral sitting x-ray at this time shows a thoracic lordosis and thoracolumbar kyphosis. He has a T11 level paralysis. *F,* Analysis of the curve by bending films shows correction to 66 degrees in the thoracic spine. Once again, note the absence of pedicles and laminae in the concavity of the thoracic curve. This area of the spine did, however, have sufficient flexibility to allow correction of his curve. *G,* A supine stretch film shows the rigidity of the lumbar curve with very incomplete correction of proper alignment of the torso over the pelvis. The arrow A points to the last normal pedicle on the right side proximally, and B to the first normal pedicle distally. Because of the translation problem in the stiff lumbar spine, it was felt necessary to attack this lumbar spine problem first to attempt to get the spine in a more centralized position. Correction of the thoracic curve without correction of the lumbar curve would increase the decompensation to the left. *H,* First stage was a Dwyer procedure on the convexity of the lumbar curve. The second stage was an anterior transthoracic fusion from T5 to T12 through a left thoracotomy. These two operations were done two weeks apart.

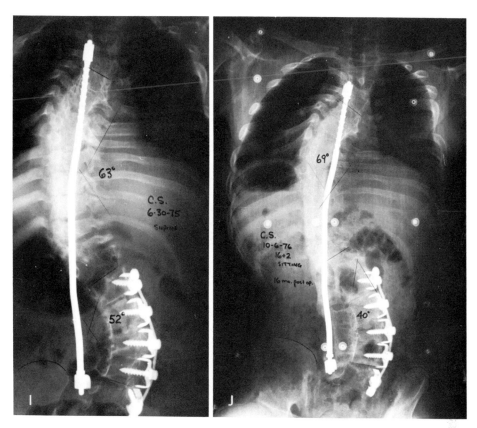

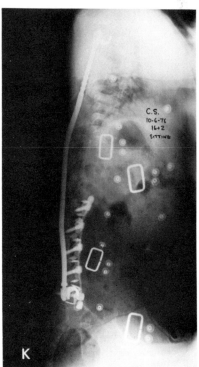

**Figure 9–23** *Continued.* *I,* The third stage was a posterior fusion and instrumentation encompassing the entire spine from T2 to the sacrum. *J,* An AP sitting x-ray 16 months following surgery shows a solid fusion and only slight residual pelvic obliquity. *K,* Lateral sitting x-ray 16 months following surgery shows a considerable improvement of the lateral outline. Note the extreme contouring of the long distraction rod, which is necessary to fit his peculiar anatomy. Postoperative management was with a bivalved polypropylene body jacket.

leg fractures, osteoporosis, genitourinary problems, and psychologic retardation. The fusion will usually be solid in six to nine months (Figs. 9–21 and 9–22).

## Results of Operative Treatment

Relatively few reports of operative treatment of myelomeningocele patients have been made, especially those showing results a year or more after treatment.

The first report was by Norton and Foley,[31] who analyzed a group of children with paraplegia and secondary spine deformity. Most of these were myelomeningocele, but some were acquired paraplegia. They reported a case of congenital lumbar kyphosis treated by excision of the cauda equina, excision of the body of L3, and interbody fusion. Although the fusion in this case failed, it is the first known report of this procedure.

In a second and more extensive article from the same institution, Kilfoyle et al.[21] reported on spine deformity in 104 children with paraplegia, 73 of these being myelomeningocele. The authors divided the problems into scoliosis, lordosis, and kyphosis. Of the 104 patients, 97 had deformities of the spine and/or pelvis. It was found important whether the patient was balanced, partially balanced, or unbalanced. Lordosis was the most common problem, with scoliosis second, and kyphosis third. All deformities tended to worsen with growth unless surgically stabilized. Correctability was lost if neglected too long. Their most cogent observation was: "Early intervention is now considered an expression of conservatism."

Sriram et al.[42] reported 33 patients operated on between 1958 and 1969 (prior to the use of the Dwyer procedure). These were patients ages 10 to 15 with severe deformities. Twenty-seven were done in one stage, and the other six in two stages. The average fusion was 11 segments. Seven patients (21 per cent) developed wound infection, but none were infected in those cases where the sac was avoided. All infected cases required rod removal and were failures. Forty-five per cent of the patients developed pseudoarthrosis. Good results were obtained in only 16 of the 33 patients (50 per cent). This article vividly pointed out the problems of spinal surgery in these patients, especially when attempting to use only the conventional posterior approach.

Hull et al.[19] reported 33 patients surgically treated with a follow-up of one year or more. Fifteen had developmental scoliosis; 10, congenital scoliosis; 8, congenital kyphosis; and 5, developmental lordosis. There was an average of 2.7 major spine operations per patient, the overall infection rate was 45 per cent, and the pseudarthrosis rate was 67 per cent. There were 3 deaths. Cast sores were noted in 5 patients. There was 51 degrees (45 per cent) average correction of kyphosis and 22 degrees (37 per cent) average correction of developmental scoliosis.

Lindberg et al.[23] reported 34 patients treated at Rancho Los Amigos. The average age at fusion was 12 years. The lordoscoliosis group (19 patients) predominated. There was 41 per cent pseudarthrosis rate and a 12 per cent infection rate. All pseudarthroses occurred prior to 1972, at which time combined anterior and posterior fusion became routine. These authors recommended a program of a) early surgery, b) anterior fusion, c) posterior fusion, and d) early return to sitting or ambulation in a well-molded plastic body jacket two to three weeks following the second surgery. Since adopting this more aggressive approach, 11 patients had been operated and there were no infections and no pseudarthroses, and all returned quickly to their preoperative functional status.

In general, the results of surgery in the myelomeningocele patient have been less than ideal, fraught with high pseudarthrosis rates and frequent infection. Despite these "negative" aspects, continued diligent efforts by spinal surgeons are gradually overcoming virtually all of the previous problems. Figure 9–23 serves as a final example to illustrate the complex problems that can occur and their solution by modern spinal surgery and orthotics.

## References

1. Baker, R. H., and Sharrard, W. J. W.: Correction of lordoscoliosis in spina bifida by multiple spinal osteotomy and fusion with Dwyer fixation. A preliminary report. Dev. Med. Child Neurol., 15 12–23, 1973.
2. Banta, J. V., Whiteman, S., Dyck, P. M., Hartleip, D., and Gilbert, D.: Fifteen year review of myelodysplasia. J. Bone Joint Surg., 58A:726, 1976.
3. Banta, J. V., and Hamada, J. S.: Natural history of the kyphotic deformity in myelomeningocoele. J. Bone Joint Surg., 58A, 279, 1976.
4. Barden, G. A., Meyer, L. C., and Stelling, F. H.: Myelodysplastics. Fate of those followed for 20 years or more. J. Bone Joint Surg., 57A:643–647, 1975.

5. Barson, A. J.: Radiological studies of spina bifida cystica. The phenomenon of congenital lumbar kyphosis. Br. J. Radiol., *38*:294–300, 1965.

6. Brown, J. Bonnett, C., Perry, J., and Sherman, R.: The surgical treatment of spine deformity in the childhood and adolescent myelodysplastic. Paper presented at the scoliosis Research Society, Hartford, 1971.

7. Bunch, W. H.: The Milwaukee brace in paralytic scoliosis. Clin. Orthop., *110*:63–68, 1975.

8. Bunch, W. H., Cass, A. S., Bensman, A. S., and Long, D. M.: Modern Management of Myelomeningocoele. St. Louis, W. H. Green, Inc., 1972.

9. Bunch, W. H., and Geist, R.: Myelomeningocoele. Current concepts in the treatment. Minn. Med., *53*:245–250, 1970.

10. Donaldson, W F.: Neural spinal dysraphism. *In* Hardy, J. M. (ed.): Spinal Deformity in Neurological and Muscular Disorders. St. Louis, C. V. Mosby Co., pp. 140–168, 1974.

11. Drennan, J. C.: The role of muscles in the development of human lumbar kyphosis. Dev. Med. Child Neurol., *12*:33–38, 1970.

12. Drennan, J. C.: Orthotic management of the myelomeningocoele spine. Dev. Med. Child Neurol. *18*(Suppl. 37):97–103, 1976.

13. Duncan, J. W., Lovell, W. W., Bailey, S. C., and Ransom, D.: Surgical treatment of kyphosis in myelomeningocoele. Paper presented at the Scoliosis Research Society, Louisville, 1975.

14. Eckstein, H. B., and Vora, R. M.: Spinal osteotomy for severe kyphosis in children with myelomeningocoele. J. Bone Joint Surg., *54B*:328–33, 1972.

15. Emery, J. L., and Lendon, R. G.: Clinical implications of cord lesions in neurospinal dysraphism. Dev. Med. Child Neurol., *14*:45–51, 1972.

16. Eyring, E., and Wankin, J.: Spinal osteotomy in myelomeningocoele kyphosis. Paper Presented at AAOS, 1971.

17. Hall, J. E., and Bobechko, W. P.: Advances in the management of spinal deformities in myelodysplasia. Clin. Neurosurg., *20*:164–173, 1973.

18. Hall, J. E., and Martin, R.: The natural history of spine deformity in myelomeningocoele. A study of 130 patients. Paper Presented to Canadian Orthopaedic Association, Bermuda, June, 1970.

19. Hull, W. J., Moe, J. H., Lai, C., and Winter, R. B.: The surgical treatment of spinal deformities in myelomeningocoele. J. Bone Joint Surg., *57A*:1767, 1974.

20. Hoppenfeld, S.: Congenital kyphosis in myelomeningocoele. J. Bone Joint Surg., *49B*:276–280, 1967.

21. Kilfoyle, R. M., Foley, J. J., and Norton, P. L.: Spine and pelvic deformity in childhood and adolescent paraplegia. A study of 104 cases. J. Bone Joint Surg., *47A*:659–682, 1965.

22. Levin, G. D.: Functional evaluation of 18 adult myelomeningocoele patients. Clin. Orthop., *100*:101–107, 1974.

23. Lindberg, C., Brown, J. C., and Bonnett, C. A.: The surgical treatment of spine deformity in myelodysplasia. Paper presented at the Scoliosis Research Society, Louisville, Sept., 1975.

24. Lorber, J.: Spina bifida cystica. Results of treatment of 270 consecutive cases with criteria for selection for the future. Arch. Dis. Child., *47*:854–873, 1972.

25. McKay, D. A.: The McKay plate for kyphosis of the spine. Paper presented at the Scoliosis Research Society, Louisville, Sept., 1975.

26. Mackel, J. L., and Lindseth, R. E.: Scoliosis in Myelodysplasia. AAOS, San Francisco, 1975. J. Bone Joint Surg., *57A*:1031, 1975.

27. Menelaus, M. B.: The Orthopaedic Management of Spina Bifida. Edinburgh and London, E. and S. Livingstone, 1971.

28. Menelaus, M.: Spinal deformities in spina bifida. J. Bone Joint Surg., *55B*:223, 1973.

29. Menelaus, M. B.: Orthopaedic management of children with myelomeningocoele: A plea for realistic goals. Dev. Med. Child Neurol. *18*(Suppl. 37):3–11, 1976.

30. Micheli, L. J., and Hall, J. E.: The management of spine deformities in the myelomeningocoele patient. Med. Ann., *43*:21–24, 1974.

31. Norton, P. L., and Foley, J. J.: Paraplegic in children. J. Bone Joint Surg., *41A*:1291–1309, 1959.

32. Park, W. M., and Watt, I.: The preoperative aortographic assessment of children with spina bifida cystica and severe kyphosis. J. Bone Joint Surg., *57B*:112, 1975.

33. Parsch, K., and Goesseus, H.: The operative treatment of spine and hip deformities in spina bifida. Acta Orthop. Belg., *37*:230–244, 1971.

34. Poitras, B., and Hall, J. E.: Excision of kyphosis in myelomeningocoele. Paper presented at the Scoliosis Research Society, September, 1974.

35. Raycroft, J. F., and Curtis, B. H.: Spinal curvature in myelomeningocoele. AAOS Symposium on Myelomeningocoele. St. Louis, C. V. Mosby Co., 1972.

36. Rose, G. K., Owne, R., and Sanderson, J. M.: Transposition of rib and blood supply for stabilization of spinal kyphosis. J. Bone Joint Surg., *57B*:112, 1975.

37. Roth, K.: Spinal deformities in myelomeningocoele: A radiologic assessment. Scoliosis (Paul R. Harrington), pp. 1–29, 1971.

38. Sharrard, W J. W.: The kyphotic and lordotic spine in myelomeningocoele. AAOS Symposium on Myelomeningocoele. St. Louis, C. V. Mosby Co., 1972.

39. Sharrard, W. J. W.: Spinal osteotomy for congenital kyphosis in myelomeningocoele. J. Bone Joint Surg., *50B*:466–471, 1968.

40. Sharrard, W. J. W., and Drennan, J. C.: Osteotomy, excision of the spine for lumbar kyphosis in older children with myelomeningocoele. J. Bone Joint Surg., *54B*:50–60, 1972.

41. Shurtleff, D. B., Goiney, R., Gordon, L. H., and Livermore, N.: Myelodysplasia: The natural history of kyphosis and scoliosis. A preliminary report. Dev. Med. Child Neurol. *18*(Suppl. 37):126–133, 1976.

42. Sriram, K., Bobechko, W. P., and Hall, J. E.: Surgical management of spinal deformities in spina bifida. J. Bone Joint Surg., *54B*:666–676, 1972.

43. Walker, G., and Cheong-Leen, P.: Spinal excision osteotomy in myelomeningocoele with special reference to internal fixation. Postgrad. Med. J., *50*:145–149, 1974.

44. Wedge, J. H., and Gillespie, R.: The problems of scoliosis surgery in paraplegic children. J. Bone Joint Surg., *57B*:396, 1975.

# Chapter 10

# SCOLIOSIS ASSOCIATED WITH NEUROFIBROMATOSIS

## INTRODUCTION

Neurofibromatosis involves both ectodermal and mesenchymal tissues of the body. Its basic entity is tumor formation in the peripheral as well as the central nervous system. Tumors in bone have not been described, although some aspects of skin and subcutaneous tissue involvement were described in 1793 by Tilseus[31] and in 1849 by Smith.[28] The first adequate histologic manifestations was described by von Recklinghausen in 1882,[23] who described the nerve tumors as neurofibromas and attached the term neurofibromatosis to the disease.

No mention of scoliosis associated with the disease was made until 1921, when Weiss, a dermatologist, reported scoliosis in neurofibromatosis.[32] Since that report the medical literature has been replete with descriptions of the various manifestations of this disease, which may involve the entire central nervous system, the skeletal system, soft tissues, and skin.

## MANIFESTATIONS AND DIAGNOSTIC FINDINGS

The most common stigmata of the disease are café au lait skin markings, which in white-skinned individuals are tan, macular, and melanotic. In blacks they appear light colored. They occur around the basal layer of the epidermis.[7] They are found in at least 90 per cent of patients exhibiting other diagnostic features of neurofibromatosis.[7] Since a few brown spots are not uncommon in normal individuals, they are considered diagnostic only when they are found in numbers greater than six.[33] Other skin manifestations are patches of thick brown rough skin, called local elephantiasis neuromatosa. There may be hemangiomatous tissue incorporated in many of these. Other manifestations of the disease are subcutaneous nodules of tumor tissue (fibroma molluscum) and variable numbers of generalized pedunculated tumors of the same type within the skin (Fig. 10–1). Other features of the disease include skeletal and soft tissue enlargement, sometimes focal such as macrodactyly, sometimes multiple and assuming major proportions (Fig. 10–2).

Hunt and Pugh in 1961[13] outlined the various bone manifestations of the disease. With some modification, these are as follows:

1) The classical type of scoliosis or kyphoscoliosis, which consists of a sharply angulated lateral curvature comprising five to eight vertebrae, which is often associated with an acute kyphosis in the same area. The kyphoscoliotic curve is usually made up of severely deformed dystrophic vertebrae. The scoliotic types without kyphosis are often less dystrophic, but all classical curves have a varying degree of scalloped margins, and the vertebrae are distinctly abnormal.

2) The ribs associated with the apical portion of the classical curve are often narrow and deformed, commonly called "penciling."

3) The vertebrae within the curve may have deep invagination visible on myelography. These are dural invasions or meningoceles and vary in degree. Occasionally an

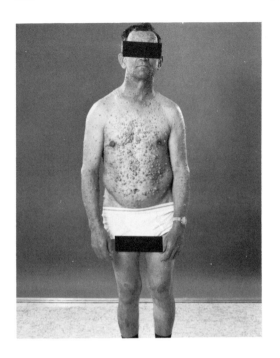

**Figure 10–1** L.C., age 45 + 6, 4/13/76. Front view of torso. Multiple skin tumors (fibroma molluscum) in a patient with a 55 degree right thoracic curve. The vertebrae showed only moderate scalloping. No kyphosis of significance. Patient was fused in 1974 with correction to 40 degrees because of pain within the curve. Severe osteoporosis was found in the spine. Harrington instrumentation could not be used, and a halo cast supplied some corrective distraction. The entire body was covered with tumors and café au lait skin markings. There was no evidence of soft tissue overgrowth.

entire vertebral body may show a filling defect on myelography. The cause is unknown. The meningocele protrusions may extend laterally beyond the spinal canal.

4) Patients with numerous café au lait skin markings or other skin manifestations may have a lesser degree of dystrophic vertebral malformations, such as marginal scalloping in a lateral curvature. These curves also tend to be shorter than idiopathic curvatures.

5) Occasionally patients with skin manifestations of the disease may have a characteristic idiopathic curvature. Congenital spine abnormalities may also be found associated with neurofibromatosis stigmata.

6) Enlarged vertebral foramina may be present, usually associated with dumb-bell tumors.

7) Congenital pseudarthrosis of the tibia is considered by many to be a manifestation of the disease. Most of these have characteristic

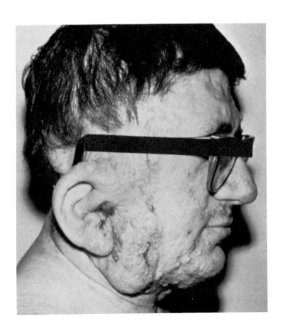

**Figure 10–2** D.D., age 27 + 6, 1967. The severely grotesque overgrowth of the right side of the face and the increased skin tumor formation have increased markedly since first seen at age 21.

skin markings. Bowing of the tibia is also occasionally found.

8) Orbital defects, particularly in the posterior superior wall.

## ETIOLOGY AND GENERAL CHARACTERISTICS

The disease is hereditary to a high degree, being transmitted as an autosomal dominant with variable penetrance. The frequency of neurofibromatosis scoliosis in the population is probably less than two per cent of all existing scolioses. There are many patients with evidence of neurofibromatosis who do not have scoliosis. Neurofibromatosis scoliosis can sometimes be diagnosed at birth, but this is rare. Malignant changes in the tumors have been variously reported as occurring in 5 per cent[12] to 10 per cent[22] of cases.

## CURVE PATTERNS AND TYPES

### Scoliosis

There are several distinct types of scoliosis. Idiopathic scoliosis is occasionally found, coincidental with café au lait skin markings, but in these patients other manifestations of neurofibromatosis are rarely found. The scoliotic spine is completely free from any stigmata of the disease, and the usual pattern is right major thoracic.

Scolioses having some of the characteristic stigmata of neurofibromatosis in the vertebral bodies do occur not associated with kyphosis of any significant degree. The vertebral bodies are deformed and have scalloped margins. Their natural history shows an almost constant tendency toward slow and steady progression. Some of these have tumors within the spinal canal that may produce paraplegia (Fig. 10–3). Some have paravertebral tumors. One patient in our series had a nonprogressive moderate sharply angulated curve at age 40.

### Kyphoscoliosis

This constitutes the most classical type of spine deformity directly associated with neurofibromatosis. It may begin as a deformity of moderate degree, but the kyphotic element soon begins to increase. The early states are correctable although the curve is of the sharply angulated short type which is so characteristic, and the vertebral bodies at first may not be severely dystrophic. Later, as progression occurs, either without treatment or with inadequate treatment, they progress rapidly. In the absence of severely distorted apical vertebrae the curve becomes more rigid, although it may still correct somewhat with halofemoral distraction (Fig. 10–4). As in all kyphoscoliosis of this origin, the curves continue to progress into adult life unless checked by an adequate spine fusion, both anterior and posterior.

Another form of kyphoscoliosis due to neurofibromatosis is characterized by extreme dystrophic deformity of many segments. This form, when occurring in a relatively flexible part of the spine (the thoracolumbar or cervical region), remains flexible and can be straightened considerably by distraction (Fig. 10–5).

Progression of the classical form of kyphoscoliosis is inevitable without adequate treatment and will lead to cord compression and paraplegia in a high percentage of these severe deformities.

### Lordosis

The incidence of lordosis with ventral angulation of the thoracic spine is low, but in our recent study of 112 cases of spine deformity associated with neurofibromatosis stigmata there were 7 cases, ranging from −22 to −48 degrees. All were corrected to a varying degree by Harrington strut bars. One case of thoracic lordosis in a 4 year old child deserves special mention.

This patient had clear evidence of neurofibromatosis, and the dystrophic thoracic vertebrae were angled anteriorly 45 degrees from a straight spine on the lateral view. Treatment was by exposure of a single lamina and joint at the upper end of the lordotic curve and the insertion of a #1254 dull hook into this joint. Another similar incision and exposure of a lamina at the lower end provided room for placement of a similar hook under the lamina. A large size threaded rod was then inserted *subcutaneously* between the two hooks. Nuts were placed on the rod to engage the hooks to

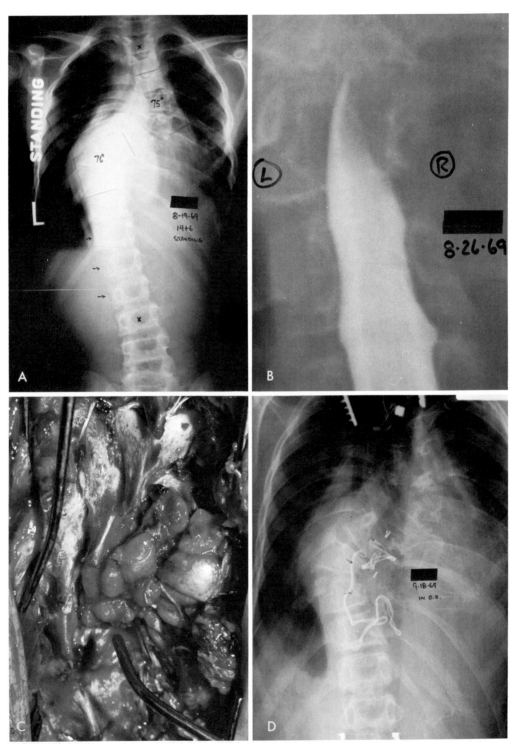

**Figure 10–3**  *A,* R. McG., 14 + 6. 8/19/69, A classical neurofibromatosis scoliosis without kyphosis. This patient was paraparetic. *B,* 8/26/69. A myelogram showed a block, probably extradural. *C,* A hemilaminectomy was done, demonstrating numerous extradural grapelike neurofibroma tumors. These were easily removed and a fusion carried out on the intact laminae. Only a posterior fusion was done because there was no kyphosis. Harrington distraction rod inserted. *D,* 9/18/69. An x-ray taken at surgery showing the appearance after removal of all tumors including ends of ribs.

*Legend continued on opposite page*

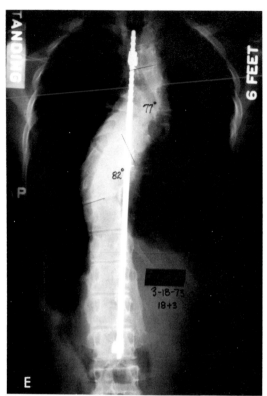

**Figure 10-3** *Continued. E, 3/18/73.* An AP x-ray taken three years after fusion shows the spine balance well maintained. This patient in 1977 developed a sarcoma and died.

provide *distraction,* and these were tightened, giving a distraction force. Periodically, as the child grew, the short incisions were reopened and the nuts tightened to provide further distraction. Between the lengthening procedure, the patient was kept fulltime in a Milwaukee brace.

The original plan of Harrington was to distract curves in the young paralytic child with a strut bar and to periodically lengthen it without fusion. This failed for two reasons. First, the complete subperiosteal exposure of the length of the curve led to new bone formation and a partial fusion. Second, he did not provide external support to the curve; as a result the hooks displaced, and the end of the rod protruded.

In the patient described, correction of the lordosis down to −16 degrees has been obtained in four years. Periodic elongation was successful for four years, but increasing scoliosis led to fusion at that time.

## TREATMENT

The treatment depends upon the type of deformity. The idiopathic curve with café au lait spots should be treated like any other idiopathic curve. The Milwaukee brace is sometimes very successful. Surgical correction is used when indicated. We have found no difference in this type from ordinary idiopathic scoliosis.

Treatment of the congenitally abnormal spine with stigmata of neurofibromatosis elsewhere should be treated as any other congenital scoliosis.

Treatment of all forms of scoliosis having any of the findings in the spine that are considered to be associated with this disease should be surgically fused at once in the best correction. This should be done at any age at which the curve is diagnosed (Fig. 10-3). Milwaukee brace treatment has been ineffectual in correcting these curves. If the child is very young and the curve is small, the brace may be tried temporarily as long as there is no progression.

In our series, 100 per cent of curves showing dystrophic changes progressed in the brace and required fusion. Only those having an idiopathic curve responded favorably in a small percentage.

If there is no kyphosis associated with the scoliosis, a posterior fusion alone will be

*Text continued on page 297*

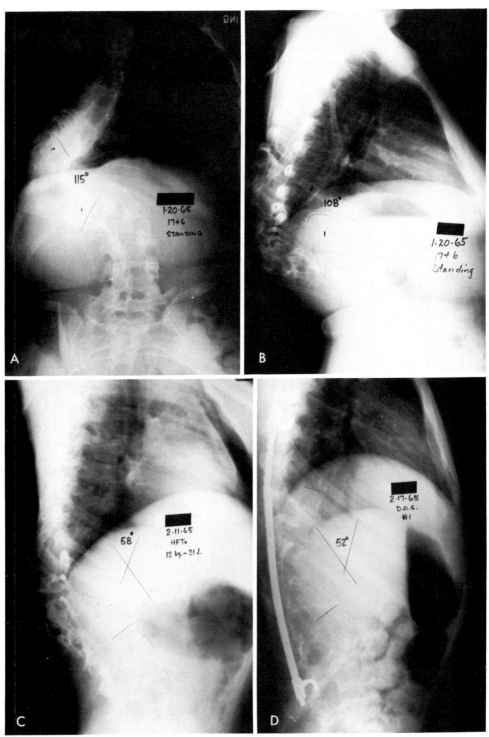

**Figure 10–4**   *A*, M.J., age 17 + 6, 1/20/65. X-ray of a classical kyphoscoliosis due to neurofibromatosis. *B*, Lateral x-ray shows the severe kyphosis. *C*, 2/11/65. Halofemoral distraction for 21 days demonstrates relative flexibility of the kyphosis. *D*, 2/17/65. Only a posterior fusion was performed with excellent correction of kyphosis maintained by a Harrington distraction strut bar.

*Legend continued on opposite page*

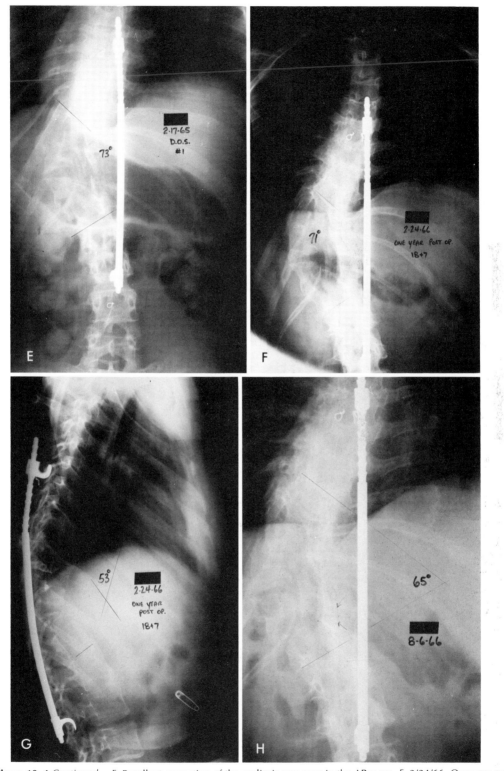

**Figure 10–4** *Continued.* *E,* Excellent correction of the scoliosis was seen in the AP x-ray. *F,* 2/24/66. One year post-operatively the correction was maintained on the AP standing x-ray. The fusion was felt to be solid. *G,* The posterior displacement of the upper hook was *not* noted. *H,* 8/6/66. X-ray sent by local orthopedic surgeon showed a probable pseud-arthrosis. Advice by letter given to explore, repair, and continue cast support.

*Legend continued on following page*

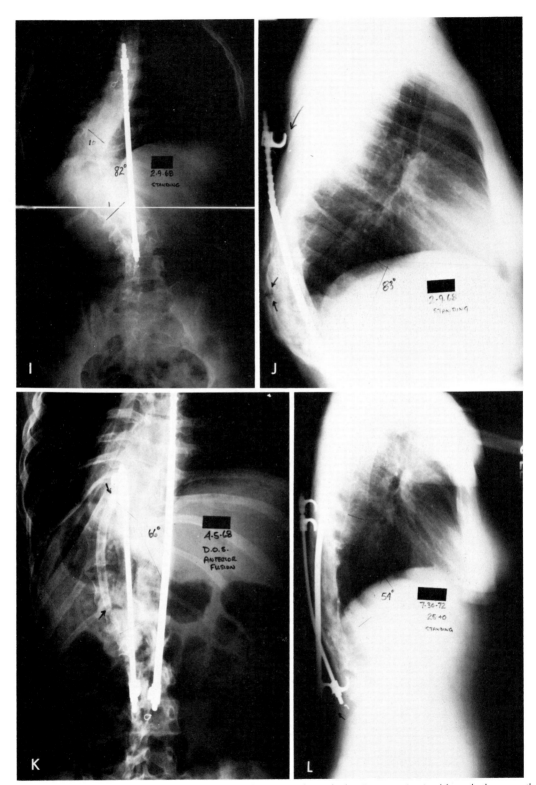

**Figure 10–4** *Continued.* *I,* 2/9/68. Cast correction after repair of pseudarthrosis was maintained for only three months. Deformity recurred and patient returned for evaluation. Loss of correction on AP x-ray is evident. *J,* Loss of correction on lateral x-ray is marked. Now 83 degrees and pseudarthrosis at apex is evident as well as complete displacement of upper hook. *K,* 4/5/68. Anterior rib strut is clearly visible with excellent recorrection on AP x-ray. *L,* 7/30/72. Lower hook of distraction rod was protruding. Rods removed and fusion explored. Found very solid and mature.

*Legend continued on opposite page*

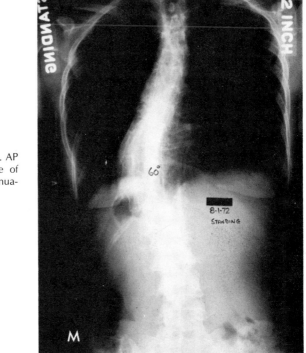

**Figure 10–4** *Continued.* M, M.J., age 25, 8/1/72. AP x-ray after instruments removed shows maintenance of correction. Further follow-up by letter indicates continuation of good result.

sufficient, making certain that the fusion is solid and mature before discarding external support. If any doubt exists as to the presence of a pseudarthrosis, exploration and repair of defects are mandatory. We do not feel that exploration must be routinely done. Harrington instrumentation should be used for stability whenever possible. If a single pseudarthrosis is present at the apical area of the curve, and the graft above and below is thick and substantial, a contraction hook assembly will close the gap and increase the potential for healing. Obviously, the fibrous tissue in the pseudarthrosis should be curetted out and abundant bone placed within and over the defect.

Kyphoscoliosis offers the most difficult problem for maintaining correction. To obtain a solid fusion, an anterior and posterior approach is necessary. If the apex is at the thoracolumbar area and distraction is effective in correcting the deformity, it may be best to do a posterior fusion as a primary stage. The kyphosis is maximally corrected with a contracting hook assembly, and the scoliosis with a distraction strut bar. Two weeks later, an

anterior fusion is performed. Failures from anterior fusion have occurred in our hands mainly because the strut graft was too short and did not extend well above and below the apical area. At least two normal vertebrae above and two below must be included.

In the thoracic spine, the kyphos is usually more rigid, and an anterior grafting must be done as the primary procedure, followed by a posterior fusion and instrumentation as a second step. The same holds true anywhere in the spine where distraction does not effectively correct the kyphosis.

Kyphoscoliosis due to neurofibromatosis must always have a two-stage procedure, both anterior and posterior. Traction preoperatively as well as postoperatively has been safe in our hands. We are familiar with one patient treated elsewhere who had a severe kyphoscoliosis with no neurologic involvement and after a short period of halofemoral distraction developed paraparesis of the lower extremities, necessitating discontinuance of the traction and immediate anterior decompression and fusion. It is well known that if the central vertebra at the apex of a congenital kyphosis

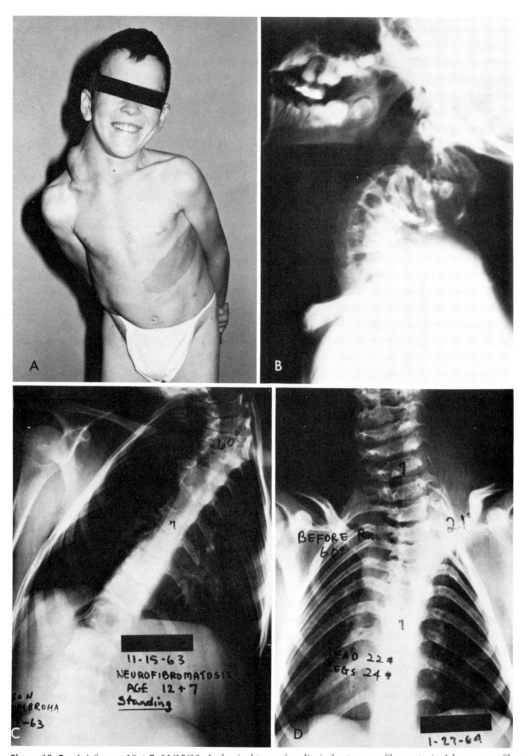

**Figure 10–5**   A, L.S., age 12 + 7, 11/15/63. A classical type of scoliosis due to neurofibromatosis. A large neurofibroma was present in the right neck. This was excised before spine treatment was undertaken. B, The dystrophic cervical vertebra produced a severe neck deformity, especially on the lateral x-ray. There were no neurologic manifestations. C, Severe thoracic scoliosis was present on the AP x-ray. D, After 10 weeks of carefully controlled halofemoral distraction, the spine straightened remarkably. The weights were gradually added after beginning with 1 kg. E, On the lateral view the extreme neck deformity also straightened. F, 8/5/70. The final result was satisfactory in spite of the loss of correction. G, For two years after surgery he was kept in a Milwaukee brace with side outriggers to keep the neck straight.

*Legend continued on opposite page*

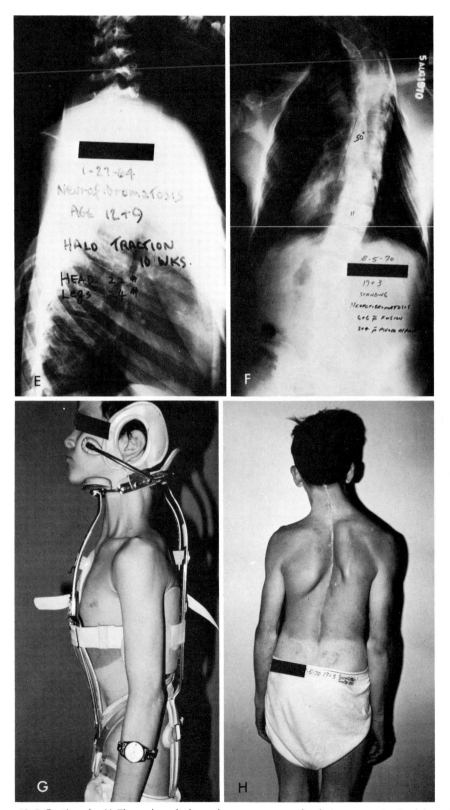

**Figure 10–5** *Continued. H,* The end result shown here seven years after fusion was maintained thereafter.

is fixed, distraction will often produce neuro-logic complications, but in kyphoscoliosis due to neurofibromatosis such fixation at the apex is not commonly found. A predistraction hyperextension view will demonstrate the mobility of the apical area.

### Paralysis and Laminectomy

There are no indications for laminectomy in the patient with progressive kyphoscoliosis with neurologic evidence of cord compression. Laminectomy has invariably been productive of or worsened the paralysis and caused rapid progression of the deformity in kyphoscoliosis.

The only indication for a laminectomy is the presence of tumors within the spinal canal. Under all circumstances, a fusion must be done at the same time or very soon after. Every effort must be made to preserve bone in doing the laminectomy. Preferably it should be a hemilaminectomy. Tumors of nerve roots may likewise require laminectomy (Fig. 10–4).

Paralytic complications should first be treated in distraction, since a good percentage improve by this means. If decompression of the cord is indicated it must be done from an anterior approach and must always be accompanied by an anterior fusion using multiple strut grafts (see Chapter 20). A posterior fusion must follow.

### Results

***Posterior Fusion Alone.*** In our series no patient with kyphoscoliosis was successfully fused by a posterior fusion alone; therefore, the combined procedure of anterior and posterior fusion is always indicated in the presence of kyphosis.

In our series, 94 per cent of patients without kyphosis were successfully fused by one procedure. Pseudarthrosis can usually be diagnosed by adequate x-ray studies at six months postoperatively and must always be repaired.

With improved technic of fusion and postoperative immobilization, the pseudarthrosis rate should be lowered to about five per cent or less.

### References

1. Adrian, C.: Ueber Neurofibromatose und ihre Komplikationen. Beitr. Klin. Chir., *31*:1–98, 1901.
2. Aegerter, E., and Kirkpatrick, J. A.: Orthopedic Diseases, 3rd ed. W. B. Saunders Co., 1968.
3. Allibone, E. C., Illingworth, R. S., and Wright, T.: Neurofibromatosis (von Recklinghausen disease) of the vertebral column. Arch. Dis. Child., *35*: 153–158, 1960.
4. Barson, A. J.: Neurofibromatosis with congenital malformation of the spinal cord. J. Neurol. Neurosurg. Psychiatry, *30*:71–74, 1967.
5. Brooks, B., and Lehman, E. P.: The bone changes in Recklinghausen's neurofibromatosis. Surg. Gynecol. Obstet., *38*:587–595, 1924.
6. Cobb, J. R.: Discussion of paper by H. R. McCarrol. J. Bone Joint Surg., *32A*:617, 1950.
7. Crowe, F. W., Schull, W. J., and Neel, J. V.: A Clinical, Pathological, and Genetic Study of Multiple Neurofibromatosis. Springfield, Illinois, Charles C Thomas, 1956.
8. Crowe, F. W., and Schull, W. J.: Diagnostic importance of café au lait spot in neurofibromatosis. Arch. Intern. Med., *91*:758, 1953.
9. Curtis, B. H., Fisher, R. L., Butterfield, W. L., and Saunders, F. P.: Neurofibromatosis with paraplegia. J. Bone Joint Surg., *51A*:843–861, 1969.
10. Enklaar, J. E.: Scoliosis in neurofibromatosis. Demonstration of 2 patients. Ned. Tijdschr. Geneeskd., *106*:2019–2020, 1962.
11. Hagelstam, L.: On deformities of the spine in multiple neurofibromatosis. Acta Chir. Scand., *93*:169, 1946.
12. Holt, J. R., and Wright, E. M.: Radiological features of neurofibromatosis. Radiology, *51*:647–664, 1948.
13. Hunt, J. C., and Pugh, D. G.: Skeletal lesions in neurofibromatosis. Radiology, *76*:1–20, 1961.
14. Kerr, J. G.: Scoliosis with paraplegia. J. Bone Joint Surg., *35A*:769–773, 1953.
15. Levin, O. L.: Recklinghausen's disease: Its relation to the endocrine system. Arch. Dermatol. *4*:303–321, 1921.
16. Marchetti, P. G.: Le Scoliosi. Aulo Gaggi Editore, 307, 1968.
17. McCarrol, H. R.: Clinical manifestations of congenital neurofibromatosis. J. Bone Joint Surg., *32A*:601–617, 1950.
18. McNairy, D. J., and Montgomery, H.: Cutaneous tumors of von Recklinghausen's disease. Arch. Dermatol. Syphilis, *51*:384–390, June, 1945.
19. Meszaros, W. T., Guzzo, F., and Schorsch, H.: Neurofibromatosis. Am. J. Roentgenol., *98*:557–569, 1966.
20. Pratt, R. T. C.: The Genetics of Neurologic Disorders. London, Oxford University Press, 1967.
21. Preiser, S. A., and Davenport, D. B.: Multiple neurofibromatosis (Recklinghausen's disease) and its inheritance, with description of a case. Am. J. Med. Sci., *156*:507–540, 1918.
22. Preston, F. W., Walsh, W. S., and Clarke, T.: Cutaneous neurofibromatosis–clinical manifestations and incidence of sarcoma in sixty-one patients. Arch. Surg., *64*:813–827, 1952.

23. Recklinghausen, F.: Ueber die Multiplen Fibrome der Haut und ihre Beziehung zu den Multiplen Neuromen. Berlin, August Hirschwald, 1882.
24. Recognition of neurofibromatosis. Leading article. Br. Med. J., 2:1025, 1966.
25. Robb-Smith, A. H. T., and Pennybacker, J.: von Recklinghausen's disease. In British Encyclopedia of Medical Practice, 2nd ed., vol. 10. London, Butterworth, and Co., Ltd., 1952.
26. Salerno, R. N., and Edeiken, J.: Vertebral scalloping in neurofibromatosis. Radiology, 97:509–510, 1970.
27. Scott, J. C.: Scoliosis and neurofibromatosis. J. Bone Joint Surg., 47B:240–246, 1965.
28. Smith, R. W.: A Treatise on the Pathology, Diagnosis and Treatment of Neuroma. Dublin, Hodg & Smith, 1849.
29. Swann, G. F.: General softening of bone due to metabolic causes: Pathogenesis of bone lesions in neurofibromatosis. Br. J. Radiol., 27:623–629, 1954.
30. Thiebierge, V.: Un cas de maladie de Recklinghausen (neurofibromatose generalisee) sans fibromes cutanes. Bull. Mem. Soc. Med. Hop. Paris, 15:143, 1898.
31. Tilseus, T. W. C.: Historia Pathologica Singularis Cutis Turpitudinis. Leipzig, S. L. Crusius, 1793.
32. Weiss, R. S.: Curvature of the spine in von Recklinghausen disease. Arch. Dermatol. Syphilis, 3:144, 1921.
33. Whitehouse, D.: Diagnostic value of the café au lait spot in children. Arch. Dis. Child., 41:316–319, 1966.
34. Wilson, P. D., Jr., Veliskakis, K., and Levine, D. B.: Neurofibromatosis and scoliosis: Significance of the short, sharp, angular spinal curve. Read at the meeting of the Scoliosis Research Society, Houston, Texas, Sept. 5–7, 1968.

# Chapter 11

# SPINE DEFORMITY FOLLOWING IRRADIATION

Since Perthes[21] first demonstrated in 1903 the occurrence of skeletal changes following irradiation of the osseous structures, considerable information, both clinical and experimental, has become available. The first microscopic studies of irradiated bones were carried out and reported by Recamier and Tribondeau in 1905.[23] These authors noted that radiation caused retarded growth, but they were unable to demonstrate any specific histologic changes. Segale, in 1920,[30] first described microscopic changes in the bones of young rats that had received radiation. He noted a disorganization of cartilage cells in the growth zones. This was later confirmed by Hoffman et al.[15] In the 1920s Phemister[22] and Ewing[11] both demonstrated that the effects of radiation on bone included decalcification and necrosis as well as dense sclerosis from radiation osteitis. From the information gathered in these earlier reports and from more recent studies by several authors,[2, 4, 10, 14, 23, 26] it has become apparent that radiation treatment shortens bones and prevents their normal maturation and that the effect is related to dose and age; that is, the younger the animal and the greater the radiation dosage, the greater will be the ultimate effect in creating deformity.

With this background of data, Engel[10] first produced scoliosis in goats, dogs, and rabbits by exposing one side of the vertebral column to radium. Arkin and Simon[2] likewise produced scoliosis in rabbits by irradiating asymmetrically the vertebral bodies with radon seeds and external irradiation.

The first clinical case of scoliosis in a human following irradiation treatment was reported by Arkin et al. in 1950.[1] They presented a patient, 19 months old, with a Wilms' tumor treated by preoperative irradiation, nephrectomy, and postoperative irradiation. This patient subsequently developed a severe structural lumbar scoliosis concave to the side of maximum irradiation. In light of the fact that Bick and Copel[7] had shown that the vertebral bodies have epiphyseal plates and grow by enchondral ossification similar to that occurring in the epiphyseal plates of long bones, the deformities produced were believed to have been caused by damage to the growth centers of the vertebral bodies exposed to the radiation. Since this original report by Arkin in 1950[1] numerous papers concerning bone changes developing after irradiation of childhood tumors have appeared.[16]

In attempting to put these reports in proper perspective, our discussion will be focused on the following questions: 1) What are the type and incidence of bony changes, particularly scoliosis and kyphosis, associated with irradiation to the axial skeleton? 2) How might these deformities be decreased or prevented? 3) What is the prognosis of untreated deformities? 4) What is the optimal treatment of irradiation-induced spinal deformity?

Although irradiation to the axial skeleton for any reason may produce the changes described, most of the discussion to follow will be based on experience collected from series of patients with Wilms' tumor or neuroblastoma, since these would apply to the majority of patients receiving irradiation in the childhood period.

## INCIDENCE

The incidence of bony changes following irradiation treatment to the spine has varied from reported series. Neuhauser and associates in 1952[20] showed that in 34 surviving patients having received irradiation to and about the spine, 21 showed radiographic changes of the vertebrae. These changes consisted of horizontal transverse lines or a "bone within a bone" appearance, gross irregularity and scalloping of the vertebral epiphyseal cartilage plate, or gross contour abnormalities of the vertebral bodies (Fig. 11–1). Other authors have confirmed these findings and in the series of Vaeth et al.,[31] they occurred in all patients receiving irradia-

tion to the spine. The initial changes appear 9 to 12 months after radiation, and it is generally believed that a dosage of 1000r to 2000r is necessary to produce these abnormalities.[29] It is important to recognize that late bony complications may not always be due to radiation effects per se but may be secondary to recurrent tumor and the reparative processes.[27]

Other effects of irradiation to the axial skeleton include hypoplasia of the ilium and the rib cage (Fig. 11–2). This abnormality developed in 60 per cent of the patients of Katzman et al.[16] These authors also found that patients with severe iliac hypoplasia secondary to radiation treatment had more severe scoliosis and vertebral body changes. Damage to the femoral head and the proximal end of the femur associated with avascular necrosis has also been reported in cases where care is not taken to exclude that area

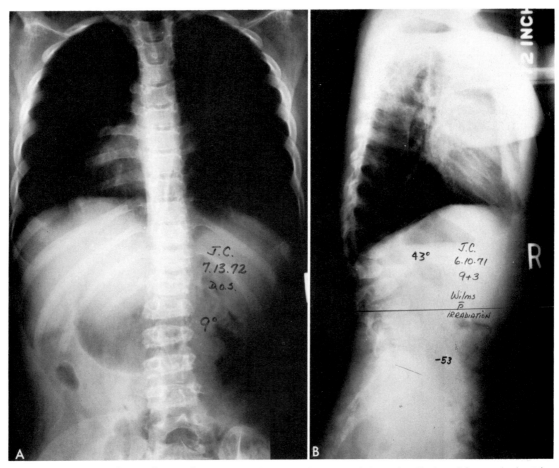

**Figure 11–1** *A* and *B*, Irradiation effects on a growing spine. Gross irregularity and scalloping of the vertebral epiphyseal cartilage plate. A "bone within a bone" appearance is visible in *B*, and scoliosis and kyphosis are present.

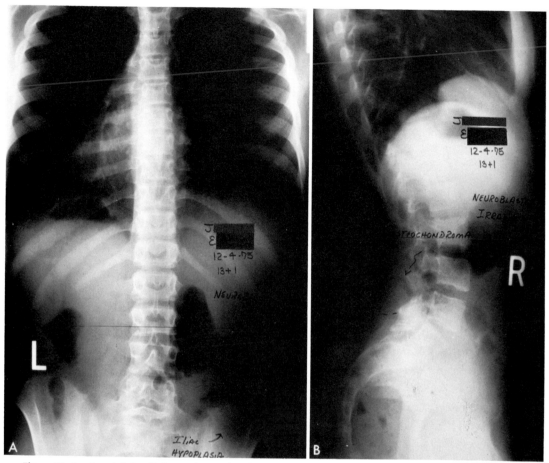

**Figure 11–2**  *A* and *B*, Irradiation to the axial skeleton may also cause iliac hypoplasia (*A*) and osteochondroma (*B*).
Hypoplasia of the ilium per se is not necessarily associated with scoliosis.

from the irradiation fields. Osteocartilaginous exostoses can be expected to develop in about 15 to 20 per cent of patients.[16, 20] Thirty-five cases of cartilaginous exostosis have been reported in the literature.[16] These are not limited to long bones but may develop in any irradiated area. Postirradiation sarcoma has also been reported.[8, 16] It is a most uncommon complication, however, and there is no reported case of malignant degeneration in the postirradiation exostosis. If a postirradiation sarcoma does arise, osteosarcoma is the most common form, with fibrous sarcoma and chondrosarcoma less frequently observed. Dosage and incidence appear to be related, with the higher doses resulting in a higher incidence.[3] This complication should not occur with doses less than 3000r.[9]

The incidence of scoliosis following irradiation to the spine is reported to be approximately 70 per cent.[16, 25, 28] The scoliotic curves are observed mainly in children who receive x-ray therapy for abdominal neoplasms such as Wilms' tumor and neuroblastoma. The primary treatment field actually lies lateral to the spine, but the spine is usually included, and due to its off-center position, an unequal absorption of radiation results. Essentially two types of deformity are seen;[26, 29] 1) a lateral flexion curve and 2) a rotary scoliosis. The lateral flexion curve is mobile, easily corrected, and associated with minimal rib deformity. The rotary scoliosis originates from changes in the laminae and the pedicles and is much more rigid. The abnormalities may be detected as early as six months after therapy.[16, 20, 28, 32] From the reported experience, therefore, it would appear that scoliosis following radiation therapy to the spine is usually not clinically significant. However, in a small percentage of patients, severe progression may occur, and treatment of the deformity is therefore necessary. Kyphosis following irradiation appears to develop less frequently than scoliosis.[16]

Recent reports by Riseborough et al.[25] have noted of 81 patients who received irradiation for Wilms' tumor, 55 developed hypoplasia of iliac wing (67 percent), 21 developed kyphosis (26 percent), and 57 developed scoliosis (70 percent). Of the 57 patients with scoliosis, 43 had curvatures less than 25 degrees; of the remaining 14, the average curvature was 46 degrees (range, 27 to 67 degrees). All were noted at follow-up to have asymmetrical or symmetrical failure of vertebral body development at the level of irradiation. Deformity only of the spine developed in 59 patients (pure scoliosis in 38, kyphoscoliosis in 19, and pure kyphosis in 2).

Our own experience parallels that reported by others. We have noted that the kyphosis or scoliosis that develops following irradiation of the axial skeleton usually does not show progressive changes until the adolescent growth spurt occurs. Patients with a relatively minimal deformity, though not requiring active treatment, must be followed until the completion of skeletal maturity and with particular care during the pubertal growth spurt.

## PREVENTION

In order to minimize the extent of orthopedic deformity of the axial skeleton following irradiation, the treatment field should be meticulously placed and documented with field roentgenograms. We feel every child subjected to irradiation of the skeletal system, should have orthopedic consultation and repeated follow-up evaluation. X-rays of the spine throughout the active growing years should be mandatory in order to document any treatable changes that are developing. It has been stated and stressed by the experimental work of Engel[10] and Arkin et al.[1] and through the clinical observation of Neuhauser et al.[20] that the entire width of the vertebra should be irradiated in order to avoid a unilateral wedging effect from epiphyseal damage secondary to irradiation. However, this has not been confirmed by the clinical report of Rubin and workers,[27] who felt that the degree of scoliosis was not related to the fields of irradiation.

It is believed by some that dosages greater than 2000r delivered to the spine will be associated with the most severe type of vertebral abnormalities.[12, 16, 20, 32] Those patients receiving less than 2000r will show the least amount of bony change. Every effort should be made to avoid including the iliac crest in the treatment field, since damage to the iliac epiphysis will appreciably decrease growth of the ilium, resulting in a hypoplastic ilium. Indirectly this could adversely affect any spinal curvature that was present. The acetabular fossa and femoral head should always be excluded from the irradiation fields. Irradiation of this area is rarely if ever necessary for the treatment of Wilms' tumor or neuroblastoma.

## PROGNOSIS

In general, the younger the child and the higher the radiation dose, the greater will be the probability and the extent of skeletal damage. Also, the higher the growth potential of a bone, the greater will be the radiation effects. This is particularly true when the epiphysis or metaphysis is affected.[20, 29, 31, 32] It is important to remember that although the likelihood that a spinal deformity will develop following irradiation for Wilms' tumor or neuroblastoma is high, the incidence of progressive deformity is only 15 to 20 per cent.[16, 27, 32] If the deformity occurs rapidly with marked vertebral body changes, one must be certain that tumor invasion of the bone has not occurred.

## TREATMENT

The management of spine deformities secondary to radiation has received little attention in the literature. Spine fusion with Harrington rod instrumentation for progressive spine deformity secondary to irradiation has been found an effective form of treatment. Recently, Riseborough et al.[25] presented a series of 81 patients with Wilms' tumor who received radiotherapy as a part of their treatment. They felt that the Milwaukee brace was of little help except perhaps as a holding device. We have likewise found the Milwaukee brace for the most part ineffective in the management of postirradiation sco-

*Text continued on page 310*

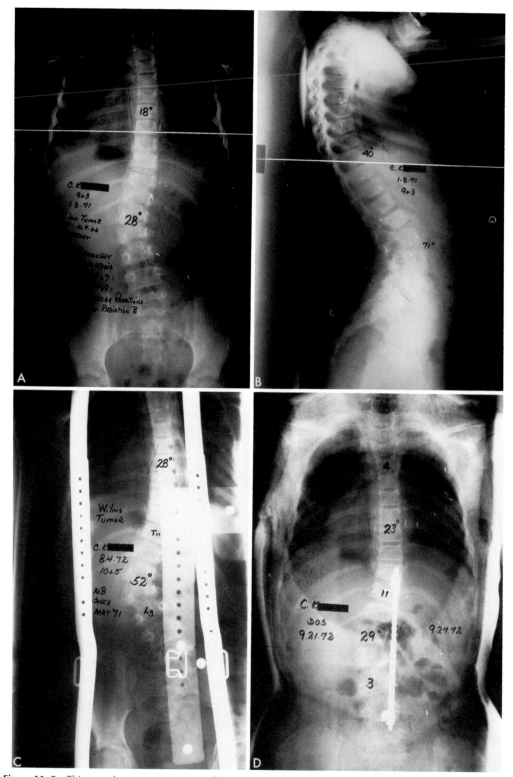

**Figure 11–3** This case demonstrates many problems and pitfalls in the management of postirradiation spine deformity. When first seen in 1971, C.K. was 9 + 3 years old and had surgery in 1966 with removal of a Wilms' tumor, receiving 3500r. Pulmonary metastases were removed by wedge resection in 1966 and 1969 (*A* and *B*). A Milwaukee brace proved ineffective in controlling the curvature (*C*). Spine fusion with Harrington rod instrumentation was carried out in September, 1972 (*D*).

*Illustration continued on following page*

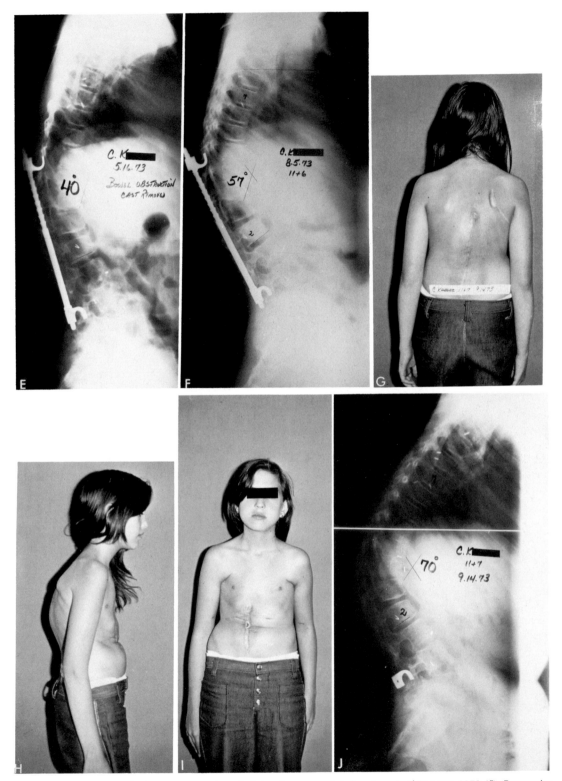

**Figure 11–3** *Continued.* A spontaneous bowel obstruction necessitated cast removal in May, 1973 (*E*). Progressive kyphosis was apparent three months later, with evidence of the upper hook protruding at skin surface (*F,G,H*). Scar contracture was visualized anteriorly (*I*). Exploration and rod removal did not reveal a pseudarthrosis. Kyphosis continued to progress, however (*J*).

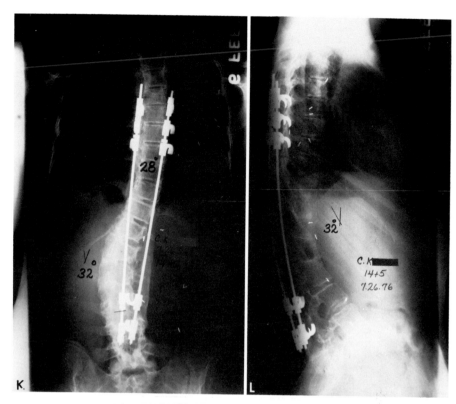

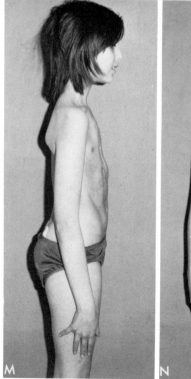

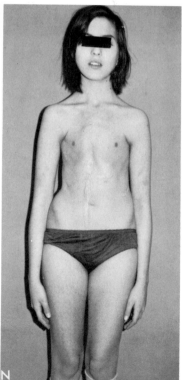

**Figure 11–3** *Continued.* Posterior osteotomy and spine fusion with Harrington rod instrumentation in October, 1973, followed two weeks later by anterior interbody spine fusion (T10–L2), resulted in excellent correction. The patient was maintained in a halo cast for six months and a Risser cast for an additional six months. Her condition three years later remains satisfactory (*K,L,M,N*). A longer posterior fusion initially with exploration of the fusion at six months might have prevented these problems. As it was, the fusion was too short and the kyphosis, aggravated by the anterior scar contracture and presumable pseudarthrosis, progressed to the point where anterior surgery was virtually essential.

liosis. Curvatures may occasionally be prevented from progressing, but more often than not structural curvatures will continue to progress in spite of bracing. Kyphosis is poorly managed in a Milwaukee brace and generally will require a combined anterior as well as a posterior spinal arthrodesis.

It is extremely important to evaluate these patients from a standpoint of soft tissue contractures. Severe contracture of the anterior abdominal soft tissues can preclude a successful result with a Milwaukee brace and may only magnify the progressive tendency of scoliosis secondary to a malformed abnormally growing spine. If patients demonstrate severe scar contracture or soft tissue contracture secondary to irradiation and have an associated scoliosis, they are not candidates for a Milwaukee brace but will require surgery (Fig. 11–3).

### PLAN OF PATIENT MANAGEMENT

Scoliosis curvatures of less than 20 degrees may be observed carefully for evidence of progression. Since only one third of these

curvatures are likely to progress, one may under these circumstances develop an attitude of watchful expectation and treat only if the curvature does demonstrate progression. Curvatures in the range of 20 to 40 degrees in a growing child should be treated with a Milwaukee brace. Although these curvatures are invariably quite stiff, progression may possibly be prevented with a Milwaukee brace. If progression continues in spite of adequate bracing, spine fusion with or without Harrington rod instrumentation should be undertaken, irrespective of the age of the patient. We have found that the bone substance in these patients is extremely poor and successful arthrodesis may not be achieved following a single operation, even with adequate amounts of autogenous iliac bone grafting. Therefore, we favor reexploring the fusion area within 6 months, adding more autogenous iliac bone and continuing the immobilization in a cast for a total period of 12 months. If patients have severe structural deformities with marked scar contracture, preoperative halofemoral distraction is often quite beneficial in overcoming the contracted skin, fascia, and subcutaneous tissues.

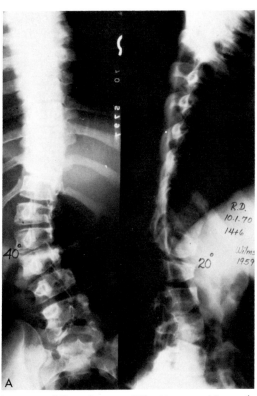

**Figure 11–4**   At the age of three years, R.D. underwent a Wilms' tumor excision on the right, receiving irradiation to the right flank area. For progressive kyphosis, he underwent spine fusion in 1971 from T12–L5 (A).

*Legend continued on opposite page*

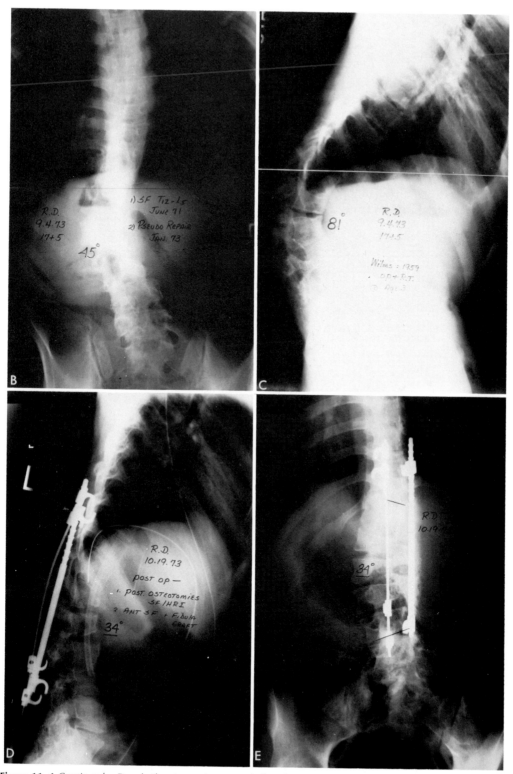

**Figure 11–4** *Continued.* Pseudarthrosis repair was carried out in 1973. However, because of progressive kyphosis, he was evaluated at the Twin Cities Scoliosis Center in September, 1973 (*B, C*). A two-stage procedure was carried out in October, 1973, consisting of a posterior osteotomy with spine fusion and Harrington rod instrumentation, followed by a second-stage anterior spine fusion (*D, E*).

*Legend continued on opposite page*

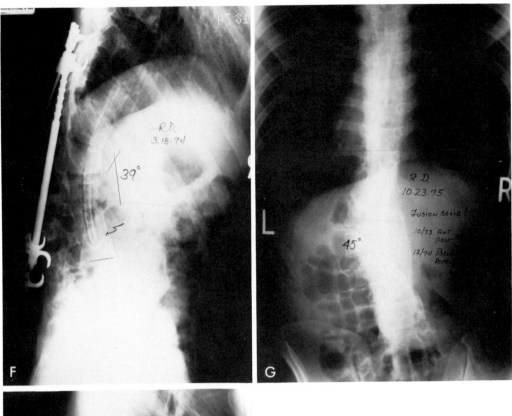

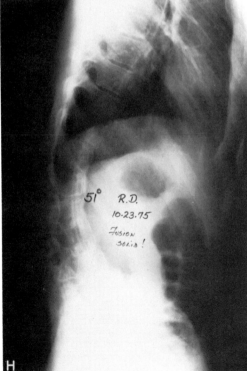

**Figure 11–4** *Continued.* Consolidation of the fusion anteriorly was slow (*F*), and the rods began to tent the skin at the lower end of the fusion. The patient was kept in the cast until December, 1974. The rods were removed and the fusion explored. Two pseudarthroses were found and repaired. The patient was kept in the cast for five more months. When last seen in October, 1975, the fusion appeared solid (*G,H*), and the clinical results were satisfactory.

*Legend continued on opposite page*

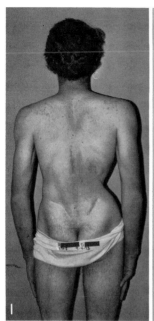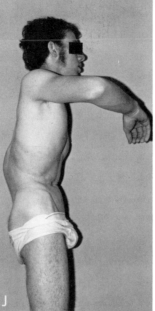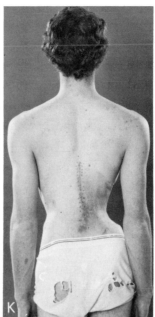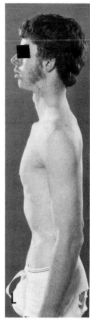

**Figure 11–4** *Continued. I* and *J,* Before treatment at the Twin Cities Scoliosis Center: *K* and *L,* after treatment.

In those patients who have a moderately increased thoracic or thoracolumbar kyphosis with an associated scoliosis, a Milwaukee brace may be tried in order to prevent progression of the curvature, but again surgery will usually be necessary. If progression continues in spite of adequate bracing, or if the kyphosis is greater than 50 degrees when the patient is first seen, spine fusion is the treatment of choice. We have found the best results in kyphosis to be a combined anterior as well as a posterior arthrodesis in order to decrease the incidence of pseudarthrosis and to obtain maximum correction of the deformity (Fig. 12–4).

## References

1. Arkin, A. M., Pack, G. T., Ransohoff, N. S., and Simon, N.: Radiation-induced scoliosis. A case report. J. Bone Joint Surg., *32A*:401, April, 1950.
2. Arkin, A. M., and Simon, N.: Radiation scoliosis. An experimental study. J. Bone Joint Surg., *32A*:396, April, 1950.
3. Arlen, M., Higinbotham, N. L., Huvos, A. G., et al.: Radiation-induced sarcoma of bone. Cancer, *28*:1087, 1971.
4. Barr, J. S., Lingley, J. R., and Gall, E. A.: The effect of roentgen irradiation on epiphyseal growth. I. Experimental studies upon the albino rat. Am. J. Roentgenol., *49*:104, 1943.
5. Bemerkungen zur Árbeit, Schulitz, K. P., and Aalam, M.: Wachstumsstorungen am Skelett nach Strahlentherapie und ihre Behandlung. Z. Orthop., *111*:249, 1973.
6. Berdon, W. E., Baker, D. H., and Boyer, J.: Unusual benign and malignant sequelae to childhood radiation therapy: Including "unilateral hyperlucent lung." Am. J. Roentgenol., *93*:545, 1965.
7. Bick, E. M., and Copel, J. W.: Longitudinal growth of the human vertebra. A contribution to human osteogeny. J. Bone Joint Surg., *32A*:803, Oct., 1950.
8. Cahan, W. G., Woodard, H. Q., Higinbotham, N. L., Stewart, F. W., and Coley, B. L.: Sarcoma arising in irradiated bone. Report of eleven cases. Cancer, *1*:3, 1948.
9. Cohen, J., and D'Angio, G. J.: Unusual bone tumors after roentgen therapy of children. Two case reports. Am. J. Roent., *86*:502, Sept., 1961.
10. Engel, D.: Experiments on the production of spinal deformities by radium. Part I. Am. J. Roentgenol., *42*:217, 1939.
11. Ewing, J.: Radiation osteitis. Acta Radiol., 6:339, 1926.
12. Frantz, C. H.: Extreme retardation of epiphyseal growth from roentgen irradiation. A case study. Radiology, *55*:720, 1950.
13. Gross, R. E., Farber, S., and Martin, L. W.: Neuroblastoma sympatheticum; a study and report of 217 cases. Pediatrics, *23*:1179, 1959.
14. Hinkel, C. L.: The effect of roentgen rays upon the growing long bones of albino rats. II. Histopathological changes involving endochondral growth centers. Am. J. Roentgenol., *49*:321, 1943.
15. Hoffman, V., Ueber Erregung und Lahmung Tierischer: Zellen durch Rontgenstrahlen. Strahlentherapie, *13*:285, 1922; *14*:516, 1923.
16. Katzman, H., Waugh, T., and Berdon, W.: Skeletal changes following irradiation of childhood tumors. J. Bone Joint Surg., *51A*:825, 1969.
17. Lattimer, J. K., Melicow, M. M., and Uson, A. C.: Nephroblastoma (Wilms' tumor). Progress more favorable in infants under one year of age. JAMA, *171*:2163, 1969.
18. Mayfield, J. K., Riseborough, E. J., Jaffe, N., and Nehme,

M.: Axial skeletal deformity in patients treated for neuroblastoma (In press.)

19. Murphy, F. D., Jr., and Blount, W. P.: Cartilaginous exostoses following irradiation. J. Bone Joint Surg., *44A*:662, June, 1962.

20. Neuhauser, E. B. D., Wittenhoy, M. H., Berman, C. F., and Cohen, J.: Irradiation effects of roentgen therapy on the growing spine radiology, *59*:737, 1952.

21. Perthes, G.: Ueber den Einfluss der Rontgenstrahlen auf Epithelial Gewebe Insbesondere auf das Carcinom. Verhandl. d. deutsch. Gesellsch. F. Chir., *32*:525, 1903.

22. Phemister, D. B.: Radium necrosis of bone. Am. J. Roentgenol. Rad. Therapy, *16*:340, 1926.

23. Racamier, D., and Tribondeau, L.: A propos de l'action des rayons X sur l'osteogenese. Comp. Rend. Soc. de Biol., *59*:621, 1905.

24. Reidy, J. A., Lingley, J. R., Gall, E. A., and Barr, J. S.: The effect of roentgen irradiation on epiphyseal growth. II. Experimental studies upon the dog. J. Bone Joint Surg., *29*:853, 1947.

25. Riseborough, E. J., Grabias, S. L., Burton, R. I., and Jaffe, N.: Skeletal alterations following irradiation for Wilms' tumor. J. Bone Joint Surg., *58A*:526, 1976.

26. Roaf, R.: Rotation movements of the spine with special reference to scoliosis. J. Bone Joint Surg., *40B*:312, May, 1958.

27. Rubin, P., Duthie, R. B., and Young, L. W.: The significance of scoliosis in post-irradiation Wilms' tumor and neuroblastoma. Radiology, *79*:539, Oct., 1962.

28. Rubin, P., Andrews, J. R., Swarm, R., and Gump, H.: Radiation-induced dysplasia of bone. Am. J. Roentgenol., *82*:206, 1959.

29. Rutherford, H., and Dodd, G. D.: Complications of radiation therapy: Growing bone. Semin. Roentgenol., *9*:15, 1974.

30. Segale, G. C.: Sull'azione biologica dei raggi Rontgene del radium sulle cartilagini epifisarie. Radiol. Med. *7*:234, 1920.

31. Vaeth, J. M., Levitt, S. H., Jones, M. D., and Holtfreter, C.: Effects of radiation therapy in survivors of Wilms' tumor. Radiology, *79*:560, 1962.

32. Whitehouse, W. M., and Lampe, I.: Osseous damage in irradiation of renal tumors in infancy and childhood. Am. J. Roentgenol., *70*:721, 1953.

# Chapter 12

# SCOLIOSIS IN MARFAN'S SYNDROME

## INTRODUCTION

Scoliosis is a common skeletal finding in patients with Marfan's syndrome. The incidence ranges from 40 to 75 per cent.[3, 4, 7, 8, 9, 11] Furthermore, the scoliosis is often severe, frequently painful, and may interfere with pulmonary function.[10]

## CLINICAL MANIFESTATIONS

Marfan's syndrome is a hereditary connective tissue defect which includes cardiovascular, ocular, and skeletal manifestations. The etiology is unknown. It is inherited as an autosomal dominant trait.[5]

Mitral insufficiency, aortic insufficiency, dissecting aneurysm of the aorta, and dislocation of the lens of the eye are classic characteristics. The skeletal manifestations are arachnodactyly, dolichomorphism, dolichocephaly, pectus excavatum, pectus carinatum, high arched palate, ligament laxity, pes planus, and scoliosis.

The differential diagnosis includes congenital contractural arachnodactyly,[1] homocystinuria,[2] and Ehlers-Danlos syndrome (Fig. 12–1).

## SCOLIOSIS

The age of onset varies considerably. Four patients in our study had the onset of their curve before age three. These curves all became quite severe.

The pattern of curvature is quite similar to idiopathic scoliosis. Curves tend to be right thoracic single major curves or right thoracic, left lumbar double major curves. In the 35 patients with Marfan's scoliosis seen by the authors, 16 had double curves, and 9 had single thoracic curves. In the 23 patients reported by Orcutt and DeWald,[7] 10 had right thoracic curves, and 8 had right thoracic, left lumbar double curves. Kyphosis is unusual, but occurred twice in our experience. Lordoscoliosis was more commonly noted and can cause significant respiratory compromise, especially if associated with pectus excavatum. Pelvic obliquity was not found.

Pain in the curve is a frequent complaint in patients with Marfan's syndrome, even in children and adolescents, and especially in adults. Pain was more common in the double major curve pattern.

The curve magnitude can range from very mild to extremely severe. Two untreated patients in our material reached 170 degrees and 185 degrees, respectively. Of the 14 patients fused by the authors, the curves ranged from 40 to 130 degrees. The average double curve was 69 degrees, the average thoracolumbar curve was 90 degrees, and the average thoracic curve was 100 degrees. Obviously, many of these patients had been neglected elsewhere and should have been operated on sooner (Fig. 12–2).

## TREATMENT

As with other structural scolioses, there are only three treatment choices: 1) observa-

*Text continued on page 321*

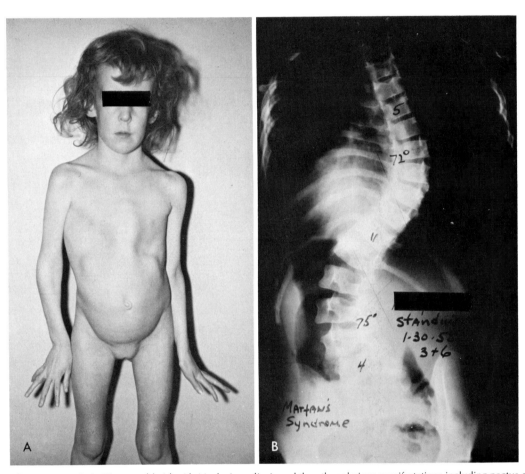

**Figure 12–1** *A,* A 3½ year old girl with Marfan's scoliosis and the other obvious manifestations including pectus carinatum, a heart murmur, and arachnodactyly. *B,* AP standing x-ray at age 3 years and 6 months showing a 72 degree right thoracic curve and a 75 degree left lumbar curve. These were progressive. She underwent spine fusion but died at age 6 of mitral insufficiency.

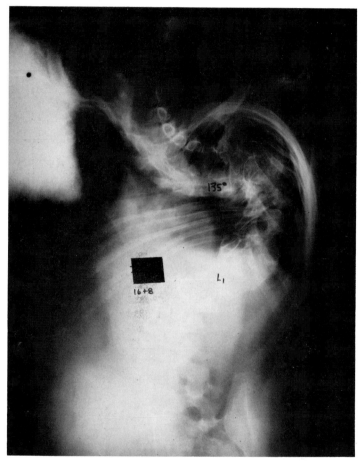

**Figure 12–2**   A 16 year old male with a 135 degree neglected curve due to Marfan's disease. He was in severe respiratory distress at this time. This amount of deformity should never be permitted to develop.

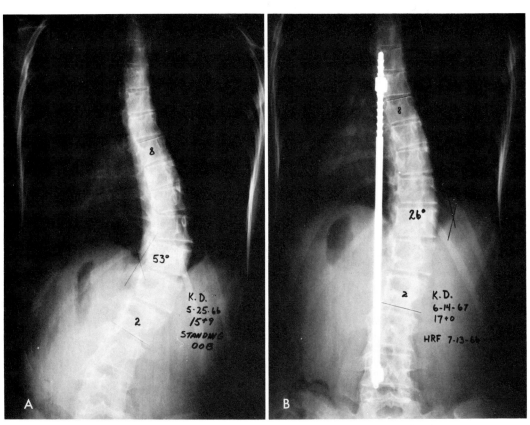

**Figure 12–3**    *A,* A 15 + 9 year old girl with a 53 degree right thoracolumbar curve. *B,* The patient underwent Harrington instrumentation and spine fusion with excellent correction and a solid fusion in a single stage without complication. This represents optimal treatment of scoliosis due to Marfan's disease.

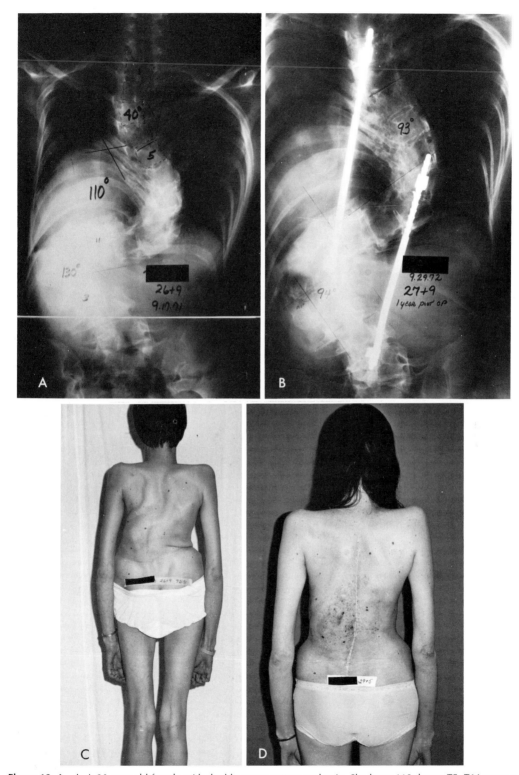

**Figure 12–4**  *A,* A 26 year old female with double curve pattern and pain. She has a 110 degree T5–T11 curve and a 130 degree T11–L3 curve. *B,* One year postoperatively, her curves measure 93 degrees and 94 degrees. The correction on x-ray has been minimal owing to the rigidity of the curves. *C,* Preoperative photograph of the patient. *D,* A postoperative photograph at age 29. She required an anterior fusion to stabilize a pseudarthrosis at the junction of the two curves. Notice the improved cosmetic appearance, despite the relatively meager correction on x-ray.

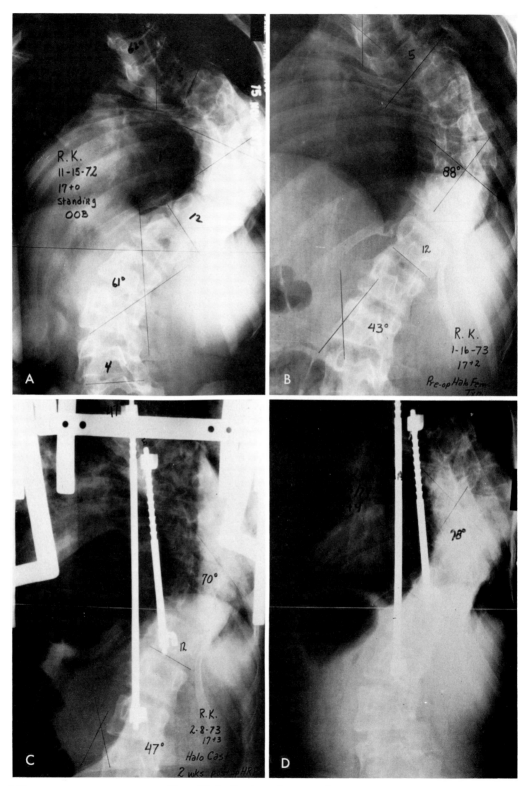

**Figure 12–5** *See legend on opposite page.*

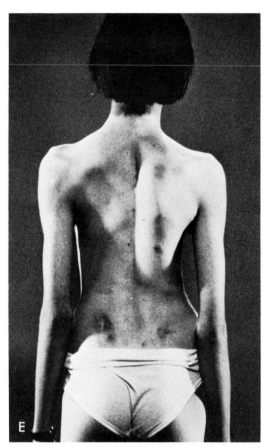

**Figure 12–5** *A,* A 17 year old male with a 123 degree right thoracic curve. He had been treated in a Milwaukee brace for seven years despite a steadily progressing curve. He had no cardiac problems. *B,* For such a severe curve, preliminary skeletal traction is advantageous. He was corrected to 88 degrees in halofemoral traction. *C,* The patient underwent Harrington instrumentation and spine fusion from T3 to L2 with correction to 70 degrees. This was maintained in a halocast. *D,* One year postoperatively. The fusion is solid and the curve measures 78 degrees. *E,* A postoperative photograph.

tion, 2) bracing, and 3) fusion. Since the curvatures in Marfan's syndrome seem similar to those in idiopathic scoliosis, it seems best to apply the same principles of treatment.

Brace treatment is less reliable in the patient with Marfan's, apparently because of the inability of the soft tissues to "stabilize." Progression can often be halted and pain controlled, but whether lasting curve control can be achieved is doubtful. Braces are satisfactory for delaying fusion in the young child with a progressive curve. The best brace is the Milwaukee brace, since most patients have thoracic or double thoracic curves. A lumbar brace might be used for a lumbar or thoracolumbar curve, but no results of such treatment have been reported (Fig. 12–3).

Surgical treatment is preferable for all

**TABLE 12–1   Results of Surgical Treatment — Marfan's**

| | | | *Combined All Curves (14 patients)* | | | |
|---|---|---|---|---|---|---|
| | *Age* | *Curve* | *Bend* | *Post-op* | *Final* | *Loss* |
| Single | 20 | 90° | 54° | 45° | 47° | 2° |
| Double | 15 | 70° | 45° | 43° | 47° | 4° |
| Avg. | 17 | 80° | 50° | 44° | 47° | 3° |

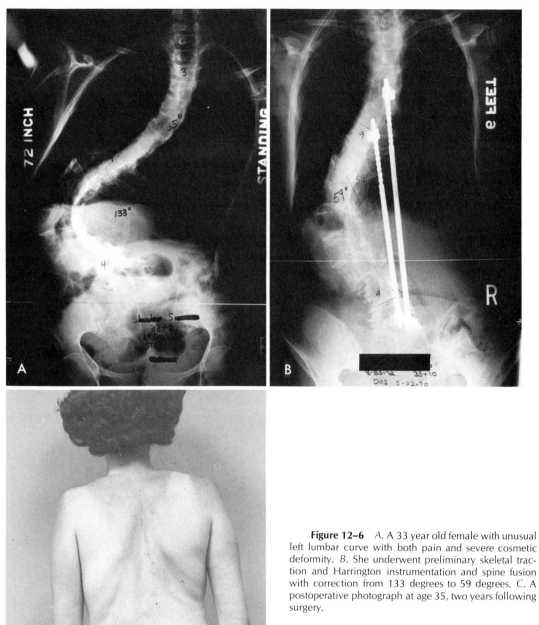

**Figure 12–6**  *A,* A 33 year old female with unusual left lumbar curve with both pain and severe cosmetic deformity. *B,* She underwent preliminary skeletal traction and Harrington instrumentation and spine fusion with correction from 133 degrees to 59 degrees. *C,* A postoperative photograph at age 35, two years following surgery.

patients with significant curves, provided that their general condition permits. Patients age 12 or older with a curve of 50 degrees or more should have surgical correction and fusion. All surgical candidates should have careful preoperative cardiovascular evaluation, searching especially for aortic aneurysmal dilation.

Patients with curves of 50 to 90 degrees are best treated by spine fusion supplemented by Harrington instrumentation. Preoperative traction or casting is not necessary. Curves greater than 90 degrees should be treated by 10 to 14 days of preoperative halofemoral traction followed by fusion with Harrington instrumentation. The selection of the fusion area is identical to that for idiopathic scoliosis. Fusion to the sacrum is *not* necessary (Figs. 12–4, 12–5).

Postoperatively, the patient should be placed in a Risser cast and ambulated at 7 to 10 days. The cast can be removed at 8 to 10 months. Pseudarthrosis seldom occurs but should be repaired if present. One patient required an anterior fusion as well as posterior pseudarthrosis repair to solve a difficult pseudarthrosis problem (see Table 12–1).

## SUMMARY

Scoliosis is very common in patients with Marfan's syndrome. The curve patterns seen are those of idopathic scoliosis, with a high frequency of double major, right thoracic, left lumbar curves. The curves are often painful and progressive. Bracing is appropriate for the small but progressive curve. All curves of 50 degrees or more should have surgical correction and fusion. A reasonable amount of correction (40 to 50 per cent) can usually be obtained without risk. Solid arthrodesis can be achieved. The patient with Marfan's syndrome should not be denied adequate care of the spine. The life expectancy of the average patient is 32 years. Some have lived into their seventies. The only contraindications to surgery are untreatable mitral insufficiency, aortic insufficiency, or aortic aneurysm.

## References

1. Beals, R. K., and Heckt, F.: Congenital contractural arachnodactyly. J. Bone Joint Surg., *53A*:987–993, 1971.
2. Brenton, D. P., and Dow, C. J.: Homocystinuria and Marfan's syndrome. A comparison. J. Bone Joint Surg., *54B*:277–298, 1972.
3. Daudon, D. P.: Contribution a l'etude du syndrome de Marfan: Les deviations vertebrales de ce syndrome a propos de 21 observations du dentre de massues. Thesis for PhD, Lyon, 1972.
4. Fauchet, R., and Stagnara, P.: Die Skoliose bei Arachnodaktylie. Z. Orthop., *113*:566–568, 1964.
5. McKusick, V. A.: Heritable Disorders of Connective Tissue. St. Louis, C. V. Mosby Co., 1972.
6. Murdoch, J. L., Walker, B. A., Halpern, B. L., Kuzma, J. W., and McKusick, V. A.: Life expectancy and causes of death in the Marfan's syndrome. N. Engl. J. Med., *286*:804–808, 1972.
7. Orcutt, F. V., and DeWald, R. L. The special problems which the Marfan syndrome introduces to scoliosis. Paper presented at the Scoliosis Research Society, San Francisco, Sept., 1974.
8. Robins, P. R., Moe, J. H., and Winter, R. B.: Scoliosis in Marfan's syndrome, its characteristics and results of treatment in 35 patients. J. Bone Joint Surg., *57A*:358–368, 1975.
9. Silman, N. A.: Propos de 16 cas de scoliosis-Marfan. Tunis. Med., *49*:93–101, 1971.
10. Wanderman, K. L., Goldstein, M. S., and Faver, J.: Cor pulmonale secondary to severe kyphoscoliosis in Marfan's syndrome. Chest, *67*:250–251, 1971.
11. Wilner, H. I., and Finby, J.: Skeletal manifestations in the Marfan syndrome. JAMA, *197*:490–495, 1975.

# Chapter 13

# KYPHOSIS-LORDOSIS: GENERAL PRINCIPLES

The management of kyphosis and lordosis has posed a major problem for the orthopedic surgeon and neurosurgeon. In the past decade, a better understanding of the types of kyphosis and lordosis, their prognosis, and indications for operative and nonoperative management has emerged. Untreated kyphosis in a growing child may lead to progressive deformity, back pain, paraplegia, and cardiopulmonary failure. Hyperlordosis may lead to cardiopulmonary failure as well, along with lumbar and thoracic back pain and compromised ambulation. Therapeutic efforts directed at prevention or even correction of these deformities have until recently been hampered not only by a lack of satisfactory surgical techniques but also by an inadequate understanding of the natural history of sagittal deformities. Furthermore, lack of agreement of the normal ranges of sagittal curvatures has compounded the problem.

At birth, the entire spine is straight or may show a slight anterior concavity from occiput to sacrum. When the infant begins to raise his head, a cervical lordosis develops. With ambulation, the pelvis tilts, and a lumbar lordosis and a thoracic kyphosis develop. Animals which walk on all fours never develop a lumbar lordosis but do develop a cervical lordosis and thoracic kyphosis.[10] Minimal wedging of the thoracic vertebrae, particularly of the apical three, develops with maturation (never greater than 5 degrees), while the lumbar vertebrae, particularly L5, develop a "reverse" wedge, which has greater height anteriorly than posteriorly.[10]

Staffel,[11] the German orthopedist, should be credited for having classified the human posture into certain groups i.e., "round," "flat," and "lordotic" categories (Fig. 13–1). Even this classic of the nineteenth century, however, lacked necessary precision in the description of normal sagittal curvatures.[1] Scheuermann,[9] along with others recognized a category of patients with increased thoracic kyphosis, but his major contribution lay in defining the radiographic cause of juvenile kyphosis: vertebral wedging. Although patients with this deformity were considered by him to have a kyphosis greater than normal, "normal" was never defined, Sørensen's major contribution,[9] published 40 years later, left the question of the normal degrees of thoracic kyphosis unanswered, although the limits of normal vertebral wedging had been precisely spelled out (<5 degrees).[3, 5]

In the past 20 years, scattered reports have been published describing normal values of thoracic kyphosis and lumbar lordosis.[2, 4, 7, 8] These are of particular interest because the figures given are remarkably similar. Roaf in 1960 stated that the normal thoracic kyphosis ranged between 20 and 40 degrees. Rocher in 1965 felt that the normal thoracic kyphosis was 35 degrees. Boseker, in 1958, carried out an unpublished x-ray study of 121 normal children at Gillette Children's Hospital in St. Paul, Minnesota. He found a normal range of 25 to 42 degrees. Normal cervical lordosis was 50 degrees. Ranges were not given, and it is apparent from these studies that further work is needed to establish normal ranges for sagittal curvatures in growing children. Until then, however, we would

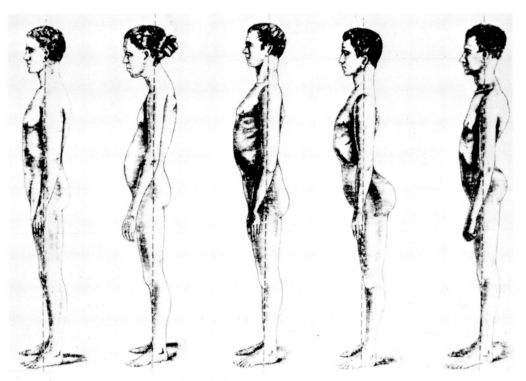

**Figure 13–1**  Types of human posture described by Staffel in 1889, as reported by Bonne.[1] Staffel should be credited for having classified human posture into groups such as the "roundback," "flatback," and the "lordotic" thoracic back.

suggest that 20 to 40 degrees be considered the normal range of thoracic kyphosis and 40 to 60 degrees the normal range for lumbar lordosis.

In order to understand the progressive nature of kyphosis and lordosis as well as the therapeutic approaches to these problems, consideration of biomechanical principles is of great importance. The stability and resting positions of sagittal curvatures are dictated by the osseous, ligamentous, and muscular components. The physiologic thoracic kyphosis is relatively more fixed than the physiologic lumbar lordosis, both clinically and radiographically.[12] In considering the biomechanics of increased thoracic kyphosis, one must think of the vertebral column divided into anterior and posterior components, the posterior elements resisting flexion and the anterior elements resisting compression. Increased deformity may occur when either of the components fails: tension on the convexity—compression on the concavity (Fig. 13–2). In viewing the upright spine from the side, it would seem obvious that the apex of the kyphosis is the most vulnerable biomechanically. Factors tending to produce flexion are

both the effects of gravity and the powerful abdominal musculature. Counteracting this moment are the spinal extensors. The exten-

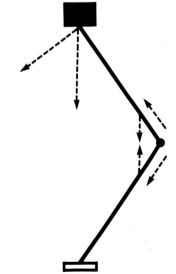

**Figure 13–2**  In considering pathomechanics of thoracic kyphosis, it is useful to think of the spine as being divided into anterior and posterior components, the posterior elements resisting flexion and the anterior elements resisting compression. Failure of either one of these components results in increasing kyphosis.

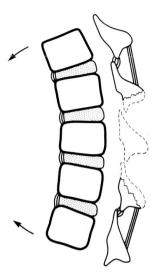

**Figure 13–3** Failure on the tension side, which results from multiple level laminectomies, will lead to increased kyphosis.

sors are quite close to the axis of flexion so they are at a significant mechanical disadvantage. Stability is maintained with the help of soft tissue support (Fig. 13–2).

Surgery that destroys posterior support (multiple level laminectomies) (Fig. 13–3) will result in a failure in tension with progressive kyphosis. Failure on the compression side may occur in osteoporosis, tumor invasion of bone, fractures, infection, or disturbed growth of the vertebral body (Fig. 13–4). These factors will all result in progressive kyphosis.

Three factors play a significant role in the progression of the kyphosis: 1) The amount of load and duration of the load (weight of the person). 2) The amount of angulation present at any given time (Fig. 13–5). This is analogous to a child sitting on a limb of a tree. As the limb begins to bend, the further from the tree trunk the child becomes, the greater the moment and the greater the likelihood that more bending will continue to occur. The moment increases as the angle increases. 3) The effect of asymmetric loading of a growth plate in a growing child: As the kyphosis increases, the retardation of the growth will be greatest on the anterior portion of the plate, causing asymmetric growth and increased kyphosis.

Lordosis in the lumbar spine more often than not mirrors thoracic kyphosis. It can also be thought of as failure in one or both of the structural columns. Lordosis usually results from alterations in muscle strength, activity, or length, i e., weakness of abdominals, spastic extensors of the spine, or hip flexion contractures. Rarely is it the primary problem except in cases of a congenital posterior bar, or following a lumboperitoneal shunting procedure for the treatment of hydrocephalus.

Correction of kyphotic deformities of the thoracic or lumbar spine may be accomplished by nonoperative means, provided that normal growth of the spine exists and the spine can be held in a corrected position while remodeling of the growth plate occurs and wedging, if present, is reversed. In fact, this is only

**Figure 13–4** Disturbed growth of the vertebral body, as seen in congenital deformity of the spine, can be thought of as representing a growth failure on the compression side. These deformities will result in the most severe degree of kyphosis, Type I (A) leading to a much greater degree of deformity than Type II (B).

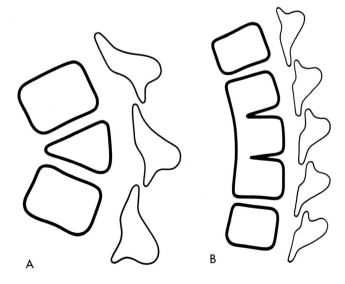

A                                    B

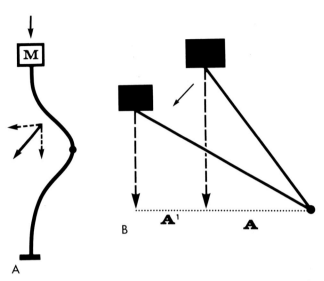

**Figure 13–5**  Factors directly related to the progression of the kyphosis are 1) amount of load and duration of load (*A*) and 2) amount of angulation present at any given time (*B*). As the angulation increases, the moment increases, and the tendency to further bending becomes greater.

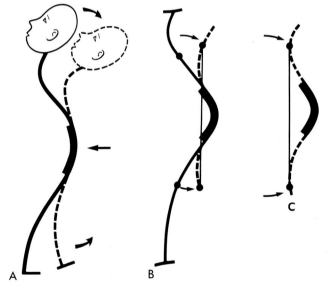

**Figure 13–6**  Correction of kyphotic deformities must be done anteriorly. Arthrodesis on the posterior or tension side is doomed to failure. The extent of anterior fusion depends upon the flexibility of the kyphosis. The flexibility may be determined by the hyperextension x-ray of the spine (*A*). Anterior fusion should encompass at least the rigid and inflexible portion of the kyphosis as noted in the heavily drawn area in *B*. With less flexibility, anterior fusion must encompass a greater area, as shown in *C*. A posterior spine fusion should encompass the full extent of the kyphosis, irrespective of the degree of flexibility.

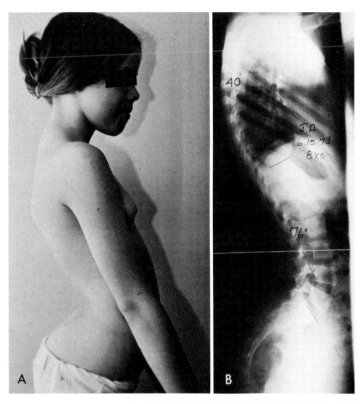

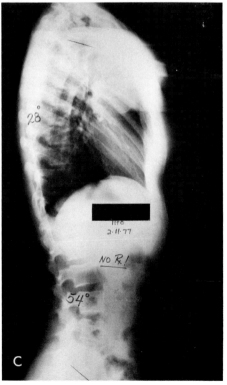

**Figure 13–7** Lumbar lordosis per se rarely requires treatment. It is usually secondary to a thoracic kyphosis, and even if it is not, it may be corrected adequately with physical therapy exercises directed at strengthening the abdominal musculature and maintaining a pelvic tilt. *B,* A severe degree of lumbar lordosis in a young growing child without evidence of neuromuscular disease. In this individual, no treatment was prescribed, not even exercises or bracing, and one can notice that 3½ years later the lordosis is spontaneously corrected, and the kyphosis is actually improved (*C*). Bracing is rarely if ever necessary for these problems.

feasible in kyphosis due to Scheuermann's disease or postural roundback. In all other kyphotic deformities, permanent correction is possible by surgery only, and this must be done anteriorly. Fusion on the tension side (posterior spine fusion with or without instrumentation) will fail unless the deformity is minimal and correction develops through overgrowth of the vertebral bodies adjoining the congenital kyphos (congenital kyphosis <50 degrees). The extent of anterior fusion depends on the flexibility of the kyphosis (Fig. 13–6). The anterior fusion should encompass at least the rigid inflexible portion of the kyphosis as visualized on a hyperextension x-ray. A posterior spine fusion is usually advisable to add strength and support to the posterior column and should encompass the full extent of the kyphosis.

Lordosis, per se, rarely requires treatment, except in situations where it is the primary deformity. This may be seen in congenital lordosis, following lumboperitoneal shunting procedures, and in achondroplasts with spinal stenosis. Mild postural hyperlordosis in a growing juvenile will respond to exercises or observation alone (Fig. 13–7). We have rarely found bracing necessary.

## References

1. Bonne, A. J.: On the shape of the human vertebral column. Acta. Orthop. Belg. *35*:567, 1969.
2. Boseker, E. H.: The determination of the normal thoracic kyphosis: A roentgenographic study of the spines of 121 "normal" children. Gillette Children's Hospital, St. Paul, MN. Presentation 1958.
3. Brudzik, G., and Wvensch, K.: Beitrag Zum Roentgenbilt Der Brustkyphsol Und Seiner Deritung. Z. Orthop. *84*:591, 1954.
4. Farfan, H. F.: Mechanical Disorders of the Low Back. Philadelphia, Lea & Febiger, 1973.
5. Fletcher, G. H.: Anterior vertebral wedging — frequency and significance. Am. J. Roentgenol. *57*:232, 1947.
6. Hall, J., and Winter, R. B.: Kyphosis. Spine (In press).
7. Roaf, R.: Vertebral growth and its mechanical control. J. Bone Joint Surg., *42B*:40, 1960.
8. Rocher, Y. R., and Perez-Casas, A.: Anatomia Funcional del Aparato Locomotor de la Inervacion Periferica. Madrid, Casa Editorial Bailly-Bailliere, 1965.
9. Scheuermann, H.: Kyphosis dorsalis juvenilis. 2. Orthop. Chir. *41*:305, 1921.
10. Sorensen, K. H.: Scheuermann's Juvenile Kyphosis. Copenhagen, Munksgaard, 1964.
11. Staffel, F.: Die Menschlichen Haltungstypen und ihre Beziehungen zer den Rückgratsverkrummungen. Wiesbaden, 1889.
12. White, A. A., Danijabi, M. M., and Thomas C. L.: The clinical biomechanics of kyphotic deformities. Clin. Orthop. (In press.)

# Chapter 14

# JUVENILE KYPHOSIS

## INTRODUCTION

Of the deformities that may develop during childhood and adolescence, kyphosis remains one of the most frequently neglected. Parents and even physicians may recognize that a child has a minimal roundback deformity of the spine and diagnose it as a problem of poor posture. This may indeed prove to be correct, but more often than not, the "poor posture" may be a manifestation of severe structural alterations in the vertebral column. Early recognition and prompt treatment of patients with roundback deformity can be expected to produce a superior result not only in correcting the deformity but also in alleviating back complaints.

Juvenile kyphosis was a poorly understood disease until 1920, when Holger Scheuermann[59] first outlined the radiographic manifestations of this deformity (Fig. 14–1). He noted that the deformity was caused by wedging of the vertebral bodies. Scheuermann's juvenile kyphosis was considered to be an abnormal degree of kyphosis developing at puberty, caused by wedge-shaped deformities of one or more vertebra, which show certain radiographic peculiarities. In 1964, K. Harry Sørenson[70] further categorized the disease process and suggested the definition of Scheuermann's disease should be a kyphosis including three central adjacent vertebrae with wedging of five or more degrees.

## ETIOLOGY AND PATHOGENESIS

The etiology of Scheuermann's disease is unknown. In fact, there are few definitive studies concerned with the early pathogenesis of this problem. Histologic material from patients during the active stages of the disease process has been described only rarely.[8, 63]

Scheuermann, in 1920, first proposed that the disease process was caused by avascular necrosis of the cartilage ring apophysis of the vertebral body.[59] With the onset of avascular necrosis of the rings, growth inhibition occurred, and subsequently kyphosis developed. However, this theory has never been verified. Bick and Copel[5, 6] noted that the limbus or ring apophysis was not connected to the growth plate and therefore contributed nothing to the longitudinal growth of the vertebrae. Any changes or alterations that occur in the limbus, therefore, would not necessarily alter the growth potential of the vertebral body.[34, 38, 40, 65, 66]

Schmorl, in 1930,[63] suggested that herniation of the intervertebral disc material through the growth plate produced the kyphosis. He believed that the changes first started as bulging of the disc material in the area of the nucleus pulposus, presumably because of developmental disturbances. Through congenital or traumatic tears in the end-plates, part of the disc material was then forced into the bony spongiosum, resulting in diminished height of the intervertebral disc. Disturbed enchondral growth ultimately produced the kyphosis. This theory has not been widely accepted. It is known that disc protrusions may occur outside the area of the kyphosis in patients with Scheuermann's disease. In addition, patients who have no evidence of Scheuermann's disease may have Schmorl's nodules, which may be noticed as an incidental finding on a chest x-ray.

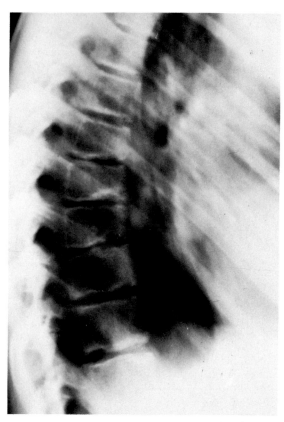

**Figure 14–1**  A classical x-ray appearance of the spine in a patient with Scheuermann's disease. Note the wedged vertebra, Schmorl's nodules, and marked irregularity of the vertebral end-plates.

Mechanical factors have been implicated in the development of kyphosis. Scheuermann[59, 60] noted that the disease, in his experience, occurred most often in young agricultural workers who were involved in heavy labor. However, Scheuermann's kyphosis is also known to occur in normal healthy schoolchildren who are not involved in physical labor.

Muscle contractures are occasionally noted in patients with Scheuermann's disease. Lambrinudi, in 1934,[39] noted tight hamstrings in many patients and felt that this was of significance in the development of the deformity. Michelle[42] believed that the contractures of the iliopsoas muscle were instrumental in producing this disease process. Although these findings are of interest, they may not be present in all patients with Scheuermann's disease, and their significance consequently remains unknown. Muscle weakness[51] and an infectious process[71] have both been suggested, but for the most part, proof is lacking.

A familial occurrence of Scheuermann's disease has been described in the past (Fig. 14–3).[70] It has not been established whether this observation is of genetic or environmental importance. We have noted many families in which a very high incidence of Scheuermann's disease has occurred, but we have also seen patients in whom there is no family history of roundback deformity or even of scoliosis.

Of interest are the questions raised in the past concerning the relationship of Scheuermann's kyphosis to endocrine or nutritional abnormalities (Fig. 14–4).[41] In 1969, Müller and Gschwend[46] noted that of 22 patients with Turner's syndrome, 11 demonstrated radiographic changes of Scheuermann's kyphosis. Patients with Turner's syndrome are known to have severe osteoporosis, not unlike that developing in the postmenopausal female.[16] Simon[67] has suggested that vitamin deficiency is instrumental in the onset of Scheuermann's disease, and Kemp and workers[36, 37] have noted an association be-

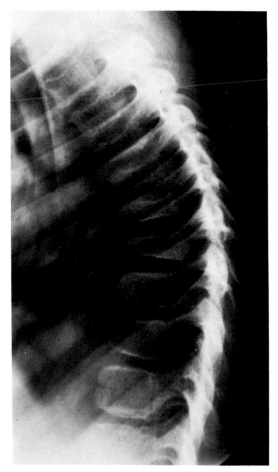

**Figure 14–2**  A patient who survived an infection with tetanus resulting in multiple compression fractures and kyphosis. Although mechanical factors have been implicated in the pathogenesis, one can see that the radiographic manifestations of these compression fractures are quite different from those seen in Scheuermann's disease. (Case kindly furnished by Dr. Peter Cockshott, McMaster University, Canada.)

tween malnutrition and the onset of kyphosis during growth. Mühlback et al.[45] and Gardemin and Herbst[24] have published work to suggest that patients with Scheuermann's disease may show alterations in bone metabolism.

Recent work in our department has suggested that many of these patients may indeed have a mild form of juvenile osteoporosis.[12] A dietary analysis suggested that a deficiency of calcium may be a common finding in these patients. Furthermore, we have been impressed with the clinical and radiologic similarity between Scheuermann's kyphosis and kyphosis in children secondary to malabsorption diseases such as nontropical sprue and cystic fibrosis. Thus it would seem

that kyphosis may occur in the adolescent period as a consequence of deficient skeletal mass, much as one would see in the adult patient, although the x-ray changes are not entirely similar.

Gross and microscopic findings from pathologic material of patients with Scheuermann's disease are of interest (Fig. 14–5).[8] Grossly, one will often find a contracted thickened anterior longitudinal ligament, which in effect acts as a bowstring across the kyphosis, serving to maintain the relative inflexibility of the deformity. The width of the disc material appears to be normal, whereas the vertebral body anteriorly is quite wedge-shaped. Histologically, one can see disruption of the endplates and extravasation of nuclear material

*Text continued on page 338*

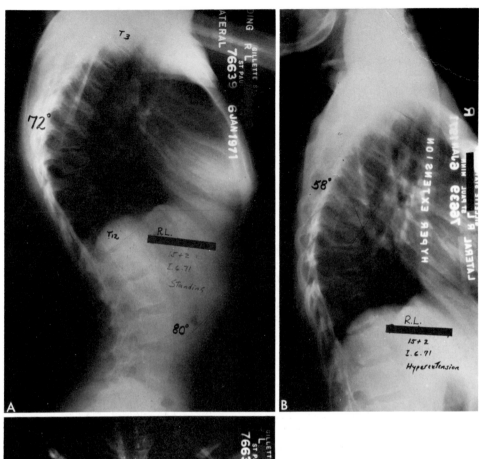

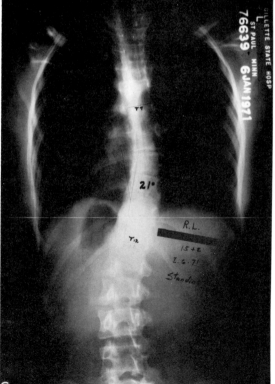

Figure 14–3 *See legend on opposite page.*

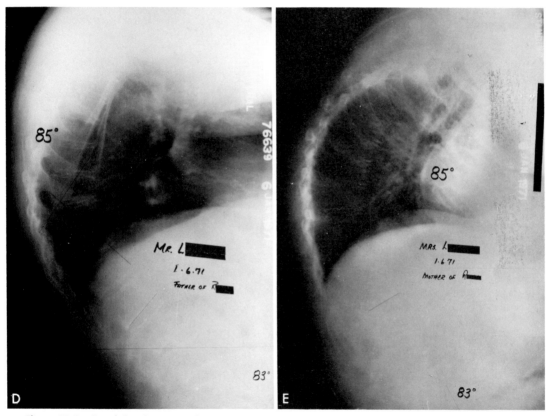

**Figure 14–3** *A* and *B*, Fifteen-year-plus-two-month-old female with Scheuermann's disease. Rigidity of kyphosis is noted by poor correctability on hyperextension x-ray. *C,* Scoliosis, though mild, is present in one third of patients. *D* and *E,* Scheuermann's disease is sometimes familial; in this case, the father and the mother are afflicted. (From Rothman, R. H., and Simeone, F. A.: The Spine, vol. I. Philadelphia, W. B. Saunders Co., 1975.)

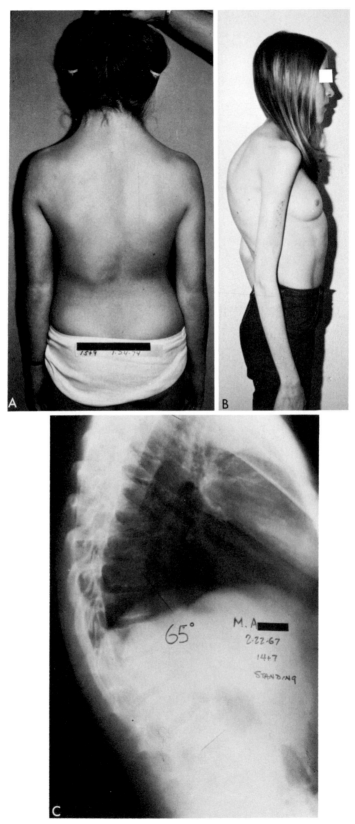

**Figure 14–4**  A relationship may exist between Scheuermann's disease and certain endocrine and metabolic disturbances. A high incidence of kyphosis is found in *A*, Turner's syndrome, *B*, cystic fibrosis, and *C*. Dilantin osteoporosis.

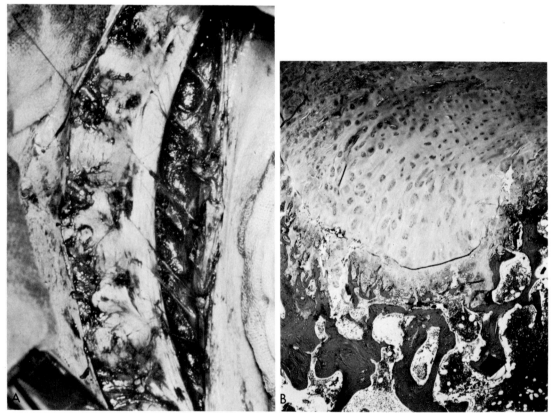

**Figure 14–5**  *A* and *B,* The anterior longitudinal ligament in patients with Scheuermann's disease is quite tight and thickened. Histologically, nuclear material can be seen disrupting the end-plate and lying in the bony spongiosum. (From Bradford, D. S. and Moe, J. H.: Scheuermann's juvenile kyphosis—a histologic study. Clin. Orthop. *11*:45, 1975.)

into the bony spongiosum of the vertebral body. We have not found evidence of avascular necrosis or inflammatory changes in bone disc or cartilage.

## CLINICAL DESCRIPTION

The reported incidence of Scheuermann's disease varies from 0.4 to 8.3 per cent of the general population, depending upon whether the diagnosis was based on radiographic or clinical criteria.[70] From a review of 1338 cases reported in the literature, the male-to-female ratio appears to be equally divided.[70] However, in recent studies on our service, we have found a female-to-male ratio of two to one.[10] The age of onset of the disease is difficult to establish, because radiographic changes typical of Scheuermann's disease are rarely demonstrable prior to age 10 to 11 years. However, by the age of 12 to 13 years, typical vertebral changes, along with wedging and kyphosis, are usually present.

## SYMPTOMS

Initial complaints relate to deformity with or without pain at the apex of the kyphosis. The incidence of these complaints varies in the series reported. Albanese[2] and Güntz[27, 28] have noted pain in only 20 per cent of their patients, while Scheuermann[60] and Nathan and Kuhns[47] reported an incidence greater than 60 per cent. Sørenson[70] has noted that pain is infrequent in the early stages of the deformity, but in the early teens, when the more florid stage of the disease is apparent, the incidence of pain rapidly increases. In his 103 patients, he found that pain was present in over 50 per cent. Furthermore, the incidence of pain was even higher in patients with a kyphosis involving the first or second lumbar vertebra (78 per cent) and in patients in whom the kyphosis had become relatively fixed (64 per cent).

## PHYSICAL EXAMINATION

On examination, an increase in normal thoracic kyphosis and lumbar lordosis will be readily apparent (Fig. 14–6).[9, 18, 44, 49, 78] The kyphosis will have lost a good deal of its mobility and will not fully correct when the patient attempts thoracic hyperextension in the prone position. The lumbar lordosis, however, is not structural except in rare circumstances and is readily correctable on forward bending. However, with forward bending the thoracic "hump" becomes very marked, as seen on the lateral view.

A minimal lateral curvature of the spine with a slight rib prominence on forward bending is noticeable in less than one half of patients. Direct tenderness with muscle spasm may be elicited over the kyphosis. Muscle tightness and apparent "contractures" are common. This is particularly true of the pectoral and hamstring groups, and it leads to forward protrusion of the shoulder girdle and limited straight leg raising. A spastic paraparesis manifested by ataxia and hyperreflexia may present on rare occasions secondary to spinal cord compression.

## RADIOGRAPHIC FINDINGS

For the radiographic evaluation of the patient with Scheuermann's disease, several views are essential (see Chapter 3). A lateral two-meter standing film of the spine with the arms held parallel to the floor and the hands resting on a support is most helpful in evaluating the kyphosis. The patient must be instructed to hold his head erect. A standing two-meter anterior-posterior x-ray is taken to rule out an associated scoliotic curvature. A supine hyperextension lateral x-ray of the thoracic spine is taken, using a polyurethane plastic wedge placed at the apex of the curvature. This facilitates the exposure and provides important information concerning the flexibility of the kyphosis. A hand x-ray may be taken in order to assess the extent of skeletal maturation. Note should also be taken of the maturation of the iliac crest epiphysis and vertebral ring apophysis. The degree of kyphosis and lordosis and the amount of vertebral wedging is then calculated. (For measuring technique, see Chapter 3.) The angles should be outlined by marking the end vertebrae which are maximally tilted into the curve. The angle from end-plate of the end vertebrae is considered to be the kyphotic angle. The sacrum is considered to be the end vertebra for the measurement of lordosis.

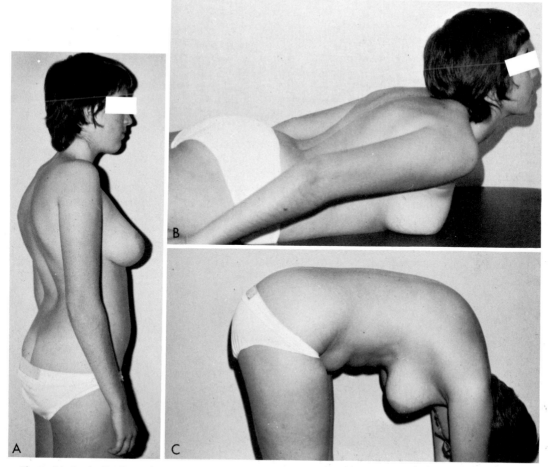

**Figure 14–6**  *A,* On physical examination, a definite increase in thoracic kyphosis and lumbar lordosis is visualized. *B,* The thoracic kyphosis does not fully correct on thoracic extension. *C,* The lumbar lordosis, on the other hand, usually corrects on forward bending.

Vertebral wedging is outlined in a similar fashion, marking lines parallel to the endplates and measuring the angle thus created.

Characteristic changes of the vertebral bodies secondary to Scheuermann's disease include vertebral wedging, Schmorl's nodules, and irregular end-plates. A mild scoliosis (10 to 20 degrees) with or without vertebral rotation is visualized in 20 to 30 per cent of patients.[10] Persistent vascular grooves may be present, but they appear to be related more to the immaturity of the vertebral body rather than to the presence or absence of Scheuermann's disease. Late radiographic changes (age 40 or more) include those associated with degenerative arthritis to the spine, such as osteophyte formation between the vertebral bodies. An anterior-posterior x-ray of the spine should be evaluated for evidence of increased interpedicular distance, which may be seen in association with spinal epidural cysts.[17]

We have found that the best radiographic criteria for the diagnosis of classical Scheuermann's disease are 1) irregular vertebral end-plates, 2) apparent narrowing of the disc space, 3) one or more vertebrae wedged 5 degrees or more, and 4) an increase beyond the normal thoracic kyphosis. Unfortunately, there are no definitive studies demonstrating the normal values for thoracic kyphosis in the growing child. From limited unpublished studies in our department, we have determined that a kyphosis greater than 40 degrees in a growing child is abnormal. The normal ranges of lumbar lordosis are unknown.

## RELATIONSHIP BETWEEN POSTURAL ROUNDBACK, SCHEUERMANN'S DISEASE (CLASSICAL), AND TYPICAL SCHEUERMANN'S DISEASE

Scheuermann's disease should be distinguished from postural roundback deformity. Children with postural roundback have only a slight to modest increase in thoracic kyphosis (40 to 60 degrees) and an accentuated lumbar lordosis. Although the kyphosis may rarely be greater, clinically it is quite mobile, easily and voluntarily correctable, and unassociated with muscle contractures. X-rays show normal vertebral body contours without vertebral wedging or end-plate irregularity (Fig. 14–7). Since radiographic changes of Scheuermann's disease may not be apparent until age 10 to 12 years, it is possible that early Scheuermann's disease could be incorrectly diagnosed as a postural roundback deformity. It is also possible that a severe untreated postural roundback might progress into Scheuermann's disease with vertebral wedging, but concrete evidence for such a progression is not available.

Finally, there is an atypical form of Scheuermann's disease that may present in two fashions: 1) vertebral body changes without wedging or increased kyphosis, 2) increased kyphosis without vertebral body changes. In the former case, patients often have back pain and spasm with radiographic changes of end-plate irregularity, disc space narrowing, and Schmorl's nodules. These changes may be completely confined to the thoracolumbar spine, even resulting in a minimal thoracolumbar kyphosis (less than 40 degrees).[20, 29, 59] In the other situation, we may

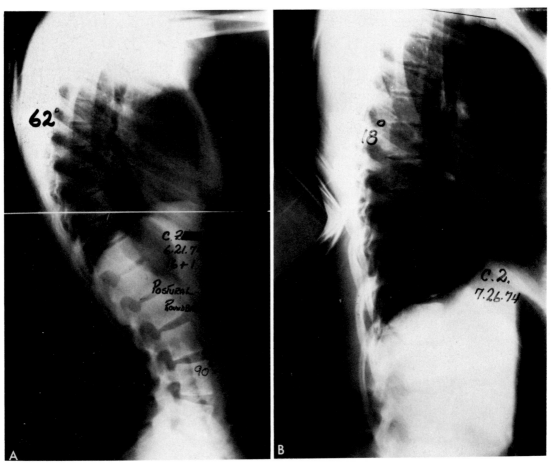

**Figure 14–7** A 16-year-old patient with postural roundback. Note mild kyphosis, with absence of vertebral body changes and marked correctability on thoracic hyperextension.

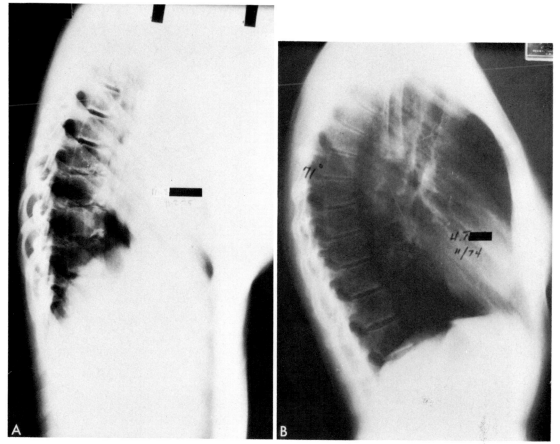

**Figure 14–8** Atypical forms of Scheuermann's disease. *A*, Vertebral body abnormalities without kyphosis. *B*, Increased kyphosis without vertebral changes.

see a structural kyphosis in a teenager, without radiographic changes of end-plate irregularity or vertebral wedging. This is not common but may present a clinical appearance of classical Scheuermann's disease. The relationship of these kyphoses to each other as well as to Scheuermann's disease is unknown. We feel that they are variations or perhaps subtypes of the same pathophysiologic condition.

## DIFFERENTIAL DIAGNOSIS

Besides differentiating Scheuermann's disease from its atypical forms and from postural roundback, other types of kyphosis should be considered.[9, 16, 70, 80]

Many authors have emphasized the problems occasionally encountered in differentiating Scheuermann's kyphosis from infectious spondylitis. However, with a thorough clinical and laboratory evaluation, as well as tomography and bone scans of the spine, a true diagnosis should be readily established. Traumatic injuries to the spine occasionally present a confusing picture, but in these cases, usually only one vertebra is involved, while in Scheuermann's disease, often more than one vertebra is affected. Multiple compression fractures of the spine can arise from severe flexion injuries, and after healing, differentiation from Scheuermann's disease may be extremely difficult, if not impossible. Osteochondrodystrophies, such as Morquio's disease and Hurler's disease, as well as post-laminectomy kyphosis, tumors, and congenital deformities of the spine, may be considered in the differential diagnosis of this group (Fig. 14–9).

Type II congenital kyphosis may be mistaken for Scheuermann's disease. In this type of kyphosis, however, anterior interbody fusion develops spontaneously, whereas in Scheuermann's disease it does not (Fig. 14–10). Osteophytes may form anteriorly, but

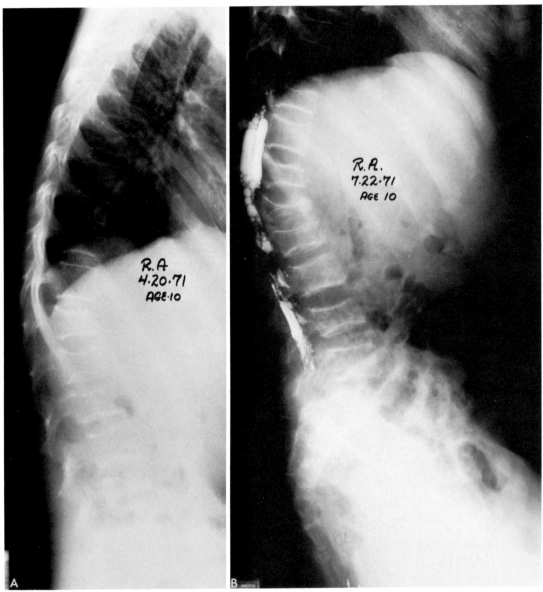

**Figure 14–9**  This 10-year-old female presented with a painful roundback deformity. Original x-rays were suggestive of Scheuermann's disease. Evaluation disclosed acute lymphocytic leukemia, which became more evident on follow-up x-rays.

bony bridging across the disc space does not develop even in the untreated adult. Lumbosacral anomalies should always be ruled out. Spondylolisthesis at L5–S1 can produce a severe lumbar lordosis and consequently a compensatory thoracic kyphosis. These patients will be completely asymptomatic except for a roundback deformity. They usually do not show the radiographic changes of the vertebrae that are characteristic of Scheuermann's disease. Finally, ankylosing spondylitis should be ruled out in the male; if the

clinical and x-ray evaluations do not furnish a reliable differentiation, HL-A tissue typing will prove helpful. Ninety-seven per cent of patients with ankylosing spondylitis will be B-27 positive.

## COMPLICATIONS OF SCHEUERMANN'S DISEASE

A kyphosis of less than 40 degrees is rarely if ever of cosmetic significance. How-

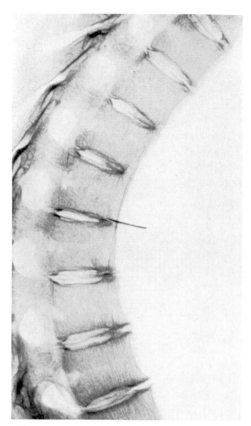

**Figure 14–10** A Type II congenital kyphosis, which may be mistaken for Scheuermann's disease. In this type of congenital deformity, spontaneous interbody fusion may develop after birth, whereas in Scheuermann's disease this does not occur, although osteophytes may arise anteriorly as a late sequela. (From Schmorl, G., and Junghanns, H.: Deformities of the Spine. New York, Grune & Stratton, 1959.)

ever, if the curvature becomes greater, the clinical deformity will be more pronounced, even in an obese individual. Deformities above 65 to 70 degrees are noticeable and, because of an increased compensatory lordosis and forward protrusion of the cervical spine, may present a cosmetically objectionable appearance. Curves of this magnitude may increase even after skeletal maturation is complete (Fig. 14–11).

Back pain, when present in a growing child with Scheuermann's disease, may be transient with or without treatment.[70] The incidence of thoracic pain in the untreated adult ranged from 10 to 42 per cent of patients.[27, 32, 33] Low back pain developing in Scheuermann's disease after the completion of growth would appear to be much more common. Güntz[27] noted that 42 per cent of 50 patients with this disease had low back pain

after they reached maturity. He stated that from the fourth decade on, Scheuermann's kyphosis predisposed to low back pain and disc degeneration. Saunders and Inman[58] and Schlegel[62] supported this concept.

Dittmar[19] reported that pain in the low back as well as in the thoracic spine was found in 89 per cent of his 36 patients. Patients with a herniated lumbar disc would be expected to have a higher incidence of Scheuermann's kyphosis than is present in the general population. Søderberg and Andrén[68] found that in 106 patients with back pain and sciatica, 46 per cent had Scheuermann's kyphosis, while a control series showed that only 13 per cent had Scheuermann's disease. Sørenson,[70] in reviewing long-term follow-up on 239 patients, noted that one-half had back pain at the site of kyphosis before they had reached the age of 20. After the age of 20, the incidence fell to one fourth of the patients. This pain did not influence the patients' working ability and only occasionally required treatment. On the other hand, Sørenson[70] found that low back pain was no more frequent in these patients than in the normal population, except for those with the long or low kyphosis (involving the first or the second lumbar vertebra).[19] Nearly all of these patients had complaints of low back pain.

Neurologic complications in Scheuermann's disease, although rare, have been outlined in the past.[12] Cord compression, presenting as a spastic paraparesis, may develop secondary to the angular deformity alone or to a herniated thoracic intervertebral disc at the apex of the curvature. One should always carefully examine the anterior-posterior x-ray of the thoracolumbar spine in patients with Scheuermann's disease to be sure that widening of the interpedicular space is not present. A spinal epidural cyst may be associated with classical radiographic changes of Scheuermann's disease and present on x-ray with widening of the interpedicular space (Fig. 14–12).[1, 17, 21]

## INDICATIONS FOR TREATMENT

Although Sørenson has suggested (notwithstanding the reports described earlier) that if Scheuermann's disease is confined to the thoracic spine, the prognosis is favorable and no treatment need be prescribed, such an outcome has not been our experience.[9, 10]

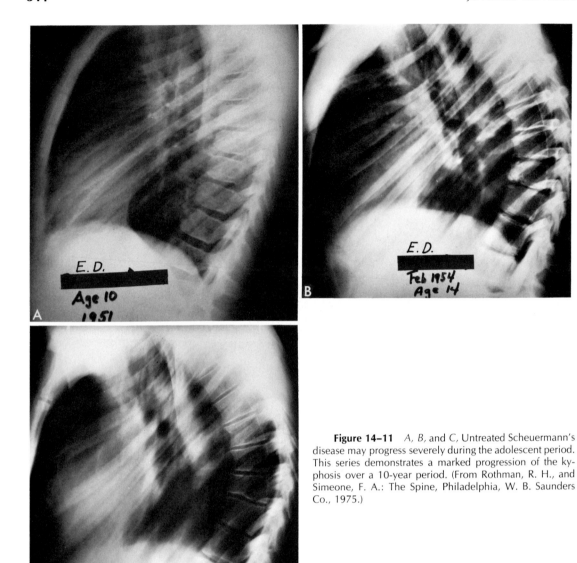

**Figure 14–11** *A, B,* and *C,* Untreated Scheuermann's disease may progress severely during the adolescent period. This series demonstrates a marked progression of the kyphosis over a 10-year period. (From Rothman, R. H., and Simeone, F. A.: The Spine, Philadelphia, W. B. Saunders Co., 1975.)

Adult patients frequently present to us with an untreated thoracic kyphosis that is not only a psychological handicap but also a source of significant and disabling thoracic back pain. The pain alone is at times difficult to manage except by spine fusion. Rarely the kyphosis may be a cause of paraplegia developing in late adolescence or early adult years. We feel that treatment of kyphosis in the growing child is therefore indicated 1) to correct the cosmetic deformity, 2) to prevent the possibility of progression of the deformity, 3) to alleviate present symptoms, and 4) to prevent further problems from untreated kyphosis.

## TREATMENT

### Nonoperative Methods

Numerous methods of treatment have been described that have enjoyed varying degrees of success (Fig. 14–13). Exercises alone have been suggested,[47, 67] but definitive evidence of improvement has been noted

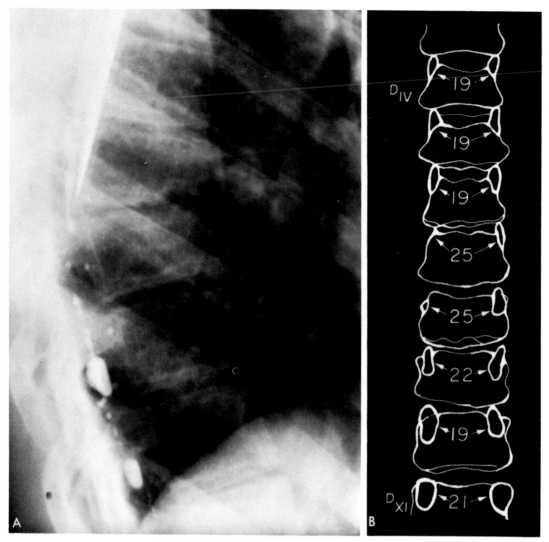

**Figure 14–12** Complications of kyphosis can include: *A,* Cord angulation or disc herniation with cord compression at the apex of the curvature; *B,* A kyphosis associated with spinal epidural cysts. In the latter instance, the diagnosis may be suspected by the presence of a widened interpedicular space. (From Rothman, R. H., and Simeone, F. A.: The Spine, vol. I. Philadelphia, W. B. Saunders Co., 1975.)

only rarely. Indeed, one study has shown that although the kyphosis improved slightly, vertebral wedging actually increased.[9] Exercise as a supplement to other forms of treatment,[13, 76] however, has been found to be beneficial and may furnish a means of correcting tightness of the hamstrings and pectoral musculature.

A therapeutic regimen comprising bed rest and the use of a plaster shell or body jacket and hyperextension treatment on a Bradford frame has been recommended.[21, 22, 34, 47, 67, 74, 79] Such combined methods of

treatment have been advocated by many authors.[24, 47, 61, 76] These techniques consist of a period of best rest or traction to decrease the muscle tightness, followed by the application of a plaster shell to straighten out the kyphosis. The plaster jacket may be used to maintain the correction until growth is complete.

A hyperextension cast applied in one or two stages has also proved to be an effective method of treatment. With the two-stage technique,[2, 21, 26, 54, 75] the lordosis is corrected first by the patient's bending forward while

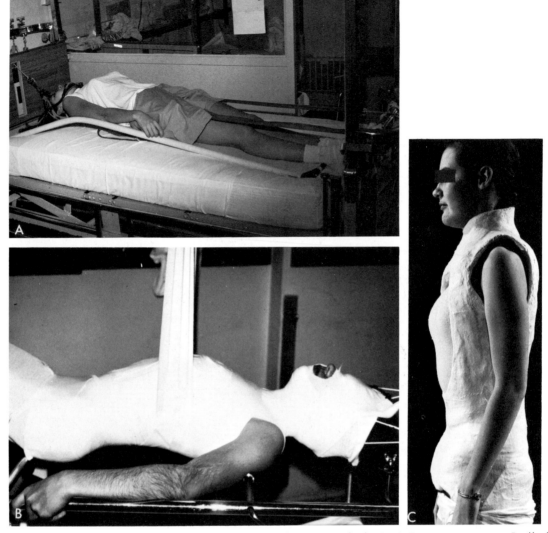

**Figure 14–13** Methods of nonoperative treatment of Scheuermann's kyphosis. *A,* Traction on a reverse Bradford frame. *B,* Positioning for hyperextension cast application. *C,* Appearance of hyperextension Risser antigravity cast. (From Bradford, D. S., Moe, J. H., and Winter, R. B.: Minn. Med., 56:114–120, 1973.)

the lower part of the plaster is applied. Then as a second stage, the plaster is extended up to the upper part of the trunk, correcting the kyphosis. The cast is changed every three months for approximately one year. Stagnara and Perdriolle[73] have noted a marked improvement in the degree of kyphosis in patients treated by this method. Other authors have likewise found bracing and casting techniques to be extremely effective in the correction of the kyphosis.[25, 48, 52, 56, 57, 72]

The use of the Milwaukee brace in the nonoperative treatment of scoliosis was first reported by Blount in 1958.[7] Moe, in 1965,[3]

reported successful results in correcting the deformity of juvenile kyphosis with the use of the Milwaukee brace. (See Chapter 15.) Recent results of the treatment of Scheuermann's kyphosis with the Milwaukee brace have been reported.[9] Vertebral wedging and kyphosis improved 40 per cent, and lumbar lordosis improved 36 per cent (Fig. 14–14).

## PLAN OF PATIENT MANAGEMENT

Following a complete and thorough history and physical examination, along with x-ray evaluation, as previously outlined, the pa-

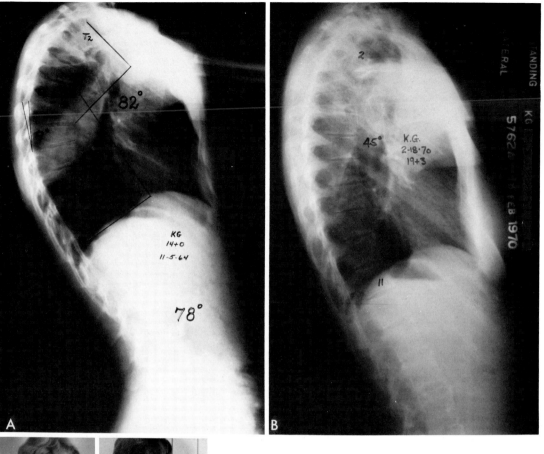

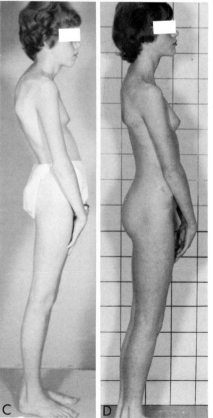

**Figure 14–14** A 14 + 0 year old female with Scheuermann's disease treated for 52 months with a Milwaukee brace. Her clinical appearance shows substantial improvement, and the x-rays demonstrate a correction from 82 to 45 degrees and reversal of vertebral wedging. (From Bradford, D. S., Moe, J. H., Montalvo, F., and Winter, R. B.: J. Bone Joint Surg., 56A:740, 1974.)

tient is fitted for a Milwaukee brace. If the curvature is rigid, demonstrating less than 15 to 20 degrees of mobility on the hyperextension x-ray, a hyperextension Risser antigravity cast, including the neck in the cast, may be used. The cast may be changed two to three times during this pre-brace period in order to obtain more correction. Once the brace is ready, it is applied, and a specific exercise program is initiated by the physical therapist. This program comprises pelvic tilting exercises to decrease lumbar lordosis, muscle-stretching exercises designed to overcome contractures, and thoracic extension exercises to build up the thoracic extensor muscle groups. Exercises are carried out in the brace as well as out of it. The patient is allowed to be out of the brace at least one hour a day for personal hygiene and bathing.

The patient should be checked with lateral x-rays of the spine in the brace at four-month intervals. If scoliosis was present, an anterior-posterior x-ray of the spine should be obtained as well with each follow-up visit. Gradual weaning from the brace (two to four hours a day out of the brace) is begun when correction of the kyphosis has been achieved (kyphosis less than 40 degrees) and vertebral wedging has approached normal (5 degrees or less). The weaning may progress to an increased time out of the brace at each follow-up interval, provided loss of correction does not occur. If correction is lost at any time during the weaning period, the time out of the brace is decreased accordingly.

It has been our experience that kyphosis and vertebral wedging are corrected usually within one year. However, it must be appreciated that there are variations in the severity of the disease, which require variations in brace management. All patients do not necessarily require full-time bracing until skeletal maturation or closure of the vertebral ring apophyses. In contradistinction to patients undergoing brace treatment for adolescent idiopathic scoliosis, patients with juvenile kyphosis may be corrected and show stability of correction before complete maturation.

Factors that may serve to limit the degree of correction obtained with the Milwaukee brace are a kyphosis of greater than 65 to 70 degrees; severe vertebral wedging averaging greater than 10 degrees; or skeletal maturation, as noted by closure of the iliac epiphyses at the time of initial treatment. Correction is still possible even though the iliac epiphyses may be closed. Indeed, correction is still possible to some degree as long as the ring apophyses of the vertebral bodies involved are still open. Consequently, some patients with a chronological age of 18 to 19 years may possibly still benefit from the brace, although the result will not be optimal.

It is important to remember that complications can arise with the use of the Milwaukee brace. One may maintain the deformity by constructing the brace in the deformed position. On the other hand, one may overcorrect the deformity, producing complete straightening of the back or even producing lordosis of the thoracic spine (Fig. 14–15). Likewise, one must repeatedly check the patient in order to be certain that a scoliotic curvature is not developing or, if one has been present, that it is not progressing. This may be overlooked as attention is directed solely to the kyphosis.

## COMMENTS ON POSTURAL ROUNDBACK

The management of patients with true postural roundback may follow the same principles as outlined for Scheuermann's kyphosis. However, if the child is a young preadolescent individual with a very supple kyphosis, exercises alone, in our experience, have proved sufficient. Frequent radiographic evaluation of the deformity, however, is mandatory. Any progression of the kyphosis, loss of complete correctability (as noted on the hyperextension lateral x-ray), or the development of vertebral wedging or other changes suggestive of Scheuermann's disease would imply that the treatment was inadequate and that a Milwaukee brace should be instituted immediately. Thus exercises alone are usually adequate treatment for postural roundback, but bracing may be useful if the patient is unable or reluctant to follow an exercise program or if the roundback deformity has not improved within six months (Fig. 14–16).

### Operative Treatment

Spine fusion for the treatment of Scheuermann's juvenile kyphosis has been mentioned only rarely in the literature.[3, 69, 73, 77] Ferguson[22] suggested that spine fusion might occasionally be indicated, but Hallock and his associates[30] believe that posterior spine fusion alone

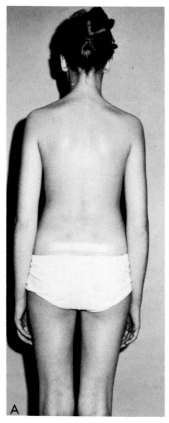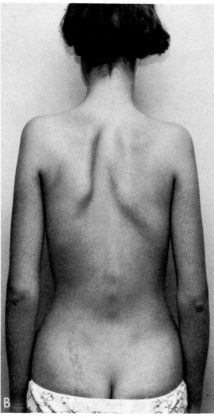

**Figure 14-15** *A* and *B,* The complication of overcorrecting the kyphosis. This 12 + 7 year old female had a 57 degree kyphosis; treated with a Milwaukee brace, the kyphosis corrected to 9 degrees. Thoracic lordosis was produced, with a noticeably poor result.

will not correct the kyphosis, unless the fusion is done over an extensive area of the spine at a very young age. Roaf,[55] on the other hand, noted that posterior spine fusion could be advantageous in correcting the deformity. Moe, in 1965,[43] presented evidence indicating that this approach is feasible. More recent work has indicated that surgery may be quite beneficial in correcting the deformity and relieving symptoms.[11]

Surgery should only rarely be necessary. The indications include a severe kyphosis in a patient who has completed growth; severe and disabling back pain in the area of the kyphosis, which is unresponsive to conservative management; and/or neurologic signs and symptoms secondary to the kyphosis. Posterior spinal fusion with Harrington rod instrumentation,[31] using the compression assembly, can be effective in correcting the deformity. However, posterior fusion alone for kyphosis greater than 65 to 70 degrees may be asso-

ciated with significant complications and loss of correction of the kyphosis with instrumentation failure (Fig. 14-17). This might well be expected in light of the problems in obtaining a solid posterior fusion over any kyphosis where the fusion mass is under tension rather than compression. Therefore, for severe kyphosis (greater than 65 degrees), we feel that anterior spine fusion followed by posterior spine fusion is the procedure of choice (Fig. 14-18).

## PLAN OF MANAGEMENT

For adult patients with severe Scheuermann's kyphosis and with symptoms that fulfill the operative indications as outlined, we initially proceed with anterior transthoracic spine fusion,[53] completely removing the intervertebral discs and dividing the anterior longitudinal ligament over the apical six or

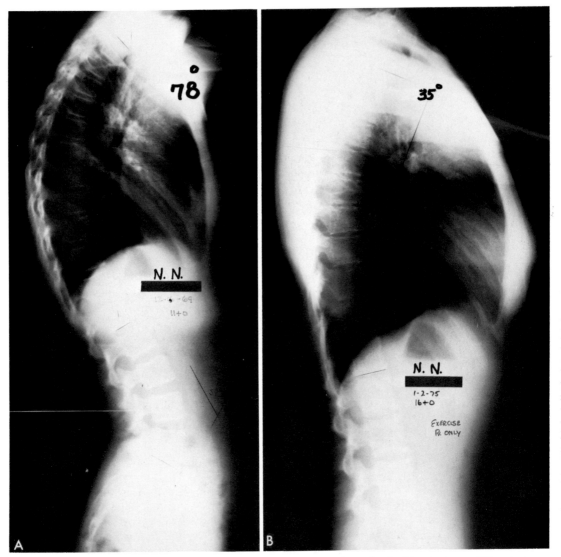

**Figure 14–16**  Exercise treatment alone is usually adequate for postural roundback. This 11 + 0 year old female demonstrates an excellent result of exercise treatment.

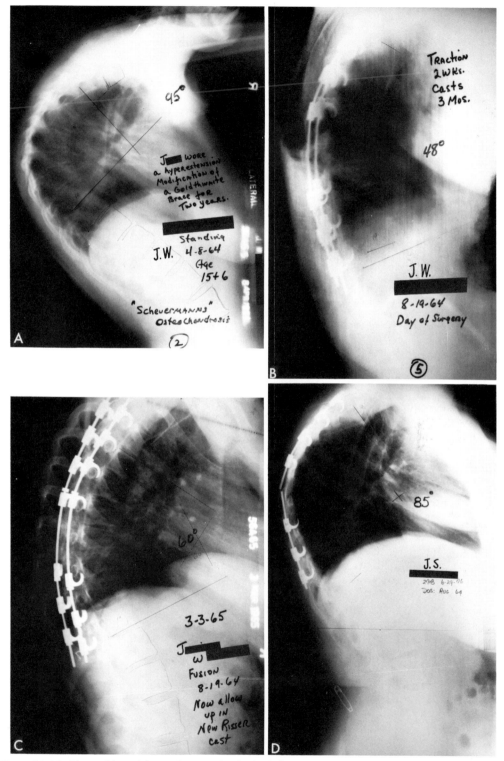

**Figure 14–17** The problems inherent in managing kyphosis by posterior correction and fusion alone. Even a severe kyphosis of 95 degrees *(A)* may be substantially corrected *(B)*. However, progressive loss of correction often results *(C)*, leading ultimately to instrumentation failure and pseudarthrosis *(D)*.

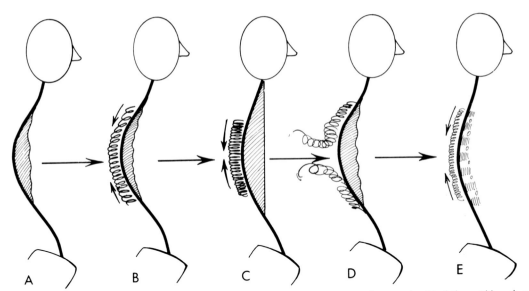

**Figure 14–18** Posterior fusion for severe kyphosis with or without instrumentation may lead to failure. Although correction is initially possible *(B)*, the lack of mobility of anterior structures (anterior longitudinal ligament), with a fusion under tensile forces *(C)*, may lead to fusion failure *(D)*. Anterior release with anterior spine fusion coupled with posterior spine fusion will result in an improved and more stable correction. (See Figure 16–20.)

seven vertebrae and bridging the intervertebral disc space with rib and/or iliac bone graft (see Chapter 20). Following the closure of the thoracotomy incision, a halo is applied. During the next two weeks, progressive distraction is carried out with the patient hyperextended in bed. Countertraction may be carried out with femoral pins if the Cotrel pelvic harness becomes too uncomfortable.

Two weeks after the anterior procedure, a posterior spine fusion and Harrington rod instrumentation, using the Harrington compression assembly, is carried out. The halo is most useful during this procedure, since the head must be lifted backward in order to approach and instrument the upper thoracic vertebrae with the Harrington compression device (Fig. 14–19). In order to obtain maximum correction and reasonable fixation, we have found it preferable to extend the fusion up to T2, placing the compression assembly over the transverse processes of T2, T3, and T4 and underneath the lamina or into the facet joints over the lower three vertebrae of the kyphosis. It is important that the fusion extend over the length of the kyphosis. If the fusion is too short, correction will be lost.

Following the completion of the spine fusion and Harrington instrumentation, the halo may be removed if the fixation is secure. One week later, the patient is placed in a Risser antigravity cast (including the neck) and ambulated. The plaster immobilization is continued for a period of nine months, with a change of plaster after five months. Early ambulation requires excellent plaster technique and repeated measurements of the curvature by x-ray. Any loss of correction must be explained, and either the patient should be kept supine or a new cast should be applied.[11] Underarm casts are not sufficient (Fig. 14–20).

If spine surgery is indicated because of spastic paraparesis secondary to cord compression, the following procedures would be employed: anterior decompression and spine fusion, followed, two weeks later, by posterior spine fusion and Harrington instrumentation. Of course, the technique of anterior spine fusion, would differ from that for Scheuermann's kyphosis (see Chapter 23). Likewise, traction between the anterior procedure and the posterior procedure must be carefully carried out in order to be certain that neurologic deterioration does not occur.

Results in treating Scheuermann's kyphosis by Harrington instrumentation and posterior spine fusion alone have for the most

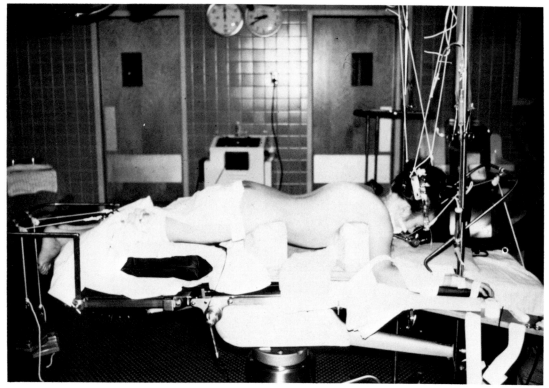

**Figure 14–19**  Use of the halo for the second-stage surgical correction of kyphosis. With gentle extension of the spine at surgery, easier access to T1 is possible.

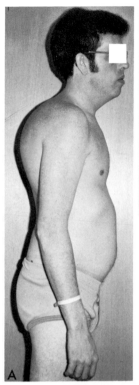

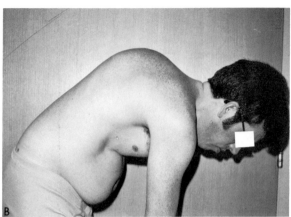

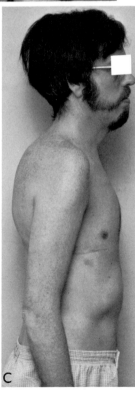

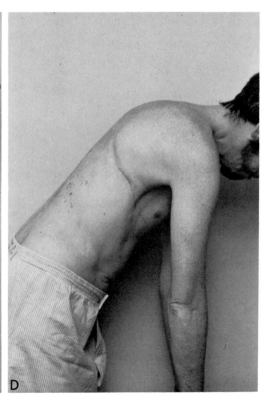

**Figure 14–20** This 35-year-old male underwent a combined anterior-posterior spine fusion for severe Scheuermann's disease with incapacitating back pain. Clinical appearance preoperatively (A and B) and 2 years postoperatively (C and D). The kyphosis of 99 degrees (E) was corrected to 55 degrees following surgery (F). He lost no significant correction over the next 1 1/2 years in spite of the fact that two hooks from one rod cut out, necessitating rod removal 1 1/2 years postoperatively (G).

*Illustration continued on opposite page*

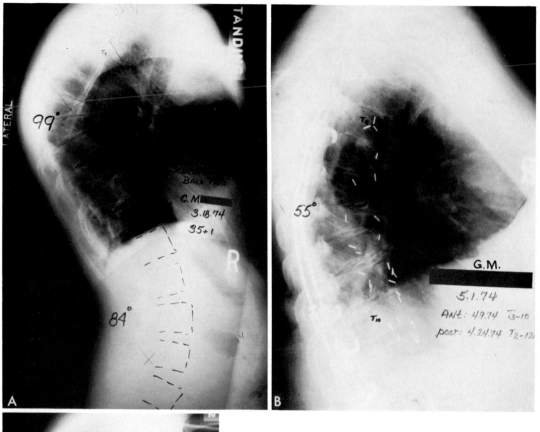

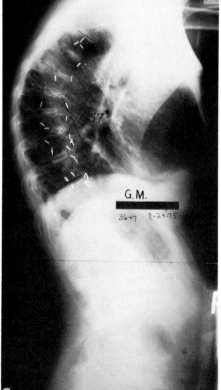

Figure 14–20   *Continued.*

part been satisfactory in relieving pain and correcting the kyphosis. A tendency to lose correction (averaging 20 degrees) in patients with kyphosis greater than 70 degrees, has led us to favor the combined anterior and posterior approach as described. With this technique, in 14 patients the average loss of correction has been only 4.5 degrees.

## References

1. Adelstein, L. J.: Spinal extradural cyst associated with kyphosis dorsalis juvenilis. J. Bone Joint Surg., 23:93, Jan., 1941.
2. Albanese, A.: Le cifosi dell'adolescenze. Arch. Orthop., 52:189, 1936.
3. Becker, K. J.: Uber die Behandlung jugendlicher Kyphosen mit einem aktiven bzw. einem kombinierten zweiteiligen akitv-passiven Reklinationskorsett. Z. Orthop., 89:464, 1958.
4. Berg, Atle: Contribution to the technique in fusion operations on the spine. Acta Orthop. Scand., 17:1, 1948.
5. Bick, E. M., and Copel, J. W.: Longitudinal growth of the human vertebra; contribution to human osteogeny. J. Bone Joint Surg., 32A:803, 1950.
6. Bick, E. M., and Copel, J. W.: Ring apophysis of human vertebra; contribution to human osteogeny. J. Bone Joint Surg., 33A:783, 1951.
7. Blount, Walter P., Schmidt, Albert C., and Bidwell, Richard G.: Making the Milwaukee brace. J. Bone Joint Surg., 40A:523, 1958.
8. Bradford, D. S., and Moe, J. H.: Scheuermann's juvenile kyphosis: A histologic study. Clin. Orthop., 110:45, 1975.
9. Bradford, D. S., Moe, J. H., and Winter, R. B.: Kyphosis and postural roundback deformity in children and adolescents. Minn. Med., 56:114, 1973.
10. Bradford, D. S., Moe, J. H., Montalvo, F. J., and Winter, R. B.: Scheuermann's kyphosis and roundback deformity, results of Milwaukee brace treatment. J. Bone Joint Surg., 56A:749, June, 1974.
11. Bradford, D. S., Moe, J. H., Montalvo, F. J., and Winter, R. B.: Scheuermann's kyphosis: Results of surgical treatment in twenty-two patients. J. Bone Joint Surg., 57A:439, 1975.
12. Bradford, D. S., Brown, D. M., Moe, J. H., Winter, R. B., and Jowsey, J.: Scheuermann's kyphosis, a form of juvenile osteoporosis? Clin. Orthop., 118:10, 1976.
13. Bradford, D. S.: Neurological complications in Scheuermann's disease. J. Bone Joint Surg., 51A:657, 1969.
14. Brocher, J. E. W.: Die Scheuermannsche Krankheit und ihre Differential diagnose. Basel, B. Schwabe and Co., 1946.
15. Brocher, J. E. W.: Die Wirbelsaulentuber Kulose und ihre Differential diagnose. Stuttgart, G. Thieme, 1953.
16. Brown, D. M., Jowsey, J., and Bradford, D. S.: Osteoporosis in ovarian dysgenesis. J. Pediatr., 84:816, 1974.
17. Cloward, R. B., and Bucy, P. C.: Spinal extradural cyst and kyphosis dorsalis juvenilis. Am. J. Roentgenol., 38:681, 1937.
18. Dameron, T. B., and Gulledge, W. H.: Adolescent kyphosis. U.S. Armed Forces Med. J., 4:871, 1953.
19. Dittmar, Otto: Die rundrückenbildung der Jugendilcher (Kyphosis juvenilis). Med. Klin., 35:1203, 1939.
20. Edgren, W.: Osteochondrosis juvenilis lumbalis. Acta Chir. Scand. Suppl., 227:1, 1957.
21. Elsberg, C. A., Dike, C. G., and Brewer, E. D.: The symptoms and diagnosis of extradural cysts. Bull. Neurol. Inst., 3:395, 1934.
22. Ferguson, A. B., Jr.: Etiology of pre-adolescent kyphosis. J. Bone Joint Surg., 38A:149, 1956.
23. Ferguson, A. B., Jr.: Roundback in children. J. Med. Assoc. Ga., 45:458, 1956.
24. Gardemin, Herbert, and Herbst, Wolfgang: Wirbeldeformierung bie der Adoleszentenkyphose und Osteoporose. Arch. Orthop. Unfallchir., 59:134, 1966.
25. Grospic, F.: Kyphosis dorsalis adolescentium. Zentralbl. Chir., 55 (I):61, 1928.
26. Gschwend, N., and Müller, G. P.: Egebnisse einer aktiv-passiven Behandlungsmethode fixierter juveniler Thorakalkyphosen. Arch. Orthop. Unfallchir., 61:55, 1967.
27. Güntz, E.: Kyphosis juvenilis sive adolescentium. Z. Orthop., 65:53, 1937.
28. Güntz, E.: Gedanken zur Begutachtung von Wirgelsäulenschäden nach orthopadischen Gesichtspunkten. Arch. Orthop. Unfallchir., 47:558, 1955.
29. Hafner, R. H.: Localized osteochondritis. Scheuermann's disease. J. Bone Joint Surg., 34B:38, 1952.
30. Hallock, Halford, Francis, K. C., and Jones, J. B.: Spine fusion in young children. A long-term end-result study with particular reference to growth effects. J. Bone Joint Surg., 39A:481, June, 1957.
31. Harrington, P. R.: Treatment of scoliosis. Correction and internal fixation by spine instrumentation. J. Bone Joint Surg., 44A:591, June, 1962.
32. Hodgen, J. T., and Frantz, C. H.: Juvenile kyphosis. Surg. Gynecol. Obstet., 72:798, 1941.
33. Hult, L.: Cervical, dorsal and lumbar spinal syndromes. Acta Orthop. Scand., 24:174, 1954.
34. Jaffe, H. L.: Metabolic, Degenerative and Inflammatory Diseases of Bones and Joints. Philadelphia, Lea and Febiger, 1972.
35. Junghanns, H.: Fur Atiologic, Prognose und Therapie des M. Scheuermann. Medizinische, 1:300, 1955.
36. Kemp, F. H., and Wilson, D. C.: Some factors in the aetiology of osteochondritis of the spine. Br. J. Radiol., 20:410, 1947.
37. Kemp, F. H., Wilson, D. C., and Emrys-Roberts, Elinor: Social and nutritional factors in adolescent osteochondritis of the spine. Br. J. Soc. Med., 2:66, 1948.
38. Knutson, F.: Observations on the growth of the vertebral body in Scheuermann's disease. Acta Radiol., 30:97, 1948.
39. Lambrinudi, L.: Adolescent and senile kyphosis. Br. Med. J., 2:800, 1934.
40. Larsen, E. H., and Nordentaft, E. L.: Growth of the epiphyses and vertebrae. Acta Orthop. Scand., 32:210, 1962.
41. Lyon, M.: Krankheiten der wirbelkorperepiphyse. Fortschr. Geb. Rontgenstr. Nuklear Med., 44:498, 1931.
42. Michelle, A. A.: Osteochondrosis deformans juvenilis dorsi. N. Y. J. Med., 61:98, 1961.

43. Moe, J. H.: Treatment of adolescent kyphosis by non-operative and operative methods. Manitoba Med. Rev., *45*:481, 1965.

44. Monnet, J. C.: Osteochondritis deformans. J. Okla. State Med. Assoc., *52*:376, 1959.

45. Mühlbach, von R., Hahnel, H., and Cohn, H.: Zur Bedeutung biochemischer Parameter bei der Beurteilung der Scheuermannschen Krankheit. Medizin und Sport, *10*:331, 1970.

46. Muller, G., and Gschwend, N.: Endokrine Storungen und Morbus Scheuermann. Arch. Orthop. Unfallchir., *65*:357, 1969.

47. Nathan, Louis, and Kuhns, J. G.: Epiphysitis of the spine. J. Bone Joint Surg., *22*:55–62, Jan., 1940.

48. Nicod, L.: Traitement de la maladie de Scheuermann et des dystrophies rachidiennes de croissance. Praxis, *46*:1619, 1968.

49. Outland, T., and Snedden, H. E.: Juvenile dorsal kyphosis. Clin. Orthop., *5*:155, 1955.

50. Overgaard, K.: Prolapses of nucleus pulposus and Scheuermann's disease. Nord. Med., *5*:593, 1940.

51. Raisman, V.: Adolescent round back deformity—A late result of poliomyelitis. Bull. Hosp. Joint Dis., *16*:94, 1955.

52. Rathke, F. W.: Pathogenese und Therapie der juvenilen Kyphose. Z. Orthop., *102*:16, 1966.

53. Riseborough, E. J.: The anterior approach to the spine for the correction of deformities of the axial skeleton. Clin. Orthop., *93*:207, 1973.

54. Risser, J. C., Lauder, C. H., Norquist, D. M., and Craig, W. A.: Three Types of Body Casts. *In* The American Academy of Orthopaedic Surgeons: Instructional Course Lectures, vol. 10, pp. 131–142. Ann Arbor, J. W. Edwards, 1953.

55. Roaf, Robert: Vertebral growth and its mechanical control. J. Bone Joint Surg., *42B*:40, Feb., 1960.

56. Romer, U.: Behandlung des Morbus Scheuermann. Schweiz. Med. Wochenschr., *97*:1615, 1967.

57. Rütt, A.: Zur Therapie der Scheuermannschen Krankheit. Beitr. Orthop., *13*:731, 1966.

58. Saunders, J. B. de C. M., and Inman, V. T.: Intervertebral disc; critical and collective review. Int. Abs. Surg., *69*:14, 1939.

59. Scheuermann, H. W.: Kyfosis dorsalis juvenilis. Ugeskr. Laeger, *82*:385, 1920.

60. Scheuermann, H. W.: Kyphosis juvenilis (Scheuermann's krankheit). Fortschr. Geb. Rontgenstrahlen, *53*:1, 1936.

61. Schildbach, Johannes: Die Entwicklung der juvenilen Kyphose. Zentralbl. Chir., *64*:2086, 1937.

62. Schlegel, K. F.: Die biologische Bedeutung der jugendlichen Kyphosen. Med. Klin., *48*:917, 1953.

63. Schmorl, G.: Die Pathogenese der juvenilen Kyphose. Fortschr. Geb. Roentgenstr. Nuklearmed., *41*:359, 1930.

64. Schmorl, G.: The Human Spine in Health and Disease. New York, Grune and Stratton, 1971.

65. Scholder, P.: Aspect morphologique des dystrophies rachidiennes de croissance de type Scheuermann. Praxis, *46*:1608, 1968.

66. Scholder, P., and Basti, H.: Vers une meilleure comprehension des lesions de Scheuermann. Schwiez. Med. Wochenschr., *50*:1979, 1968.

67. Simon, R. S.: The diagnosis and treatment of kyphosis dorsalis juvenilis (Scheuermann's kyphosis) in the early stage. J. Bone Joint Surg., *24*:681, July, 1942.

68. Söderberg, Lennart, and Andrén, Lars: Disc degeneration and lumbago-ischias. Acta Orthop. Scand., *25*:137, 1955.

69. Soeur, R.: A propos de la pathogenie et du traitment du dos rond de l'adolescent. Acta Orthop. Belg., *24*:146, 1958.

70. Sørenson, K. H.: Scheuermann's juvenile kyphosis. Copenhagen, Munksgaard, 1964.

71. Sorrel, E., and Delahaye, A.: Growing pains simulating Pott's disease. Presse Med., *32*:737, 1924.

72. Stagnara, P., DuPelous, J., and Fauchet, R.: Traitement orthopedique ambulatoire de la maladie de Scheuermann en periode d'evolution. Rev. Chir. Orthop., *52*:585, 1966.

73. Stagnara, P., and Perdriolle, R.: Elongation vertebrale continue par platre à tendeurs. Possibilities therapeutiques. Rev. Chir. Orthop., *44*:57, 1958.

74. Stein, H., and von Zahn, L.: Zur Pathogenese, Fruhdiagnose und Prophylaxe des Morbus Scheuermann. Dtsch. Med. Wochenschr., *81*:200, 1965.

75. Steindler, Arthur: Post-Graduate Lectures on Orthopedic Diagnosis and Indications. Springfield, Ill., Charles C Thomas, 1952.

76. Stracker, O.: Zur Behandlung der Kyphosis adolescentium-Scheuermann. Wien. Med. Wochenschr., *99*:48, 1949.

77. Vidal-Naquet, G.: Un cas de resection des apophyses epineuses pour une cyphose dorsal douloureuse. Bull. Mem. Soc. Chir. Paris, *27*:571, 1935.

78. Wassman, K.: Kyphosis juvenilis Scheuermann. Acta Orthop. Scand., *21*:65, 1951.

79. Watermann, H.: Die Kyphosis Adolescentium und die Notwendigkeit ihrer Erkenntnis in der Unfallbegutachtung. Arch. Orthop. Unfallchir., *24*:179, 1927.

80. Williams, E. R.: Observations on the differential diagnosis and sequelae of juvenile vertebral osteochondrosis. Acta Radiol. Suppl., *116*:293, 1954.

# Chapter 15

# TECHNIQUES IN BRACING

## HISTORICAL BACKGROUND

Nonoperative corrective appliances have been used for many years in the treatment of scoliosis and other spinal deformities. Hippocrates, one of the first to write on the subject, described an apparatus for the forcible reduction of the deformity, but it did not appear to be very effective.[26] Paul of Aegina, one thousand years later, attempted to reduce spinal deformity by bandaging the body to splints.[7] Ambroise Paré, in 1579,[44] was the first to attempt trunk support by anterior and posterior metal plates, made by armorers (Fig. 15–1). By the eighteenth century, scoliosis became more recognized as a pathologic entity. Exercises, vertical halter traction, and braces of ingenious design were used to overcome the deformity and prevent progression. Some of these braces included head caps and halters.

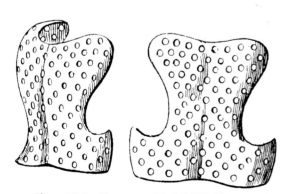

**Figure 15–1** The corset of Paré (1579). These anterior and posterior metal plates were the first external support used. (From Rothman, R. H., and Simeone, F. A.: The Spine, W. B. Saunders Co., 1975. Reprinted with permission.)

In 1847, Edward Lonsdale of London wrote a treatise on the treatment of lateral curvatures of the spine.[31] He advocated a special support, which consisted of a spring-supported pad against the rib prominence (Fig. 15–2). Unfortunately, he showed no end results of his treatment. The first carefully fitted supports were made about 1895, by Friedrich Hessing of Augsburg (Fig. 15–3).[25] He established a great reputation and had many brace shops in Germany. Albert Hoffa[27] used this brace, and he emphasized the need for concomitant exercises to furnish active correction.

In 1875, with the advent of plaster of Paris jackets,[47, 48, 59] new methods for correction were devised. By the end of the nineteenth century, the plaster of Paris jacket had become an accepted method of holding correction of a curvature. Wüllstein included the head and neck in the jacket and combined multiple pressure pads against bony prominences (Fig. 15–4).[59] Lewis Sayre used vertical head suspension to apply the cast (Fig. 15–5).[50] Other frames for applying casts using both vertical and horizontal distraction were designed by Bradford and Brackett.

At the turn of the century, most braces relied on passive support with axillary crutches, elastic bands for rib pressure, and even weights and pulleys. These included the passive correction brace of Steindler (Fig. 15–6) and later the ingenious lever system of Barr–Buschenfeldt (Fig. 15–7).[7] An active brace was first proposed by Spitzy, who placed sharp buttons under the chin and occiput (Fig. 15–8).[54] The patient had to actively maintain elongation of the spine or suffer

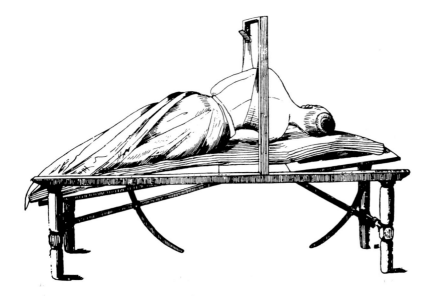

**Figure 15–2** The spinal support of Lonsdale (1847) provided a pad for pressure against the rib prominence.

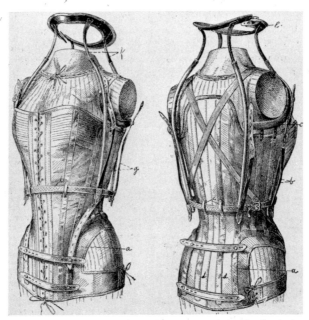

**Figure 15–3** An example of the first carefully fitted spinal support, made by Hessing in Augsburg. Note the similarity of the brace to the brace of Ponte in Figure 15–27.

pain. There was no passive support. Not surprisingly, the brace proved unpopular.

A landmark in the control and correction of scoliosis was the development of the Milwaukee brace.[4, 6, 8] This was originally designed by Blount and Schmidt as a substitute for the distraction plaster jacket to obtain passive correction and fixation following surgery (Fig. 15–9). They substituted a circular metal neck ring with occipital and chin pads for the plaster collar. A molded leather pelvic girdle replaced the plaster girdle. The two sections were joined by metal uprights, and adjustable localizer pads were added. After numerous refinements, it began to be used for nonoperative care of scoliosis in the mid-1950s.

At the present time, the corrective devices used for the nonoperative treatment of spine deformities can be grouped into the Milwaukee brace category and various underarm braces and body jackets.

## BRACING OBJECTIVES

All orthoses are applied to control spinal curvatures. The control can be in the juvenile years till either adequate spine growth has occurred or the curve progresses in the orthosis. In the adolescent the orthosis is designed to prevent the curve from increasing. Recently there have been studies of patients with idiopathic scoliosis treated in the Milwaukee brace, and reviewed after being out of the brace from 5 to 10 years.[10, 16] In the majority of cases, the final curves were about the same as the initial curve. Thus in general, the brace controls curves and prevents small curves from increasing but does not permanently change large curves into small ones.

## BRACING PRINCIPLES

Before discussing the techniques of bracing, certain basic principles are important in the understanding and application of bracing techniques.

1) All orthoses exert force through the skin over a variable area. This pressure must be exerted over the soft tissues. There cannot be localized, direct pressure on bony prominences, as local ischemia and pressure sores will result.

2) The forces applied to correct a curve can be divided into distractive forces and lateral forces. With larger curves, a lateral corrective force is biomechanically ineffective, and distractive force becomes more important. Similarly, with smaller curves, distractive forces are of minimal use, whereas laterally directed forces are very important.

3) The vertebral column is inaccessible to direct force, and thus the forces have to be applied indirectly. Lateral forces are transmitted via the ribs in the thoracic spine and via the paraspinal muscles overlying the transverse processes in the lumbar spine. Because the ribs normally slope downward, the corrective force must be applied to the rib going to the vertebra below the apex. As the curves become larger, the ribs become more oblique, making it difficult, if not impossible, for the force to be transmitted through the ribs to the spine. The force applied to these ribs may cause an increased obliquity of the rib rather than a correction of the deformity. With a paralytic rib "droop," a lateral force may not be transmitted to the spine at all but may cause more rib droop and decreased lung space.

4) In correcting a deformity and maintaining normal body balance, all orthoses use three or more corrective forces. A force is applied to the apex of the deformity, with counterforce points on the opposite side of the body. The patient's muscle tone and righting reflex can provide a force component in response to the orthosis.

5) To help achieve contact of the corrective force with the lumbar transverse processes, the vertebral column must be controlled so that the spine does not move forward, away from the posterolateral force. Thus all orthoses are made to control lumbar lordosis. The abdominal apron, plus the brace extending low over the buttocks, plays a role in controlling lordosis.

6) Orthoses work by active and passive correction of the deformity, active correction occurring only in patients with effective trunk muscle function. Generally speaking, to be effective in correcting and holding the deformity, the orthosis must be worn full-time until growth ceases, with reduced wearing only in special circumstances. Constant supervision of the orthosis and its fit is necessary in order to make appropriate readjustments for growth and correction.

7) Weaning from the brace is carried out

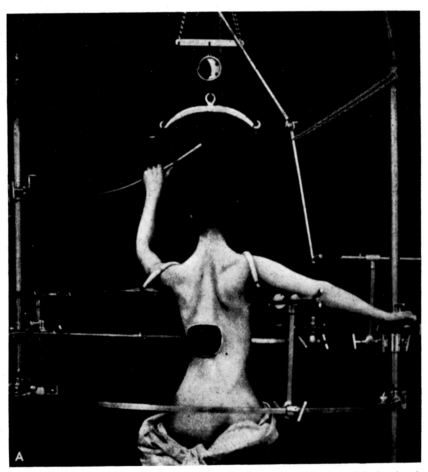

**Figure 15–4**   Wullstein cast. Note the multiple pressure points and incorporation of the head and neck.

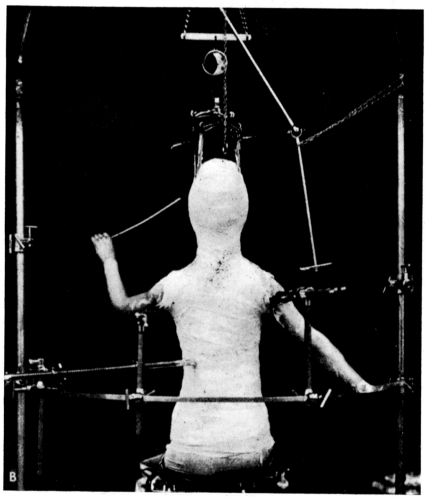

**Figure 15-4**  *Continued.*

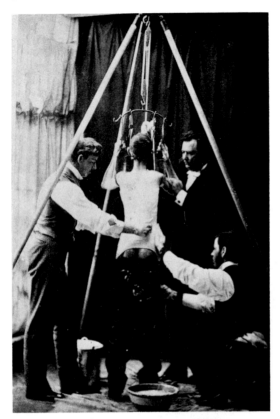

**Figure 15–5**  Plaster application technique of Sayre for scoliosis correction using vertical head suspension.

**Figure 15–6**  Passive correction brace of Steindler.

**Figure 15–7**  Passive brace of Barr-Buschenfledt, using a system of corrective levers.

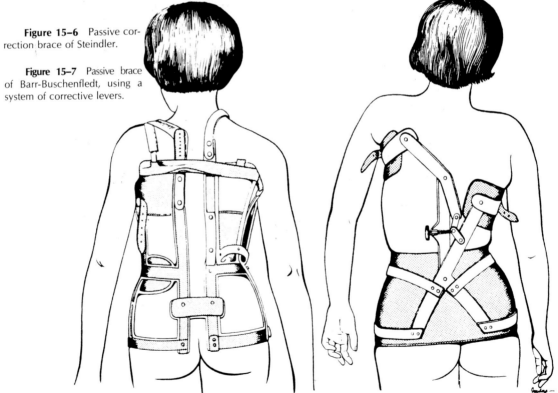

Figure 15–6                                              Figure 15–7

on a set schedule (Table 15–1). A little understood principle is the stability that usually occurs with long-term bracing of spine deformities. When an idiopathic scoliotic is braced, some correction may be maintained after the brace is discontinued. Very little is known about how a curve "stabilizes." It is unknown whether changes occur in the intervertebral disc, facet joint capsules, intervertebral ligaments, rib vertebral articulations, or muscles to cause a curve to stabilize. Do changes occur in one of the above areas, or is a combination of changes important? Some basic research is being done to explain these changes, but as there are so many unknown factors, much more pertinent study is necessary.

8) In respiration, the ribs move in a "bucket handle" manner, increasing the anteroposterior and transverse diameters of the thoracic cage. Any correcting pad applied to the ribs may prevent expansion in that area. More extensive restriction of chest expansion by a circumferential brace will further de-

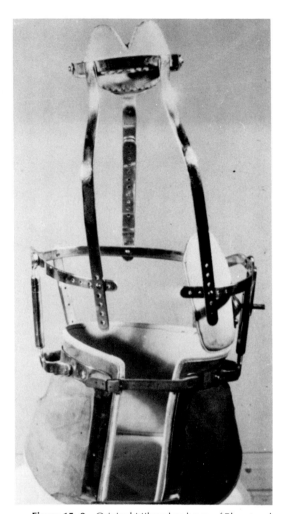

**Figure 15–9** Original Milwaukee brace of Blount and Schmidt.

crease chest expansion and pulmonary function. This defeats one of the purposes of the brace; to control the curvature *without* any restriction of chest expansion and pulmonary function.

9) Corrective devices are fitted to growing children. During the growth of the thorax, any constant circumferential compression will retard normal rib growth and lead to a deformed chest wall and a "tubular thorax."

10) Pressure against the developing breasts will prevent normal maturation. This compression must be prevented in order to allow normal breast growth.

11) Excessive mandibular pressure must be prevented. This pressure will result in restriction of normal mandibular growth and dental deformities.

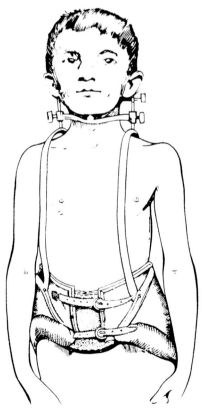

**Figure 15–8** Active brace of Spitzy. Sharp buttons under the chin and occiput forced the child to pull away from the buttons, giving elongation and active correction.

In summary, an orthosis to be maximally effective should have certain features. It must be lightweight, aesthetically acceptable, and easily applied. Such a device will allow full participation of the patient in all activities. At the same time, the deformity must be maximally controlled. The design of the orthosis must allow full chest expansion and thus maintain respiratory function.

## BRACE MANUFACTURE

Many braces are available for the treatment of spine deformities. Since our experience has been primarily with the Milwaukee brace, and since the best statistical results have come from the use of the Milwaukee brace[10, 16, 34, 53] the majority of this discussion will center around the Milwaukee brace.

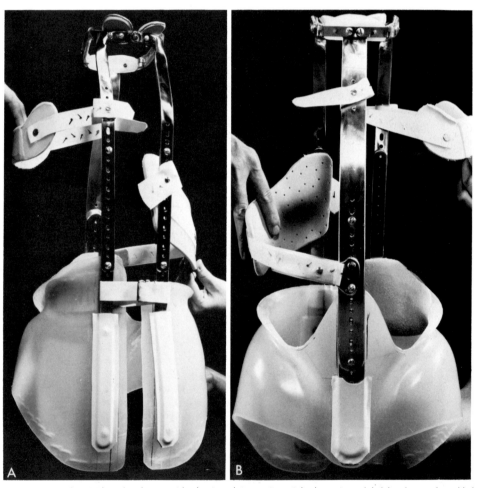

**Figure 15-10**   Modern Milwaukee brace with plastic pelvic section, right thoracic pad, left lumbar pad, and left axillary sling. Note that brace cannot stand unsupported due to length of pelvic section posteriorly. A, Posterior view, showing parallel posterior uprights and pelvic girlde extending upward on left to support the lumbar pad. B, Anterior view, showing anterior outrigger for thoracic pad, abdominal apron, and molded throat mold.

## Milwaukee Brace

The Milwaukee brace was designed originally by Blount and Schmidt[4, 6, 8] of Milwaukee in 1945, and consists of a molded, well fitting pelvic section, two posterior uprights and a single anterior upright which connect the pelvic section to the neck ring. The neck ring has a throat mold and two occipital pads. Appropriate lateral pads are fitted to the uprights to correct the specific deformity (Fig. 15–10).

### PELVIC SECTION MANUFACTURE

The first step in brace manufacture is forming the pelvic section. This is fitted individually to each patient and is manufactured in one of two ways: (a) through the formation of a negative and positive, according to the patient's size and, (b) prefabricated pelvic sections.

***Manufacture Using a Positive.*** To create a positive, a negative impression is taken of the patient. This may be taken supine or standing. Supine molds are taken in patients with paralytic deformities unable to stand without collapse of the spine, and in small children where anesthesia is used. The mold is usually taken in a frame with the patient standing with knees bent and supported from behind by a cross bar. The arms are supported at shoulder level by a bar on the frame, and occasionally head halter traction is used in

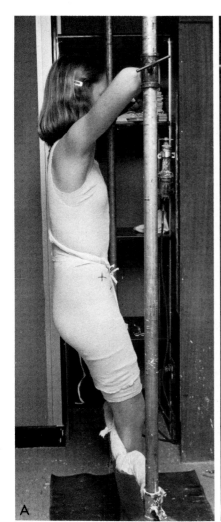
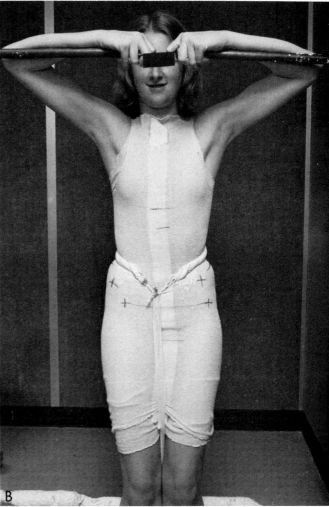

**Figure 15–11**  *A and B,* Standing mold being taken for Milwaukee brace. Patient stands in special frame with knees bent and arms supported overhead. Note the double layer of stockinette with the bony prominences marked.

addition. This position for taking the positive decreases lumbar lordosis and the distractive force corrects the curve (Fig. 15–11). Measurements are taken using such bony landmarks as the pubis, anterior superior iliac spines and xiphoid. In addition, these landmarks are marked on the two layers of stockinette covering the patient. The negative is taken with careful but deep molding above the iliac crests. The cast is wrapped from below the trochanters to the axillae. Once this mold has set, guide points and vertical lines are accurately marked, the cast is removed, fitted together and re-united with plaster.

The inferior margin is then trimmed using a horizontal guide line. Next the lower end of the negative is sealed, and the whole cast is filled with plaster, thus obtaining a positive mold. This basic positive mold is further modified. These modifications consist of skiving of the abdominal area to give adequate control of lumbar lordosis. In addition, more plaster or additional padding is added over the lower ribs and the anterior superior iliac spine area to distribute the forces away from these bony prominences. In the concavity of the lumbar curvature, plaster is added which in the final pelvic section gives an area into which the curve can move (Fig. 15–12).

The modified positive is now covered to form the pelvic section. Leather was used in the original brace and is still used in many centers. We prefer to use thermo-labile plastic for the pelvic section. Orthoplast is still used for small children as it is easy to work with on very small braces but disintegrates too rapidly for most patients. In larger children and adolescents vitrathene or polypropylene is used, which is heated and molded on the positive. (See book, The Milwaukee Brace[5] for exact technique.) The technique used in the Twin Cities for the Milwaukee brace pelvic section is vacuum forming of polypropylene to the positive (Fig. 15–13). Once the plastic has hardened, it is removed from the positive, appropriately trimmed, leaving adequate length posteriorly on the buttocks to hold the lumbar lordosis. Anteriorly it is trimmed to just above the pubis and sufficiently at the thighs to allow 100° of hip flexion. An abdominal apron is left extending to just below the xiphoid. The uprights are fitted using the previous measurements and the neck ring is applied. Finally, the appropriate pads are added.

### Manufacture Using A Prefabricated Pelvic

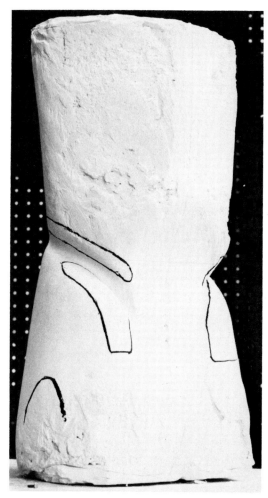

**Figure 15–12** Modified positive of patient. Note the skived abdominal area and areas over the bony prominences and above the iliac crest indentation where excess plaster has been added.

***Section.*** Investigations have been made into a series of sizes of prefabricated pelvic sections that can be fitted to most patients and thus eliminate the need for making each girdle separately from a positive. This reduces the time and ultimately may cut the cost of brace manufacture.[11, 23]

When fitting a prefabricated pelvic section, the patient is first measured, and after referral to a chart of sizes, the pelvic section is trimmed and, where necessary, modified by heating to fit the patient (Fig. 15–14). The remainder of the brace manufacture is the same as described earlier. Depending upon the number of sizes available, up to 80 per cent of patients can be fitted with a prefabricated girdle.

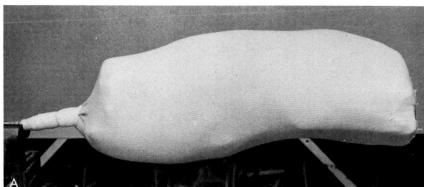

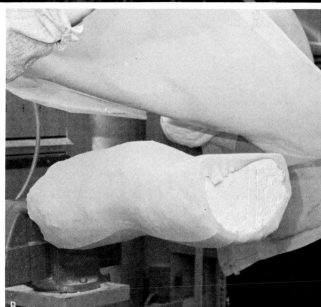

**Figure 15–13** Vacuum forming technique for pelvic section. *A,* Modified positive is covered with stockinette, and the ends are sealed. On the left the positive is attached by a hollow rod to the compression pump. *B,* A sheet of polypropylene, heated to 425° F., is placed over the positive. *C,* Diagram to show the principle of vacuum forming. The rod holding the positive has a hole (a) just above the plaster and is connected to the compression pump. Once the plaster has been sealed on all sides, making the space between the polypropylene and plaster airtight, a vacuum force is applied, using the pump. Air is removed from between the plastic and plaster, making the plastic mold to the positive.

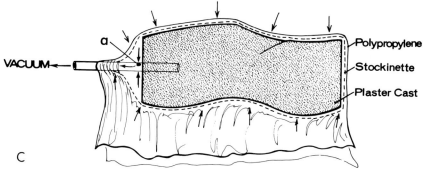

C

*Legend continued on following page*

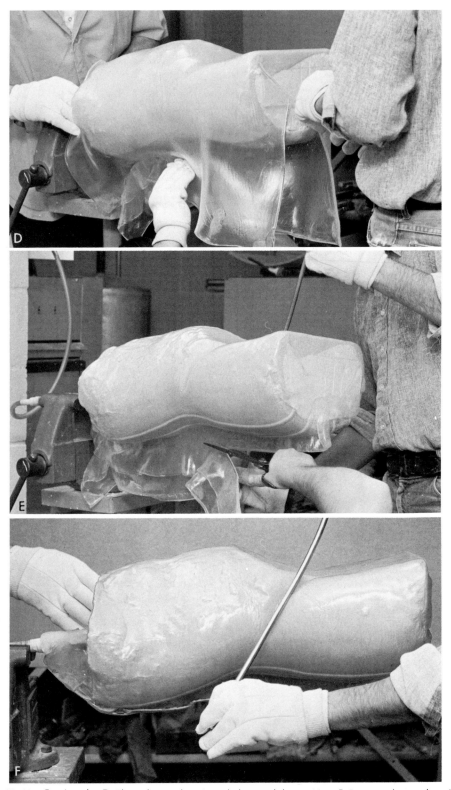

**Figure 15–13**   *Continued.*   *D,* The polypropylene is sealed around the positive. *E,* Excess polypropylene is trimmed, and a metal rod is used to contour the iliac crest indentation. *F,* Another view of the molding above the iliac crest using a metal rod.

*Legend continued on opposite page*

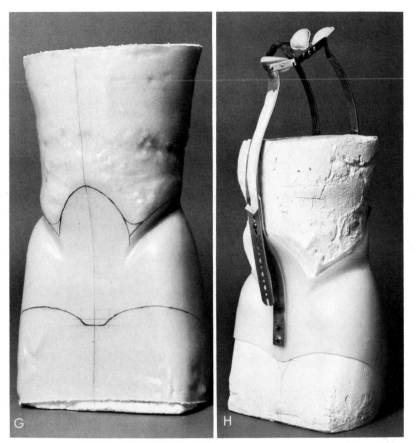

**Figure 15–13** *Continued.* *C,* Completed brace is now marked and removed from the positive for trimming. *H,* Milwaukee brace near completion. Uprights and neck ring have been added to the trimmed pelvic section.

***Milwaukee Brace Pads.*** The Milwaukee brace operates on two principles. The first of these is the three-point principle, the three points usually being one side of the pelvic section, the thoracic pad over the convexity of the thoracic curve, and the lateral aspect of the neck ring on the opposite side. The axillary sling acts as an active assist to centralize the neck in the neck ring. The neck ring induces balance by using the patient's righting reflex and active muscle tone. With a lumbar curve, the lumbar pad is applied to the convexity of the curve, either with a thoracic pad on the opposite side or with the neck ring on the opposite side being the third force point (Fig. 15–15). The force point on the pelvic girdle stabilizes the brace. Occasionally, an extension over the trochanter is necessary for this stabilization if listing occurs in the brace (Fig. 15–15*B*). The second principle of correction is distraction. Distraction is applied by the occipital pads, which fit under (not behind) the occiput. Each time the patient looks upward, the spine is elongated.

THORACIC PAD. Different corrective pads are used for various curves. A thoracic pad is used for mid and low thoracic curves (Figs. 15–10 and 15–16). It is situated laterally for scoliosis and posterolaterally for kyphoscoliosis, and the lateral force is applied to the ribs leading toward the apex of the curve. The pad may be situated at varying levels on the thorax, depending on the horizontal or oblique anatomic configuration of the ribs. The pad is usually placed just lateral to the posterior upright. It is attached to the anterior upright by an outrigger and posteriorly to the near (ipsilateral) posterior upright by a strap that goes under and around the upright, in this way being closely applied to the chest wall. To give an effective force vector, the anterior outrigger is long when used for kyphoscoliosis and short for sco-

*Text continued on page 376*

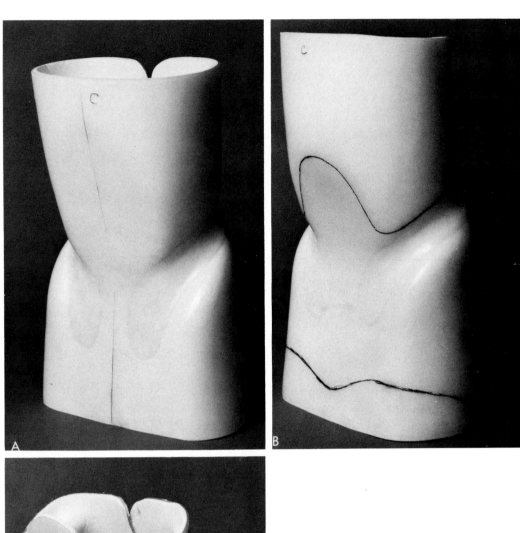

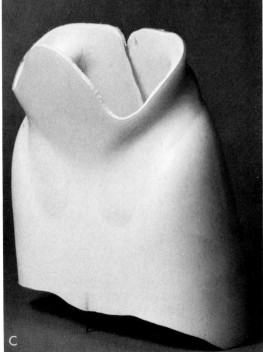

**Figure 15–14** Formation of pelvic section from prefabricated pelvic section. *A,* Prefabricated pelvic section. Note that enough length exists to make a pelvic section or TLSO. *B,* Once the correct size is chosen, it is fitted to the patient and marked for trimming. *C,* The trimmed pelvic section is shown. The edges are smoothed and the uprights fitted as in Figure 15–13*H.* Note that the pelvic section cannot stand upright without support.

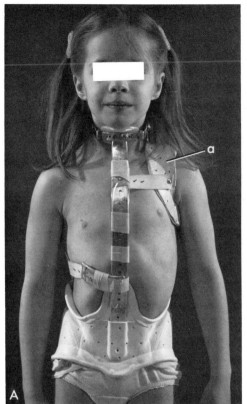

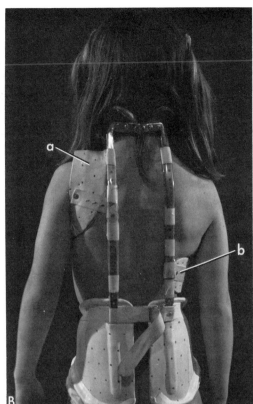

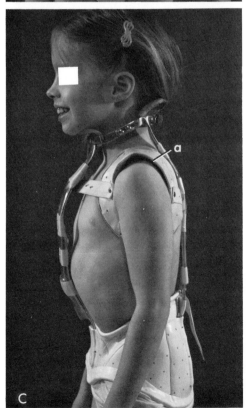

**Figure 15–17** *A, B,* and C. Patient fitted with a left shoulder ring (a) and right oval pad (b). Note the snug fit of the shoulder ring. It is attached to the uprights by nylon straps, but an elastic strap may be used anteriorly. The direction of the straps will depend on the force required. The oval pad is attached by an outrigger anteriorly and is applied to the lower right ribs. Note the clearance of the anterior upright, allowing full chest expansion. (From Winter, R. B., and Moe, J. H.: Clin. Orthop., *102*:72, 1974, with permission.)

liosis. The upper part of the pad fits over the inferior tip of the scapula and helps to control the scapular protrusion while aiding in correction of the rib prominence. The oval thoracic pad is used for pressure on the lower ribs in the thoracolumbar curves, and is attached in the same manner as the thoracic pad (Fig. 15–17). It is often used in conjunction with a lumbar pad for thoracolumbar curves.

AXILLARY SLING. An axillary sling fits into the axilla, with straps extending cranially and medially (Figs. 6–10 and 6–19). It is used

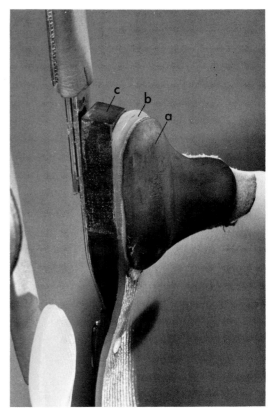

**Figure 15–19** Close-up of lumbar pad. Pad (a) is attached to the pelvic section, and the polypropylene (b) extends to support the pad. Note the bolster (c) between the posterior upright and pelvic section, giving additional support to the lumbar pad.

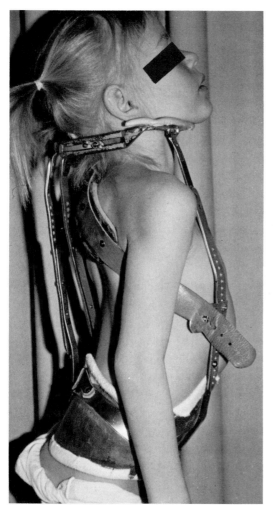

**Figure 15–18** Poorly fitting Milwaukee brace. The pelvic section is very short posteriorly, giving no control of lumbar lordosis and allowing the brace to stand upright unaided. The anterior upright is close to the chest, preventing normal chest expansion. The chin rest is fitted with marked pressure against the mandible. The neck ring is horizontal and the posterior uprights far from the torso. The thoracic pad is incorrectly fitted.

to keep the neck in the middle of the neck ring in initial fitting of the Milwaukee brace. It is placed on the side opposite to the thoracic pad. With the force exerted by the thoracic pad, the patient is forced laterally in the brace, producing irritating pressure of the neck against the neck ring. The axillary sling counteracts this force. After four to six months of brace-wearing, the body's righting reflex counteracts this tendency, and use of the axillary sling can be discontinued. Thus, the axillary sling is *not* used to elevate a shoulder, nor to treat a curve, but merely to keep the patient well centered in the neck ring.

LUMBAR PAD. The lumbar pad is attached to the inside of the lumbar portion of the pelvic section with Velcro so it can be adjusted easily (Figs. 15–10 and 15–19). It presses against the transverse processes via the paraspinal muscles and is situated just posterolateral to these muscles, at the apex of the lumbar curve. The lumbar pad must lie below the twelfth rib and above the iliac crest. Occasionally the pelvic section plastic is not strong enough to hold the lumbar pad firmly against the patient, and a bolster must be placed between the pelvic section and the posterior upright. In thoracolumbar curves, the lumbar pad is used in conjunction with an oval low thoracic pad on the same side.

TRAPEZIUS PAD. A trapezius pad is used for correction of high thoracic curves with prominence of the first ribs. The force is exerted through the trapezius muscle and first two ribs downward and medially onto the vertebrae (Fig. 15–16). The pad is attached via two straps directed caudally and medially, the posterior strap passing to the far (contralateral) posterior upright. The anterior strap may be elastic. A molded shoulder ring is occasionally used for the treatment of certain high thoracic and cervicothoracic curves. The shoulder ring is attached via two straps directed medially or medially and caudally, the exact direction depending on the force vector required to correct the curve (Fig. 15–17).

In summary, the way in which corrective pads are applied to the brace depends on the curve patterns:

1) Thoracic curve. This is the commonest curve pattern and is treated with a thoracic pad and an axillary sling on the opposite side.

2) Single high thoracic curve. Trapezius pad.

3) Thoracolumbar curve. Low thoracic oval pad and lumbar pad on the same side.

4) Lumbar curve. Lumbar pad.

5) Cervicothoracic curve. Molded shoulder ring, with addition of face and head support in some cases (see below).

6) Double thoracic curves. In these cases, a combination of the trapezius pad and thoracic pad is used.

7) Double curves—thoracic and lumbar. A thoracic pad and a lumbar pad.

USE IN KYPHOSIS. In kyphosis, the pressure is applied posteriorly, either through padded posterior uprights or through kyphosis pads. The force is directed through the paraspinal muscles to the vertebrae at or below the apex of the deformity (Fig. 15–20). These pads are thickened, and the uprights

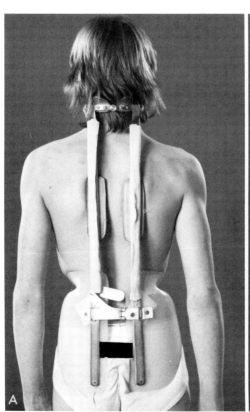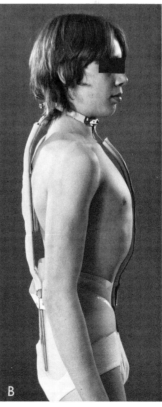

**Figure 15–20** *A and B,* Patient fitted with kyphosis pads. The kyphosis pads fit the kyphosis closely, and there is sufficient chest room anteriorly. Note that the occipital pads are lower than for scoliosis, reducing any tendency to push the head forward.

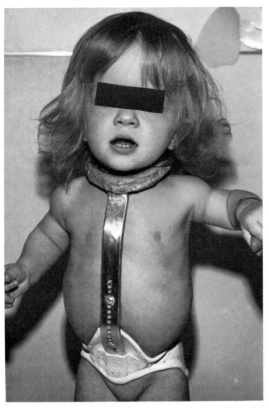

**Figure 15–21** Padded neck ring and orthoplast pelvic section as used in infants. (From Winter, R. B., and Moe, J. H.: Clin. Orthop., *102*:72, 1974.)

realigned to apply a constant force as the kyphosis corrects in the brace. Most patients with thoracic kyphosis have a forward-protruding head. Only the Milwaukee brace neck ring restores the head to the proper alignment above the shoulders and hips. Braces that reach only as far as the sternum do not provide either distraction or repositioning of the head. Furthermore, the apex of the typical thoracic kyphosis is most often at T7, and the third point for effective correction must be higher than the upper sternum. Only a kyphosis with the apex at the lower thoracic area or thoracolumbar area will respond to a brace without a neck ring (see Fig. 15–15C and *D*).

*Modifications.* In certain cases, modifications of the basic Milwaukee brace are necessary to fit the patient's specific needs. Normally the pelvic section is not lined, but in cases where the bony prominences are marked or there is concern about skin sensation, the girdle can be lined with a synthetic spongy material such as Alimed, Pelite, or Plastazote. In very young children a neck ring with the usual throat mold and occipital pads is not feasible, so a padded neck ring is used (Fig. 15–21). With Sprengel's deformity, the neck ring must be contoured to the shoulders so that there is no pressure against the base

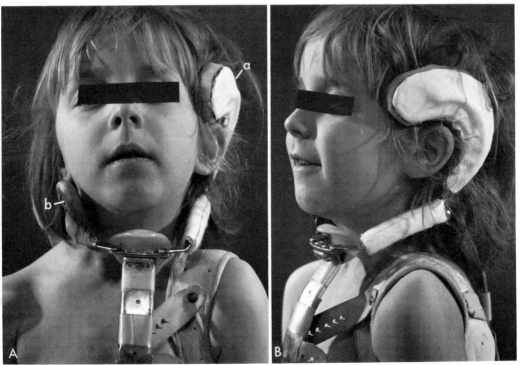

**Figure 15–22** *A* and *B*, Patient fitted with padded head support on left (a) and chin support (b) for head control in cervicothoracic and high thoracic curves.

of the neck. In young children with cervico-thoracic curves and head tilt, usually of congenital origin, the brace is modified by adding a lateral face-and-head support to obtain and maintain an upright position of the head (Fig. 15–22). Occasionally, the brace is attached to a halo for holding the head. This device is used usually postoperatively for high cervicothoracic curves (Fig. 15–23). In Scheuermann's disease, when the pectoral muscles are tight, shoulder outriggers are fitted for protrusion of the shoulders (Fig. 15–24.) In myelodysplasia, the pelvic section has to be modified with an opening to allow for care of the ileal diversion; an adequate area should be cut out over the collecting bag site (Fig. 15–25).

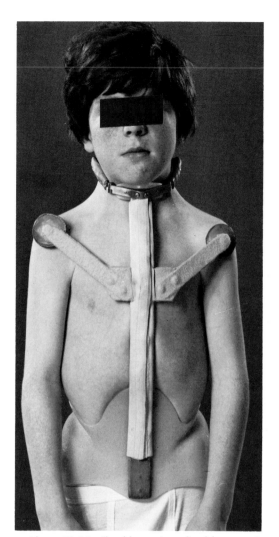

**Figure 15–24** Shoulder outrigger fitted for protrusion of shoulder. This is sometimes useful in Scheuermann's disease with tight pectoral muscles.

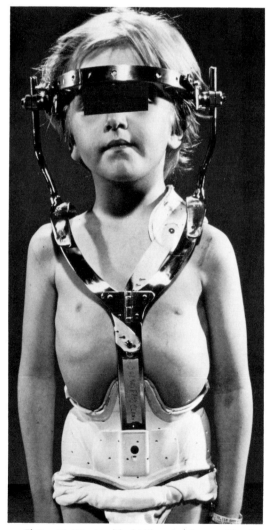

**Figure 15–23** Modified Milwaukee brace with adaptation to fit halo.

## TLSO

The TLSO (thoracolumbosacral orthosis) is used for flexible thoracolumbar or lumbar curves (Fig. 15–26). With this orthosis, the three points are the lateral aspect of the pelvis, a lumbar pad over the apex of the curve, and the thoracic extension on the opposite side.[23] Occasionally, the lateral aspect of the pelvis gives insufficient support, and the pelvic section is lengthened into a trochanteric extension, which gives a more distal force point (see Fig. 15–15B). The force system is very similar to that of the brace used by Dr. Alberto Ponte of Italy (Fig. 15–27)[46] or by Levine.[29]

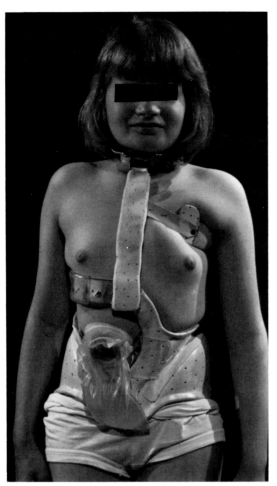

**Figure 15–25**　Adaptation of pelvic section to accommodate ileal conduit collection bag.

The TLSO may either be formed on a positive or be prefabricated. Manufacture is the same as for the Milwaukee brace pelvic section (p. 367). Our initial experience shows that this brace is effective for flexible mild lumbar or thoracolumbar curves but is not satisfactory for thoracic or double structural patterns. We have found that curves with the apex above T12 do not respond consistently to the brace, and we do not recommend its use for these curves.

As with the Milwaukee brace, there is no restriction of chest mechanics in the TLSO. Due to absence of the uprights and neck ring, there is little alteration of the patient's activities.

The Kalibis splint (Fig. 15–28) is a simple TLSO used in the neonatal period for severe thoracolumbar scoliosis until the baby is large enough to fit a Milwaukee brace (6 to 9 months of age). The splint works on a three-point principle, with a thoracic pad and two points of counterpressure on the opposite side—a shoulder ring and the lateral aspect of the pelvic section.

## Body Jacket

A body jacket is a circumferential body orthosis extending from the pelvis to upper thorax with or without extensions over the shoulder and around the neck (Fig. 15–29). In the strict orthotic terminology, they are also thoracolumbosacral orthoses, but their design, indications, and application differ from those of the TLSO described previously. The body jacket is used for the nonoperative treatment of neuromuscular spine deformity in cases where the use of the Milwaukee brace is difficult and not of greatest benefit, e.g., polio, cerebral palsy, muscular dystrophy, certain cases of myelomeningocele, and spinal cord trauma. These deformities tend to be long curves that are flexible and collapsing. The body jacket, as it is lightweight and can be removed for skin care, is also used as the postoperative support in certain cases of these neuromuscular deformities. It must be emphasized that for such neuromuscular problems, the body jacket plays a purely passive supporting role. The conventional TLSO cannot be used, since it requires a righting reflex and active muscle power in the trunk, which are not present in paralytic curves. Because the mold is taken in a corrected position on a Risser frame, correction occurs while the patient is in the jacket, but this correction is due to passive support given by the jacket. It is not effective for cervicothoracic or upper thoracic curves and is best for lumbar and thoracolumbar curves.

Recently, Cockrell and Risser[19] and Murphy[36] have presented preliminary results of the treatment of idiopathic scoliosis using a molded polycarbonate (Lexan) plastic underarm "localizer" brace. Bunnell and MacEwen[14] have a large number of patients with idiopathic scoliosis treated with an orthoplast body jacket. A similar brace, the Lyonnaise brace, manufactured from a rigid plastic and also lacking a thoracic window, is used extensively in France for the nonoperative treatment of idiopathic scoliosis (Fig. 15–30).[43] These orthoses have been shown to decrease pulmonary function and, because of their rigid circumferential nature, can lead to significant chest wall deformity.[32, 55]

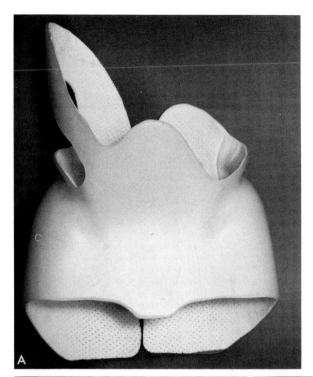

**Figure 15–26** *A, B,* and *C,* Thoracolumbosacral orthosis (TLSO). Underarm brace used for flexible lumbar and thoracolumbar curves has a built-in lumbar pad posteriorly on the right with support of the brace in this area. The brace extends into the axilla on the right for counterpressure.

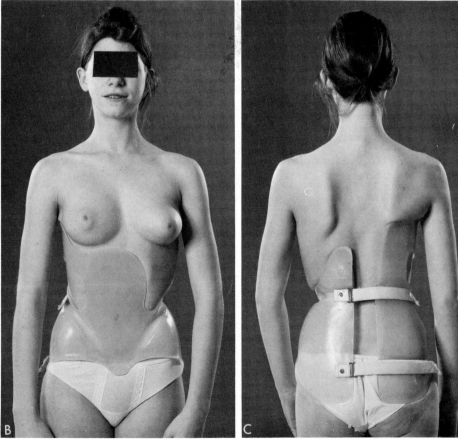

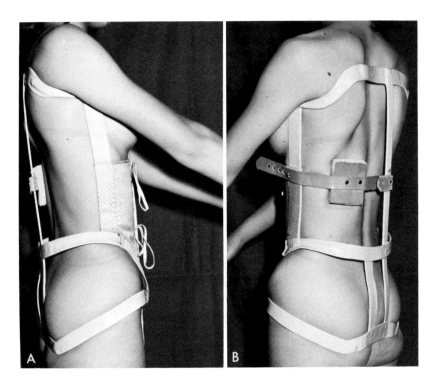

**Figure 15–27** *A* and *B,* Underarm brace used by Dr. Ponte in Italy. Note similarity to spinal support of Hessing shown in Figure 15–3. (With permission from Dr. A. Ponte.)

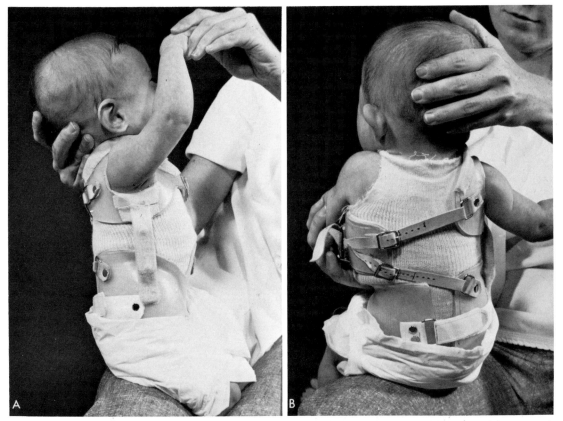

**Figure 15–28** *A* and *B,* Modified Kalibis splint. This has a molded pelvic section, shoulder ring, and thoracic pad, working on a simple three-point correction system.

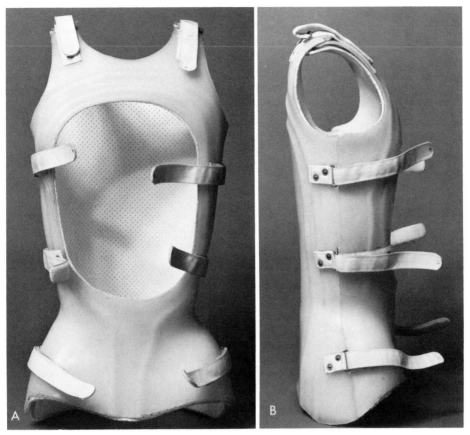

**Figure 15–29**   A and B, Polypropylene molded body jacket. Well-fitting side-closing brace with two half-shells interlocking laterally. Note the large thoracic window anteriorly to allow full chest expansion and thus limit restriction of pulmonary function.

The body jacket used at the Twin Cities Scoliosis Center is currently made out of polypropylene (Fig. 15–29). It consists of anterior and posterior shells, which interlock laterally and are fastened with Velcro straps. There is a large anterior thoracic window to allow maximal chest expansion. The jacket is lined with a plastic sponge material (Alimed, Pelite, or Plastazote). The brace is manufactured after a supine negative mold is taken in the fully corrected position on a Risser frame and then formed into a positive mold. The vacuum-forming technique is also used for manufacture of this brace.

## BIOMECHANICS

Biomechanical studies have been performed on the fitted Milwaukee brace to evaluate the forces exerted by the brace. A dynamometer was first used by Schultz and Galante[52] and implanted in the mandibular and occipital pads to evaluate the traction force in the brace. Using the old chin rest,[18, 22, 35] the total traction force has been recorded as 1.13 to 1.94 KP (kilo ponds; 1 kilo pond = 9.8 newtons, the weight of a 1 kilogram mass). Walking raised the force slightly, to 2.1 KP, and in the supine position a further increase to 2.8 to 5 KP was noted. In the right recumbent position, there was a similar increase, and maximal forces were found with movement away from the thoracic pad in the "shift" maneuver (4.4 to 6.4 KP). With exercise, deep breathing, or coughing, increased forces on the chin rest and occipital pads were recorded. These forces against the chin rest were so large that growth changes in the mandible and face resulted. There is a shortening of the lower third of the face, a depression of the premolars and molars, and deflection of the maxillary anterior teeth.[1, 15, 28, 30, 42]

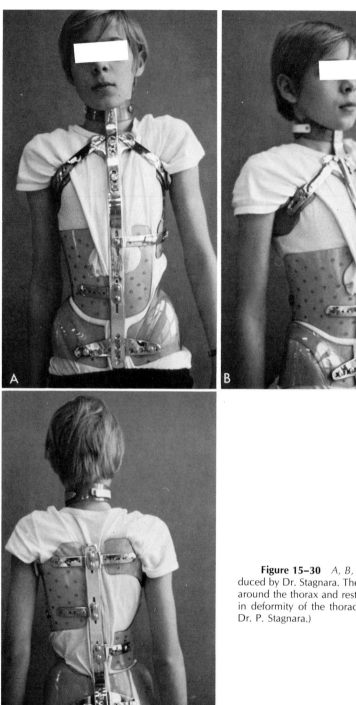

**Figure 15–30** *A, B,* and *C,* Lyonnaise brace, as introduced by Dr. Stagnara. The molded plastic brace fits tightly around the thorax and restricts chest expansion and results in deformity of the thoracic cage. (With permission from Dr. P. Stagnara.)

The growth changes on the face and mandible were initially treated with orthodontic braces and appliances.[12] The flat chin rest was then changed to a shaped throat mold that fits within the rami of the mandible and exerts minimal force on the soft tissues of the floor of the mouth. Simultaneously, more space was permitted, as the chin rest was set 1 to 2 centimeters lower. Dynametric studies of this modified Milwaukee brace showed a marked reduction in the traction forces[35] to 0.4 KP standing (the maximal force on lateral shift was 1.2 KP). The previously reported facial and dental changes do not occur with this throat mold.[15, 20, 42, 45]

The forces in the thoracic pad have also been measured in the Milwaukee brace, with both the chin rest and the throat mold.[18, 22, 35] There is no difference in the forces with these two devices; the forces were 3.8 KP standing and increased to 5.7 KP with a 21 to 30 degree major curve and to 6.5 KP with a 41 to 50 degree curve.[35] The traction forces did not increase with curve increase, demonstrating that the lateral force is more important than the distractive forces. With the new throat mold, distractive forces are not present. The application of these forces has been shown by Nachemson and Elfstrom[38] to be effective in reaching the spine. Using a Harrington distraction rod with a force gauge, the forces applied to the rod were evaluated in a patient in various positions with and without a holding cast or Milwaukee brace. The lowest loads recorded were in patients in the Milwaukee brace. The brace had a superior force-relieving effect compared to their holding cast. They also found that chin-pad distraction was not necessary to obtain a corrective force, but the thoracic pad force with a proximal counter point was most effective.

Andriacchi et al.[2] have developed simulation studies conducted in mathematically modeled analogues. Their findings confirm the observations of Nachemson and Elfstrom that traction forces are not important and that the use and application of corrective pads are effective in correcting the major curve and controlling the spine in the brace. This model was tested on Milwaukee brace patients, with 80 per cent accurate prediction of brace outcome.

Nachemson and Morris,[39] on measuring intradiscal pressures in vivo, found pressures of 10 to 15 kg./cm. in normal discs in the sitting position, with a 30 per cent decrease in standing and a 50 per cent decrease in the reclining position. When an inflated corset was worn, the pressure in the discs decreased by 25 per cent. These data demonstrate that the increased intra-abdominal and intra-thoracic pressures resulting from the abdominal apron of orthoses decrease the load on the discs. The possible role of this effect in correction of scoliosis is unknown. Waters and Morris also showed that a brace changes the electromyographic activity of the erector spinae muscles very little. The activity of the abdominal muscles was significantly decreased while wearing a corset or brace.[56]

No biomechanical studies are available regarding the forces in the TLSO or body jacket. Further studies of the biomechanics of all spinal orthoses are necessary for a better understanding of their application to the treatment of spine deformities.

Investigations are under way in a number of centers to evaluate the energy requirements in the Milwaukee brace. Nash et al.[40] evaluated the pulmonary function of patients on initial presentation and after brace fittings. Initially, they found increased oxygen consumption and an increased respiratory rate. This improved in 19 per cent of patients after brace fitting and was unchanged in 43 per cent. In the remaining 38 per cent, a further increase in oxygen consumption and respiratory rate was noted. These changes did not correlate with the curve magnitude and were static after six months of brace wearing. The initial results of Cochran and Garrett,[17] in a similar study, indicate somewhat higher energy requirements in a patient while wearing the brace as compared to the same exercise without the brace. This increase is at an acceptable level with current brace design, providing the fit is adequate.

## FITTING AND APPLICATION

### Correct Milwaukee Brace Fit (Figs. 15–16, 15–17, 15–18)

When the brace has been fabricated, it is fitted to the patient and adjustments made. The pelvic section fits snugly over the pelvis, with the indentation above the iliac crest and without any pressure on the crest or anterior or posterior iliac spines. The fit should be comfortable, with a two to four centimeter gap between the two halves of the pelvic sec-

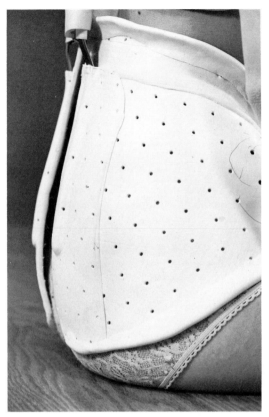

**Figure 15–31** Correct length of pelvic section posteriorly. While sitting on a firm chair or bench, the brace should clear the seat by 1–2 cm.

usually 30 degrees. The neck ring is positioned so that the head is directly above the torso, with the ear over the center of the shoulders and greater trochanter. The throat mold is fitted below the floor of the mouth within the rami of the mandible, so that it is located two centimeters below the mandible at rest and one centimeter anterior to the larynx (Fig. 15–32). The occipital pads are fitted below the occiput and should never push the head forward. In kyphotic deformities, these pads are fitted slightly lower than for scoliosis. Occipital pads assist in better positioning of the head.

The positioning of the corrective pads is important for maximal control and correction of the deformity (see Figs. 15–16 and 15–17). The pad placement is determined clinically and may be verified once the initial standing

tion posteriorly. When sitting on a firm chair, the posterior portion of the pelvic section should clear the chair by two centimeters (Fig. 15–31). Anteriorly over the thighs, full hip flexion to 100 degrees is allowed, and no pressure on the thighs in the sitting position should be present. When the pelvic portion is too long anteriorly or posteriorly, the brace is forced upward against the mandible in sitting. When this occurs, the brace should not be shortened, but rather the pelvic portion should be trimmed. Note that a properly designed Milwaukee brace cannot stand upright by itself.

The posterior uprights are parallel and vertical and should be close to but not applying pressure to the thorax (see Figs. 15–16 and 15–17). The anterior upright is positioned just far enough from the thorax to permit full chest expansion on inspiration but need not be any farther away. The neck ring is angled, being higher posteriorly, but may vary depending on individual anatomy. The angle is

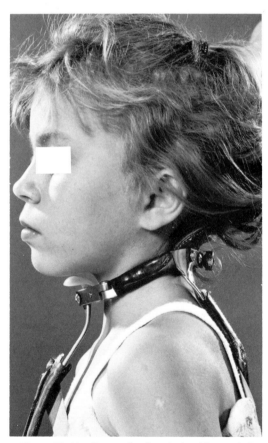

**Figure 15–32** Correct fit of neck ring. The neck ring slopes upward posteriorly; the molded plastic throat piece fits closely to the neck and is within the rami of the mandible and 1–2 centimeters below the soft tissue of the floor of the mouth. The occipital pads fit under the occiput and lie just below the skull.

x-ray is taken in the brace. Some of the pads are visible on the radiograph, and the position of others is indicated by holding screws or radio-opaque markers incorporated in the pad. The lumbar pad is fitted between the twelfth rib and iliac crest, so that pressure is exerted through the lateral part of the paraspinal muscles. The thoracic pad is centered on the rib that goes to the apex of the thoracic curve and is positioned just under or a little lateral to the posterior upright, over the thoracic prominence.

If the thoracic rounding is in the upper range of normal (normal being 20 to 40 degrees) or above, the vertebral margin of the thoracic pad is placed *under* the posterior upright and the anterior outrigger is relatively long. This positioning gives a significant anterior component of the force vector exerted by the pad. If the thoracic rounding, on the other hand, is in the lower range of normal or there is thoracic lordosis, it is necessary to minimize the anterior component by placing the pad lateral to the posterior upright and shortening the anterior outrigger. The amount of rotational prominence is also considered when determining pad placement. The upper part of the thoracic pad overlies the lower end of the scapula. The kyphosis pads are applied just below the apex of the kyphosis (see Fig. 15–20).

The positioning of the other pads is verified on clinical grounds. The axillary sling should be comfortably positioned in the axilla, with an upward and medial vector. This pull should not be so excessive as to raise the shoulder, and the medial pull should be sufficient to counteract the force of the thoracic pad and keep the head centered in the neck ring. The trapezius pad and shoulder ring are fitted as discussed on page 377.

## APPLICATION

In the majority of cases there is no need for a period of "weaning" into the brace. The brace is applied to the patient and the fit checked by the physician, who evaluates the pelvic section, uprights, neck ring, and pads, using the criteria described earlier. Once these initial adjustments have been made, the brace is worn "full-time" — that is, 23 out of

every 24 hours. Only in very young children and in patients with disturbed or absent skin sensation is a gradual program of brace application necessary.

The brace is always worn over a T-shirt, body stocking, or piece of tubular stockinette, the material being preferably seamless. No wrinkles should be present in the material when fitted, as this causes areas of increased skin pressure. When removed for the hour each day, the plastic of the pelvic section should be washed and thoroughly dried. The skin is checked for areas of excess pressure, which usually appear over the bony prominences. The skin areas over the iliac crests and under the pads are usually red immediately upon removal of the brace, but this should disappear rapidly. The skin in these areas is gradually toughened by the use of the brace. Ointments and lotions should never be used to treat the skin.

Once the brace is fitted and all initial adjustments made, return clinic visits are made every three to four months. In addition to checking the progress of the correction with an upright radiograph, constant adjustments in brace height and pad position and placement are necessary to correct for growth and curve improvement.

## EXERCISES

An integral part of any good brace program is played by activity and exercises. All sports and activities can be performed in the brace, with only three exceptions: 1) Contact sports, i.e., football and hockey; 2) gymnastics — trampolining and tumbling; 3) water skiing and swimming. Swimming is the only sport allowed out of the brace. This is a good exercise for general muscle toning and spine muscles, because of the absence of gravity in the water. One to two hours daily is allowed out of the brace specifically for swimming.

In addition, specific therapeutic exercises are used. These exercises are designed to maintain muscle tone and help to correct the deformity. Full details of the exercise programs for scoliosis and kyphosis have been described in The Milwaukee Brace by Blount and Moe[5] and will not be repeated here.

## WEANING

Weaning *from* the brace causes more problems for the physician and patient than does application of the brace. Guidelines have been published by Winter and Moe[57] regarding when to start weaning, at what rate to wean, and when to end weaning. The data are constantly changing as our knowledge of brace treatment increases.

At the present time, we feel that most patients are removed from the brace too early, because the physician yields to the natural desire to be a "good guy." This is usually a disservice to the patient.

Generally, the patient should be kept in the brace full-time until the ring apophyses have fused to the vertebral bodies in the area of the scoliosis. Patients who have been in the brace for at least two years and who show stable correction can sometimes be weaned earlier; the program may be individualized according to the patient's correction and stability (see below).

Weaning progresses in regular small increments, increasing the time out of the brace as stability is shown. An x-ray is taken after two hours out of the brace. If no significant loss of correction has occurred, two hours out of the brace is permitted. Three months later, an x-ray is taken after four hours out of the brace. If no significant loss of correction occurs (up to 3 degrees), four hours each day is allowed out of the brace. The physician should not permit additional time out of the brace unless it has been demonstrated that no loss of correction occurs during that period out of the brace ("stability test").

The weaning program is continued at three-month intervals, advancing to eight, and then twelve hours out of the brace. The final step is wearing the brace at night only. This night wear is generally well-tolerated by the patient and should be continued for a minimum of one year. The average weaning program is summarized in Table 15–1.

In Scheuermann's disease, a more rapid weaning program is sometimes possible and is outlined in Chapter 14, page 348.

The schedule described may seem overly strict, but practical experience has shown that this is necessary. In patients properly selected for nonoperative treatment, early weaning and uncooperative wearing have been the prime causes of failure.

**TABLE 15–1    Recommended Wearing Program**

| Full time | Generally until ring apophyses fuse* | |
|---|---|---|
| 2 hr/day out | 3 months | |
| 4 hr/day out | 3 months | |
| 8 hr/day out | 3 months | 2 years |
| 12 hr/day out | 3 months | |
| Nights only | 12 months | |

*With complete exclusion of iliac epiphysis, at least two years of brace wearing, and stability of correction, weaning probram can be initiated earlier.

## INDICATIONS AND CONTRAINDICATIONS

The general indication for brace application is a flexible curve in a growing child. The main purpose of the brace is to prevent progression of the curve; a secondary purpose is to gain improvement of the curve. A patient has to be actively growing to benefit from brace treatment—once growth has been completed, with closure of vertebral ring apophyses, a brace is ineffective.

The use of braces in scoliosis varies, depending on numerous factors, including etiology of deformity, age of child, maturity of child, magnitude of deformity, and flexibility of curve. Use of braces is discussed fully in other chapters in relation to specific conditions.

There are only a *few* absolute contraindications to bracing: 1) congenital scoliosis due to a unilateral unsegmented bar; 2) congenital kyphosis; 3) classic neurofibromatosis; 4) myelomeningocele kyphosis of the acute angular type; 5) thoracic lordosis; and 6) large scoliotic curves (over 45 degrees) in the adolescent patient.

In addition to the factors just named, successful brace use requires 1) a cooperative patient with supportive and encouraging parents. Children from nonstable home environments generally do poorly; 2) an orthotist with training and experience in the fabrication and fitting of braces; and 3) a treating orthopedist who is interested, enthusiastic, and knowledgeable about brace use.

## COMPLICATIONS

Complications of brace therapy are unusual. The most common problem is psychological.[3, 37, 41] Very positive attitudes of the orthopedic surgeon, therapist, and orthotist are necessary. The family, physician, and ancillary help must be supportive to the child in this time of stress. When the brace is rejected by the patient for psychological reasons, its use is discontinued. In some cases, a cast is used temporarily in the hope that this treatment will be accepted by the patient. The patient often rejects or refuses to undergo this treatment as well, in which case the curve is watched carefully. For progressive curves, surgery is performed. If the brace was applied to a curve that is borderline for surgery initially, surgery is performed when the brace is rejected.

The next most common complication is pressure sores. These are usually due to poor brace construction or fit. Local care of the sore alone will be unsuccessful without brace adjustment or modifications.

Skin irritation can occur under the pelvic section or pads and may be due to excess perspiration or allergy. Some patients perspire excessively; excess perspiration also occurs in very hot and humid climates. Perspiration can result in skin irritation, and this can be reduced with daily cleaning of the plastic. The moisture problem can be reduced with repeated changing of the underclothing, perforation of the plastic girdle, or use of astringents. If the skin irritation persists, removal of the brace for a day or two will usually clear the skin eruption. True allergy to the plastic or leather can occur. If true allergy exists, lining of the girdle with one of the synthetic foams—Alimed, Pelite, or Plastazote—or with moleskin or changing of the girdle material (plastic to leather) will usually cure the allergy.

A more common problem is numbness of the front of the thigh. This is due to pressure on the anterior femoral cutaneous nerve. Adequate relief in the region of the anterior superior iliac spine will relieve pressure on this nerve.

Dental deformities were the most common complication seen with the old Milwaukee brace using the chin rest. The forces on the mandible caused shortening of the lower third of the face, depression of the premolars and molars, and deflection of the maxillary anterior teeth.[1, 15, 28, 30, 42] The development of the throat mold, which removes all pressure from the mandible, occurred at the same time that lowering of the chin rest was initiated. This new mold prevents excessive mandibular pressure and has made dental changes and deformities a thing of the past as long as the brace is properly fabricated and applied.

Other complications that have been seen (but these are rare) include vascular obstruction of the duodenum and brachial plexus palsy. The latter is due to pressure of the neck ring on the brachial plexus and neuropraxia of the upper trunk. This condition usually results from the patient's sleeping in a lateral position with poor pillow support or from absence of an axillary sling and disappears after the brace is adjusted or the sleeping position altered.

### References

1. Alexander, R. G.: The effects on tooth position and maxillofacial vertical growth during treatment of scoliosis with the Milwaukee brace. Am. J. Orthod., 52:161, 1966.
2. Andriacchi, T., Schultz, A., Belytschko, T., and DeWald, R.: Milwaukee brace correction of idiopathic scoliosis; A biomechanical analysis, presented at the annual meeting of the Orthopaedic Research Society, San Francisco, February, 1975. J. Bone Joint Surg., 57A:582, 1975.
3. Bengtsson, G., Fallstrom, K., Jansson, B., and Nachemson, A.: A psychological and psychiatric investigation of the adjustment of female scoliosis patients. Acta. Psychiatr. Scand. 50:50, 1974.
4. Blount, W. P.: Scoliosis and the Milwaukee brace. Bull. Hosp. Joint Dis., 19:152, 1958.
5. Blount, W. P., and Moe, J. H.: The Milwaukee Brace. Baltimore, The Williams and Wilkins Co., 1973.
6. Blount, W. P., Schmidt, A. C., Keever, D. D., and Leonard, E. T.: The Milwaukee brace in the operative treatment of scoliosis. J. Bone Joint Surg., 40A:511, 1958.
7. Blount, W. P.: Bracing for scoliosis. Orthotic Etcetera, B617-92, L617. p. 306, 1966.
8. Blount, W. P., Schmidt, A. C., and Bidwell, R. G.: Making the Milwaukee brace. J. Bone Joint Surg., 40A:523, 1958.
9. Blount, W. P.: Non-operative Treatment of Scoliosis. Symposium on the Spine, American Academy of Orthopaedic Surgeons, Cleveland, 1967. St. Louis, C. V. Mosby, Co., 1969, p. 188.
10. Blount, W. P., and Mellencamp, D.: Long-term results of idiopathic scoliosis treated with the Milwaukee brace. Clin. Orthop., 126:47, 1977.

11. Bonnett, C., Brown, J. C., Workman, A., and Tosoonian, R.: An easier way to make a Milwaukee brace. Orthop. Review, 5:47, 1976.

12. Bunch, W.: Orthodontic position treatment during orthopaedic treatment of scoliosis. Am. J. Orthod., 47:174, 1961.

13. Bunch, W.: The Milwaukee brace in paralytic scoliosis. Clin. Orthop., 110:63, 1975.

14. Bunnell, W. P., and MacEwen, G. D.: Use of orthoplast jacket in the non-operative treatment of scoliosis; presented at Annual Meeting of Scoliosis Research Society, Louisville, Kentucky, September, 1975. J. Bone Joint Surg., 58A:156, 1976.

15. Caldwell, P. B.: An evaluation of the modified Milwaukee brace. M.S.D. thesis, University of Baylor Dental College, 1972.

16. Carr, W., Moe, J. H., Winter, R. B., Lonstein, J. E., and Bradford, D. S.: Results of idiopathic scoliosis treated with the Milwaukee brace—interim report. In preparation.

17. Cochran, G. V. B., and Garrett, A.: Effects of the Milwaukee brace on energy consumption during physical activity of patients with idiopathic scoliosis. Orthopaedic Research and Educational Fund, Journal of Abstracts, December, 1975.

18. Cochran, G. V. B., and Waugh, T. R.: The external forces in correction of idiopathic scoliosis. In Proceedings of Scoliosis Research Society. J. Bone Joint Surg., 51A:201, 1969.

19. Cockrell, R., and Risser, J.: Plastic body jacket in the treatment of scoliosis. Exhibit at the Annual Meeting of the American Academy of Orthopaedic Surgeons, Las Vegas, Nevada, 1973.

20. Currier, G. G.: Dentofacial changes in scoliosis patients treated with the new Milwaukee brace. M.S.D. thesis, The University of Washington, 1971.

21. Edmonson, A. S., and Morris, J. T.: Follow-up study of Milwaukee brace treatment in patients with idiopathic scoliosis. Clin. Orthop., 126:58, 1977.

22. Galante, J., Schultz, A., DeWald, R. L., and Ray, R. D.: Forces acting in the Milwaukee brace on patients undergoing treatment for idiopathic scoliosis. J. Bone Joint Surg., 52A:498, 1970.

23. Hall, J. H., Miller, M. E., Shumann, W., and Stanish, W.: A refined concept in the orthotic management of scoliosis. Orthotics and Prosthetics, 29:7, 1975.

24. Hardy, J. H., and Dennis, M.: An evaluation of Milwaukee brace failures. Presented at the Annual Meeting of the Scoliosis Research Society, Wilmington, Delaware, September, 1972. J. Bone Joint Surg., 55A:439, 1973.

25. Hessing, F., and Hasslauer, L.: Orthopadische Therapie. Berlin, Urban and Schwarzenburg, 1903.

26. Hippocrates: On the Articulation. In Adams, F. (trans.): The Genuine Works of Hippocrates, vol. 2. London, Sudenham Society, 1849.

27. Hoffa, A.: Lehrbuch der Orthopadischen Cirurgie. Stuttgart, Verlag von Ferdinant Enke, 1898.

28. Howard, C. C.: A preliminary report of infraocclusion of the molars and premolars produced by orthopaedic treatment of scoliosis. Int. J. Orthod., 12:434, 1926.

29. Levine, D.: Results of underarm brace treatment of idiopathic scoliosis. Paper presented at American Academy of Orthopaedic Surgeons, course on Scoliosis. Indianapolis, Indiana, May 4, 1976.

30. Logan, W. R.: The effect of the Milwaukee brace on the developing dentition. Dent. Practice, 12:447, 1962.

31. Lonsdale, E. F.: Observation on the Treatment of Lateral Curvature of the Spine. London, J. Churchill, 1847.

32. Michel, C. R.: Lyon non-operative treatment. Paper presented to the Scoliosis Research Society and the Groupe d'etude de la Scoliose. Lyon, France, 25 September, 1973.

33. Moe, J. H.: The Milwaukee brace in the treatment of scoliosis. Clin. Orthop., 77:18, 1971.

34. Moe, J. H., and Kettleson, D. N.: Analysis of curve pattern and preliminary results of Milwaukee brace treatment in 169 patients. J. Bone Joint Surg., 52A:1509, 1970.

35. Mulcahy, T., Galante, J., DeWald, R., Schultz, A., and Hunter, J. C.: A follow-up study of forces acting on the Milwaukee brace on patients undergoing treatment for idiopathic scoliosis. Clin. Orthop., 93:53, 1973.

36. Murphy, J.: The Lexan jacket in the conservative treatment of scoliosis—a comparison of results obtained with the Milwaukee brace. Presented at the Annual Meeting of the Western Orthopaedic Association, Honolulu, Hawaii, October, 1974. J. Bone Joint Surg., 57A:136, 1975.

37. Myers, B. A., Friedman, S. B., and Weiner, I. B.: Coping with a chronic disability: Psychosocial observations of girls with scoliosis treated with a Milwaukee brace. Am. J. Dis. Child., 120:175, 1970.

38. Nachemson, A., and Elfstrom, G.: Intravital wireless telemetry of axial forces in Harrington distraction rods in patients with idiopathic scoliosis. J. Bone Joint Surg., 53A:445, 1971.

39. Nachemson, A., and Morris, J. M.: In vivo measurements of intradiscal pressure. J. Bone Joint Surg., 46A:1077, 1964.

40. Nash, C. L., Vega, G. E., and Brown, R.: Oxygen consumption studies in idiopathic scoliosis patients undergoing Milwaukee brace treatment. Presented at the Annual Meeting of the Scoliosis Research Society, Wilmington, Delaware, September, 1972. J. Bone Joint Surg., 55A:439, 1973.

41. Neff, J., Feminine identity concerns of girls undergoing correction of scoliosis. Maternal Child Nursing Journal, 1:9, 1972.

42. Northway, R. O., Alexander, R. G., and Riolo, M. L.: A cephalometric evaluation of the old Milwaukee brace and the modified Milwaukee brace in relation to the normal growing child. Am. J. Orthod., 65:341, 1974.

43. Ollier, M.: Technique des platres et Corsets de Scolioses. In Corset Lyonnais, p. 87, Masson et Cie, 1971.

44. Pare, A.: Opera Ambrosii Parie. Paris, Afud Jocabum Du-Puys, 1582.

45. Persky, S. L., and Johnson, L. E.: An evaluation of dentofacial changes accompanying scoliosis therapy with a modified Milwaukee brace. Am. J. Orthod., 65:364, 1974.

46. Ponte, A.: A brace for the non-operative treatment of lumbar and thoraco-lumbar curves. Presented at the Annual Meeting of the Scoliosis Research Society, San Francisco, September, 1974.

47. Risser, J. C.: The application of body casts for the correction of scoliosis. Am. Acad. Orthop. Surgeons, Lect., 12:255, 1955.

48. Risser, J. C., Lauder, C. H., Norquist, D. M., and Craig, W. A.: Three types of body casts. Am. Acad. Orthop. Surgeons, Lect., *10*:131, 1953.

49. Risser, J. C.: Treatment of scoliosis during the past 50 years. Clin. Orthop., *44*:109, 1966.

50. Sayre, L. A.: Spinal Disease and Spinal Curvature. London, Smith-Elder & Company, 1877.

51. Schraudebach, T., Rossler, H., and Dennert, R.: Erfahrungen Mit Dem Milwaukee-Korsett Im Rahmen Einer Skolioseambulanz. Z. Orthop., *112*:1265, 1974.

52. Schultz, A. B., and Galante, J. O., Measurement of forces exerted in the correction of idiopathic scoliosis using three-component dynamometers. Experimental mechanics, 9:419, 1969.

53. Shufflebarger, H. L., and Keiser, R. P.: Milwaukee brace treatment of idiopathic scoliosis: A review of one hundred and twenty-three completed cases. Clin. Orthop., *118*:19, 1976.

54. Spitzy, H.: Scoliosis. *In* Lange, Fritz: Lehrbuch der Orthopadie. Jena, G. Fixcher, 1928.

55. Stagnara, P.: Lyon non-operative treatment. Paper presented to the Scoliosis Research Society and the Groupe d'etude de la Scoliose. Lyon, France, 25 September, 1973.

56. Waters, R. L., and Morris, J. M.: Effect of the spinal support on the electrical activity of muscles of the trunk. J. Bone Joint Surg., *52A*:51, 1970.

57. Winter, R. B., and Moe, J. H.: Orthotics for spinal deformity. Clin. Orthop., *102*:72, 1974.

58. Winter, R. B., Levine, D. B., Edmonson, A., Mullen, M., Tupper, J., and Gilespie, R.: Preliminary results—a field test of the Boston prefabricated Milwaukee brace pelvic section. Presented at the Annual Meeting of the Scoliosis Research Society, Louisville, Kentucky, September, 1975. J. Bone Joint Surg., *58A*:156, 1976.

59. Wüllstein, L., and Schulthess, W.: Die Skoliose in inrer Behandlung und Entstchung Nach Klinishen und Experimentellen Studien. Z. Orthop. Clin., *10*:178, 1902.

# Chapter 16

# COMPLICATIONS OF TREATMENT

Corrective spine surgery is a major undertaking, and some of the techniques used are the most complex in orthopedics. Complications are inherent in this as in all types of surgery. A thorough knowledge of the occurrence of complications and their recognition and prevention is essential for the care of the scoliotic patient. Complications are classified as those related to nonoperative therapy and those related to operative therapy. The latter group is divided into intraoperative and postoperative groups and the latter subdivided into immediately postoperative (early) and occurring late.

## NONOPERATIVE PROBLEMS

### Traction

With the use of traction for correction of rigid deformities there are complications due to the traction device (halo, femoral pins, pelvic pins) and those occurring as a result of traction (neurologic, pressure sores).

#### HALO

**Infected Pins.** This is the most common problem found with the use of the halo.[27, 28] The skin surrounding the halo pin becomes infected, with resultant edema, erythema, drainage, and tenderness. The drainage increases with extension of the infection. The infection can spread to the underlying skull, with osteitis and osteomyelitis.[48] With the resorption of bone that occurs from the infection, the halo pins become loosened, and if continually tightened, skull penetration can occur. The infection can extend intracranially and a subdural or even intracerebral abscess may result.[47]

Prevention of pin site infection depends on daily pin care. This is performed by the nurses at least twice daily, and if the patient is discharged in a halo cast, the parents must be adequately instructed in pin site care. The hair around the site of scalp penetration is cut short to allow visualization of the pin-scalp junction. This area is thoroughly cleaned with alcohol or peroxide solution, removing all crusting or exudate. An iodine-containing solution such as Betadine is then applied to the area. In addition, the entire scalp and hair are washed twice weekly, with more frequent washing in patients with oily scalps. With this daily care, pin loosening rarely occurs, and tightening of the pins is usually necessary the day after halo application only. A painful pin site indicates loosening or infection.

When the pin site becomes infected, the pin is removed and reinserted in an adjacent halo pin hole, using local anesthesia after thorough shampooing of the hair (see halo application, p. 265). Local care of the infection is usually sufficient. When the infection is more extensive, with marked cellulitis, systemic antibiotics are given after the drainage has been cultured.

If osteomyelitis is present as a result of an extensive infection, adequate debridement is necessary. With severe infection or continued drainage, symptoms of headache, visual changes, seizures, or drowsiness should alert one to the presence of intracranial spread with an intracranial (subdural or intracerebral) abscess. After removal of the halo pin, these abscesses are appropriately treated.

*Halo Slippage.* When properly applied below the maximal diameter of the skull, halo slippage is rare. When it does occur, reapplication of the halo is necessary. Slippage is more common when large distractive forces are being used or in uncooperative patients. It can be prevented by increasing the skull fixation through use of six or eight halo pins.

### FEMORAL PINS

*Pin Tract Infection.* With motion of the pin in the thigh, drainage is common and infection frequent. With the use of plaster of Paris to incorporate the femoral pins, the motion has been eliminated, and drainage and infection are now unusual. When these problems do occur, the pin is removed and the infection treated with local care. Because the infections are usually mild, they respond to such care. With more extensive involvement and systemic manifestations, appropriate systemic antibiotics are added.

*Pin Loosening.* Occasionally, with very osteoporotic bone or with poor insertion technique, the femoral pin may cut out of the bone. Pain with the distraction is present and the pin is not rigid in the bone. If doubt exists, a radiograph will confirm that the pin is not in the femur. The pin is removed and reinserted, care being taken to place it in the distal femoral diaphysis, not the metaphysis.

### HALOPELVIC TRACTION

Since the original description of the halopelvic apparatus,[7] numerous complications have been described with the use of this technique.[16, 28, 29, 32, 43, 44, 53]

*Lacerated Peritoneum or Bowel.* During insertion of the pelvic pin, it is possible for the peritoneum or large bowel to be traumatized when the pin enters the iliac fossa. This penetration, which can result in peritonitis, can be prevented by positioning the patient on the side for the pin insertion. With dissection

on the inner table of the iliac wing, the path of the pin is fully visualized. Penetration of the iliacus muscle, peritoneum, and/or bowel is then most unlikely.

*Infected Pelvic Pins.* The most common halopelvic problem reported by O'Brien[28, 29] was pin tract infection, occurring in 50 per cent of the reported series. Pelvic pin drainage is very common, but the drainage is usually sterile. When the drainage becomes profuse and purulent, gross infection is present. No true osteomyelitis of the ilium has been reported, but the infection has persisted in some cases, with a systemic infection occurring in one of our patients. With infection, the bone around the pelvic pin is resorbed, and loosening occurs.

The chance of infection can be lessened with meticulous pin site care after the incisions for the application have healed. Twice daily cleaning with alcohol or peroxide solution and application of an iodine solution (Betadine) will keep the pin sites clean. With increased drainage and infection, the patient's activities should be restricted and systemic antibiotics started. With rest and local care, the infection usually can be controlled. With persistent infection, removal of the pelvic pin is necessary, with change to a halo cast in cases where fixed distraction is still required.

*Pin Breakage.* The pelvic pin may break either within the crest or between the skin and pelvic hoop. In the latter case, readjustment of the hoop to maintain fixation to the two pelvic pins is necessary. Intrapelvic breakage has not been reported, but should it occur, consideration must be given to removal of the apparatus if the treatment is near completion. Otherwise the broken pin should be removed and a new one inserted.

*Osteoporosis.* The bony tissue between the halo and pelvis are rigidly immobilized by the halopelvic apparatus. Osteoporosis of these tissues is thus inevitable and is shown radiographically after prolonged distraction. This results in difficulty in firm seating of the instrumentation used in the subsequent spinal fusion. Reduction of the immobilization time to the minimum necessary will help to reduce osteoporosis.

*Cervical Spine.* Cervical spine problems have been found in a high percentage of patients undergoing halopelvic distraction. Changes occurred in 32 of 77 patients in O'Brien's series.[28, 29, 43, 44] The abnormal radiologic findings included: 1) Degenerative changes of the facet joints of the cervical spine.[44] The joint space became diminished with erosions and cystic lesions in the bone adjacent to the joint. These changes were seen in patients both in the apparatus and after removal. 2) Avascular necrosis of the proximal pole of the dens has been found and is probably due to interruption of the blood supply to this area via the apical and alar ligaments. These changes were evidenced by cystic areas and irregularity of contour of the proximal end of the dens and adjacent sclerosis.[43] 3) With prolonged strong distraction, a large amount of separation is found at the atlantoaxial joint. This chronic subluxation is found on followup using flexion extension radiographs. 4) With prolonged distraction the cervical spine is straightened, with loss of cervical lordosis, and in some cases true cervical kyphosis occurs. With the straightening of the cervical spine, radiographically the facet joints are seen to open posteriorly. 5) With rapid distraction, avulsion of the ring apophysis from the inferior surface of the second cervical vertebra has been described in one patient.

The factors related to these changes have been evaluated by Tredwell and O'Brien.[44] The older the patient being treated, the greater is the incidence of these changes; and the longer the period of immobilization, the greater the incidence of radiologic changes. With greater distractive forces approaching 60 per cent of body weight, cervical spine changes were more common. The important factors causing these changes are acute rapid distraction, excessive lengthening, and prolonged immobilization. These changes also occur in the apparatus without distraction. They are permanent and result in loss of range of motion. This was found in half of the patients one year after removal of the halopelvic apparatus.

Prevention of these cervical spine changes is usually possible by avoiding acute rapid distraction, excessive lengthening, and prolonged immobilization. Gardner et al.[11] reported on electronic measurement of forces in the halopelvic apparatus. Using this technique and a maximal distractive force of 40 to 50 per cent of body weight and a maximal traction time of two to three months, a series of patients are being investigated to see whether the incidence of cervical spine changes is reduced. In addition, routine cervical spine radiographs during the course of therapy would monitor some changes in the cervical spine, and some permanent sequelae may be prevented.

## NEUROLOGIC PROBLEMS

The most feared complication of distraction (halofemoral or halopelvic) is paralysis, which may be quadriplegia, paraplegia, or cranial or peripheral nerve loss.

*Paraplegia/Quadriplegia.* Quadriplegia or paraplegia can occur as a result of traction or surgery. It may be complete or partial, and flaccid at first and spastic later.

Spinal cord lesions have been reported with the use of both halofemoral and halopelvic distraction but are much more common with the latter.[23, 29, 30] The majority of reported cases occur when distraction is applied to a kyphotic deformity and especially when distraction is used postoperatively after fusion or a releasing procedure (osteotomy or wedge excision of rigid deformities). In a severe deformity, the spinal cord occupies the shortest route in the spinal canal, being situated along the concavity of the deformity. In kyphosis, it is thus stretched anteriorly against the vertebral bodies (Fig. 16–1).

The vascular anatomy of the spinal cord is very important in the pathogenesis of these lesions. Because of the high incidence of paraplegia following surgery for severe scoliosis in adults, Dommisse[8, 9] investigated the blood supply of the spinal cord and size of the spinal canal. He described a "critical vascular zone of the spinal cord" from approximately the fourth to the ninth vertebral segment. In this area the blood supply of the cord is poorest, with the fewest feeding vessels and cord perforators. In addition, the spinal canal is narrowest in this area. Breig[1] demonstrated that the spinal cord shortens and lengthens to accommodate changes in length of the spinal canal in flexion and extension of the spine. In the thoracic area there was the least amount of increase possible (1 centimeter), while the cervical spinal cord showed up to 2.8 centimeters increase in length. This increase occurred by unfolding the neurones in the cord and by the natural elasticity of tissues.

In severe kyphosis, the spinal cord is taut anteriorly over the vertebral bodies.[48] With the use of distraction such as halofemoral or halopelvic, the cord is in danger, as it lies parallel to the axis of the traction force. The cord becomes pulled even tighter against the vertebral body. Where there is less elasticity combined with a critical vascular supply (thoracic area), the blood supply becomes interrupted, with paraparesis or paraplegia resulting (see Fig. 16–1). A lesser lesion, such as bladder paralysis, can occur and must be recognized as due to the traction. A similar effect is seen during the use of the Harrington distraction rod intraoperatively with correction of scoliosis (see p. 403).

Prevention of paraplegia and quadriplegia is paramount. It is necessary to recognize "cords at risk" where possible vascular changes due to the deformity, rigid kyphosis, or diastematomyelia exist. In these cases distraction should *not* be used with kyphosis; distraction is safe only if there is flexibility. In cases where cord compression due to kyphosis is already present, distraction may increase the neurologic loss. Thus, if some flexibility of the kyphosis is present as shown on hyperextension x-ray, the correcting force should be hyperextension, *not distraction.*

Constant monitoring of neurologic function is necessary with patients in distraction. With loss of function—paresis or paralysis—immediate decrease or cessation of traction force is necessary for recovery to occur. This recovery will occur if the lesion is recognized and traction is promptly released. Delay may result in permanent paralysis.

***Cranial Nerve Lesions.*** Cranial nerve palsies can occur during the use of distraction. The most common of these is abducent palsy with loss of lateral gaze. This paralysis is often unilateral, but bilateral palsy has been reported.[23, 28, 41] Palsies of the lower cranial nerves can occur; namely, the tenth, eleventh, or twelfth, with weakness of tongue motion and difficulty with speech or swallowing and recurrent laryngeal nerve palsy with speech difficulties.[28] In addition, traction can affect the medulla with respiratory palsy and respiratory arrest. Cases of the latter are reported, and we have a case of rapid distraction during application of a cast in a patient with congenital scoliosis resulting in respiratory arrest. Immediate release of traction and removal of the cast resulted in return of spontaneous respiration.

Traction will cause elongation of a nerve with a vertical course. The lower three cranial nerves, after exiting from the brain stem, run upward to leave the skull via the jugular and hypoglossal foramina. The abducent nerve also runs upward, has a long intracranial course, and, like the three lowest cranial nerves, it passes over a bony prominence; the apex of the petrous temporal bone. With elongation of the nerve fibers the deformation obliterates the vessels, the venules being the first affected, as shown by Lundborg and Rydervik.[20] This results in an interruption of conduction with preservation of anatomical continuity, and has been termed neuropraxia by Seddon.[34] If complete loss of conduction

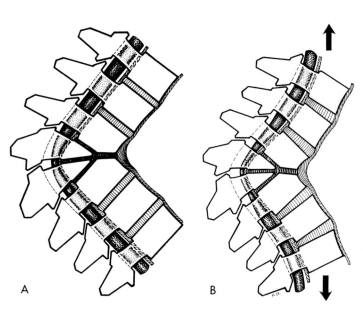

**Figure 16–1** The effects of traction on congenital kyphosis. A, Type I congenital kyphosis with two hemivertebrae at the apex of the deformity. Note that the spinal cord is tented over the apex of the kyphosis. B, Longitudinal traction is applied. The apical area is rigid, and no correction occurs. The spine adjacent to the apex lengthens, and the kyphosis improves. As the apical area is unchanged, the spinal cord is pulled against the apical bone with paralysis resulting.

occurs, paralysis is the result, but if the loss is partial, paresis occurs. The palsies are temporary, and recovery is rapid with release of distraction, but complete recovery may take up to one year, as in one case described by O'Brien.[28]

***Brachial Plexus Lesions.*** Traction can also result in neuropraxia of cervical plexus roots, the ones commonly affected being the cervical fifth and sixth roots and the first thoracic nerve root. The lesions occur singly or in combination, the upper roots being involved due to their nearly vertical course. The first thoracic nerve is thought to be involved where it crosses the first rib, the distraction pulling the nerve against the rib.

The pathogenesis is similar to that described with the cranial nerves, i.e., a vascular compression due to elongation in nearly vertical nerves. Seddon[34] has shown that the nerve fibers are affected in order of their size, motor fibers being thus affected first. Clinically, motor weakness is common, and sensory loss is minimal. With immediate release of traction, recovery is usually rapid and complete.

***Prevention.*** Prevention of nerve or cord "stretch" is by recognition of high risk cases, such as rigid kyphosis or curvatures. In addition, excessive traction can be monitored with sequential cervical spine radiographs, especially with the use of the halopelvic apparatus. Neurologic complications of traction can be prevented by careful daily neurologic examination. All patients must have an evaluation of cranial nerves, brachial plexus, and spinal cord function. Lateral eye motion is tested as well as tongue motion, speech, and swallowing. Upper extremity motion must be tested completely on both sides. Toe motion is tested. All of the above is done daily by the physician and three times a day by the nursing staff. An occasional early symptom is burning in the upper or lower extremity, which is followed soon afterward by paresis. When present, a complete neurologic examination is essential. Another early sign is bladder paralysis. This can be difficult to diagnose in a patient kept supine, as positional difficulty in voiding can occur. Normally, inability to void due to position is accompanied by a sensation of bladder distention. With bladder paresis, a loss of the sensation of bladder distention occurs, and the muscle paralysis allows overdistention.

Whenever neurologic loss occurs, the traction is reduced or discontinued. With early detection of this complication and prompt decrease of the distraction, return of function is usually rapid and complete.

## PRESSURE SORES

As has been well shown in large spinal cord injury units, this formerly common problem can be prevented. A patient in bed in traction has decreased mobility. A large number of these patients have decreased skin sensibility. With prolonged, constant pressure on the skin over bony prominences such as the sacrum or scapulae, skin circulation is decreased and skin breakdown occurs. Constant attention to the skin is necessary to prevent pressure sores. The patient is placed on a foam mattress with a central cut-out area to hold a pressure relieving pad. The patient is turned every two hours, day and night, being positioned sequentially supine and on both sides. The skin is inspected for areas of redness, which are the first signs of increased pressure. These areas are massaged to restore skin circulation and watched carefully. If skin breakdown is imminent, the pressure is further decreased with the use of a foam donut. Pads placed directly over a prominence only increase the pressure on that prominence.

## THROMBOPHLEBITIS[42]

With the increase in the number of complex adult spine deformities being treated, the incidence of thrombophlebitis has increased also. It can occur either preoperatively or postoperatively. Thrombophlebitis may present with the classical signs of fever, pain, and muscle tenderness, or the first sign may be a pulmonary embolus (Fig. 16–2). Prevention of this complication is by maintaining venous flow in the lower extremities. Antiembolic stockings are worn by all patients and regular leg exercises encouraged. Aspirin or other antithrombotic medication is used in most adults. The best prevention is to minimize the use of traction and to decrease the time patients spend in bed by careful selection of candidates for halofemoral traction and by the use of early ambulation postoperatively. The Cotrel hip traction straps may be used in place of femoral pins, and foot, knee, and hip motion is stressed. Casts extending to the legs should be avoided if at all possible.

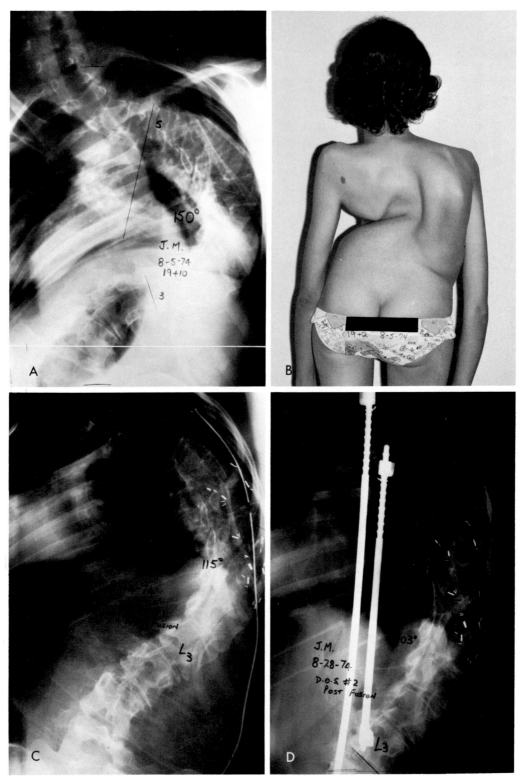

**Figure 16–2**   *See opposite page for legend.*

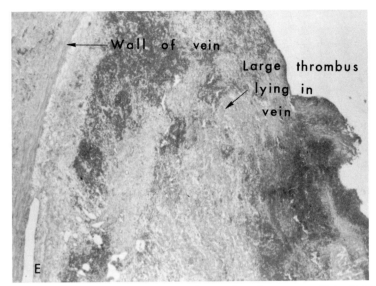

**Figure 16–2** *A,* J.M. presented at the age of 19 years and 2 months with an untreated infantile idiopathic scoliosis. An anteroposterior spine x-ray shows a 150 degree right thoracic scoliosis. *B,* Clinical photograph on presentation shows the severe right thoracic curve with a marked deformity. *C,* Treatment consisted of halofemoral traction for one week followed by an anterior disc excision. This anteroposterior x-ray on the day of the anterior fusion shows the areas of osteotomy and reduction of the curve to 115 degrees. *D,* Two weeks of halofemoral traction was followed by a posterior releasing procedure with insertion of distraction rods. This x-ray shows the two rods in place with slight additional correction to 103 degrees. *E,* An additional two weeks of traction was used to further correct the curve. A spinal fusion was planned, but on the morning of that day the patient suddenly died. An autopsy showed pelvic vein thrombosis and pulmonary embolism. This photomicrograph shows a hypogastric vein with a large intraluminar thrombus.

## Cast

### PRESSURE SORES (Fig. 16–3)

The most common cast complication is a pressure sore. Any constant excessive pressure by the cast on a localized area, especially over bony prominences, results initially in erythema with pain. With continued pressure the circulation to the skin is impaired, and breakdown occurs; at this time pain decreases, as the sensory nerve endings are also ischemic. The pressure sore starts as a

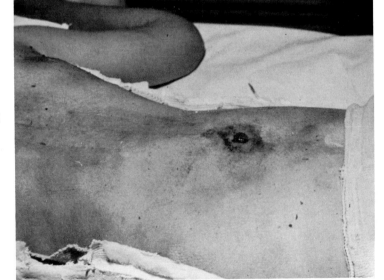

**Figure 16–3** Pressure sore found under a cast.

superficial partial skin defect, which extends deeper to the subcutaneous tissue and the underlying muscle or bone. The area becomes infected superficially, and there is a serous or purulent discharge. This drainage and associated malodor are often the first signs of a pressure sore in the anesthetic patient. The common sites are over bony prominences — sacrum, iliac spines, scapula, clavicles, or due to a sharp edge or irregular area of the cast.

With careful attention to details in cast application, the incidence of pressure sores can be radically reduced. All bony prominences in very thin patients are adequately padded. The padding is ineffective if placed over the prominences, as pressure is still present over the apex or edge of the bone. The central area of the felt padding must be removed by excision or relieved by cutting it radially, and the center of the felt pad is placed over the bone prominence. Felt padding is applied on either side of the sacrum in thin patients. With cast application, a smooth well-fitting plaster is applied, with no pressure placed over prominences. In this way the pressure of the cast is distributed over a large area and not localized. The edges of the cast must all be skived and all loose plaster removed, leaving a smooth gentle edge.

In the first few days after a cast is applied, all skin under the cast should be inspected frequently for erythematous or tender areas. The plaster in these areas is relieved at once, and if necessary, a felt pad is added. The pad must *not* be placed over the bony prominences but on the sides or around it. In cases with a sharp kyphosis or rib prominence the cast must be windowed over the prominence for skin inspection. This skin inspection is performed by the family after the patient is discharged from the hospital.

When a pressure area develops, the cast must be windowed widely over the area of skin breakdown. This window is left out, and support is provided on the sides of the deformity. This is treated with local care; debridement when necessary, cleansing with Zephiran, alcohol, or peroxide, and dressing with an iodine solution (Betadine) and a sterile gauze pad. With relief of pressure exerted by the cast and local care, the pressure sore usually heals without difficulty. Vigilance will prevent pressure sores. Any suggestion of pressure (either pain or redness) must be evaluated carefully and treated rapidly. The common sites of pressure are just under the edge of the cast, over the sacrum, and over the rib hump. These areas must be adequately undercut during cast application and the undercutting extended if redness ensues.

## FEMORAL CUTANEOUS NERVE IRRITATION

Occasionally the cast causes compression of the femoral cutaneous nerve, with resultant paresthesia or anesthesia of the anterior thigh. Compression is relieved by skiving the cast over the anterior superior iliac spine to provide adequate room for the nerve.

## VASCULAR COMPRESSION OF DUODENUM[10, 12, 15, 35, 37]

Vascular compression of the duodenum ("cast syndrome") is an obstruction of the third part of the duodenum by the superior mesenteric artery. It has been reported in patients with scoliosis, multiple trauma, burns, or conditions requiring application of body casts or spica casts. In scoliosis, the syndrome occurs in cases with correction of the curve by a cast, Harrington instrumentation, Milwaukee brace, or traction. As a result of correction of the curve, the angle between the superior mesenteric artery and aorta is narrowed. The third part of the duodenum, which lies in the angle, is pinched and compressed, and obstruction results (Fig. 16–4A).

The syndrome presents as a high intestinal obstruction with nausea and vomiting. There is minimal bowel distention, since the obstruction is high, but epigastric fullness may develop as the stomach distends. The abdomen is soft, with tenderness in the epigastrium to deep palpation. Bowel sounds are usually normal, and flatus and stools are still passed. The diagnosis may be difficult in the postoperative period after spine fusion and Harrington instrumentation, because there may be nausea and vomiting due to analgesics and distention due to ileus or aerophagia. Enlargement of the stomach accentuates the downward pressure on the duodenum. Prolonged vomiting will result in dehydration and hypovolemia, and loss of electrolytes causes hypokalemic alkalosis. If untreated, shock, oliguria, gastric rupture, and death can occur.

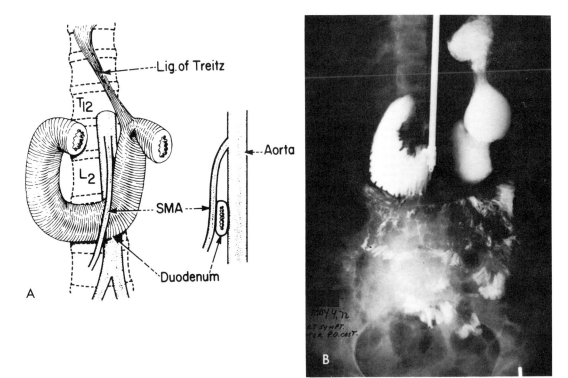

**Figure 16–4** Vascular compression of the duodenum. *A*, Diagrammatic representation of the third part of the duodenum to show the site of the duodenal compression. The third part of the duodenum passes between the superior mesenteric artery (SMA) anteriorly and the aorta and vertebral column posteriorly. Any reduction of the angle between the SMA and aorta will compress the duodenum. (From Skandalakis, J. E., et al., Contemp. Surg., *10*:33, 1977, with permission.) *B*, C. W., a 16-year-old girl with idiopathic scoliosis and a 60 degree right thoracic curve. In a preoperative cast this was corrected to 19 degrees, and on the day of surgery the correction was 20 degrees. One week later a postoperative cast was applied, and she was ambulated. A day later she presented with nausea and vomiting. A Gastrografin swallow showed obstruction of the third part of the duodenum. The cast was removed and the patient kept supine with nasogastric suction to decompress the stomach. The obstruction resolved with this therapy, and a second postoperative cast was applied without recurrence of the obstruction.

Early diagnosis and management of vascular compression of the duodenum is essential. Initial general measures include oral intake restriction, nasogastric suction, and administration of intravenous fluids. Fluid intake and output must be carefully monitored and serial electrolyte level measurements performed. Specific measures consist of positioning the patient in the left lateral position and with the foot of the bed raised. This position occasionally relieves symptoms, but if the problem persists, removal of the cast, traction, or brace becomes necessary. Simply windowing the cast over the abdomen is ineffective. Usually with these techniques the obstruction spontaneously regresses after 48 to 72 hours of nasogastric suction. Careful restarting of oral fluids, followed by soft solids and then a regular diet can be given. Delay in diagnosis and treatment leads to an intractable obstruction requiring surgery. Occasionally an obstruction does not improve with adequate early nonoperative means, but the need for surgery has been markedly reduced by prompt recognition and early treatment.

Radiographic studies confirm the diagnosis. A plain film of the abdomen may show major gastric and duodenal distention with little gas in the remainder of the bowel. Contrast studies using Gastrografin demonstrate the obstruction of the third part of the duodenum, with delay in gastric emptying. The proximal duodenum is dilated and usually shows increased peristaltic activity or reverse peristalsis (Fig. 16–4*B*). A six-hour followup study may show that some contrast medium has passed, indicating partial obstruction. If surgery is necessary, a side-to-side duodenojejunostomy is performed. Other techniques to relieve the obstruction, such as release of the ligament of Treitz or gastrojejunostomy, have been found to be less effective.

The most effective treatment for vascular obstruction of the duodenum is early prompt recognition and adequate nonoperative therapy. In this way the general metabolic effects of the obstruction and vomiting will be reduced and the need for surgical intervention decreased.

### Braces

Problems related to the use of braces, especially the Milwaukee brace, have been fully discussed in Chapter 15. These complications include: psychologic problems, pressure sores, skin irritation, dental deformities, and vascular compression of the duodenum.

## OPERATIVE COMPLICATIONS

### Intraoperative Complications

#### CARDIAC ARREST

Cardiac arrest occurs intraoperatively due to anoxia, blood replacement problems, or air embolism. Anoxia is the most frequent cause of cardiac arrest. An adequate endotracheal airway must be present, with adequate ventilation of both lungs. Insertion of the endotracheal tube too deeply will cause it to enter the right mainstem bronchus. Before turning the patient, the anesthesiologist must ensure that the aeration of the lungs is equal and adequate. The airway must be securely fastened, so that it will not come out when the patient is prone. A patent airway must be maintained throughout the procedure, with the use of suctioning to remove excess secretions or mucous plugs that can obstruct the endotracheal tube.

Scoliosis surgery, if not done with great care, can result in a substantial blood loss. Occasionally, even with careful technique the loss may be significant. In our experience this problem occurs more frequently in patients with paralytic scoliosis or those who have been in a Milwaukee brace for nonoperative therapy preoperatively. Trauma to the intercostal artery during posterior fusion, to the gluteal artery during bone graft removal, or the iliac vessels during anterior lumbar approach will result in rapid excessive blood loss. The loss must be minimized by careful technique and must be accurately measured by weighing all sponges and calculating suction drainage. Blood replacement must be neither inadequate nor excessive. Inadequate replacement leads to hypovolemia, shock, cardiac arrest, or cerebral ischemia. Excessive transfusion will raise the central venous pressure, resulting in cardiac decompensation, acute pulmonary edema, and cardiac arrest. Volume replacement is very critical in children and in patients who are below normal size for their age (those with paralytic diseases and multiple congenital anomalies). The blood volume of the patient should be calculated using body weight.

When blood loss is approximately 10 per cent of circulating volume, a transfusion should be started. With loss of greater than 80 per cent of blood volume, replacement becomes less accurate, and all hemostatic elements are markedly depleted. With large volumes of transfusion, the serum potassium level rises due to the high level of potassium in stored blood, and this hyperkalemia can cause cardiac arrest. The cardiac effect can be diminished with calcium chloride injections, which reduce cardiac sensitivity. Another problem with old stored blood is the transfusion of microemboli, which can result in a "shock lung syndrome."[2, 4] To prevent these emboli from reaching the circulation, micropore filters[4, 38] are used to clear the blood. The filters should be changed when large volumes of blood replacement are necessary. In addition, the blood needs to be warmed, as rapid administration of large volumes of cold blood can result in hypothermia, cardiac cooling, and cardiac arrest.

A rare cause of cardiac arrest is air embolism.[5] Air can enter the circulation through the intravenous line if the blood storage container or fluid bottle becomes empty without a control filter. This situation is especially likely to occur if the blood is being transfused under pressure. A rare route of entry of the air is through the exposed decorticated bone, especially with large venous channels. The air enters the circulation during expiration, when the interosseous intravascular pressure falls; there is also a fall during the "wake up test" if the patient becomes very light. Vigilance in watching the blood administration system is necessary, as is the maintenance of positive pressure with expiration.

When an intraoperative cardiac arrest

occurs, the incision is rapidly packed with gauze sponges and closed using towel clips. The patient is then turned over, and resuscitative measures are carried out. When resuscitation is complete, the wound can be irrigated and sutured with the patient on the side.

## SPINAL CORD INJURY

This complication may result from direct injury to the spinal cord or from excessive traction on the cord. During decortication, a gouge may slip and injure the spinal cord or tear the dura. Direct injury can also occur during anterior fusion, disc excision, or cord decompression. In cases where there are large laminar defects — in spina bifida deformities or neurofibromatosis with erosion of the lamina or bone graft, or in postlaminectomy patients — the spinal cord can be injured during the exposure. Careful surgical technique can prevent these injuries. The possibility of laminar or graft defects must always be considered during the exposure when the anatomy appears unusual.

Cord injury due to distraction or surgery is always the greatest fear of the scoliosis surgeon. Paraplegia was almost nonexistent in the days of plaster cast correction. Since the advent of Harrington instrumentation, forceful distraction technique, and the treatment of severe rigid deformities, paraplegia has been more commonly reported.[3, 21, 30, 31, 39, 52] The neurologic loss can be associated with Harrington instrumentation, posterior fusion, or osteotomy.

With the use of distraction during Harrington instrumentation, the distractive force is placed on all tissue, including the spinal artery. The interruption of vascular supply to the cord is thought to be the cause of the paralysis or paraplegia, similar to that described in relation to traction complications (p. 395). Added evidence has been presented by Ponte, who described two cases where paraplegia associated with hypovolemia developed in the postoperative period after spinal fusion and Harrington instrumentation. While arrangements were made for emergency rod removal, the blood volume and blood pressure were restored with blood transfusions, and the paraplegia disappeared.[31] With the use of Harrington instrumentation, paraplegia can be present when the patient awak-

ens from the anesthetic, or the neurologic loss can develop in the first 24 hours (usually within 8 to 12 hours) postoperatively. In this delayed type, paraparesis may progress to paraplegia. The paraparesis can present with muscle weakness, bladder paralysis, or sensory changes, usually paresthesiae of a burning or tingling nature (Fig. 16–5).

Paraplegia is more frequent in congenital scoliosis,[21] probably due to the common condition of spinal dysraphism or cord tethering by bony spurs, fibrous bands, or a tight filum terminale. It is thus preferable *not* to use Harrington instrumentation to gain excessive correction in congenital scoliosis. After osteotomies have been performed and a period of traction used to correct the deformity, application of Harrington instrumentation to gain additional correction sometimes results in paraplegia. The use of the instrumentation in these cases is to maintain the correction obtained with traction. A high incidence of paraplegia also occurs with instrumentation in severe rigid curves.[40] In all these cases the paraplegia may be present when the patient awakens from surgery, or it may develop later. Excessive distraction in congenital scoliosis and after osteotomies should be avoided. Preoperative traction should be used to obtain the correction; the Harrington instrumentation should be employed only to maintain this correction.

The technique developed by Vauzelle and Stagnara of Lyon, France, is most helpful in assessing spinal cord function.[45, 46] It consists of partially awakening the anesthetized patient after insertion of the Harrington rod. The patient is then requested to move the fingers and then the toes. If toe motion occurs voluntarily, the cord is functioning. If not, the rods should be loosened and the test repeated. If loosening does not result in return of function, the rod is removed. The patients seldom remember any part of this episode. All but one case of a "positive wake up test" (i.e., ability to move the toes) in Stagnara's experience have been in curves greater than 120 degrees,[40] but our experience shows that this positive test can occur in a curve of 57 degrees (Fig. 16–6). Another method of monitoring cord function is that of cortical evoked potentials, as described by Nash et al.[26] Both of these tests help to prevent the occurrence of patients waking up paraplegic from the anesthesia, but it is of no value in the

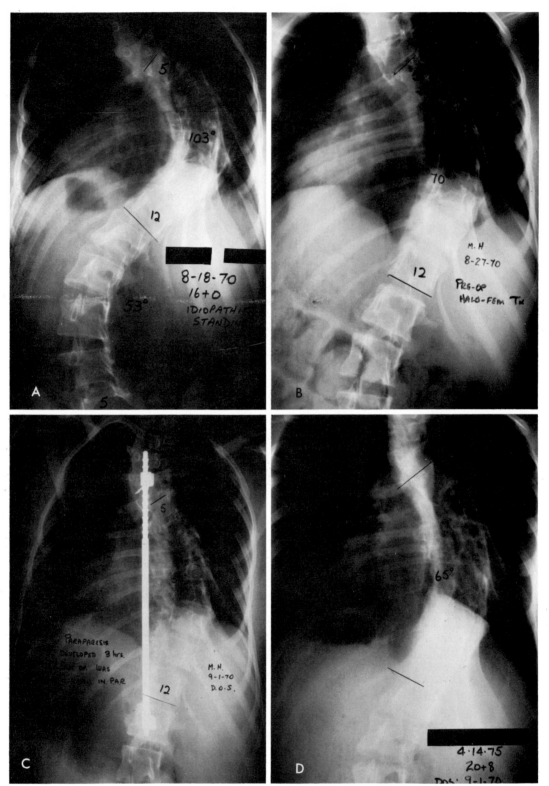

**Figure 16–5** *A,* Postoperative paralysis. This 16-year-old girl presented with a 103 degree right thoracic idiopathic scoliosis. *B,* After two weeks of halofemoral traction the curve was reduced to 70 degrees. *C,* Spine fusion and Harrington instrumentation was performed. Correction to 55 degrees was obtained. On awakening the patient was neurologically normal. Three hours later paraparesis developed. Immediate reoperation and removal of instrumentation was carried out with complete neurologic recovery. *D,* Four and a half years postoperatively this anteroposterior radiograph shows a solid fusion and a 65 degree right thoracic curve. Note that the use of the "wake-up test" would *not* have prevented this complication.

**404**

patient who awakes from the anesthetic with normal cord function and develops paraplegia later.

All patients should be monitored carefully every hour during the postoperative period for a minimum of 24 hours. Early diagnosis of paraplegia is essential. If it develops, the patient must be *immediately* returned to surgery and the instrumentation removed. Laminectomy is unnecessary unless there is a specific reason to suspect the presence of a bone fragment or a hematoma in the spinal canal. It has been shown that there is a direct correlation between the recovery from paraplegia and the interval between its onset and removal of the Harrington instrumentation.[21] With a delay after onset of paraplegia of three hours or less, the chance of recovery is excellent, but if the delay is over six hours, the chance of recovery is slight. MacEwen[21] reviewed the experience of the Scoliosis Research Society and found that with paraplegia occurring on awakening from the anesthetic, the likelihood of recovery is minimal.

Rarely, paraplegia can also follow a posterior spine fusion when Harrington instrumentation is not used. It is more common with congenital kyphosis or where a neurologic deficit existed preoperatively.[21] In these cases the blood supply of the spinal cord is just sufficient but critical. With the trauma of surgery, even with gentle technique the circulation is decreased and paraplegia results. This complication may be prevented by using the anterior approach in severe congenital kyphosis. When neurologic defects are present preoperatively, the compression of the spinal cord should be relieved by anterior cord decompression.

Spinal osteotomy can also be complicated by paraplegia. A previous spine fusion may be osteotomized or a wedge excision performed to correct severe deformities. Paraplegia complicating these procedures may present postoperatively after a latent period. This paralysis may be caused by compression of the spinal cord by a hematoma, abscess, or edema. Careful monitoring of the patient must continue well into the postoperative period. When detected, prompt exploration is necessary to expose the spinal cord in the area of the osteotomy. Any hematoma, abscess, or other compression is removed. As cord edema with obstruction of the cord capillaries may play a role in this paraplegia, systemic steroids are given to decrease edema and hasten the recovery.

## NERVE ROOT COMPRESSION

A complication found after wedge osteotomies to correct a lumbosacral hemivertebra is compression of a nerve root when the wedge is closed. This complication may also occur with posterior wedge osteotomies to restore lumbar lordosis. During the wedge closure the nerve roots are exposed and observed. Rarely the root can be compressed by a Harrington hook. The root lesion may be a neuropraxia, where gradual and complete recovery is usual without active treatment. With increasing deficit or complete initial motor loss, the root should be surgically explored and decompressed.

## DURAL TEAR

Direct trauma to the dura during the surgical procedure results in a dural laceration with a leak of spinal fluid. This can be accompanied by trauma to the spinal cord or cauda equina. Care during exposure and decortication is necessary at all times. When the dura is lacerated, bone must be removed to adequately visualize the tear. The dura is separated and the contents inspected for damage. Careful suture of the dura is then performed. When this type of closure is not possible, the defect is closed using a fascial graft.

## PNEUMOTHORAX

A pneumothorax can occur during surgery for one of three reasons. The respirator can malfunction, forcing air into the lungs and not allowing escape. The result is a tension pneumothorax (Fig. 16–7). A pulmonary bleb (congenital or emphysematous) can rupture spontaneously, also resulting in a tension pneumothorax. During the surgical procedure, the pleura can be punctured directly. This is more likely to occur when ribs are being resected as part of the surgical procedure. The pneumothorax can present intraoperatively as a cardiac arrest or as difficulty with maintenance of aeration. Postoperatively the patient demonstrates respiratory distress and anoxia. Whenever the pneumothorax is significant, as confirmed by radiography, chest tubes should

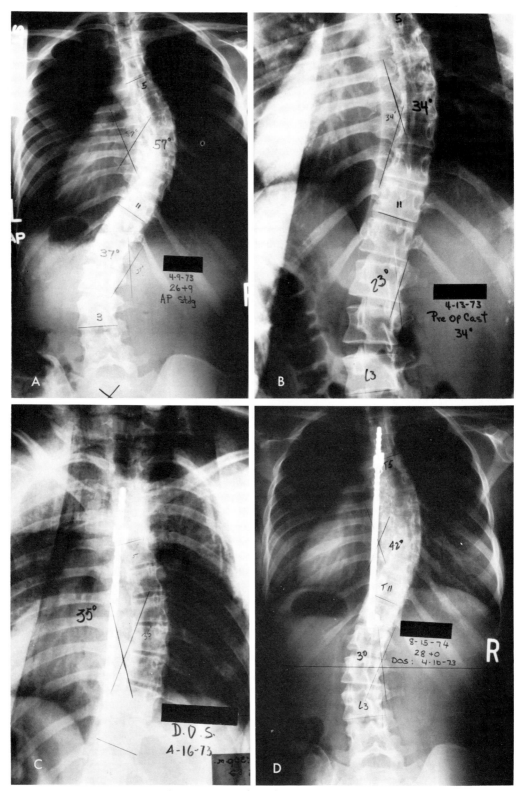

**Figure 16–6** *See legend on opposite page.*

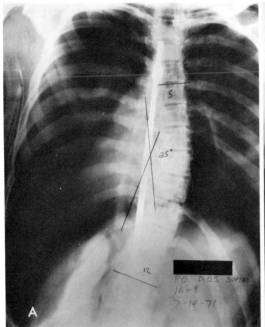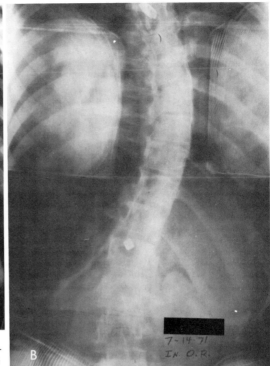

**Figure 16–7**   A, S.C., a 14-year-old female who underwent a spinal fusion with Harrington instrumentation. In the recovery room she became cyanotic, and a chest x-ray revealed a large left pneumothorax. B, In reviewing the intraoperative marker x-ray, it is seen that the pneumothorax is present at this stage. On reviewing the case with the anesthesiologists, it was learned that for the early stages of the case there was respirator malfunction with a short expiratory phase and thus a build-up of positive pulmonary pressure. This pressure probably ruptured an area of congenital bulla formation. A chest catheter connected to underwater drainage was inserted.

be inserted immediately and connected to closed underwater drainage.

## HEMOTHORAX

Hemothorax can occur from rupture of a vessel—either the intercostal along the rib or transverse process or a segmental vessel around the vertebral body. Laceration of the vessel can result from penetration by an instrument or during osteotomy of the transverse processes to correct rib prominence. The laceration and blood loss usually go undetected until severe hypotension and/or cardiac arrest develops. A chest radiograph will aid in the diagnosis of hemothorax. When a large progressive hemothorax is present, thoracotomy must be performed immediately and the lacerated vessel ligated.

## GLUTEAL ARTERY LACERATION

The superior gluteal artery can be lacerated by an osteotome or gouge at the greater sciatic notch during the process of obtaining the iliac bone graft. With a subperiosteal exposure and carefully seated Taylor retractor, the area of the sciatic notch may be adequately protected. When the artery is lacerated, packing with gauze sponges rarely

**Figure 16–6**   A, Positive "wake-up test." This 26 + 9 year old female presented with an idiopathic scoliosis and a right thoracic curve. The anteroposterior x-ray shows a right thoracic curve of 57 degrees. A supine right side bending film showed flexibility to 33 degrees. B, After 10 days of Cotrel traction, the curve was reduced to 42 degrees. A preoperative cast was applied, and the anteroposterior x-ray shows correction in the cast to 34 degrees. C, Spine fusion and Harrington instrumentation was performed. After distraction was applied, the anesthesia was lightened and toe motion to verbal command tested. The patient was unable to move her toes. After decreasing the distraction by one notch, toe motion occurred. The effect of distraction was again tested by increasing the distraction; no motion resulted. The distraction was again decreased by one notch, and toe motion to verbal command returned. This anteroposterior x-ray in the recovery room showed correction to 35 degrees. Neurologic function was normal. D, Standing anteroposterior x-ray 16 months postoperatively showed a solid fusion and a right thoracic curve of 42 degrees.

controls the hemorrhage. An attempt at ligating the artery by enlarging the incision and removing bone in the area of the sciatic notch is occasionally successful. If these attempts are unsuccessful the back wound is rapidly approximated using towel clips and the patient turned supine. A laparotomy is necessary to adequately visualize the vessel for ligation.

### EXCESSIVE BLOOD LOSS

Blood loss during spinal surgery may be excessive. It can occur in patients with paralytic diseases, congenital heart diseases, those who have been in the Milwaukee brace, and occasionally, for no obvious reason. The hemorrhage may be excessive throughout the whole procedure or only with decortication. In our experience, coagulation studies have not been useful in demonstrating the cause. Careful technique, with meticulous subperiosteal exposure, will minimize the blood loss. Occasionally the hemorrhage is so extensive that the procedure must be terminated, the wound closed, and the fusion completed two weeks later.

With anterior approaches, major arteries such as the the aorta, inferior vena cava, or iliac vessels may be lacerated with a sudden large hemorrhage. The laceration is visualized and sutured. Whenever the vertebral body is entered for an osteotomy, anterior cord decompression, or placement of a rib strut, the vascular channels may bleed profusely. This must be controlled by the liberal use of bone wax, especially during a major resection of vertebral body.

### BONE FRACTURE

During insertion of the Harrington hooks in the facet joint, lamina, or over the transverse process, it is possible to fracture the hook placement site. This problem is more common when the bone is osteoporotic or with small weak bone found in young or severely paralyzed patients. It can be avoided by the use of careful technique in hook insertion. In addition, excessive corrective forces with the Harrington instrumentation must be avoided. The use of more than one Harrington rod will help to distribute the corrective forces over four rather than two hook placement sites.

During the osteotomy of previously fused spines it is possible to fracture the posterior elements, pedicle, or vertebral body. Occasionally with anterior insertion of the Dwyer apparatus in correction, the vertebral body can fracture. This is prevented by careful technique and the avoidance of excess corrective forces, especially in osteoporotic bone.

With soft bone and difficulty in obtaining fixation of instrumentation in the bone, methyl methacrylate can be used for Harrington hook or Dwyer screw fixation.

### PERITONEAL/BOWEL LACERATION

During anterior exposure of the lumbar spine a retroperitoneal approach is used, and the peritoneum can be lacerated during the exposure. All lacerations should be closed with catgut suture. Rarely the intra-abdominal contents may be traumatized, with perforation of a loop of bowel and contamination of the retroperitoneal space. The laceration must be sutured and copious amounts of lavage used to irrigate the operative field.

## Early Postoperative Complications

### PULMONARY PROBLEMS

Pulmonary problems with respiratory distress are a major postoperative complication of spine surgery. All patients undergoing spine surgery have a postoperative decrease in respiratory function, which is more marked with the anterior approach. This decrease is especially significant in patients who have a respiratory deficit preoperatively. For this reason, preoperative evaluation of pulmonary function should be performed routinely. If not a routine procedure, evaluation is necessary for all patients in whom there is any suspicion whatsoever that there may be a deficit of pulmonary function. Preoperative preparation involves instruction in respiratory exercise and blow bottles and practice in the use of the respirator for IPPB (intermittent positive pressure breathing).

Postoperative atelectasis presents as temperature elevation, tachypnea, and restlessness. Vigorous coughing or tracheal suctioning usually expels the obstructing mucous plug. If this is unsuccessful, lavage of the endotracheal tree with a bronchoscope may be necessary.

Patients who have poor cough reflex

postoperatively due to muscle weakness, sedation, or postoperative pain have postoperative hypoventilation and anoxia. Tachypnea, restlessness, and fever are the clinical manifestations. When the hypoventilation occurs, or in patients where preoperative deficits are present with weak respiratory muscles, the endotracheal tube is not removed postoperatively until gas exchange is normal. Strong narcotics are not used so that respiratory depression is minimized. In our center the use of LDC (Levo-Dromoran Combination), which is a combination of Levorfan (a synthetic morphinate) and Dromoran (a respiratory stimulant), has given excellent pain relief without respiratory depression. If necessary, respiratory support is used at this time. Usually after 48 to 72 hours the use of respiratory depressants is decreased and the nasotracheal tube can be removed. If necessary, the tube can be left in for up to seven days. Tracheostomy with this regimen is rarely necessary. In patients with marked paralysis of respiratory muscles, a tracheostomy may be performed preoperatively. The patient is then maintained on a positive pressure respirator with the tracheostomy for several weeks postoperatively (Fig. 16–8).

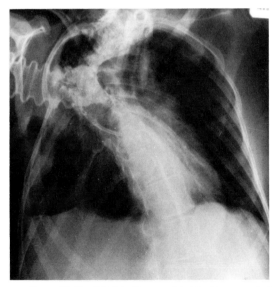

**Figure 16–8** K.J. This 13-year-old girl with congenital kyphoscoliosis underwent a transthoracic cord decompression and anterior fusion for progressive neurologic loss. Postoperative course was complicated by respiratory problems, and she had to be maintained on a respirator. The chest tubes could not be removed till the twelfth day. The x-ray shown was taken two days later and shows a large area of pneumothorax on the right base.

With adequate preoperative evaluation and postoperative care, respiratory complications are rare.

More unusual respiratory complications are pneumothorax (Fig. 16–8) (p. 405) and shock lung (see p. 402). Accurate diagnosis and appropriate therapy are necessary for these problems.

## NEUROLOGIC PROBLEMS

Paralysis occurring in the postoperative period may be related to either distraction or the surgical procedure. These events are discussed in full on pages 395 and 403.

Acute hydrocephalus can occur after surgery on a child with myelodysplasia. The acute problem can follow the excision of a nonfunctioning spinal cord during the posterior approach for correction of congenital kyphosis. Any surgical procedure performed on these children can disturb the balance of cerebrospinal fluid formation and absorption, resulting in an acute build-up of cerebrospinal fluid pressure. It is also possible for the ventriculoperitoneal shunt catheter to be disturbed during an anterior approach to the spine, causing acute hydrocephalus. The child presents with restlessness, stupor, and papilledema. Prompt diagnosis followed by neurosurgical consultation and an emergency shunting procedure is then necessary.

## WOUND INFECTION

Wound infection has been more common in scoliosis surgery than in other areas in orthopedic surgery. This may be related to the size of the wound and the muscle trauma and hematoma that predispose to an infection. In our experience an overall incidence of 9.3 per cent was noted, and certain correlations were found.[19] The infection rate was higher 1) with certain types of deformity (myelodysplasia), 2) when there was a pre-existing urinary tract infection, 3) with a large number of visitors in the operating room, or 4) in cases where Harrington instrumentation was used. The infection rate in adult patients was 20 per cent. No correlation between blood loss, operating time, and the number of levels fused was found.

The incidence of infection may be markedly decreased by 1) attention to surgical technique, with careful subperiosteal expo-

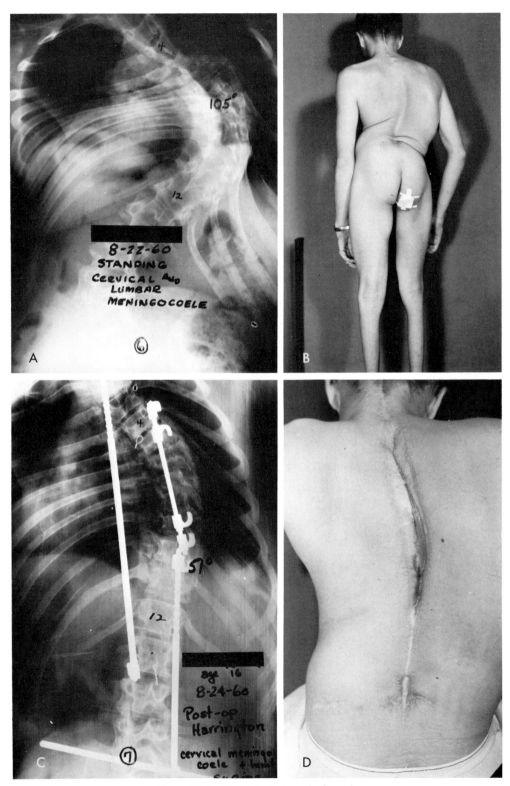

**Figure 16–9** *See opposite page for legend.*

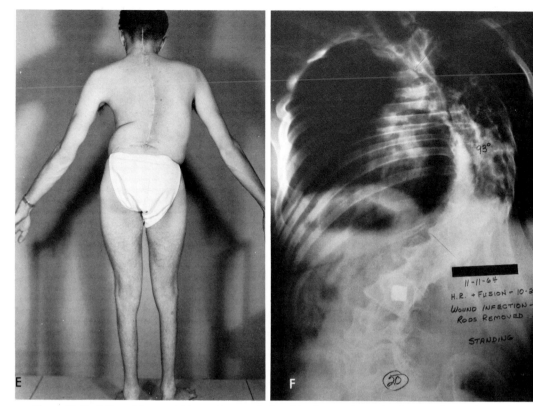

**Figure 16–9**  C.Y., a 16-year-old boy with a cervical and lumbar meningocele. On presentation the standing antero-posterior x-ray showed a 105 degree right thoracic scoliosis (A). A posterior view (B) shows the deformity and the scars of the surgical closure of the meningoceles. A pressure sore is present over the right ischial tuberosity. C, Posterior spine fusion and Harrington instrumentation was performed with correction to 51 degrees. On the third postoperative day the temperature was elevated and the wound showed local signs of inflammation. Purulent drainage began the following day. After a culture was taken the wound was treated with local opening and packing. The wound was then debrided and packed open. The infection gradually cleared and the wound became clean and granulated and then epithelialized. Total hospitalization was four months. D, On readmission 5 months postoperatively for a cast sore, sinuses were found communicating to the rods. The instrumentation was removed and the wound packed open and then skin grafted a month later. This posterior view nearly two years postoperatively shows the poor cosmetic result with a wide scar. The scar was revised and this posterior view (E) shows the result four years after the fusion and 2½ years after the scar revision. F, Anteroposterior spine x-ray with a solid fusion and a final 93 degree curve. (A, C, and F from Lonstein, J. E., Winter, R. B., Moe, J. H., and Gaines, D., Clin. Orthop. 96:222, 1973, with permission.)

sure to reduce the blood loss and amount of muscle trauma plus excision of all necrotic tissue prior to wound closure, 2) proper operating room technique, with reduction in operating room traffic and talking, and attention paid to proper preparation and draping routines, and 3) the use of prophylactic antibiotics during and for 48 hours after surgery. The routine use of prophylactic antibiotics has reduced our infection rate from 9.3 to 1.6 per cent. A dramatic decrease in this complication has also been found in adult cases, where the infection rate has fallen from 20 per cent to 1.6 per cent. Similar results have been reported by others.

If an infection develops, prompt diagnosis and early aggressive therapy are necessary.

Any temperature elevation is viewed with suspicion and the wound is inspected for erythema, edema, and tenderness. When an infection is suspected, a culture is obtained by aspiration away from the incision after surgical preparation of the wound area. If the wound is highly suspicious, one should *not* wait for culture results. When an infection is diagnosed or possibility is high, the patient is taken to surgery. The entire wound is opened down to the bone graft and debrided and irrigated thoroughly. Further cultures are taken, and after complete debridement, irrigation and suction tubes are inserted. Neither the bone graft nor the instrumentation is removed, and the wound is closed as if it were a primary closure of a clean wound, with all

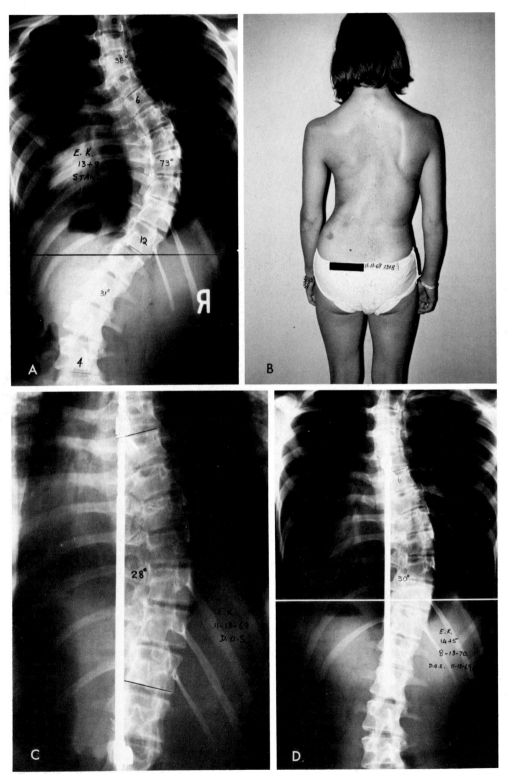

**Figure 16–10** *See opposite page for legend.*

**Figure 16–10** E.K. a 13 + 8 year old girl was first seen with a right thoracic curve of 73 degrees (A), which corrected to 46 degrees on supine side bending. B, Posterior view of her back. C, The patient underwent spine fusion and Harrington instrumentation from T5 to L2. This supine anteroposterior x-ray on the day of surgery shows correction to 28 degrees. On the third postoperative day the patient had a persistent fever and a wound hematoma, which was aspirated and cultured. The culture was negative. The fever persisted, and there was minimal sanguinous wound drainage. A wound infection was diagnosed, and wound debridement with evacuation of a large hematoma was performed. The wound was closed over irrigation-suction tubes. The culture grew gram-positive bacilli of the bacillus species, and the patient was continued on parenteral antibiotics and antibiotics in the irrigation. The irrigation-suction tubes were removed after nine days, and the patient was placed in a postoperative cast and ambulated the following day. Additional hospitalization for treatment of the infection was 10 days. D, The cast was removed nine months later. A standing anteroposterior x-ray shows correction to 30 degrees maintained. An oblique view showed a pseudarthrosis at the T11–T12 level, which was repaired, the wound being closed prophylactically over irrigation-suction tubes. The infection did not recur. E, Clinical view five years postoperatively shows the cosmetic improvement and a well-healed scar. The fusion is solid with no loss of correction. (A from Lonstein, J. E., Winter, R. B., Moe, J. H., and Gaines, D., Clin. Orthop., 96:22, 1973, with permission.)

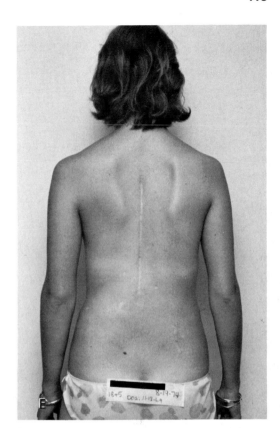

considerations for cosmetic healing of the skin. The irrigation and suction system is continued for a total of three to five days. If the patient is afebrile, the wound benign, and the sedimentation rate and white cell count falling, the irrigation is discontinued and all the tubes are connected to suction and are removed after 24 hours. The tubes are left in longer only if the temperature remains elevated and the wound still shows local signs of infection. Culture of the suction drainage or tubes is of no benefit. The treatment of infection with packing and local care is condemned, since the infection is inadequately controlled, the hospitalization prolonged, and the cosmetic result poor (Figs. 16–9 and 16–10).

Antibiotics are started in large doses preoperatively and continued intravenously for 10 days postoperatively. The patient is then placed on an appropriate oral antibiotic for six weeks. It must be emphasized that the bone graft and Harrington instrumentation should not be disturbed. After treatment for the infection, the scoliosis care continues. With this regimen the infection has been treated and the outcome of both the scoliosis fusion and the infection are good (Fig. 16–10).

## GENITOURINARY TRACT PROBLEMS

Urinary retention is common in the postoperative period in scoliosis patients. Urecholine 2.5 and 5.0 mg. subcutaneously every six hours is administered to stimulate the bladder. If this is unsuccessful the patient is catheterized. If catheterization is necessary, we prefer *not* to use an indwelling catheter but rather to use intermittent catheterization technique every six hours, with careful sterile preparation of the urethral outlet. Using this technique, the incidence of urinary tract infection is minimized.[13, 18] With symptoms of infection or a persistent postoperative fever, the urine is cultured and if an infection is found, appropriate chemotherapy is given.

## GASTROINTESTINAL TRACT PROBLEMS

Ileus rarely occurs today, since morphine is no longer used postoperatively. It is customary for bowel sounds to be present on the evening of surgery and almost always on the following day. Some patients, especially very anxious ones, have a problem with postoperative distention. This is due to air swallowing (aerophagia) and is aggravated by the use of IPPB treatments. In these cases, stopping the IPPB plus occasional use of a nasogastric tube will cure the distention.

Postoperative nausea and vomiting may be indicative of vascular compression of the abdomen. This subject is discussed in full on page 400.

### BLOOD REACTIONS AND HEPATITIS

With the extensive use of blood replacement in scoliosis surgery, problems with transfusion frequently occur. Mild allergic transfusion reactions (hives) are common, but anaphylaxis is rare in our experience. With skin eruptions the patient is given Benadryl intramuscularly and the transfusion stopped. Occasionally difficulty is encountered in crossmatching blood for the patient, especially when prior surgery has been performed. The formation of antibodies makes it difficult to obtain compatible blood. This problem can be decreased with the use of autologous predeposit transfusions. In routine cases in patients over 10 years of age, three units of blood are drawn from the patient at weekly intervals starting three weeks preoperatively and stored and retransfused at the time of surgery.[22] This amount of blood is usually sufficient for routine fusion. When extreme difficulty is experienced in obtaining compatible blood, the autologous blood can be taken and frozen, allowing storage for months if necessary.

Hepatitis is a severe complication following blood transfusions. In our center, this problem is rare. A high standard of service by local blood transfusion services or the Red Cross helps to minimize this problem. When hepatitis incidence is high, the routine use of gamma globulin has been shown to decrease this rate.[25]

### HOOK DISLODGEMENT

Upper hook dislodgement can occur in the early postoperative period. It commonly occurs in restless, uncooperative patients (for example, those with cerebral palsy or mental retardation). It can also occur in cases of unrecognized thoracic kyphosis, where the rod is not adequately contoured (Fig. 16–11). This dislodgement is usually diagnosed when the postoperative cast is applied and a loss of correction found as compared with the day of surgery. Occasionally a lateral x-ray film is necessary to confirm the position of the hook. Rarely will the diagnosis be made early, but rod protrusion through the wound or sudden discomfort at a hook site can occur (Fig. 16–12). The dislodgement is treated by reinsertion of the hook, usually at a level higher than the initial site. Adequate bending to accommodate the kyphosis is performed.

Prevention of this complication is by recognition of kyphosis or abnormal roundness of the thoracic spine on a lateral standing x-ray. The Harrington distraction rod can then be bent to the normal contour of the spine, reducing the forces on the hook placement sites. Uncooperative patients should be placed in a cast immediately postoperatively. While still anesthetized, the patient is moved onto a Risser frame and a cast applied.

### Late Postoperative Complications

### INFECTION

Late infections are those making their appearance after the patient is discharged from the hospital. Infection may become evident several months to years after surgery and usually presents as a small draining sinus. The patient is usually afebrile with minimal wound reaction. The sinus usually goes down to the fusion mass and Harrington instrumentation.

The treatment is the same as that for an early infection. A culture is taken and the wound is opened in its entirety and all scarred and necrotic material debrided. If the fusion is not solid and is less than six months old, the rod and fusion mass are not disturbed. If the infection is marked around the rod, with a large amount of granulation tissue, it may be necessary to temporarily remove the rod, curette the rod bed, and reinsert a new sterile rod. If the fusion is completely solid and at least six months have elapsed since surgery, the rod can be permanently removed. Following complete debridement and irrigation, the wound is closed cosmetically after irrigation and suction tubes are inserted. These are left in place for five to seven days, after which they are connected to suction equipment and then removed 24 hours later. Intravenous antibiotics are started as soon as the drainage is cultured. After 10 days of intravenous therapy, appropriate oral antibiotics are used for six weeks.

Local care of the draining sinus must be condemned. Placing the patient on antibiotics and inserting a wick drain in the sinus is inadequate care, and the infection will persist. Complete and thorough debridement is mandatory.

## PSEUDARTHROSIS (Fig. 16–13)

Pseudarthrosis is an accepted complication of scoliosis surgery. The pseudarthrosis rate has been lowered from levels of as high as 50 per cent to less than 2 per cent by advances in scoliosis care, particularly the use of facet joint fusions, autogenous iliac cancellous bone graft, early mobilization, adequate casts, and early ambulation postoperatively. Pseudarthroses are more common in the lumbar spine, at the thoracolumbar junction (T11–L1), and the lumbosacral junction (L4–S1). They also occur more commonly in certain conditions—paralytic curves, neurofibromatosis, or kyphoscoliosis—and in adult patients. When a significant kyphotic deformity is treated with posterior fusion alone, the fusion mass is under distraction and pseudarthroses are common.

Early recognition of pseudarthroses is important. Routine supine oblique radiographs are taken of the fusion area at five to six months postoperatively (at the time of cast change) and again when the cast is removed, usually at nine months postoperatively. The fusion mass is examined for any defects crossing it, and all visible facet joints are evaluated. A facet joint that is easily visible and not obliterated indicates an area of weakness, and defects in the fusion mass pass through these unfused joints. In addition, the area of the pseudarthrosis is commonly very tender to palpation and percussion. There may be no loss of correction, as the cast and Harrington instrumentation support the spine and maintain the correction. If a pseudarthrosis is noted on either of these evaluations, exploration of the graft is carried out. In patients fused while actively growing, other clues to the presence of pseudarthrosis may be present. The weak area in the graft allows the graft to elongate, and if Harrington rods are present, the rod is "pulled" out of the lower hook. In addition, the disc space opposite the pseudarthrosis is wide as growth continues, but the other discs become narrowed as vertebral body growth continues at the expense of the disc space.

If a pseudarthrosis has been undetected and the patient is allowed to go without a cast, loss of correction will present as loss of height and increase in the scoliosis. Occasionally the fusion mass is wide so that increase in scoliosis does not occur, but loss of correction giving kyphosis results. The instrumentation used (Harrington or Dwyer) will initially maintain correction when a pseudarthrosis is present, but eventually, with the constant motion a fatigue fracture of the metal occurs (Fig. 16–14). Occasionally pain is experienced in the fusion area, with a region of extreme tenderness. With a suspected pseudarthrosis at any time, careful oblique radiographs are taken, followed by surgical exploration and reinforcement of the fusion.

A clue to an area of pseudarthrosis is found in the exposure to the fusion mass. When the fusion is solid, the periosteum covering it can be stripped off with ease, using a periosteal elevator. In the area of pseudarthrosis the periosteum is firmly adherent to the fibrous tissue in the fusion defect, making exposure of the area difficult. Sometimes the defect is not easily visualized, and it is necessary to decorticate the entire fusion mass before the pseudarthrosis will be evident. The fibrous tissue is curetted from the defect, allowing the unfused facet joints to be visualized. It is usually not necessary to add additional iliac bone, the local bone from the fusion mass being sufficient to place over the decorticated area of pseudarthrosis. If the pseudarthrosis is very loose, or if there is insufficient local bone in the fusion mass for the pseudarthrosis repair, additional iliac bone is added.

In disorders for which the pseudarthrosis rate is high (paralytic curves, especially those fused to the sacrum, neurofibromatosis, kyphoscoliosis, and fusion in adults), routine exploration of the fusion mass is performed six months after the initial fusion procedure. The fusion mass is exposed in its entirety and all defects visualized. It is cleaned of fibrous tissue, and additional iliac bone graft is added. Even if there is no obvious pseudarthrosis, the fusion mass is sometimes explored and additional bone added on a prophylactic basis. The

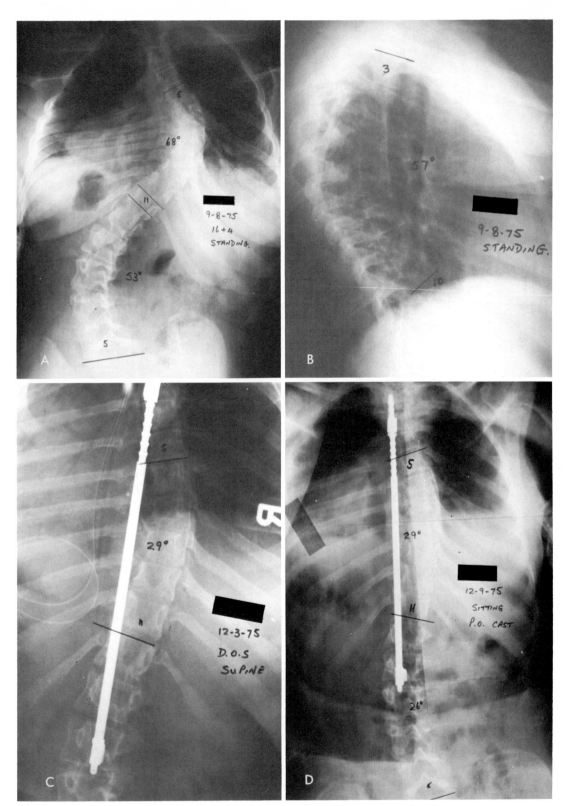

**Figure 16–11**    P de S. a 16 year and 4 month old girl with cerebral palsy presented with scoliosis. *A,* The anteroposterior x-ray shows a right thoracic curve of 68 degrees and a left lumbar curve of 53 degrees. The right thoracic curve was flexible. A lateral x-ray (*B*) shows a thoracic kyphosis of 57 degrees. A posterior spinal fusion with Harrington instrumentation was performed from T3 to L2. *C,* The anteroposterior x-ray shows that the correction obtained on the day of surgery was 29 degrees. Six days later a cast was applied and a sitting anteroposterior x-ray (*D*) shows that the correction has been maintained.

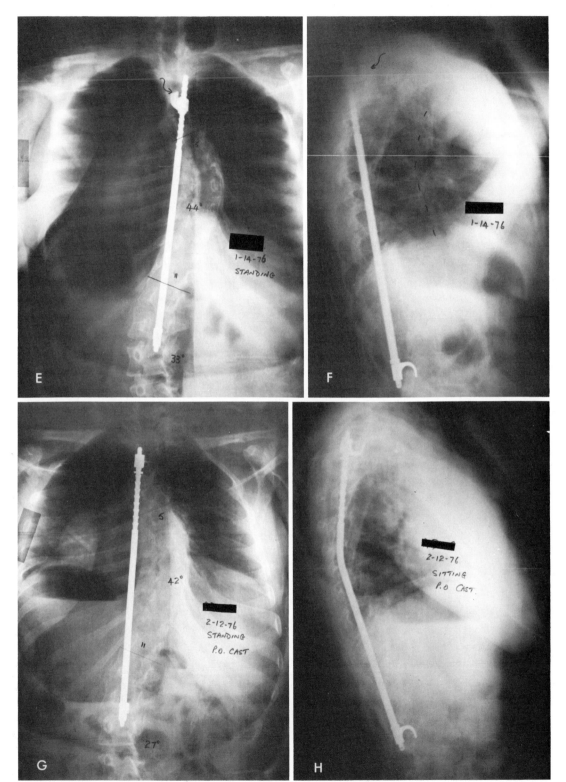

**Figure 16–11** *Continued.* A month later at a clinic visit the standing anteroposterior x-ray (*E*) showed a loss of correction in the right thoracic curve to 44 degrees, and the upper hook was displaced. A lateral standing x-ray (*F*) confirmed this displacement. Note that the rod was *not* contoured to conform to the thoracic kyphosis. The patient was reoperated upon and the hook reinserted after contouring the rod to the kyphosis. The fusion was progressing well. An anteroposterior standing x-ray (*G*) shows that the original correction could not be achieved. The lateral x-ray (*H*) shows the contoured rod in place.

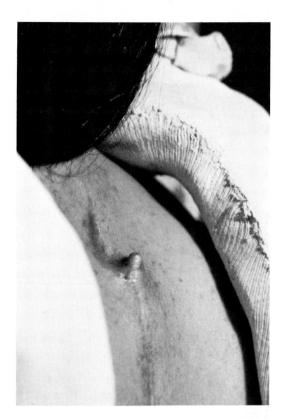

**Figure 16–12** Clinical photograph of a patient in a halo cast showing the upper end of the Harrington distraction rod tenting the skin. The upper hook had cut out, and the rod became palpable. Operative reinsertion was necessary.

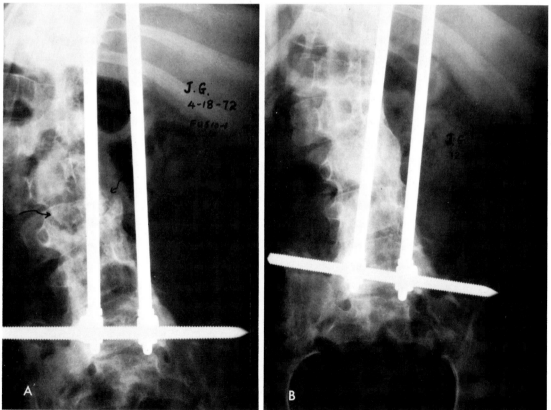

**Figure 16–13** *A,* J.G. This thirteen-year-old boy with post-traumatic paraplegia and scoliosis had a long posterior spine fusion with Harrington instrumentation on 4/13/71. A year postoperatively there was no loss of correction, but the oblique view shown demonstrates a pseudarthrosis in the fusion mass. *B,* The pseudarthrosis was repaired, and this oblique view 20 months after the repair shows a solid fusion mass.

patient is then placed in a cast for an additional six months of immobilization, for a total cast time of one year. Using this procedure, the pseudarthrosis rate has decreased, and the need for exploration and refusion after the period of postoperative casting is unusual.

## INSTRUMENTATION BREAKAGE

Failure of the instrumentation (Harrington or Dwyer) is often a complication related to pseudarthrosis. An area of pseudarthrosis will have motion, and even without any loss of correction, this constant motion will lead to metal fatigue, and breakage of the instrumentation (see Fig. 16–14). It is thus axiomatic that broken instrumentation suggests a pseudarthrosis, as it is not the metal but the fusion that has failed. Rarely a Harrington strut bar will break within a solid fusion, since rods are not firmly fixed. With the Dwyer cable the breakage process is gradual, and initially an unraveling of an area of cable is seen. At first a few cable strands break, and eventually the whole cable breaks. This breakage is always opposite a disc space that is not solidly fused and obliterated.

Whenever a pseudarthrosis and instrumentation breakage occur, exploration and refusion are necessary. If only an anterior fusion and Dwyer instrumentation are performed, the addition of a posterior fusion is necessary. The posterior fusion is of the whole curve and reinforces the anterior fusion.

The frayed cable in the area of cable breakage or the frayed cable present left at the end of the anterior fusion can cause a problem. Constant motion of the great vessels over the cable can erode the vessel, resulting in aneurysm formation or rupture. The cut end of the cable at the end of a fusion should be either covered with a metal bead or buried in the psoas muscle. Early detection and prompt treatment of cable breakage is necessary to prevent problems with broken cable.

## LENGTHENING OF THE CURVE ("ADDING ON")

By "adding on" we mean an extension of the curvature to include vertebrae that originally were not a part of the curve. This may occur as a result of improper selection of the fusion area. All vertebrae that are rotated in

the same direction as the apical vertebra should be included in the fusion area. A curve may end at the twelfth thoracic vertebra, but rotation may continue in the same direction to the second or third lumbar vertebra. In this case the fusion should include all rotated vertebrae and not follow the arbitrary rule to fuse one above and one below the curve. If these rotated vertebrae are not included in the fusion area, adding on may occur (Fig. 16–15).

Adding on can occur even with proper selection of the fusion area. In patients fused before the adolescent growth spurt and not controlled in the Milwaukee brace following fusion, this complication may be seen. As the original curve extends, it adds on adjacent unfused vertebrae, and the curve thus becomes longer. The use of the Milwaukee brace in a "young fusion" usually controls lengthening of the curve.

## BENDING OF THE FUSION

In addition to adding on, a fusion of the spine performed before the adolescent growth spurt may bend if unprotected in a Milwaukee brace. The fusion mass is living bone and, if solid, does not increase in length but rather, with the stresses placed on it, tends to remodel. The bone on the convexity is subject to tension forces and undergoes microfractures. The result is bending of the fusion and increase in the curvature. Bending is prevented by good surgical technique, providing a strong thick fusion mass, and protection of the fusion by the Milwaukee brace through the adolescent growth spurt. Occasionally, bending can occur even with protection of the brace. If bending occurs and produces an excessive loss of correction, this is treated by osteotomy of the fusion mass, recorrection and refusion.

## STUNTING OF TRUNK GROWTH

Extensive fusion at a young age produces shortening of trunk height, since the fusion mass does not elongate. Long-term follow up studies by Moe and Sundberg[24] and Winter[49] of patients undergoing fusion before the age of 10 showed the average lengthening of the fusion mass to be 1 mm. in five years. Over half of the patients showed no increase, and the maximal increase was 8 mm., in only two

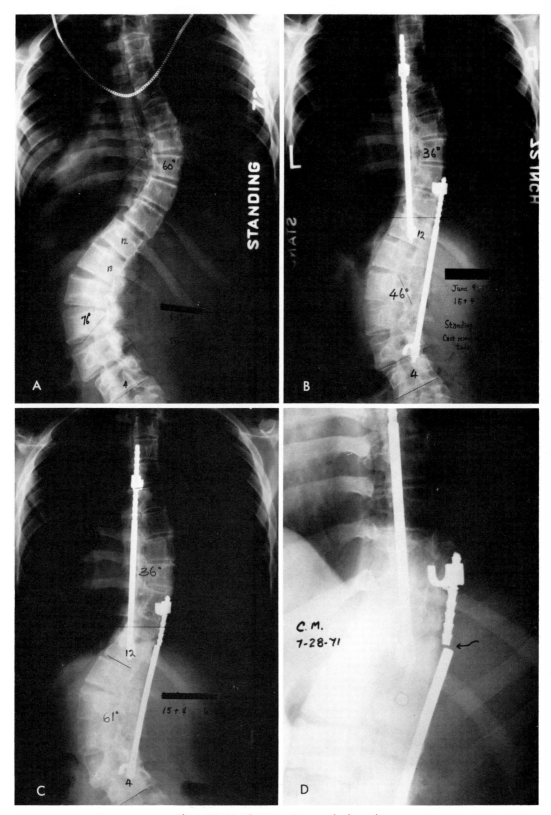

**Figure 16–14**  *See opposite page for legend.*

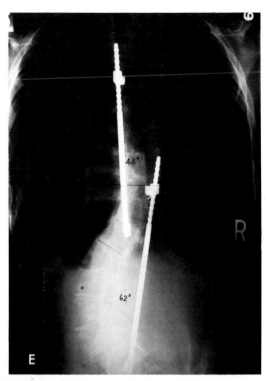

**Figure 16–14**   *A,* C.M., a 14 + 4 year-old girl, presented with a severe idiopathic scoliosis. The anteroposterior standing x-ray shows a right thoracic T6–T12 curve of 60 degrees and a left lumbar T12–L4 curve of 76 degrees. *B,* The patient underwent spine fusion and Harrington instrumentation from T5 to L3. This anteroposterior standing x-ray when the cast was removed nine months later shows correction to 36 degrees for the right thoracic curve and 46 degrees for the left lumbar curve. Oblique views showed a solid fusion. Note that owing to an error in counting the vertebrae in surgery, the fusion went to L3 when it should have gone to L4. *C,* A year later an anteroposterior standing x-ray showed loss of correction in the lumbar curve to 61 degrees. The lower distraction rod had broken at the junction of the rod and the ratchets with a pseudarthrosis were visible at this level. *D,* An oblique view shows the broken rod and the pseudarthrosis. *E,* The pseudarthrosis was repaired and the lower rod replaced with the fusion extended to L4. The standing anteroposterior x-ray 2½ years later shows a solid fusion with maintenance of correction in the lumbar curve and a loss of seven degrees in the thoracic curve.

patients.[49] These studies were done by inserting metal markers at the top and bottom of the fusion area and measuring them by standardized radiographs at yearly intervals. These were cases where it was absolutely necessary to perform a fusion in a young child. It is understood that with a severe progressive deformity in a child, a short, straight, fused spine is better than an even shorter crooked spine, which would have resulted if the fusion were not performed. In these situations, fusion in the young could not be avoided or delayed with the use of the Milwaukee brace until significant growth had occurred. In congenital scoliosis the area involved does not have normal growth potential, and if a long fusion is necessary, stunting of growth is due mainly to the underlying deformity, and the fusion stabilizes the area, preventing progression.

*LORDOSIS*

Lordosis in the area of the fusion is caused by a posterior epiphysiodesis effect with continuance of vertebral body growth anteriorly. It is most evident in very long fusions in children who received a thin posterior fusion at a young age. The amount of lordosis varies from patient to patient. In our experience, this problem has occurred infrequently.[24] The thicker the posterior fusion mass, the less likely is it that the growth forces will be able to bend it. If this becomes a significant problem in the growth spurt, anterior epiphysiodesis may have to be considered to arrest anterior growth and thus stop the progression; if already severe, osteotomy and recorrection may be necessary.

Another cause of lordosis is the position of the patient while bone graft incorporation occurs. When a Harrington distraction rod is

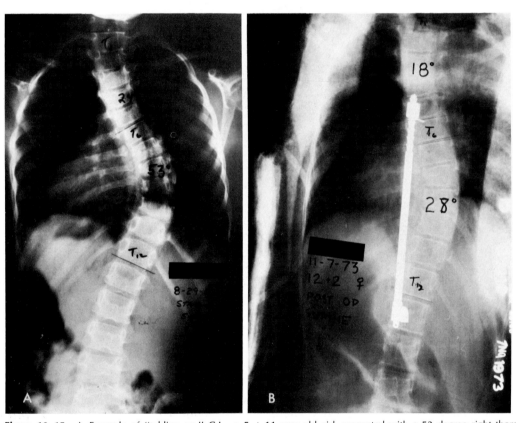

**Figure 16–15** *A,* Example of "adding on." C.L., a 5 + 11 year-old girl, presented with a 53 degree right thoracic scoliosis. The patient had congenital hand anomalies. *B,* The patient was treated with a Milwaukee brace. The control of the curve was good until she reached her adolescent growth spurt. A spine fusion with Harrington instrumentation was performed on the right thoracic curve. The supine anteroposterior x-ray on the day of surgery shows correction to 28 degrees.

*Legend continued on opposite page*

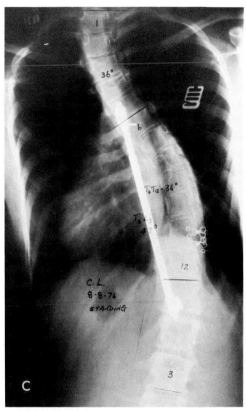

**Figure 16–15** *Continued.* C, Nearly three years later this anteroposterior standing x-ray shows that the right thoracic fusion is solid with a loss of 8 degrees since the day of surgery to 36 degrees. The patient is out of balance and the curve now extends to L3, with the T6–L3 curve measuring 47 degrees. If the previous x-ray (*A*) is studied, it will be seen that L1 and L2 are parallel to T12 and it is not until L3 that the compensatory curve begins. Also, L3 is vertically located above S1, whereas L1 and L2 are deviated to the right. Retrospectively the fusion should have extended to L3.

placed in a flexible thoracic spine, the normal kyphosis is eliminated, and fusion occurs in a straight position. This situation may be prevented by contouring the Harrington instrumentation to conform to normal thoracic kyphosis. The use of compression Harrington instrumentation produces thoracic lordosis. When no instrumentation is used, the position at the time of casting dictates the shape of the fused area. If at the time the cast is applied, a localizer is used pushing upward from behind, with the paient positioned on the cast table, normal thoracic kyphosis will be eliminated when the spine is flexible. In these patients, the back should be allowed to sag while the cast is applied in order to maintain normal thoracic kyphosis.

## LOSS OF LUMBAR LORDOSIS (Fig. 16–16)

A disturbing complication of fusion of the lumbar spine is flattening of the spine with elimination of lumbar lordosis. This problem was rare before the use of Harrington instrumentation and occurs when a straight distraction rod is inserted from the sacrum to T12 or above, causing the normal lumbar lordosis to disappear. In addition, the forces on the spine during the healing process can result in true kyphosis in the lumbar area or kyphosis just above the end of the fusion. The patient thus has a tendency to lean forward and must compensate by hyperextending the thoracic spine and by knee flexion, resulting in marked fatigue and an awkward gait.

Prevention of this complication is by preservation of lumbar lordosis. If fusion to the sacrum is necessary, a contoured rod is used to preserve the lordosis. As the ordinary rod has a tendency to rotate, a square-ended rod has been designed that has a hook with a square hole, which allows the contoured rod to maintain its position. Adding a compression assembly to the convexity of the curve will

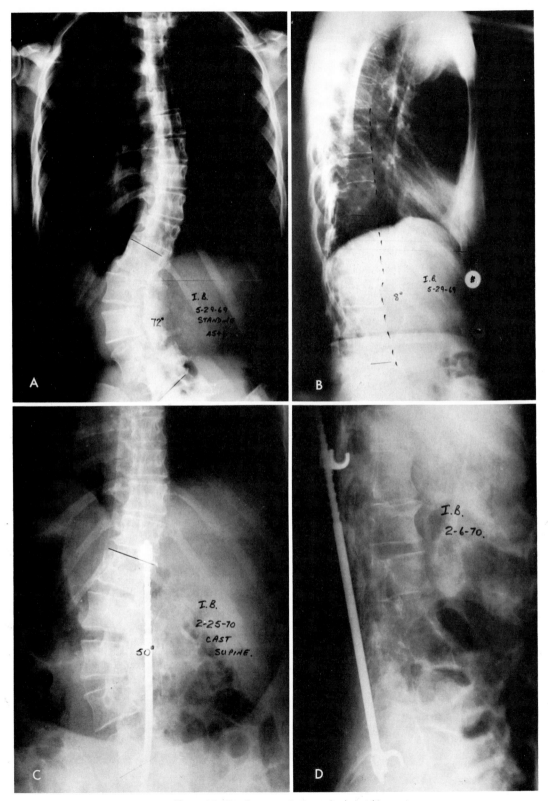

**Figure 16–16** *See opposite page for legend.*

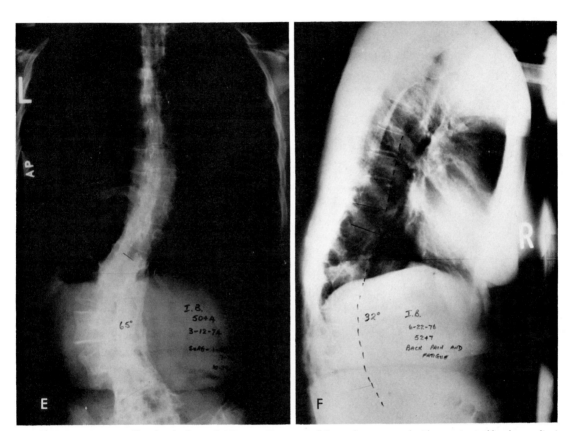

**Figure 16–16**   Loss of lumbar lordosis. *A*, I.B., age 45 years and 6 months, presented with an untreated lumbar scoliosis and severe low back and lumbosacral pain. The standing anteroposterior x-ray shows a 72 degree left lumbar curve with rotatory subluxation of L3 on L4 and facet hypertrophy and arthrosis on the right side. *B*, The lateral x-ray on presentation shows a very flat spine with 8 degrees of kyphosis in the lumbar area and lumbosacral lordosis. *C*, Patient underwent a posterior fusion and Harrington instrumentation from T11 to the sacrum. This anteroposterior x-ray, one month after the fusion, shows correction to 50 degrees. *D*, The lateral x-ray 12 days postoperatively shows the straight Harrington rod in place. *E*, A pseudarthrosis developed, which was repaired in July, 1970. The fusion became solid, and the rod caused persistent difficulties and was removed on 10/29/71. The anteroposterior x-ray four years after the initial fusion shows a solid fusion with a 65 degree curve. The patient was pain-free. *F*, The patient developed the gradual onset of mild aching back pain with fatigue in the back at the end of the day. In addition, she noted progressive forward stoop, which was more noticeable at the end of the day. A lateral x-ray taken on 6/22/76 shows an increase in the lumbar kyphosis to 32 degrees with a noticeable forward stoop.

preserve the lordosis. A spine fused with loss of lumbar lordosis is treated by rod removal and a closing wedge osteotomy of the fusion mass with Harrington compression instrumentation to regain lumbar lordosis.[6]

## References

1. Breig, A.: Biomechanics of the Central Nervous System. Almquist and Wiksell, Stockholm, 1966.
2. Brown, L. P., and Stelling, F. H.: Fat embolism as a complication of scoliosis fusion. J. Bone Joint Surg., 56A:1964, 1974.
3. Buchner, H., Pink, P., and Reinisch, H.: Funfjahrige erfahrungen mit dem Harrington-Stab bei der operativen Behandlung der Skoliose. Arch. Orthop. Unfallchir., 80:343, 1974.
4. Connel, R. S., and Swank, R. L.: Pulmonary microembolism after blood transfusions. Ann. Surg., 177:40, 1973.
5. Curtis, B. H.: Air embolism as a complication of spine fusion. J. Bone Joint Surg., 54A:201, 1972.
6. Denis, F., and Moe, J. H.: Iatrogenic loss of lumbar lordosis. Paper presented at annual meeting of Scoliosis Research Society, Ottawa, Canada, Sept. 4, 1976.
7. Dewald, R. L., and Ray, R. D.: Skeletal traction for the treatment of severe scoliosis. J. Bone Joint Surg., 52A:233, 1970.
8. Dommisse, G. F.: The blood supply of the spinal cord. J. Bone Joint Surg., 56B:225, 1974.
9. Dommisse, G. F.: The Arteries and Veins of the Human Spinal Cord from Birth. Edinburgh, Churchill Livingstone, 1975.
10. Evarts, C. M., Winter, R. B., and Hall, J. E.: Vascular compression of the duodenum associated with the treatment of scoliosis. J. Bone Surg., 53A431, 1971.
11. Gardner, A. D., O'Brien, J. P., and Hodgson, A. R.: Accurate electronic measurement of the forces applied to the spine during halo-pelvic traction. Paper presented at the Annual Meeting of the Scoliosis Research Society, Louisville, Ky., September, 1975.
12. Gray, S. W., Akin, J. T., Milsap, J. H., and Skanalakis, J. E.: Vascular compression of the duodenum. Contemp. Surg., 9:37, 1976.
13. Guttmann, L., and Frankel, H.: The value of intermittent catheterization in the management of traumatic paraplegia and tetraplegia. Paraplegia, 4:63, 1966.
14. Hardy, R. W., Nash, C. L., and Brodkey, J. S.: Follow-up report: Experimental and clinical studies in spinal cord monitoring. The effect of pressure, anoxia and ischaemia on spinal cord function. J. Bone Joint Surg., 55A:435, 1973.
15. Hughes, J. P., McEntire, J. D., and Setze, T. K.: Cast syndrome. Arch. Surg., 108:230, 1974.
16. Kalamchi, A., Yau, A. C. M. C., O'Brien, J. P., and Hodgson, A.: Halo pelvic distraction apparatus. J. Bone Joint Surg., 58A:1119, 1976.
17. Keim, H. A., and Weinstein, J. D.: Acute renal failure— a complication of spine fusion in the tuck position. J. Bone Joint Surg., 52A:1248, 1970.
18. Lapides, J., Diokno, A. C., Silber, S. J., and Lowe, B. S.: Clean, intermittent self catheterization in the treatment of urinary tract disease. J. Urol., 107:458, 1972.
19. Lonstein, J., Winter, R., Moe, J., and Gaines, D.: Wound infection with Harrington instrumentation and spine fusion for scoliosis. Clin. Orthop., 96:22, Oct., 1973.
20. Lundborg, G., and Rydevik, B.: Effects of stretching the tibial nerve of the rabbit. A preliminary study of the intraneural circulation and the barrier function of the perineurium. J. Bone Joint Surg., 55B:390, 1973.
21. MacEwen, D. G., Bunnell, W. P., and Sriram, K.: Acute neurological complications in the treatment of scoliosis. J. Bone Joint Surg., 57A:404, 1975.
22. McCollister, E. C.: Intraoperative autotransfusion in surgery for scoliosis—a preliminary report. J. Bone Joint Surg., 56A:1764, 1974.
23. Moe, J. H.: Complications of scoliosis treatment. Clin. Orthop., 53:21, 1967.
24. Moe, J. H., and Sundberg, B.: A clinical study of spine fusion in the growing child. J. Bone Joint Surg., 46B:784, 1964.
25. Morgenstern, J. M., Hassmann, G. C., and Keim, H. A.: Modifying post-transfusion hepatitis by gamma globulin in spinal surgery. Orthop. Rev., 4:29, June, 1975.
26. Nash, C. L., Schatzinger, L., and Lorig, R.: Intraoperative monitoring of spinal cord function during scoliosis surgery. J. Bone Joint Surg., 56A:1765, 1974.
27. Nickel, V. L., Perry, J., Garrett, A., and Heppenstall, M.: The halo. J. Bone Joint Surg., 50A:1400, 1968.
28. O'Brien, J. P.: The halo pelvic apparatus. Acta Orthop. Scand. (Suppl.), 163:79, 1975.
29. O'Brien, J. P., Yau, A. C., Smith, T. K., and Hodgson, A. R.: Halo pelvic traction. J. Bone Joint Surg., 53B:217, 1971.
30. Pinto, W. C.: Complications of surgical treatment of scoliosis. Israel J. Med. Sci., 9:837, 1973.
31. Ponte, A.: Postoperative paraplegia due to hyper-correction of scoliosis and drop in blood pressure. Scoliosis Research Society, Gothenberg, Sweden, 1973. J. Bone Joint Surg., 56A:444, 1974.
32. Ransford, A. O., and Manning, C. W. S. F.: Complications of halo-pelvic distraction for scoliosis. J. Bone Joint Surg., 57B:131, 1975.
33. Risser, J. C., and Norquist, D. M.: A followup study of the treatment of scoliosis. J. Bone Joint Surg., 40A:555, 1958.
34. Seddon, H. J.: Peripheral nerve injuries. M.R.C. Special Report Series, No. 82. Her Majesty's Stationery Office, 1954.
35. Shalding, B.: The so-called superior mesenteric artery syndrome. Am. J. Dis. Child., 130:1371, 1976.
36. Simurda, M. A.: Arteriovenous fistula and neurological sequelae of spinal fusion. Paper presented to Canadian Orthopedic Association, Bermuda, June, 1958. J. Bone Joint Surg., 51B:193, 1969.
37. Skandalakis, J. E., Akin, J. T., Milsap, J. H., and Gray, S. W.: Vascular compression of the duodenum. Contemp. Surg., 10:33, 1977.
38. Solis, R. T., and Gibbs, M. B.: Filtration of microaggregates in stored blood. Transfusion, 12:245, 1972.

39. Stagnara, P.: Utilization of Harrington device in the treatment of scoliosis. Chapchal, G. (ed.): Symposium in Nijmegen, Netherlands, 1971, p. 61. Stuttgart, George Thieme, 1973.

40. Stagnara, P.: Personal Communication, 1975.

41. Telfer, R. B., Hoyt, W. F., and Schwartz, H. S.: Crossed eyes and halo pelvic traction. (Letter to Editor.) Lancet, 2:922, 1971.

42. Tillberg, G.: Prophylaxis of postoperative venous thrombosis. Acta Orthop. Scand. (Suppl.), *158*:3, 1974.

43. Tredwell, S. J., and O'Brien, J. P.: Avascular necrosis of the proximal end of the dens. J. Bone Joint Surg., *57A*:201, 1972.

44. Tredwell, S. J., and O'Brien, J. P.: Apophyseal joint degeneration in the cervical spine following halo-pelvic distraction. Paper presented at the Annual Meeting of the Scoliosis Research Society, Louisville, Ky., September, 1975.

45. Vauzelle, C., Stagnara, P., and Jouvinroux, P.: Functional monitoring of spinal cord during spinal surgery. J. Bone Joint Surg., *55A*:441, 1973.

46. Vauzelle, C., Stagnara, P., and Jouvinroux, P.: Functional monitoring of spinal cord during spinal surgery. Clin. Orthop., *93*:173, 1973.

47. Victor, D. I., Bresnan, M. J., and Keller, R. B.: Brain abscess complicating the use of halo traction. J. Bone Joint Surg., *55A*:635, 1973.

48. Weisl, H.: Unusual complications of skull caliper traction. J. Bone Joint Surg., *54B*:143, 1972.

49. Winter, R. B.: The effects of early fusion on spine growth. *In* Zorab, P. A. (ed.): Scoliosis and Growth. Edinburgh, Churchill Livingstone, 1971.

50. Winter, R. B., Moe, J. H., and Wang, J. F.: Congenital kyphosis. J. Bone Joint Surg., *55A*:223, 1973.

51. Zielke, K., and Pellin, B.: Das Neurologische Risiko der Harrington—operation. Arch. Orthop. Unfallchir. *83*:311, 1975.

52. Zielke, K., and Pellin, B.: Halo-pelvic traction—Minderung ihrer Gefahren durch Vereinfachung der Anwendung. Z. Orthop., *112*:351, 1974.

# Chapter 17

# ADULT SCOLIOSIS

## INTRODUCTION

In our treatment center the number of adolescent patients requiring treatment is decreasing. This is related to the early detection programs in schools, with the early diagnosis of progressive deformities. This allows early bracing, and the need for surgical correction has decreased. In addition, many orthopedic surgeons nationwide have been trained to treat spine deformities. Newer techniques have made treatment of adult deformities possible. Therefore, the number of adult patients referred for evaluation and treatment of spine deformities has gradually increased. These factors make the consideration of the adult with a spine deformity important.

## PRINCIPLES

The first question that arises is, "What constitutes an adult?" By definition, an adult is an individual who has completed growth, and all the growth centers are fused. With reference to the spine, the iliac epiphyses have completed their excursion and fused (Risser 5),[27] and the vertebral ring apophyses have fused. An arbitrary age of 20 is not applicable, as a large number of people reach adulthood at 18 while some show growth activity into the early 20s.

Before discussing the evaluation and treatment of spine deformities in the adult, the reader is referred to Chapter 4, page 56 for a discussion of studies of the natural history of scoliosis in the adult years. The studies of Chapman et al.;[5] Bergofski et al.;[2] Nilsonne and Lundgren;[22] Nachemson;[20, 21] Collis and Ponseti;[6] Drummond et al.;[9] Ghavamian;[12] and Coonrad and Feierstein[7] are important. It is agreed that curves over 60 degrees often progress in adulthood. Those in the thoracic area over 60 degrees cause reduced respiratory capacity and if over 90 degrees cause an increased mortality rate with working disability from back pain or respiratory compromise.[2, 3, 4] The thoracolumbar and lumbar curves show a greater tendency for progression, and there is a high incidence of back pain in this group.[18] In addition, the work capacity of these patients is decreased, with definite psychologic disturbances.[1] These facts concerning the natural history are important and must be borne in mind when evaluating the adult with a spine deformity. In general, in the younger adult, treatment is directed toward the *prevention* of future problems, with principles similar to those in the adolescent. In the older adult the treatment is directed toward the correction of existing problems associated with the deformity.

Patients presenting for treatment in adulthood usually have deformities due to idiopathic scoliosis. The second most common group are the neuromuscular deformities, mainly poliomyelitis. Patients with congenital deformities rarely present for initial treatment as adults. Two broad categories of adults with spine deformities present for treatment—those who have not had previous surgical treatment (untreated group), and those who have had previous surgery (re-operation group). The adult with untreated deformity will be discussed here; those adults needing re-operation are discussed in Chapter 18.

**429**

## PRESENTATION

The adult patients presenting for treatment vary in age from 18 to 80, most being between 20 and 40 years of age. The majority of these patients are women, matching the greater incidence of curves requiring treatment in adolescence. The presenting complaints are pain, curve progression, cardiopulmonary decompensation, and cosmesis.

### Pain

There are only a few studies discussing the treatment of adult scoliosis,[8, 13, 17, 19, 23, 24, 29, 30, 33, 36] with additional studies of the treatment of severe curves over 90 or 100 degrees.[31, 32, 34] In all of these, pain is the most common presenting symptom. Thirty-nine per cent of Kostuik's 107 cases had pain alone, while an additional 24 per cent had pain and progression.[17] In the series of Dawson et al., from this center, 55 per cent of the 82 patients required treatment because of pain.[8] Ponder and co-workers evaluated 132 patients over age 20 requiring surgery, and the prime indication for treatment was pain.[24] This agrees with the authors' experience that the main reason that an adult seeks evaluation and treatment is pain. This fact differs from the opinions of Nachemson[20, 21] and Collis and Ponsetti,[6, 26] who found in their series of untreated scoliosis an incidence of pain equal to that of the general population. We cannot agree with their findings.

The symptom of pain is commonest in lumbar or thoracolumbar curves when these are single curves. In the double curve pattern pain occurs at the junction of the two curves. It also occurs with thoracic curves—either kyphosis or scoliosis. The pain is mechanical in nature and probably of discogenic origin and/or caused by facet arthrosis. The patient usually awakes pain-free or with a mild backache. As the day progresses the ache and back fatigue increase. The ache also becomes more severe, and the site of the pain is at or just below the apex of the curve. On lying down the pain and ache rapidly disappear. With the passage of time the pain becomes more severe and occurs more frequently, and less activity is necessary to aggravate the pain. The pain decreases the patients' activities and then markedly changes the lifestyle as a period of rest is required daily because of the severe

pain. Analgesics, which once helped control the pain, are now ineffective.

Rarely the pain is radicular. Such pain is due to nerve compression on the concavity of the fractional lumbosacral curve that is present below a large lumbar scoliosis. The degenerative arthrosis and lumbosacral curve both narrow the neural foramen with nerve root compression. This radicular pain may exist alone but more commonly is present in association with back pain due to the lumbar curve.

### Progression[14, 15]

This is rarely the main indication for surgery. Progression usually coexists with pain. Fifty-five per cent of Kostuik's cases had progression, half of these being associated with pain.[17] Progression is determined by the patients, who note a gradual loss in height coincident with an increase in the deformity. In adults being followed, serial radiography will show curve progression (Fig. 17–1). To diagnose progression, a definite increase of 5 to 10 degrees must be seen on x-ray reevaluation. If the patient is seen for the first time, any previous x-rays must be obtained for comparison. This initial x-ray in adulthood must *always* be compared with the most current film to show progression. As most curves increase 1 to 3 degrees each year, careful measurement and periodic x-rays over a number of years are necessary to show true curve increase. Measurement of the patient's height should be done at each visit.

### Cardiopulmonary Decompensation

The main reason for correcting curvatures is prevention of pulmonary compromise and secondary cardiac failure. If patients present with pulmonary decompensation, correction and stabilization of the curvature will prevent progressive deterioration of pulmonary function. Surgical correction may cause an increase in the volumetric studies, as well as an increase in the arterial partial pressure of oxygen, due to decreased shunting with straightening of the curve. If cor pulmonale is present, a decrease in pulmonary artery pressure may follow the straightening of the curve by traction and stabilization by fusion. It is rare for cardiopulmonary failure to be the main in-

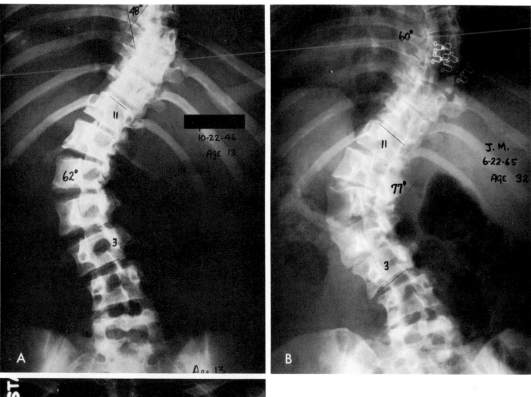

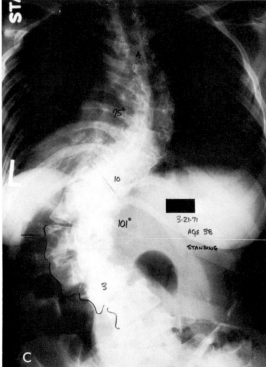

**Figure 17–1** J.McM. This patient was first seen with this 62 degree left lumbar idiopathic curve. She was treated with exercises and a Steindler brace. The brace was discontinued at age 17, and the curve measured 65 degrees. *B,* The patient married and had three children. Shortly after the birth of her third child, she noted the onset of mild aching low back pain. An x-ray at this time showed that the curve had increased to 77 degrees  Three years later the pain was more severe and started radiating into her left leg. The curve increased three degrees during these three years. *C,* The pain became more severe. It was an ache in the low back, and the patient had to rest for a while each afternoon. There was now pain in both legs with numbness and paresthesiae. She had lost two inches in height since age 18. She was referred for treatment to the Twin Cities Scoliosis Center. Anteroposterior x-ray on presentation showed a 101 degree T10–L3 left lumbar curve and a 75 degree T4–T10 right thoracic curve. Note the rotatory subluxation of L2 on L3. The marked arthrosis is seen on the concavity of the lumbar curve.

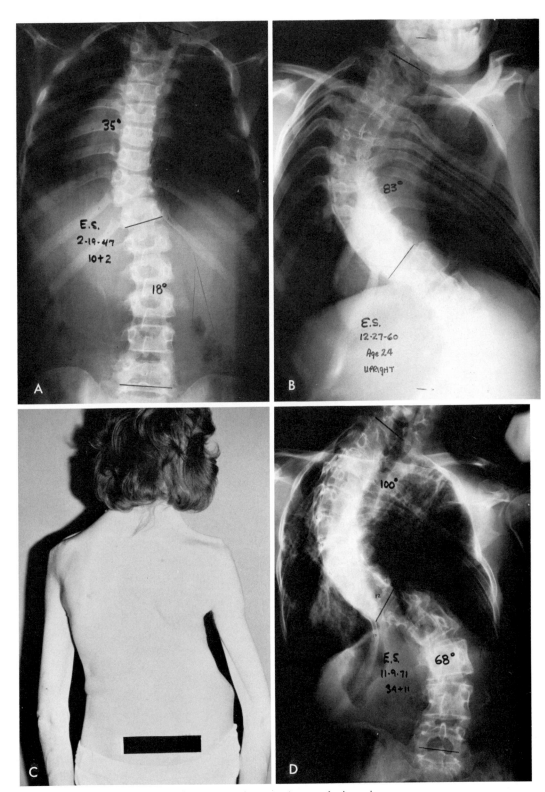

**Figure 17–2**   *See opposite page for legend.*

dication for treatment in scoliosis — it was the indication in only 15 of the 82 patients reported by Dawson (Fig. 17–2).

As respiratory failure is one of the problems that can be prevented by the treatment of scoliosis, serial pulmonary function tests should be part of the follow-up routine in a non-operated adult. A change in the curve, pain symptoms, or pulmonary function deterioration thus may become the indication for surgery.

## Cosmesis

While cosmesis alone is very rarely an indication for surgical treatment, and is usually present in conjunction with pain or progression, the patient is affected far more by cosmesis than the treating physician usually realizes. If this is discussed with the patient a year or two after surgery, the extreme psychologic effect of the preexisting deformity on the patient will be appreciated. In the past, too little attention has been paid to cosmesis and the psychologic effect of the curve.

## PATIENT EVALUATION

Patient evaluation is the first step in the care of the adult with scoliosis. A thorough history and physical examination, aided by adequate x-ray, pulmonary function tests, and ancillary tests to assess the patient's general condition allow rational decisions to be made.

## History

Why is the adult seeking evaluation? If there is pain, what is the nature of the pain; what is its site, radiation, and severity? What activities aggravate the pain, and what must be done to obtain relief? Are any analgesics necessary, and if so what type and how often? Is daily rest necessary to cope with the pain? What activities have been restricted because of the pain? The aim is to determine how the pain has affected the patient's activities and lifestyle and whether these effects are progressive.

Has any increase in the deformity been noted? Is there recent or progressive loss of height? Are any previous x-rays available for comparison with current films to document the change in the curve? As this is the only valid method of documenting progression, these previous x-rays must be obtained for comparison whenever possible.

The effect of the spine deformity on cardiorespiratory function must be documented. Any tiredness, dyspnea, tachycardia, or palpitations with effort are important. Some of these symptoms normally accompany increasing age with decreasing sports participation. It is important to determine whether these changes are static or show deterioration in cardiac or respiratory function. In addition to these specific questions, the general health of the patient is determined.

With the physical examination, the deformity, any complications, and the patient's general health are evaluated. (See Physical Examination, Chapter 3, page 14.)

A set of scoliosis films are taken and evaluated as described on page 22, Chapter 3. The curves in adults may be larger, with many over 100 degrees. They generally show rigidity as evidenced by minimal correction with side bending or traction. The facet joints show bone build-up and sclerosis on the concavity of the curve due to facet arthrosis or spontaneous fusion. In addition, in the lumbar spine, the degenerative changes are often

**Figure 17–2** A, E.S. This patient first presented at Gillette Hospital at the age of ten with a 35 degree left thoracic curve. There are hemivertebrae on the left at T3 and T10. Suspension treatment was given. Three years later the curve had increased to 40 degrees. Surgery was recommended, but the family refused treatment. B, Eleven years later the patient had a child and after delivery went into cardiac failure. This was treated medically with reversal of the failure. An upright chest x-ray showed that the curve had increased to 83 degrees. C, The patient presented 11 years later at the age of 35. She had noticed increasing fatigue during the previous year. In addition, she noted a sudden increase in her shortness of breath, and she felt that her heart rate was unsteady. A clinical view of her back showed a very thin female with a left thoracic scoliosis and decompensation to the left of 2.5 cm. She was in mild right heart failure. D, An anteroposterior standing x-ray shows a left thoracic curve of 100 degrees and a compensatory right lumbar curve of 68 degrees. The thoracic curve was rigid, correcting to 95 degrees on left side bending. Pulmonary functions showed vital capacity of 525 cc. (20 per cent of predicted normal). The $PaO_2$ was 58 and the $PaCO_2$, 50 mm Hg. Cardiac catheterization revealed a significant increase in the pulmonary wedge pressure. For treatment see Fig. 17–9.

accompanied by a rotatory subluxation at or below the center of the curve.

The lateral view is important, as apparent kyphosis often accompanies the scoliosis. The vertebral rotation must be assessed on the anteroposterior and lateral views. What often appears as kyphosis clinically in the thoracolumbar or lumbar areas is *not* true kyphosis but is a prominence caused by extreme vertebral rotation. This differentiation is important to make if the use of Dwyer instrumentation is contemplated. A view that is useful in curves over 100 degrees is the derotation view of Stagnara (plan d'election). This shows the true magnitude of the lateral curvature and shows the vertebral anatomy, allowing identification of any congenital anomalies as well as facet ankylosis (Fig. 3–27, p. 43).

The pulmonary function tests are important as an assessment of the effects of the curve on respiratory function and in the preoperative evaluation of the patient. In cases where no clear-cut indication for surgery exists, the pulmonary function tests will demonstrate any changes present as a result of the deformity. When significant reduction is present or serial tests show progressive deterioration, a more definite indication for surgery is present.

## TREATMENT

The indications for treatment in the adult presenting with a spine deformity are pain, progressive deformity, cardiorespiratory decompensation, and, rarely, neurologic problems. Where these indications exist alone or in combination, the decision is easy. In the young asymptomatic adult, the older asymptomatic adult, and the adult with only moderate pain, the decision is more difficult. The question here is not "What *can* be done?" but "What *should* be done?"

The young asymptomatic adult, under the age of 25, should be evaluated using similar criteria to those used to evaluate an older adolescent. In general this means critical evaluation for curves under 60 degrees. If pulmonary functions are definitely decreased, surgical treatment is indicated. Curves over 60 degrees are treated surgically. Asymptomatic curves under 60 degrees should be x-rayed yearly to see whether they are

progressive. Some cases of markedly decompensated lumbar or thoracolumbar curves are an exception. These usually require fusion even if they are only 45 degrees.

Asymptomatic curves in patients over 25 years of age pose a problem in decision making. If the curve is over 90 to 100 degrees, all evidence indicates that progressive curve deterioration and cardiopulmonary decompensation will occur.[3] These patients should have correction and stabilization on the basis of the curve magnitude. The only possible exception is where the curve is completely rigid on traction and side bending, and the pulmonary functions are satisfactory. If doubt exists, yearly evaluation with serial pulmonary function testing is suggested.

The patient with pain can be a problem in making a decision. Evaluation should exclude all the possible causes of low back pain caused by pathology intrinsic or extrinsic to the spine. The patient is the one who must decide whether the pain is severe enough and modifying his life enough that he wants surgical correction, knowing all the dangers and possible complications. Nonoperative treatment can be used with reevaluation to see whether the symptoms become worse.

The treatment choice is either nonoperative and operative. The choice is more difficult than the technique.

### Nonoperative treatment

Nonoperative treatment is used for: a) Mild complaints of pain, b) older patients with pain, or c) atypical pain patterns. The first factor is the exclusion of all other possible causes of back pain. An adult with an atypical pain pattern may require myelography, discography, and psychological testing for full evaluation.

Analgesics and anti-inflammatory medications are used when mild back discomfort is present. In cases where the origin of the pain is obscure, facet blocks using a local anesthetic and steroid injection are often useful. In elderly patients or those with mild painful curves, a brace often gives enough support to relieve the pain. In cases where there is facet arthrosis and a curve, with symptoms that are severe and not typical, a trial of immobilization in a body cast will determine whether stabilization will relieve the pain. There is little role for physical therapy in the non-operative treatment. Patients benefit from immobilization, *not* mobilization.

## Operative treatment

Before discussing the approaches available for the treatment of the adult with spine deformities, certain principles are important. The series on the treatment of adult scoliosis of Dawson et al.,[8] Stagnara,[30, 34] Pellin and Zielke,[23, 36] Kostuik et al.,[17] Gui and Savini,[13] and Ponder et al.[24, 25] show that the mortality and morbidity rates are high (Fig. 17–3). The incidences of thrombophlebitis, pulmonary emboli, infection, pseudarthrosis, and neurologic and psychologic problems are higher than those reported in adolescent scoliosis surgery. This is because the patients are older and generally not as healthy, with larger, more rigid curves. Healing is prolonged and general recuperation slower. Prolonged bed rest is often necessary, as multiple surgical procedures are required. Casts are not tolerated as well, as they tend to interfere with normal activities and a normal sex life.

## PRINCIPLES

Certain differences exist in the treatment of adult spine deformities compared to treatment of adolescents that are important. The aim is to correct the spine as much as is safely possible and to stabilize it in the corrected position. In general, postoperative immobilization for 12 months is necessary. Because of the high pseudarthrosis rate we frequently plan on exploration of the fusion and augmentation after six months, adding additional autologous iliac bone. The patient is immobilized for an additional six months in either a cast or a bivalved polypropylene body jacket. At six months, if the fusion appears very solid on x-ray, augmentation is not performed, but a new cast is applied.

Surgery in the adult is technically more difficult than in children and adolescents. The exposure is more difficult and takes longer, as the periosteum is not as thick. The bone often tends to be softer, and hook dislocation is more common. Because of the rigid nature of the curves, two distraction rods are often required for adequate stabilization. True kyphosis and rotatory kyphosis are common,

and thus the rods have to be contoured to fit the curve. Contouring is especially important in the lumbar spine to maintain the lumbar lordosis. If flattening occurs in this area, with elimination of lordosis, a stooped posture with leaning forward may occur (see Chapter 18).

When instrumenting curves over 100 degrees, the distraction rod usually lies over the ribs on the concavity of the curve. Often the ribs at the apex of the accompanying kyphos have to be removed subperiosteally to allow rod placement.

When a kyphosis is present, a contracting Harrington assembly is added to stabilize the kyphos. The lateral x-ray must be carefully studied to be able to appreciate the deformity in two planes. If the kyphosis is significant it may be necessary to perform an anterior fusion to stabilize the spine.

The important question with lumbar curves is whether it is necessary to fuse to the sacrum. If at all possible, fusion to the sacrum should be avoided, the fusion usually stopping at L4. This decision is based on the flexibility of the fractional lumbar curve, and especially the quantity of arthrosis between L4 and S1. If on a side bending x-ray of this curve, L5 or L4 is nearly parallel to S1 and the arthrosis is minimal, the fusion does not need to be extended to the sacrum. If on the other hand a significant residual tilt and L4–S1 arthrosis exists, and lumbosacral pain is a major symptom, fusion to the sacrum is necessary. When this is done, it is important to place the lower hook on the sacrum on the concavity of the fractional curve to prevent decompensation due to the distraction rod. This rod needs to be contoured to the existing lordosis, as a straight rod will flatten the lumbar spine.

## TECHNIQUES

The techniques applicable for untreated adult scoliosis are: 1) fusion and Harrington instrumentation, 2) traction followed by fusion and Harrington instrumentation, 3) facetectomies and a second stage spinal fusion, 4) combined anterior/posterior fusion, and 5) nerve root decompression.

***Posterior Fusion and Harrington Instrumentation.*** This is the most common procedure performed on the untreated adult scoliosis patient, especially in young adults. Previously we used preoperative traction fairly routinely in curves that showed moderate flexibility (20

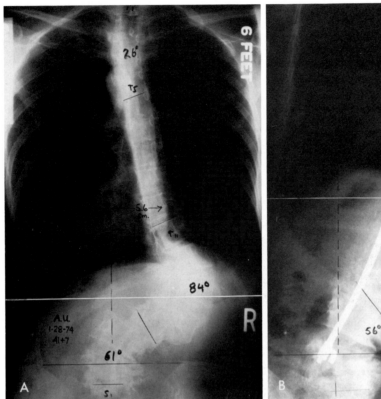

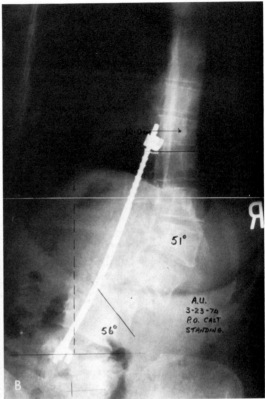

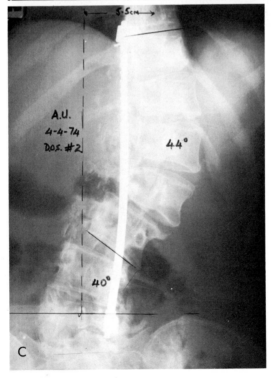

**Figure 17–3** This example demonstrates the problems and difficulties encountered in the treatment of the adult scoliosis patient. A, This 41 + 7 year old female presented idiopathic scoliosis that was first noted in adolescence and not treated. She had noted recent increase in her curve with a loss of height of four inches. There was constant severe back pain for which analgesics were necessary. This antero-posterior x-ray shows a T11 to L3 right thoracolumbar curve of 84 degrees and an L3 to S1, left lumbar curve of 61 degrees. The thorax is markedly shifted to the right, the deviation of T12 to the midsacral vertical being 5.6 cm. Clinically, the patient was deviated 3 cm. to the right. Note the rotatory subluxation at L2–L3 and L3–L4. The thoracolumbar curve corrected to 60 degrees on side bending and the lumbar curve to 54 degrees. B, A posterior spinal fusion was performed from T10 to L5, the lower hook being placed on the left on the convexity of the lumbar curve. A postoperative Risser cast was applied. There was a loss of correction in both curves, and the tilt to the right was increased. The patient felt that she was tilting to the right. C, Because of the increased tilt and decompensation due to the incorrect placement of the lower hook, it was moved to the concavity of the lumbar curve. This x-ray on the day of the second procedure showed correction of the curves to 44 degrees and 40 degrees with better balance, which was maintained in the postoperative cast.

to 40 per cent correction on side bending). For the length of time traction is used (10 to 14 days) the additional correction obtained was not sufficient to warrant this period of bed rest. In addition, the complications of traction with osteoporosis, atelectasis, and venous thrombosis are more likely to occur. We have had two patients die of pulmonary emboli while in traction. For these reasons we tend to follow the principles of Harrington and Dickson,[24, 25] who state that the patient is healthiest on admission and any bed rest places him in a less optimal condition. With the use of the Harrington outrigger, possible additional correction is obtained intra-operatively.

After full preoperative evaluation including pulmonary function testis, EKG, serum electrolytes, and medical consultation, surgery is performed. The technique, described in Chapter 20, uses autogenous iliac bone, a Harrington outrigger, and two parallel distraction rods for the larger and more rigid curves (Fig. 17–4). One week later a postoperative cast is applied, and the patient is ambulated. Six months later the cast is removed and the fusion evaluated using supine oblique views (Fig. 17–4). When doubt exists as to the fusion mass an exploration and augmentation of the fusion with iliac bone from the unused iliac crest is carried out. Immobilization in a cast or bivalved body jacket is continued for an additional six months. Some patients may need to be weaned out of their support over an additional six to nine months, this applying especially to patients with neuromuscular deformities.

***Preoperative Traction and Spinal Fusion.*** Traction is commonly used in adults for multiple stage procedures between the separate operations (see below). The types of traction used are a halo combined with femoral pins or Cotrel straps. Halopelvic distraction is used when it is mandatory to ambulate the patient.[16] Another form of traction we are using more often is the halo wheelchair. The patients are up in the chair during the day, and placed in halo-Cotrel traction or inclined bed traction at night.

We have found preoperative traction most useful in attempting to assess the operability of a patient in cardiopulmonary failure (see below) and correcting pelvic obliquity where anterior fusion and Dwyer instrumentation are not planned. In some cases of moderately rigid curves, traction is occasionally used prior to spine fusion and Harrington instru-

mentation. The basic goal of traction is to obtain a healthier, more functional patient, not a "prettier" x-ray, with more correction.

***Facetectomies and Fusion.*** In rigid curves, especially those over 90 degrees, correction prior to spinal fusion is desired. This gives a more vertical fusion mass, under compressive forces, leading to early incorporation of the bone graft. Traction alone in these rigid curves is ineffectual, and to obtain correction, the facets must be excised and osteotomized, allowing motion to occur. After obtaining correction by traction, the spine is fused at a second procedure (Fig. 17–5).

After full preoperative evaluation a halo is applied and the spine exposed over the whole length of the proposed fusion area. All facets are excised and any interlaminar bony bridging osteotomized (see Chapter 20 for full description of technique). The patient is then placed in traction for two weeks using halofemoral, halo-Cotrel, halopelvic, or the halo wheelchair. At the second procedure the spine is exposed and a spinal fusion with iliac bone graft and Harrington instrumentation performed. The majority of correction occurs in traction, the second operation merely stabilizing this correction. It is much safer to obtain correction with the patient awake, as sudden excess stretch on the spine and cord can lead to paraplegia. After the fusion, the course is the same as described in the section Posterior Fusion and Harrington Instrumentation, with immobilization for one year and reinforcement after six months.

In Europe, with widespread socialized medicine, the period of traction between the various stages is prolonged and can be up to 4 to 6 months.[30-34] In many cases this gives increased correction at the expense of spine osteoporosis and skin problems due to traction.

***Combined Anterior/Posterior Fusion.*** An anterior approach is used in the adult with kyphosis, neuromuscular thoracolumbar or lumbar curves, or, rarely, idiopathic lumbar or thoracolumbar curves. Dwyer instrumentation is used in these lumbar or thoracolumbar curves. In addition the spine is fused posteriorly, using iliac bone and Harrington instrumentation. In cases with combined fusions, the fusion rate is high and six-month reinforcement rarely indicated (Fig. 17–6).

The indication for an anterior approach in kyphosis or neuromuscular curves is well accepted. The role of anterior fusion and Dwyer instrumentation in the adult is impor-

*Text continued on page 443*

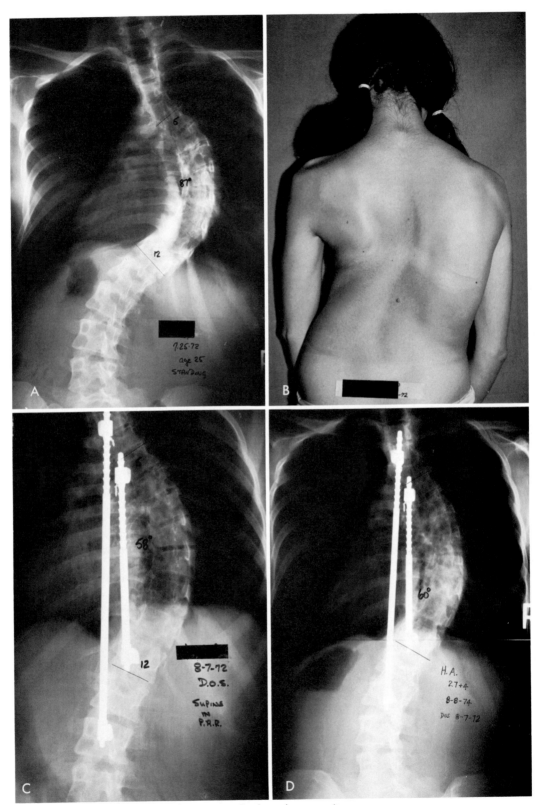

**Figure 17–4** *See legend on opposite page.*

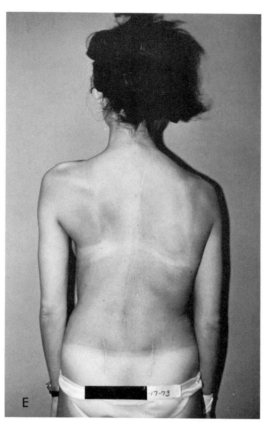

**Figure 17–4** A, H.A. This 24 year old female presented with a six month history of back pain and slight shortness of breath. Her idiopathic scoliosis was diagnosed at age 13 and treated with exercises. This anteroposterior x-ray shows an 87 degree right thoracic curve which was rigid, correcting to only 76 degrees on side bending. The patient localized her pain to the thoracolumbar area. B, Clinical view of her back shows the decompensation to the right of 3.5 cm. There is a 5.5 cm. right thoracic prominence. Pulmonary functions showed mild restrictive disease with a vital capacity of 80 per cent of predicted normal. C, After one week of Cotrel traction the curve corrected to 67 degrees. A spine fusion was performed from T3 to L2, using two distraction rods, as the curve was rigid. Correction to 58 degrees was obtained. Autologous bone from both iliac crests was added. Cotrel transverse osteotomies were performed on the right. D, Two years later, the fusion was solid with only a two degree loss of correction since the day of surgery. E, Clinical view of her back one year postoperatively shows that she is well compensated, with the plumbline falling in the gluteal cleft. The thoracic prominence is 4.2 cm.

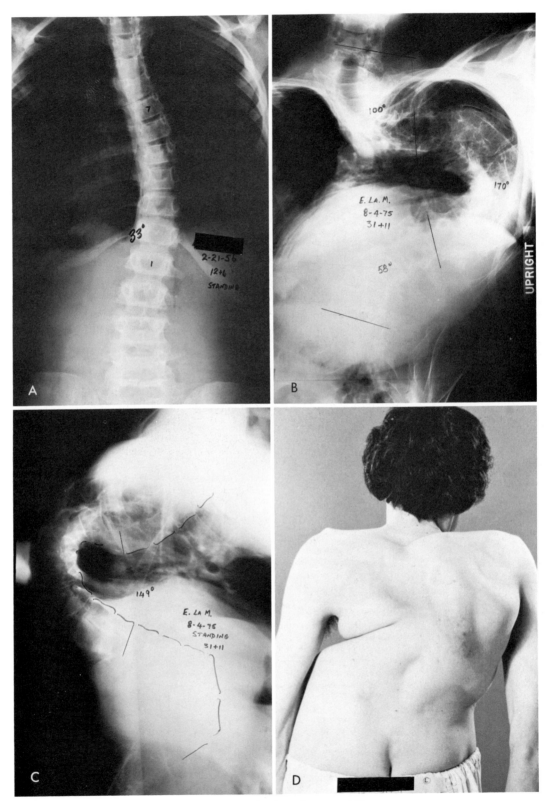

**Figure 17–5**   *See legend on page 442.*

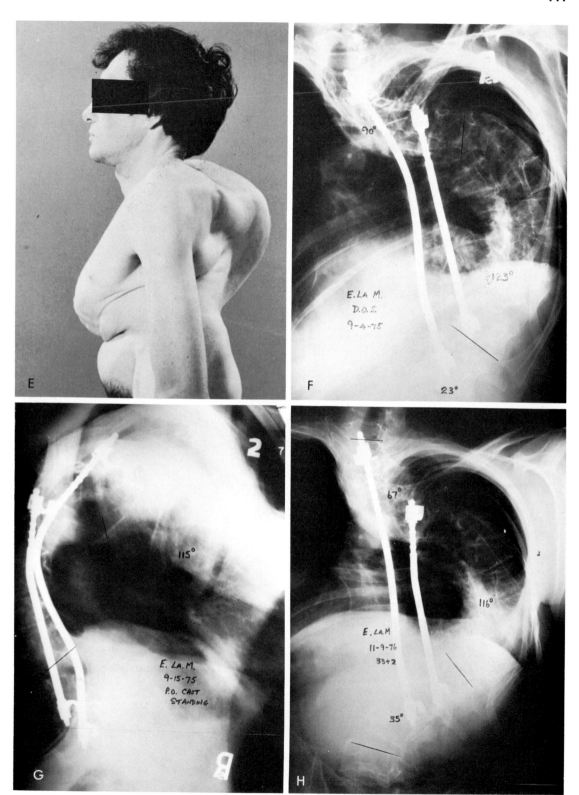

**Figure 17–5**   *See legend on following page.*

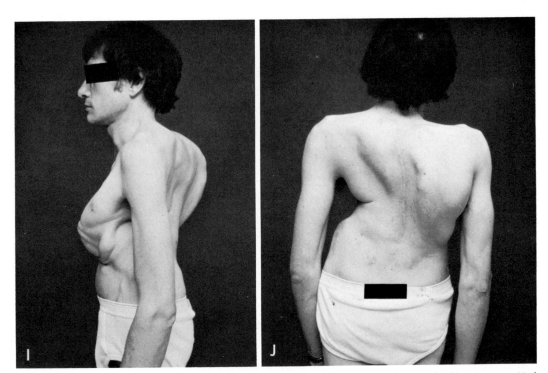

**Figure 17–5**  *A,* E.LaM. This patient was first seen at age 12½ with a T1–L1, 33 degree right thoracic curve. He had polio at the age of 9 and was left with residual abdominal muscle weakness. A Lohman fascial transplant was performed. The family did not seek further follow-up for his back. *B,* The patient presented again at the age of 32. He had noted increase in his curve, with a loss of five inches in height since age 18. There has been increasing tiredness and shortness of breath over the past four to five years, but recently this has become worse. A standing anteroposterior x-ray shows a high left thoracic curve of 100 degrees, a right thoracic curve of 170 degrees, and a left lumbar curve of 58 degrees. With traction the right thoracic curve corrected to 138 degrees. *C,* Standing lateral x-ray shows the marked kyphosis of 149 degrees. Note the marked rotation in the thoracic spine. *D,* Clinical view of the back shows the marked thoracic prominence measuring 7.2 cm. He is decompensated 1 cm. to the right of the gluteal cleft. The marked shortening of the thorax is well demonstrated. *E,* Side view shows the marked rotatory prominence with thoracic kyphosis. *F,* Pulmonary functions showed marked restriction with a vital capacity of 39 per cent of predicted normal and a $PO_2$ of 73.8 mm. of mercury. Treatment consisted of application of a halo and pelvic hoop with taking of bilateral iliac grafts at the same time. The distracting rods were applied and the patient ambulated. Ten days later, the spine was exposed from T5 to L3, and all the facets were excised. Two weeks later, after additional traction, a posterior fusion was performed from T3 to L4 using two Harrington distraction rods. This supine anteroposterior view on the day of surgery shows a right thoracic curve of 123 degrees, maintaining the correction obtained in traction. *G,* A halo cast was applied, and the patient was ambulated. There was no loss of correction. A lateral standing x-ray in the cast shows correction of the kyphosis to 115 degrees. The contouring of the rods is seen. The longer rod is contoured for the thoracic kyphosis and to maintain the lumbar lordosis. *H,* Six months later, the fusion was explored and pseudarthrosis at the thoracolumbar junction identified and cleared of fibrous tissue. The entire fusion mass was decorticated with the bone being placed at the apex of the kyphosis and over the areas of pseudoarthrosis. He was placed in a bivalved polypropylene jacket and ambulated. This anteroposterior view eight months later shows correction maintained. *I,* Side view postoperatively. The brace is worn during the day with gradual weaning over six months. This protection allows maturation of the graft to occur. Patient feels that his endurance has increased. He does not have any shortness of breath and is playing racquetball. *J,* A view of the back shows the marked improvement with lengthening of the thorax. The height gain is 10.5 cm.

tant. This allows correction of the lumbar curve and adds to the internal stability. When using the Dwyer instrumentation in adult idiopathic scoliosis it is important to study the lateral x-ray. The curve is accompanied by marked rotation and a clinical "kyphosis." It is important to differentiate rotatory kyphosis from true kyphosis, as Dwyer instrumentation is contraindicated in the presence of true kyphosis but can be used with a rotatory prominence. In addition, the amount of flexibility present is important. If the curve is rigid, with fused facet joints, a posterior releasing procedure is necessary prior to the anterior approach. There are two ways of treating this problem. The posterior facet releasing procedure can be accompanied by a posterior fusion with iliac bone but no instrumentation. Two weeks later the anterior fusion and Dwyer instrumentation are performed, followed by ambulation in a cast (Fig. 17–7). The alternate approach is to release the facets, do the anterior Dwyer fusion, and add a third stage posterior fusion with Harrington instrumentation.

A halo is applied at the same time as the first procedure when traction is necessary between the stages. Unless a halo cast is to be used for postoperative immobilization, it is removed after the second stage. If possible the patient is placed in a halo wheelchair and *not* kept supine. Unless a releasing procedure is necessary as a first stage, traction is not used in the usual idiopathic case. Active use of blow bottles plus leg motion is encouraged to prevent complications of bed rest. Prophylaxis against thrombophlebitis using aspirin or anticoagulants should be considered if bed rest is to be prolonged.

***Nerve Root Decompression.*** Nerve root decompression either is a part of the fusion operation or is a separate procedure. When there is true radicular pain, usually related to the nerve root on the concavity of the fractional lumbar curve, this nerve root needs to be decompressed. Usually the radicular pain is associated with back pain due to the lumbar curve, and the root decompression is a part of the total procedure involving spine fusion and Harrington instrumentation.

Rarely, in older adults, the only problem is the radicular pain. In these cases Epstein et al. have only decompressed the nerve root with excellent results, a spinal fusion not being

indicated.[11] We have little experience with this procedure alone.

### *CARDIOPULMONARY FAILURE*

As the problems associated with patients with cardiopulmonary failure differ from those above, a special note is necessary. These patients are in an extremely high risk surgical group and need careful preoperative evaluation and preparation. The aim is to reverse the cor pulmonale and prevent its return. Evaluation consists of pulmonary function tests and pulmonary artery wedge pressure determination. An internist helps with the patient's care with diuretics and digitalis. The important thing to determine is whether correcting the curve will improve respiratory functions and cor pulmonale. After thorough evaluation the patient is placed in traction. During the stage of failure the patient can be placed in traction sitting in bed. Progressive elongation may result in considerable improvement in the lung function.

With the cardiac failure controlled, repeat pulmonary functions and pulmonary wedge pressure tests are performed. The respiratory functions must improve, with decrease in pulmonary artery wedge pressure, before surgery can be safely considered. For this to occur, a prolonged period of traction is often necessary, as improvement is gradual. In some cases there is no response to a trial of traction, and surgical stabilization is not possible. Rarely the traction may aggravate the cardiac failure.

With improvement in the pulmonary functions and control of the cor pulmonale, a posterior spinal fusion is performed (Figs. 17–8 and 17–9). The best immobilization postoperatively is a Milwaukee brace or halo cast with no chest compression. The holding cast or brace should be as lightweight as possible and *must never* compress the thoracic cage.

The long-term prognosis in this group of patients depends on the permanent changes in the lung parenchyma, such as interstitial fibrosis and alveolar collapse. It is sometimes possible to correct and stabilize the scoliosis with resultant improvement in the respiratory and cardiac failure. However, if the lung changes are irreversible, improvement is not possible, and death from cor pulmonale will occur within a few years (Fig. 17–9).

*Text continued on page 452*

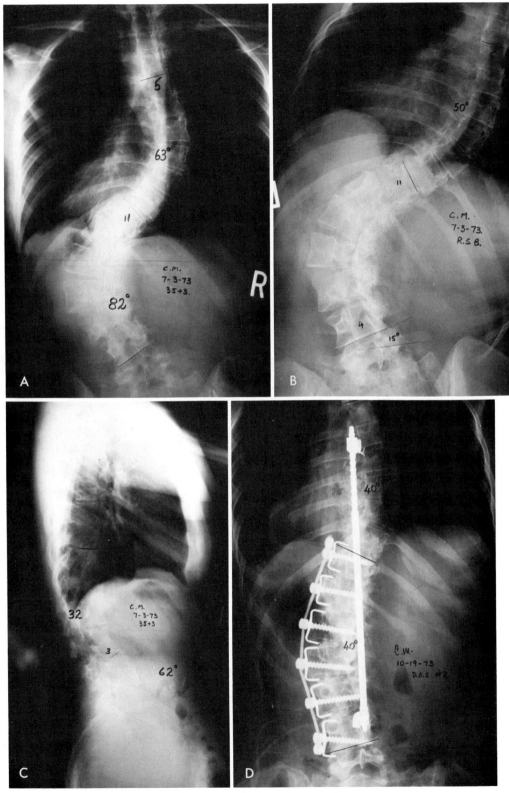

**Figure 17–6** *See legend on opposite page*

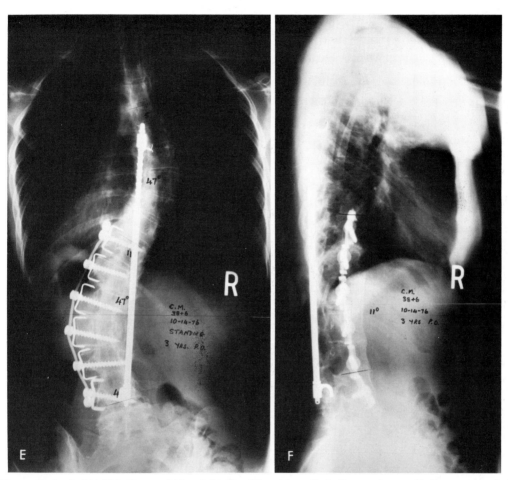

**Figure 17–6**  *A,* C.M. This 35 year old female had her idiopathic scoliosis diagnosed at age 13. She was treated with a period of casting followed by a thoracic spine fusion. She had an eight year history of pain in the thoracolumbar and left lumbar areas. This pain had become worse and had reduced her activities. In addition, there had been a 4 cm. height loss. This standing anteroposterior x-ray shows a T5–T11 right thoracic curve of 63 degrees and a T11–L4 left lumbar curve of 82 degrees. Note the marked arthrosis in the lumbar facet joints. The lumbar curve corrected to 53 degrees on side bending. *B,* A right side bending view showed that the thoracic curve corrected to 50 degrees, indicating that the fusion is not solid. L4 is nearly parallel to the pelvis, making fusion to the sacrum unnecessary. (She had no pain in the L4–S1 area.) *C,* A standing lateral view shows a thoracolumbar "kyphosis," which is rotatory in nature. *D,* Treatment consisted of an anterior fusion and Dwyer instrumentation from T11 to L4. Two weeks later a posterior fusion was performed from T5 to L4, two pseudoarthroses being present. This supine view on the day of the second procedure shows two balanced curves of 40 degrees. *E,* Three years later the patient is pain free and does not feel that her activities are restricted in any way. An anteroposterior standing x-ray shows a solid fusion and two balanced curves of 47 degrees, a loss of seven degrees in each curve. *F,* A lateral standing view shows the solid anterior fusion with reduction of the kyphosis to 11 degrees.

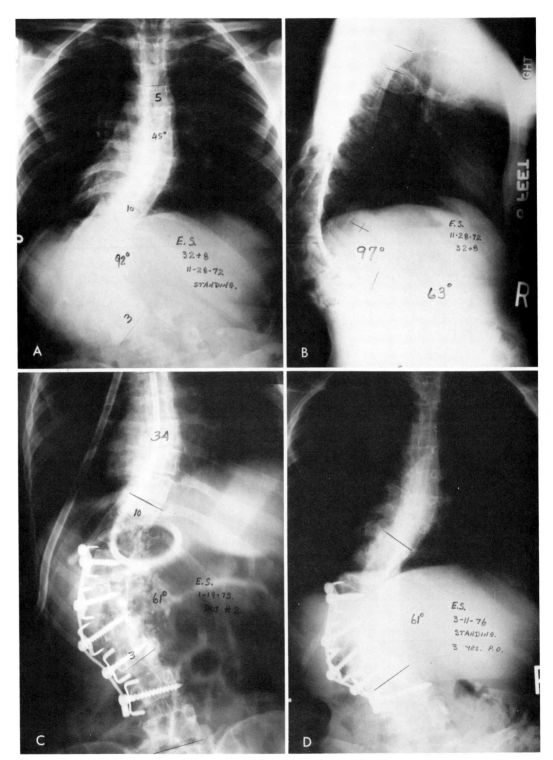

**Figure 17–7**   *See legend on opposite page.*

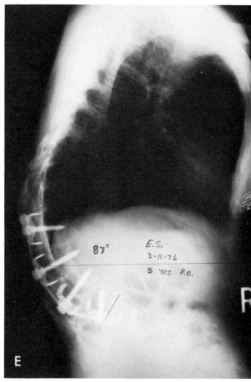

**Figure 17–7** *A,* E.S. A 32 year old female presented with idiopathic scoliosis which was first noted at age 13. She was treated with exercises, vitamin E, and a high protein diet. There has been a gradual increase over the past 14 years with a height loss of 2.5 cm. There is progressive tiredness in the back. This anteroposterior x-ray shows a T5–T10 right thoracic curve of 45 degrees and a T10–L3 left thoracolumbar curve of 92 degrees. The thoracolumbar curve corrected to 64 degrees on side bending. *B,* A lateral x-ray shows a thoracolumbar kyphosis of 97 degrees. The kyphosis is due to rotation as the vertebrae are seen in an anteroposterior projection. *C,* Treatment consisted of halofemoral traction application followed by facet excision and posterior fusion from T10 to L4. Two weeks later an anterior fusion with Dwyer instrumentation was performed from T12 to L4. The Dwyer apparatus can be used, as there is no kyphosis, the prominence being rotatory. The Dwyer should have gone up to T11. *D,* The patient was placed in a Risser body cast for nine months. Three years postoperatively, this anteroposterior x-ray shows a solid fusion with no loss of correction. The patient is asymptomatic and very happy with her appearance. *E,* A lateral view three years postoperatively. The kyphosis measures 87 degrees. The interbody fusion is well seen. A third stage posterior instrumentation should have been done to prevent this kyphosis.

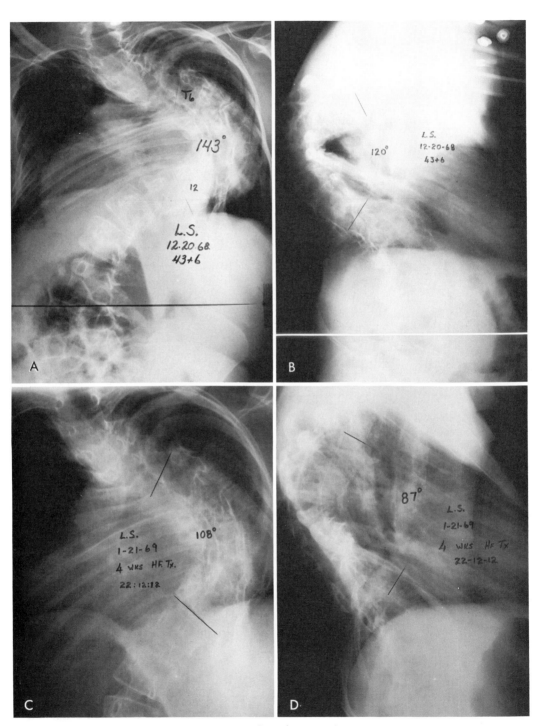

**Figure 17–8**   *See legend on opposite page.*

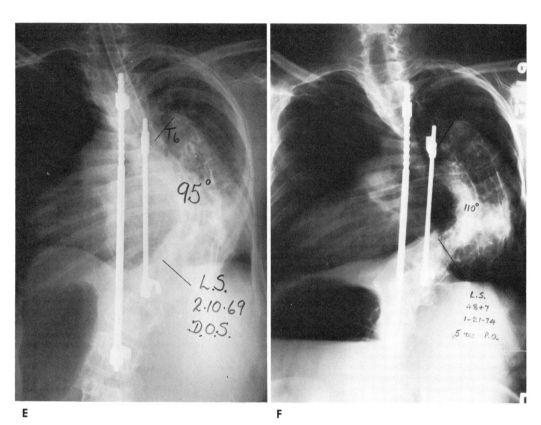

E                       F

**Figure 17–8**  *A,* L.S. is a 43 year old female who had polio at the age of 13. She was fitted with a back brace, which she wore until the age of 21. She had four uncomplicated pregnancies and presented with a six month history of increasing shortness of breath and ankle swelling. Examination revealed her to be in right-sided heart failure. The anteroposterior standing x-ray revealed a T6–T12 right thoracic curve of 143 degrees. The curve was rigid, correcting only to 130 degrees on right side bending. *B,* The standing lateral view shows a thoracic kyphosis of 120 degrees, with marked rotation of the spine. Pulmonary functions revealed a vital capacity of 850 cc. with a $PaO_2$ of 40 and a $PaCO_2$ of 54 mm. mercury. With inhalation of oxygen, the $PaO_2$ rose to 58. *C,* The patient was placed in halofemoral traction. The following table shows the result of traction:

|         | Traction     | Curve  | $PaO_2$ | $PaCO_2$ |           |
| ------- | ------------ | ------ | ------- | -------- | --------- |
| 1/9/69  | 20 lbs head  | 123°   | 76      | 64       | (3L O2)   |
| 1/21/69 | 24 lbs head  | 108°   | 51      | 49       |           |
| 2/7/69  | 30 lbs head  | 103°   |         |          |           |

The x-ray shows the correction after four weeks of traction. *D,* The kyphosis after four weeks of halofemoral traction was reduced to 87 degrees. *E,* A posterior spinal fusion was performed on 2/10/69, using two Harrington distraction rods. The correction obtained on the day of surgery was 95 degrees. The patient was ambulated in a halo cast, total cast time being 10 months. *F,* Five years postoperatively, the fusion is solid, and the thoracic curve is 110 degrees, 15 degrees loss since the day of surgery. There have been no changes in her pulmonary functions since six months postoperatively. The vital capacity is 1400 cc. with a $PaO_2$ of 54 and a $PaCO_2$ of 44 mm. mercury. The pulmonary arterial wedge pressure is increased and decreases after 15 minutes of breathing oxygen. The patient has to breathe oxygen for a few hours daily.

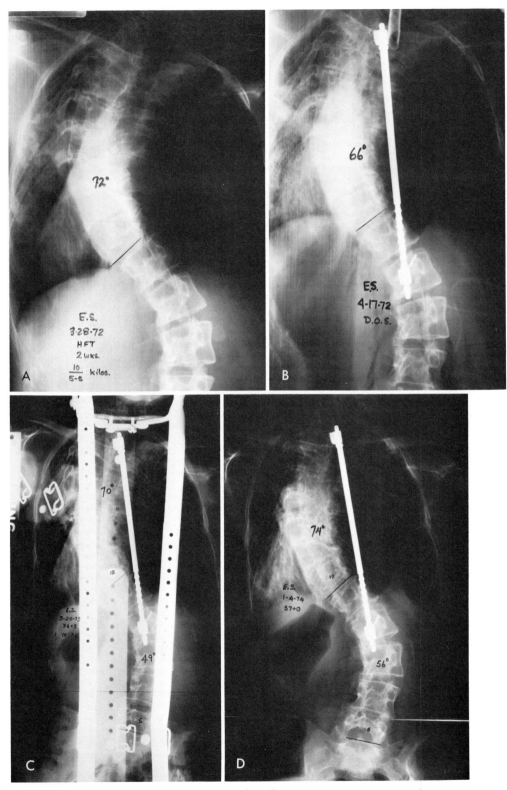

**Figure 17–9**   *See legend on opposite page.*

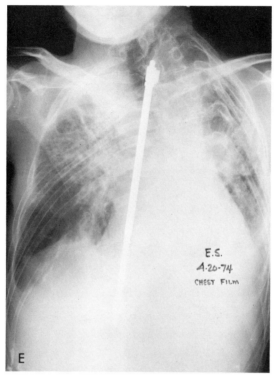

E.S.
A.20.74
CHEST FILM

E

**Figure 17–9** For history and presentation, refer to Fig. 17–2. *A,* E.S. Treatment consisted of halofemoral traction application and distraction to see whether there was any change in pulmonary functions with curve improvement. The cardiac failure was also treated medically. After two weeks of traction this x-ray shows correction of the scoliosis to 72 degrees. *B,* After an additional two weeks of traction, repeat pulmonary functions showed increase in the vital capacity to 700 cc. The $PaO_2$ had increased to 67 mm. Hg (previously 58 mm. Hg), and the $PaCO_2$ fell slightly to 46 mm. Hg (previously 50 mm. Hg). Repeat cardiac catheterization showed a significant reduction in the pulmonary arterial wedge pressure. With improvement in all the tests, fusion was indicated. Posterior spinal fusion was performed a week later from T2 to L2. This anteroposterior x-ray on the day of surgery shows correction to 66 degrees. *C,* The patient was placed in a halo cast and ambulated. Six months later she was admitted in cor pulmonale. After treatment x-rays showed a marked degree of pulmonary fibrosis. A Milwaukee brace was fitted and worn full-time. One year postoperatively this anteroposterior x-ray in the brace shows the curve of 70 degrees. *D,* Use of the brace was gradually decreased but not discontinued. The correction was maintained, being 74 degrees as shown on 1/4/74. Repeat pulmonary function showed the vital capacity to be 600 cc. The $PaO_2$ had fallen to 46, and the $PaCO_2$ was unchanged at 51 mm Hg. *E,* Patient was admitted six weeks later in cor pulmonale. This was treated, and two months later readmission was necessary for severe cor pulmonale. The chest x-ray demonstrates the severe degree of pulmonary fibrosis present. Patient died 11 days later, and the autopsy showed that both lungs were small, and microscopically there was generalized interstitial pulmonary fibrosis.

In general, we have had good response in the patients with post-poliomyelitis curves and poor response in the shorter more rigid curves of infantile idiopathic and congenital origin.

## References

1. Benetsson, G., Fällström, K., Jansson, B., and Nachemson, A.: A psychological and psychiatric investigation of the adjustment of female scoliosis. Acta Psychiatr. Scand., 50:50, 1974.
2. Bergofsky, E. H., Turino, G. M., and Fishman, A.P.: Cardiorespiratory failure in kyphoscoliosis. Medicine, 38:263–317, 1959.
3. Bjure, J., and Nachemson, A.: Non treated scoliosis. Clin. Orthop., 93:44–52, 1973.
4. Boyer, A.: Etude de la restriction ventilatoire des scolioses adultes avant et apres traitement chirurgical. Doctoral thesis; Univ. of Claude Bernard; Lyon, 1973.
5. Chapman, E. H., Dill, B. D., and Graybiel, A.: The decrease in functional capacity of the lungs and heart resulting from deformities of the chest pulmocardiac failure. Medicine, 18:167–202, 1939.
6. Collis, D. K., and Ponsetti, I. V.: Long term follow-up of patients with idiopathic scoliosis not treated surcally. J. Bone Joint Surg., 51A:425–445, 1969.
7. Coonrad, R. W., and Feierstein, M. S.: Progression of scoliosis in the adult. J. Bone Joint Surg., 58A:156, 1976.
8. Dawson, E. G., Moe, J. H., and Caron, A.: Surgical management of scoliosis in the adult. Scoliosis Research Society, 1972. J. Bone Joint Surg., 55A: 437, 1973.
9. Drummond, D. S., Fowles, J. V., Ecoyer, S., Roy, L., and Kerner, M.: Untreated scoliosis in the adult. J. Bone Joint Surg., 58A:156, 1976.
10. Duriez, J.: Evolution de la scoliose idiopathique chez l'adulte. Acta Orthop. Belg., 33:547–550, 1967.
11. Epstein, J. A., Epstein, B. S., and Lavine, L. S.: Surgical treatment of nerve root compression caused by scoliosis of the lumbar spine. J. Neurosurg., 41: 449–454, 1974.
12. Ghavamian, T.: Future of minor scoliotic curves of the spine. Exhibit, AAOS, Washington, D.C., 1972.
13. Gui, L., and Savini, R.: The surgical treatment of scoliosis in the adult. Ital. J. Orthop. Traum., 1:191–208, 1975.
14. Keim, H. A.: Scoliosis can progress in the adult. Orthop. Rev., 3:23–28, 1974.
15. Kolind-Sorensen, V.: A follow-up study of patients with idiopathic scoliosis. Acta Orthop. Scand., 44:98, 1973.
16. Kostuik, J.: Halo-pelvic traction in the surgical management of adult scoliosis. J. Bone Joint Surg., 55B: 232, 1973.
17. Kostuik, J. P., Israel, J., and Hall, J. E.: Scoliosis surgery in adults. Clin. Orthop., 93:225–234, 1973.
18. Leidholt, J., and Ballard, A.: The disability of lumbar curves in adulthood. J. Bone Joint Surg., 56A:444, 1974.
19. Marchetti, P. G.: Le Scoliosi. Bologna, Aulo Gaggi, 1968.
20. Nachemson, A.: A long term follow-up study of nontreated scoliosis. J. Bone Joint Surg., 50A:203, 1969.
21. Nachemson, A.: A long term follow-up study of nontreated scoliosis. Acta Orthop. Scand., 39:466–476, 1968.
22. Nilsonne, U., and Lundgren, K. D.: Long-term prognosis in idiopathic scoliosis. Acta Orthop. Scand., 39:456–465, 1968.
23. Pellin, B., and Zielke, K.: Scolioses sévères de l'adulte et du grand adolescent—41 cas opérés. Rev. Chir. Orthop., 60:623–633, 1974.
24. Ponder, R. C., Dickson, J. H., Harrington, P. R., and Erwin, W. D.: Results of Harrington instrumentation and fusion in the adult scoliosis patient. J. Bone Joint Surg., 57A:797–801, 1975.
25. Ponder, R. C., Dickson, J. H., Harrington, P. R., and Erwin, W. D.: Results of Harrington instrumentation and spinal fusion in the adult idiopathic scoliosis patient. A.A.O.S., San Francisco, March, 1975.
26. Ponseti, I. V.: The pathogenesis of adult scoliosis. In Zorab, P. A. (ed.): Proceedings of Second Symposium on Scoliosis Causation. Edinburgh, E & S Livingstone, 1968.
27. Risser, J. C.: The iliac apophysis: An invaluable sign in the management of scoliosis. Clin. Orthop., 11: 111–119, 1958.
28. Sicard, A., Lavarde, G., and Chaleil, B.: La greffe vertébrale dans les scolioses de l'adulte. J. Chir. (Paris), 93:517–526, 1967.
29. Sicard, A., Lavarde, G., and Chaleil, B.: Seventy instances of adult scoliosis treated with spinal fusion. Surg. Gynecol. Obstet., 126:682, 1968.
30. Stagnara, P.: Scoliosis in adults. Surgical treatment of severe forms. Excerpta Med. Found. International Congress Series No. 192, 1969.
31. Stagnara, P., Jouvinroux, P., Peloux, J., Pauchet, R., Mazoyer, D., and Callay, C.: Cyphoscolioses essentielles de l'adulte. Formes sévères de plus de 100°. Redressement partial et arthrodése. XI Sicot Congress, 206–233, Mexico City, 1969.
32. Stagnara, P., Fleury, D., Pauchet, R., Mazoyer, D., Biot, B., Vauzelle, C., and Jouvinroux, P.: Scolioses majeures de l'adulte superieures a 100°—183 cas traites chirurgicalement. Rev. Chir Orthop., 61: 101–122, 1975.
33. Stagnara, P.: Scoliose de l'Adulte chirurgie du rhumatisme. In D'Aubigne, R. M. (ed.): Chirurgie du Rhumatisme. Paris, Masson et Cie, 1971.
34. Stagnara, P.: Utilization of Harrington's device in the treatment of adult kyphoscoliosis above 100 degrees. Fourth International Symposium, 1971. Nijmegen. Stuttgart, Georg Thieme Verlag, 1973.
35. Vanderpool, D. W., James, J. I. P., and Wynne-Davies, R.: Scoliosis in the elderly. J. Bone Joint Surg., 51A:446–455, 1969.
36. Zielke, K., and Pellin, B.: Ergebnisse Operativer Skoliosen-und Kyphoskoliosen-behandlung beim Adoleszenten Uber 18 Jahre und Beim Erwachsenen. Z. Orthop., 113:157–174, 1975.

# Chapter 18

# SALVAGE AND RECONSTRUCTIVE SURGERY

The term "salvage and reconstructive surgery" refers to operations on patients who have had a previous spine fusion. The majority of patients have idiopathic or post-poliomyelitis spine deformity and have generally undergone one or more previous surgical procedures. These patients account for 31 per cent of Kostuik's series of 107 patients.[4, 5] Eleven of the 132 adult cases reported by Ponder et al. had had previous spinal fusions,[11, 12] as had 29 of Stagnara's series of 183 patients[15] and 8 of Pellin and Zielke's 41 cases.[10]

## PROBLEMS

The necessity for further surgery is based on the following problems, one or more being present in a single patient.

### Pseudarthrosis

The most common cause of problems is pseudarthrosis, either single or multiple. The commonest sites are the thoracolumbar and lumbosacral areas. Loss of correction and pain may occur at these sites. Radiographically, a distinct defect is seen crossing the fusion mass, sometimes with hypertrophic callus. These defects are best seen on oblique films of good quality.

### Loss of Correction

Many of the curves seen had fusions prior to the use of instrumentation. In some, metal reaction, infection, and instrumentation failure necessitated rod removal. If the fusion is poor and pseudarthroses are present, loss of correction with curve increase occurs. This may also occur in children who have a fusion without instrumentation and the fusion mass is not protected during growth with a Milwaukee brace. Remodeling of the bone occurs with subsequent curve increase.

In many cases, loss of height occurs, but on x-ray, the scoliosis is unchanged. An unrecognized kyphosis may be the cause. This points out the importance of appreciating all spine deformities in three dimensions and not confining the evaluation to the anteroposterior x-ray.

### Short Fusion

The patient may present years after the original fusion with an increasing deformity due to a curve that is now longer than the original curve. This is almost always due to an incorrect choice of fusion levels at the original procedure but may rarely occur despite proper selection of the fusion area. Most of the loss occurs at these additional levels, the discs opening on the convex side of the spine above or below the fusion. This is often accompanied

**453**

by a pseudarthrosis. Bending of the fusion may occur in the young even though the fusion is solid. In addition, if the lateral x-ray is not viewed, the scoliosis fusion is of correct length but stops superiorly in the middle of a thoracic kyphosis. The spine bends forward over the top of the fusion. A good example is shown in Figure 7–32, p. 182.

In children, the original fusion length was often adequate, but even with protection in a brace, the curve length increases, making the fusion of insufficient length at the end of growth.

### Loss of Lumbar Lordosis[2, 9]

This problem, appreciated more recently, is due to the use of a straight distraction rod throughout the lumbar spine. This rod flattens the lumbar spine with a resultant loss of lumbar lordosis. This deformity is particularly the result of fusion extending to the sacrum with obliteration of the normal lumbosacral angulation. It is often accompanied by a pseudarthrosis at the lumbosacral area. The result is a bending forward of the whole trunk. If hyperextension at the hips is possible, this may compensate for the loss of lordosis, but it may be necessary to stand with hip and knee flexion. In cases of poliomyelitis with hip flexion contractures and weak quadriceps muscles, this compensatory method is impossible — the patient leans forward. In addition, because of this forward stoop, support (canes or crutches) is necessary. If the lumbosacral area is not fused and the joint is normal, this will allow the patient to stand normally.

### Pain Below Fusion

Occasionally with fusions extending to L3, L4, or L5, pain develops below the fusion. These cases are difficult to evaluate, as it is often unclear whether the pain is due to facet arthrosis or disc degeneration. Careful evaluation is necessary to formulate a rational approach to therapy.

### PRESENTATION

The reasons for presentation in these cases are pain, progression of deformity, cardiopulmonary problems, or more commonly, a combination of symptoms.

### Pain

The common site of pain is at the area of pseudarthrosis with occasionally very localized tenderness. This is mechanical pain, which is relieved by bed rest and worsened with being upright, usually increasing in intensity the longer the patient is up. The pain tends to be progressive and is associated with loss of correction and loss of function.

A second type of pain is found in patients with loss of lumbar lordosis. In the morning, the patient is usually straight, can stand erect, and is pain-free. As the day progresses, a noticeable forward stoop develops, which gets worse and is accompanied by back fatigue, which also becomes worse as the day progresses. This is due to the effort of the back muscles to try to maintain the upright posture. In order to remain upright the patient must bend the knees, and the knee pain is a common presenting complaint.

The third type of pain occurs below a solid fusion and is due to disc degeneration or facet changes. This is evaluated as described in Chapter 3. This problem can often be treated by nonoperative means but may require extension of the fusion distally.

### Progression

Curve increase with loss of height is common in these cases. The progression is often accompanied by obvious increased deformity. This is confirmed when the x-rays at the time of the previous surgical procedures are compared with current x-rays. It is mandatory to obtain these x-rays for comparison so that the nature of the change will be documented, i.e., increase at the pseudarthrosis, bending above the fusion, or development of kyphosis.

### Cardiopulmonary Failure

Previously treated adults may have cardiopulmonary failure as a presenting symptom, usually in conjunction with progression. These cases are extremely difficult to treat, as correction of the deformity is rarely possible without osteotomizing the fusion mass. The latter often cannot be done because of the cor pulmonale or respiratory failure. In desperate circumstances, an osteotomy can be performed using local anesthetic.

## Loss of Function

Usually a marked functional loss is associated with the above changes. Patients who were independent ambulators now need canes or crutches for balance. Some poliomyelitis patients cannot ambulate owing to the severe unbalance and are confined to a wheelchair. Exercise tolerance decreases, and the activity level changes. All these tend to change an active person into a semi-invalid.

## PATIENT EVALUATION

The patient evaluation is the same as that described in Chapter 3. The x-rays show an area of fusion with or without Harrington instrumentation. Pseudarthroses are commonly present and easily seen on anteroposterior and oblique x-rays. When comparing the current x-ray with previous films at the time of the previous surgical procedures, loss of correction or lengthening of the curve will be diagnosed. It is essential to evaluate the lateral view to appreciate the deformity in three dimensions.

## TREATMENT[1, 4, 5, 7, 8, 10, 11, 12, 13, 15]

The common treatment for this group of patients is operative. The only exceptions are patients with a solid fusion with pain below the fusion. In these cases, it must be decided whether nonoperative treatment of bracing, analgesics, and facet blocks is sufficient to relieve symptoms or whether extension of the fusion distally is necessary.

The operative approaches available for these cases are: a) Pseudarthrosis repair; b) extension of fusion; c) single or multiple osteotomies of the fusion mass followed by traction and a second-stage fusion; d) osteotomy of fusion mass and stabilization in one stage; and, e) anterior fusion.

It is essential when evaluating the patient and x-rays that the broad aims of therapy are borne in mind. The object is to obtain a solid pain-free fusion with a level pelvis and both thorax and head in balance over the sacrum. In general, a single stage procedure is preferable to multiple stages, if both can achieve the same result. One of the deciding factors is the pelvic level and balance of head over sacrum

on admission. If these are present with lesser curves, a simple pseudarthrosis repair or extension of fusion is preferable to multiple osteotomies and second-stage fusion. In severe deformities, the danger of cord stretching and paralysis is lessened by a multiple stage procedure.

## Pseudarthrosis Repair (Fig. 18-2)

When a pseudarthrosis exists with symptoms or loss of correction, repair is indicated. Often the diagnosis is difficult to make on a single anteroposterior view, and oblique x-rays, or tomograms are helpful. If the spine is well balanced with minimal loss of correction but primarily painful, the pseudarthrosis alone is repaired. It is identified at surgery as an area of firm adherence when stripping the periosteum. This is cleaned using sharp dissection. The area of the pseudarthrosis is curetted free of all fibrous tissue and autogenous iliac bone and local graft bone added. To immobilize this area all other Harrington instrumentation is removed, and two compression rods are used across the area of pseudarthrosis. Distraction rods alone should be avoided in the lumbar spine. At the lumbosacral area, it is difficult to obtain fusion when a pseudarthrosis is present. Above, there is a solid fusion column and below, a mobile pelvis—here, compression rods are invaluable, and it is often advantageous to add bilateral trochanteric extensions to the holding cast or brace to help immobilize the pelvis.

Often pseudarthroses occur in combination with loss of correction and a decompensated curve, and here it is used as one of the sites of osteotomy (see below).

## Extension of Fusion (Fig. 18-2)

When the original fusion is too short, either due to incorrect choice of fusion levels or due to "adding on," an extension of the fusion is necessary. That can be either a single procedure with Harrington instrumentation, or part of a corrective procedure using osteotomies of the previous mass. Instrumentation is used from the end of the current curve, including the vertebrae that had "added on."

*Text continued on page 461*

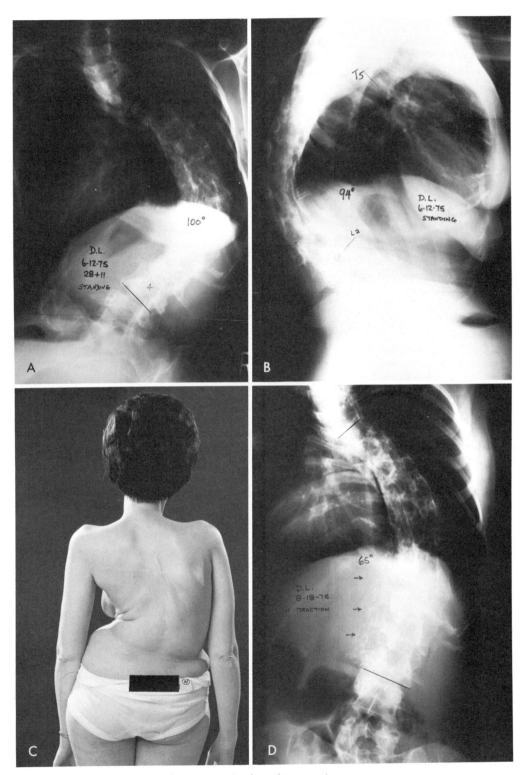

**Figure 18–1** *See legend on opposite page.*

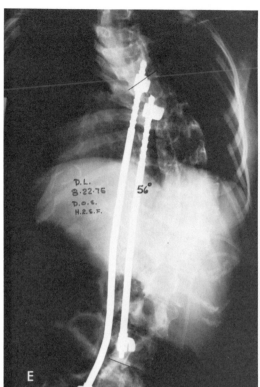

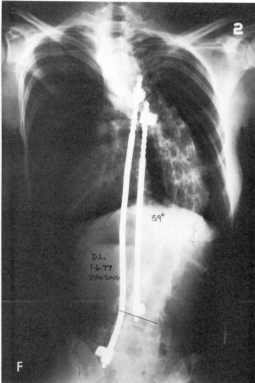

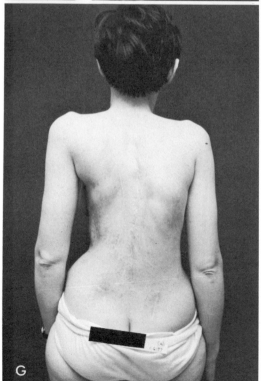

**Figure 18–1** *A,* D.C.: A 29 year old female had polio at the age of 6, with residual spine problems and a left foot drop. At age 10, a spinal fusion was performed in two stages using autogenous tibial struts. For the past few years there has been progressive back and right rib-cage pain. The curvature has progressed, and there has been a loss of height of 5 cm. An anteroposterior standing spine x-ray shows the previous fusion from T6 to approximately L2 or L3. The original curve has lengthened and now extends from T6 to L4 and measures 100 degrees. On right side bending it is rigid and corrects to 90 degrees only. *B,* A lateral standing view shows 94 degrees of thoracic kyphosis, with marked vertebral rotation. *C,* Back view shows clinical decompensation to the left of 4.0 cm. The rib prominence is sharp, measuring 7.5 cm. *D,* Treatment consisted of halofemoral traction application, followed by multiple osteotomies of the previous fusion mass, followed by correction in distraction. After 10 days of traction the curve was 65 degrees. The areas of the osteotomies are well seen. *E,* A posterior spinal fusion was performed from T3 to the sacrum using two distraction Harrington rods. This photo shows the correction on the day of the fusion. After ambulating for six months in a Risser cast, the fusion mass was explored, an L5–S1 pseudarthrosis repaired, and additional autogenous iliac bone added. The new cast was removed after an additional five months' immobilization, the fusion now being solid but not mature. Immobilization in a bivalved body jacket was continued full-time for six months during the day thereafter. *F,* One year later the fusion was solid and mature, the curve measuring 59 degrees. Gradual weaning from the body jacket was carried out over the next three months. *G,* Clinical view of the back shows the marked improvement in compensation. The height gain is 5.5 cm.

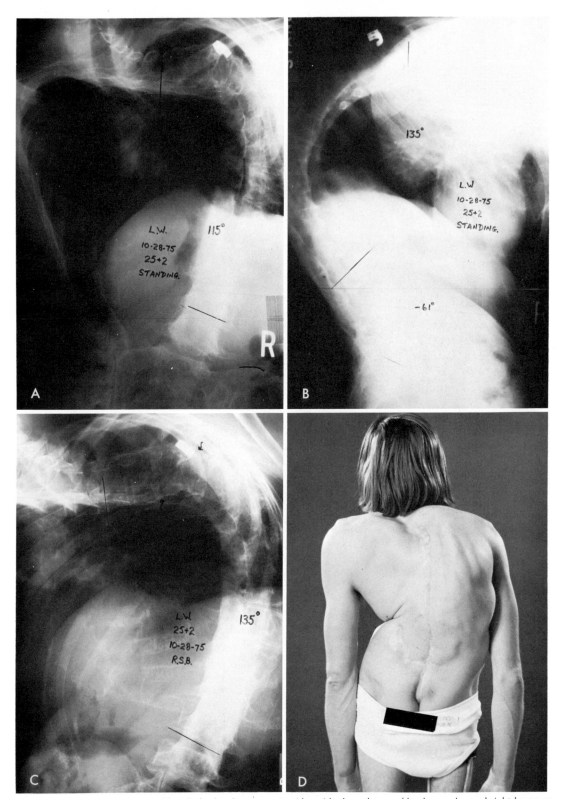

**Figure 18–2**  *A,* A 25 year old male had polio at age 7 with residual weakness of back muscles and right lower extremity. Has had numerous surgical procedures on his leg and wears an above-knee orthosis. Spine deformity, diagnosed at age 9, was treated initially with a brace. At age 14, he had a spine fusion, and during the next 5 years had an additional 8 spine procedures for recurrent pseudarthroses and infections, including removal of Harrington instrumentation. For the past few years he has had pain in the upper part of his back, which is worse at the end of the day. He feels that his deformity has increased, with his ribs impinging on his pelvis and a loss of height of 7 cm. Exercise tolerance has decreased. Standing anteroposterior x-ray shows a T4–L4 right thoracic curve of 115 degrees. A hook is still present in the upper thoracic area, with acute bending of the spine in the area of the hook. There is a solid fusion below this.

*Legend continued on opposite page*

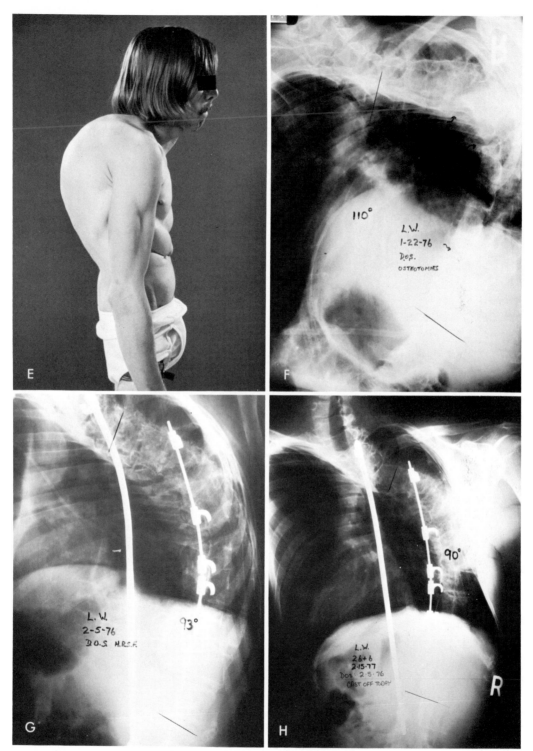

**Figure 18–2** *Continued  B,* Lateral standing view shows 135 degrees of thoracic kyphosis. This is not true kyphosis; there is much vertebral rotation seen in anteroposterior projection. *C,* Right side bending view: thoracic curve measures 135 degrees, more than standing view because the view supine is oblique, not truly anteroposterior. Large oblique pseudarthrosis is visible in area of hook, where a large amount of acute lateral bending occurs. *D,* Decompensation is 4 cm. to the left with impingement of ribs on left against iliac crest. *E,* Clinical side view shows severe thoracic kyphosis. Vital capacity is 2.5 liters (46% predicted normal) with a PaO$_2$ of 76 and PaCO$_2$ of 36 mm. Hg. *F,* Treatment consisted of halo application and multiple osteotomies of spine, the uppermost being in the area of the pseudarthrosis. X-ray taken on day of surgery shows osteotomies. *G,* After 2 weeks of halo-Cotrel traction, spine was fused from T1–L4 using contoured distraction rod for the scoliosis and compression rod for the kyphosis. Correction of scoliosis was 93 degrees. Halocast was worn for 6 months, followed by reinforcement of the fusion. No active infection occurred. Closure after each stage was over irrigation and suction tubes. Keflin was given orally for 3 months. *H,* Risser cast was worn for 6 months. On removal of cast, fusion was solid and correction maintained at 90 degrees.

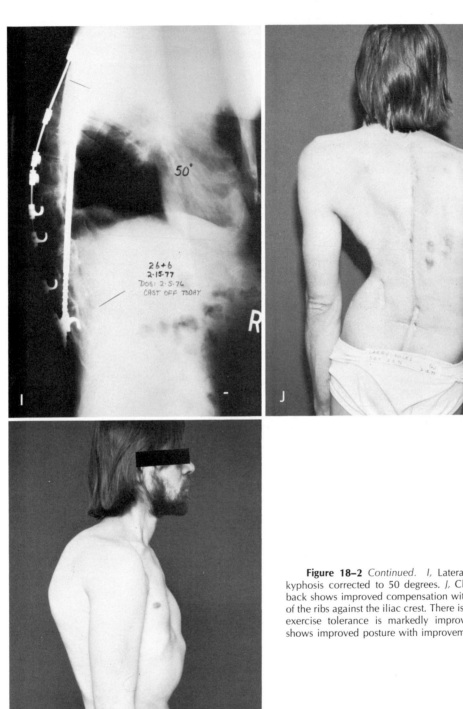

**Figure 18–2** *Continued.* *I,* Lateral view shows the kyphosis corrected to 50 degrees. *J,* Clinical view of the back shows improved compensation with no impingement of the ribs against the iliac crest. There is no back pain, and exercise tolerance is markedly improved. *K,* Side view shows improved posture with improvement in kyphosis.

## Osteotomies Plus Traction Plus Fusion[3, 6, 7, 8, 13, 14, 16]

The commonest problem requiring reconstruction is one with pseudarthroses, loss of correction, and lengthening of the curve. There is usually a marked decompensation and often some pelvic obliquity and a poor fusion mass. The aim of treatment is to realign the spine with a level pelvis, with thorax and head balanced above the sacrum. In assessing the problem, the amount of kyphosis must be appreciated. In congenital spine deformities, and where spontaneous interbody fusion is suspected, laminography will show open disc spaces — sites at which osteotomies can be performed.

The treatment regimen consists of halo application and multiple osteotomies of the fusion mass under one anesthetic. The areas of pseudarthrosis are cleaned of all fibrous tissue and widened into an osteotomy. The sites of the osteotomy depend on the curve present, one being situated at the apex of the

kyphosis or scoliosis with others at intervals above and below the apex. (For technique refer to Chapter 20.) Good motion must be obtained at each level. Multiple osteotomies are safer than a single osteotomy. The patient is now placed in traction, either halo femoral or halo-wheelchair. Halofemoral traction is invaluable for cases with pelvic obliquity where asymmetric traction or a unilateral femoral pin is necessary to level the pelvis.

After two weeks of traction, a spine fusion is performed using two distraction rods and one compression rod, the exact choice depending on the deformity present. In general, the instrumentation maintains the correction obtained with traction, excess traction being dangerous for spinal cord function. Iliac bone is added to aid in the fusion process. After approximately one week of additional traction, a cast is applied, either a halo cast or a Risser cast. Adults may tolerate a halo cast with less difficulty than a Risser cast (Figs. 18–1 and 18–2).

*Text continued on page 465*

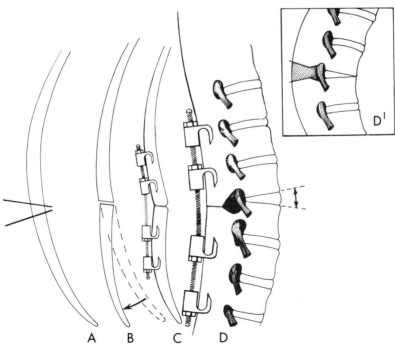

**Figure 18–3** Technique of lumbar closing wedge osteotomy for restoration of lumbar lordosis. *A, B,* and *C* show schematic representation of the osteotomy. *A,* The fusion mass is shown with the wedge of bone, the osteotomy being wider posteriorly. *B,* After the bone has been removed, the fusion mass inferiorly corrects, closing the wedge. *C,* The osteotomy is compressed and closed using two Harrington compression systems, the hooks being placed in the fusion mass. *D ',* Close-up of area of osteotomy. Note that the disc space is closed anteriorly. The wedge of bone has been removed, the apex of the wedge being anterior. The osteotomy is performed at the level of the intervertebral foramen, the nerve roots being visualized. Note that the osteotomy is undermined to prevent pinching of the dura when the closure occurs. *D,* The osteotomy is closed completely. The disc space opens anteriorly at the level of the osteotomy.

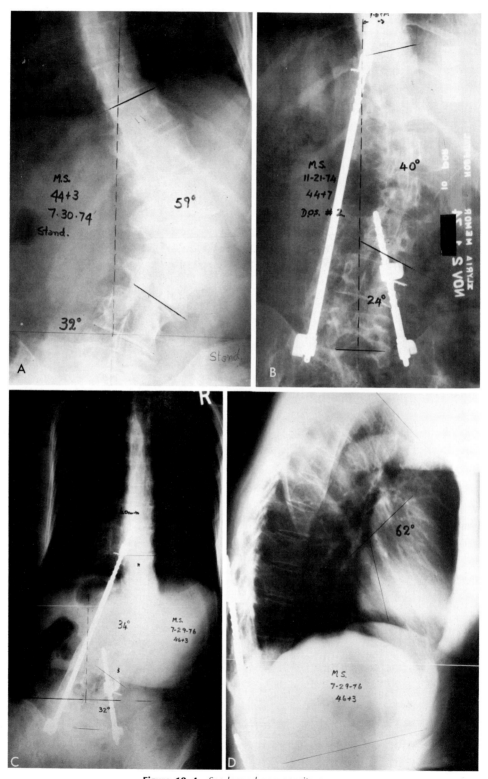

**Figure 18–4** *See legend on opposite page.*

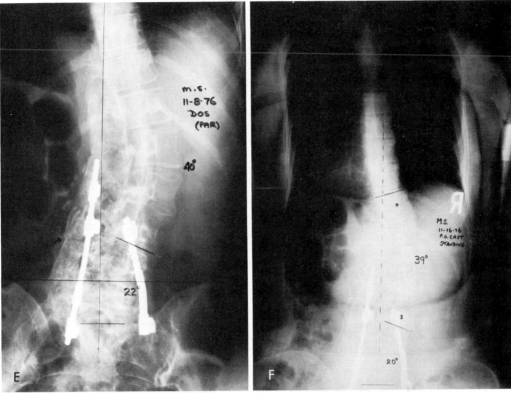

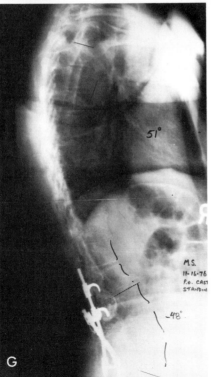

**Figure 18–4** *A,* M.S.: A female with idiopathic scoliosis that was diagnosed at age 16. She was asymptomatic and not treated. She had no problems till the age of 43, when she started having severe back pain with increasing deformity and loss of height. This standing antero-posterior x-ray shows a T11–L3 right lumbar curve of 59 degrees. *B,* Treatment consisted of posterior fusion from T10 to the sacrum. Note that the lower hook on the left was placed on the convexity of the fractional lower lumbar curve. Postoperatively the patient had a pulmonary embolus and was treated with heparin and Coumadin. On standing the patient was decompensated to the right. Because of the decompensation, reoperation was necessary, and a short distraction rod was placed from L3 to the sacrum to restore the balance, as this view demonstrates. The patient was ambulated in a cast for five months. *C,* The patient presented to the Twin Cities Scoliosis Center a year later. She complained of being deviated to the right. There is discomfort in the upper thoracic spine which is worse at the end of the day. At the end of the day, she felt as if she was deviating more to the right and forward. This anteroposterior standing x-ray shows the marked deviation to the right. The fusion is solid. *D,* Lateral standing x-ray shows the straight rod in the lumbar area with a flat lumbar spine. There is a kyphosis of 62 degrees. *E,* Surgery consisted of a lumbar wedge osteotomy, the osteotomy being fashioned to correct both the deviation to the right and the flattened lumbar spine. The supine anteroposterior view on the day of surgery shows the site of the osteotomy, which has been closed using a compression rod on the left and a distraction rod on the right. *F,* An underarm cast was applied. An anteroposterior standing x-ray in the cast shows the correction of the list. *G,* A lateral standing x-ray in the cast shows the restoration of the lumbar lordosis with improvement of standing balance.

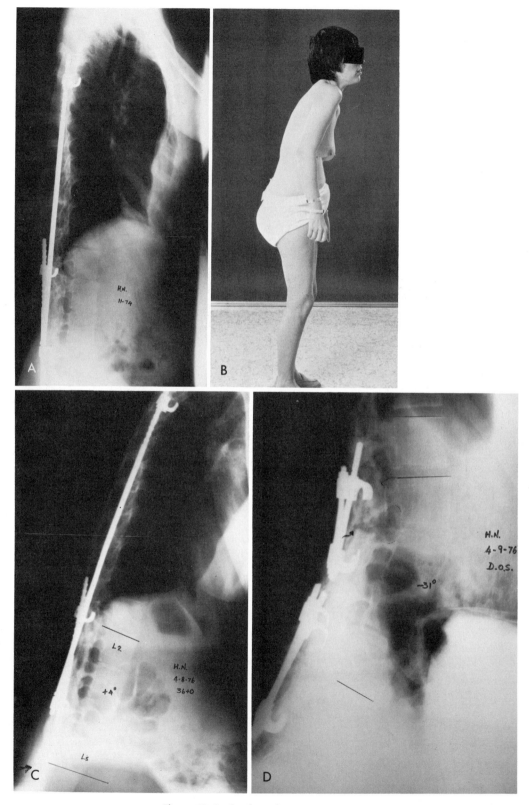

**Figure 18–5**    *See legend on opposite page.*

After six months, the cast is removed and the fusion mass assessed radiographically. If any doubt exists about the incorporation of the bone fusion, or with longer curves, exploration of the fusion area with augmentation using autogenous iliac bone and pseudarthrosis repair is performed. The fusion area is immobilized for a further six months in a cast or bivalved polypropylene body jacket.

## Osteotomy and Fusion in One Stage

In certain cases where the deformity is in one area, it is possible to perform a closing wedge osteotomy at one level with closure of the osteotomy at one stage. The typical example of this is the treatment of loss of lumbar lordosis with forward stoop. Here the fusion mass is widely osteotomized, making the osteotomy slightly wider posteriorly (Fig. 18–3). It is essential to undermine the two edges of the osteotomy to prevent pinching the dural sac when the osteotomy is closed. In addition, the nerve roots are visualized so that they do not become compressed between the pedicles when the osteotomy is closed. Two compression rods are inserted, with the hooks placed in the fusion mass and the osteotomy closed. The surrounding bone is decorticated and either local or iliac bone added. Immobilization for six months is usually sufficient to achieve a solid arthrodesis (Figs. 18–4 and 18–5).

In rare cases, a lateral decompensation is present following a posterior fusion, the main site of deformity falling at one level. In these cases, a single closing wedge osteotomy using compression and distraction instrumentation will correct the deformity (Fig. 18–4).

## Anterior Fusion

In reconstructive surgery, anterior spinal fusion has two roles. First, in the presence of kyphosis that was previously unrecognized, or where a poor anterior fusion was performed, a repeat anterior approach with fusion of sufficient length is necessary. Often a combination of ribs, fibula, and iliac crest bone is necessary. It must be borne in mind that cortical bone incorporates very slowly in adults, and iliac bone is the best graft for rapid incorporation.

In certain cases in adults, numerous attempts at posterior pseudarthrosis repair fail. In these cases, to achieve a solid fusion, an anterior approach with an interbody fusion should be performed at the level of pseudarthrosis. The latter should also be explored posteriorly, with excision of fibrous tissue and additional cancellous bone. Using this combined anterior and posterior approach, these persistent pseudarthrosis problems are usually solved.

The most difficult pseudarthroses to repair are those at the lumbosacral junction. Here there is a long lever arm of fused spine above the pseudarthrosis with a mobile pelvis below it. Numerous attempts at repair are common. The use of fibrous tissue excision, iliac bone plus compression instrumentation posteriorly, and anterior interbody fusion will help to ensure an adequate fusion.

## SUMMARY

In general, the adult case of salvage of reconstructive surgery has had numerous previous procedures with varying degrees of success. Each case needs to be evaluated individually and the correct treatment program chosen for that patient. There is no

---

**Figure 18–5** *A*, H.N.: This female had polio at the age of 12. She was asymptomatic till 1973, when she had back pain that was significant and progressive. The right thoracic curve of 60 degrees was treated with a posterior fusion from T4 to the sacrum. This standing lateral view one year postoperatively shows a very straight spine with loss of the normal lumbar lordosis. *B*, Two and one half years postoperatively, at age 36, she presented to the Twin Cities Scoliosis Center with progressive difficulty with ambulation. She felt stooped forward, the stoop increasing in the evening with aching that got worse as the day progressed. The side view shows the marked forward stooping posture. The knees are bent to allow a more upright posture. *C*, A lateral standing x-ray with her knees straight shows the loss of lumbar lordosis and the forward stoop of the whole spine. *D*, Treatment consisted of a closing wedge osteotomy of the lumbar spine with closure using bilateral compression Harrington rods. In addition, the pseudarthrosis was repaired and immobilized with two Harrington compression rods. After six months' immobilization in an underarm cast, the osteotomy and pseudarthrosis were solid. The posture is upright with no tendency to stooping forward.

patient as appreciative as one who after years of pain, reduced function, and a miserable life can now resume all the activities he or she desires.

## REFERENCES

1. Dawson, E. G., Moe, J. H., and Caron, A.: Surgical management of scoliosis in the adult. Scoliosis Research Society, 1972. J. Bone Joint Surg., 55A: 437, 1973.
2. Doherty, J.: Complications of fusion in lumbar scoliosis. Scoliosis Research Society, Wilmington, Delaware, 1972.
3. Herbert, J. J.: Vertebral osteotomy. Technique, indications and results. J. Bone Joint Surg., 30A:680–689, July, 1948.
4. Kostuik, J.: Halo-pelvic traction in the surgical management of adult scoliosis. J. Bone Joint Surg., 55B: 232, 1973.
5. Kostuik, J. P., Israel, J., and Hall, J. E.: Scoliosis surgery in adults. Clin. Orthop., 93:225–234, 1973.
6. Law, W. A.: Osteotomy of the spine. J. Bone Joint Surg., 44A:1199–1206, Sept., 1962.
7. Meiss, W. C.: Spinal osteotomy following fusion for paralytic scoliosis. J. Bone Joint Surg., 37A:73–77, 1955.
8. Moe, J., and Welch, J. A.: Post fusion spinal osteotomy.

Presented at Gillette Children's Hospital, Dec. 18, 1971.
9. Moe, J. H., Groebler, L., and Winter, R. B.: Loss of lumbar lordosis. In preparation.
10. Pellin, B., and Zielke, K.: Scolioses severes de l'adulte et du grand adolescent—41 cas operes. Rev. Chir. Orthop., 60:623–633, 1974.
11. Ponder, R. C., Dickson, J. H., Harrington, P. R., and Erwin, W. D.: Results of Harrington instrumentation and fusion in the adult scoliosis patient. J. Bone Joint Surg., 57A:797–801, 1975.
12. Ponder, R. C., Dickson, J. H., Harrington, P. R., and Erwin, W. D.: Results of Harrington instrumentation and spinal fusion in the adult idiopathic scoliosis patient. A.A.O.S., San Francisco, March, 1975.
13. Schmidt, A. C.: Osteotomy of the fused scoliotic spine and use of halo traction apparatus. In Symposium on the Spine. St. Louis, C. V. Mosby Co., 265–282, 1969.
14. Smith-Peterson, M. N., Larson, C. B., and Aufranc, O. E.: Osteotomy of the spine for correction of flexion deformity in rheumatoid arthritis. J. Bone Joint Surg., 27–1:1–11, January, 1945.
15. Stagnara, P., Fleury, D., Fauchet, R., Mazoyer, D., Biot, B., Vauzelle, C., and Jouvinroux, P.: Scolioses majeures de l'adulte supérierures à 100°—183 cas traités chirurgicalement. Rev. Chir. Orthop., 61:101–122, 1975.
16. Von Lackum, W. H., and Smith, A. DeF.: Removal of vertebral bodies in the treatment of scoliosis. Surg. Gynecol. Obstet., 57:250, 1933.

# Chapter 19

# CAST TECHNIQUES

## INTRODUCTION

Early medical writings contain many descriptions of crude and ingenious devices for distraction and straightening of spinal curvatures. There is no evidence that such devices were helpful until the introduction of plaster of Paris body casts during the latter part of the nineteenth century.[7, 8, 9, 10] Bradford and Brackett described correction on a distraction frame and holding of correction with a body cast. The correction was rarely maintained. Not until the technique of spinal fusion was introduced by Hibbs in 1911 was there any method for prolonged maintenance of correction.

Great strides have been made in the technique of cast correction. Risser perfected the turnbuckle cast in 1927[7] and combined the technique of distraction and lateral pressure with his "localizer cast" in 1952. This cast was used with early postoperative ambulation and is a widely used and effective method of maintaining correction obtained at fusion.[8] Dr. Yves Cotrel of Berck-Plage, France, developed the E.D.F. (elongation, derotation, flexion) cast, which in principle is similar to Risser's localizer cast.[2, 3]

The casts used at the Twin Cities Scoliosis Center embody some of the principles of the Risser and Cotrel casts.

### Risser "Localizer" Cast (Fig. 19–1)

This cast extends from the mandible and occiput to the buttocks, sometimes being cut down to a low neck or shoulder straps. It is applied supine on a Risser frame, a well-

molded pelvic portion being applied first. Traction is now applied via a disposable head halter and the pelvic section, and the remainder of the cast is applied with careful molding around the mandible, occiput and

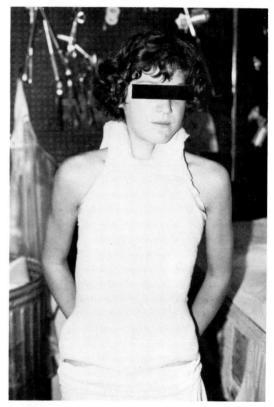

**Figure 19–1** Risser "localizer" cast for lumbar curves with shoulder straps. The cast is applied in two sections with careful molding around the pelvis and upper thorax. A localizer device presses against the convexity of the curve. The cast is extended to the mandible and occiput for thoracic curves. (Published with permission of Dr. J. Risser.)

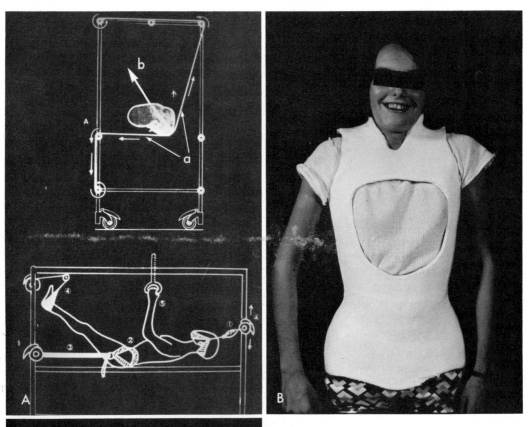

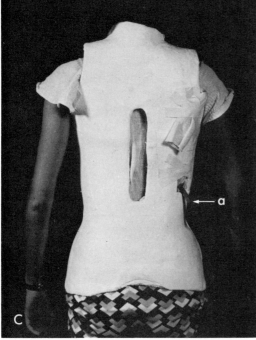

**Figure 19–2**   *A,* Cotrel, E.D.F. (elongation, derotation, flexion) principle. The patient is positioned on a special frame and placed in longitudinal traction using a head halter and pelvic straps. The hips are flexed. After the cast has been applied a derotation strap (a) is added, which passes under the patient and then overhead on the side of the convexity of the curve. Tension in this strap gives a derotating corrective vector (b) on the rib prominence. *B and C,* The cast is applied in one piece on the Cotrel frame. There is a large chest window anteriorly and a smaller window posteriorly over the concavity of the curve. In addition an inflatable bladder (a) is added over the convexity to correct the rotational prominence. (Published with permission of Dr. Y. Cotrel.)

upper thorax. A localizer device is attached that presses against the convexity of the curve, thus correcting the curve. The cast is trimmed and finished allowing hip flexion to 100° and adequate arm function. The fit over the thorax is loose to allow chest expansion.

### Cotrel E.D.F. Cast (Fig. 19–2)

The Cotrel E.D.F. cast is applied on a special frame, which is basically a Risser frame with an overhead attachment with numerous correcting pulleys. The patient is placed supine in traction using a Cotrel head halter (see page 528) and muslin straps passing around the waist, in much the same manner as the Cotrel pelvic straps (see page 528). The cast is applied in one piece, without adding a mandibular/occipital piece. Derotation straps are used, which pass under the patient and are attached to the frame next to

and above the patient, creating a lateral and derotating force against the convexity of the curve. Additional straps correct shoulder elevation and help maintain torso balance. Correction is obtained by adjusting the traction and the tension in these straps with the aid of the ratchets and pulleys. The cast is trimmed, giving shoulder straps, an anterior chest window, and a posterior window on the concavity of the curve. In addition, an inflatable bladder is added over the convexity of the curve to correct the rotational prominence.

Dr. Stagnara of Lyon, France, uses similar principles in his distraction cast and postoperative cast (Figs. 19–3 and 19–4).[6]

### Risser-Cotrel Cast

The cast used at the Twin Cities Scoliosis Center is a combination of the two casts and techniques above. It is basically a Risser cast

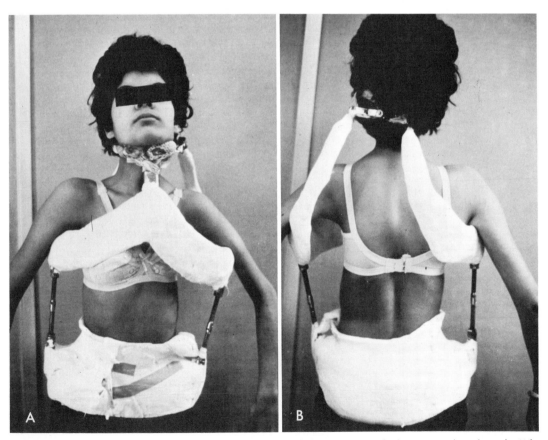

**Figure 19–3** Distraction cast as used by Dr. Stagnara. Gradual distraction is applied over a number of months. When maximal correction is obtained, the two parts of the cast are attached and the turnbuckles removed. (Published with permission of Dr. P. Stagnara.)

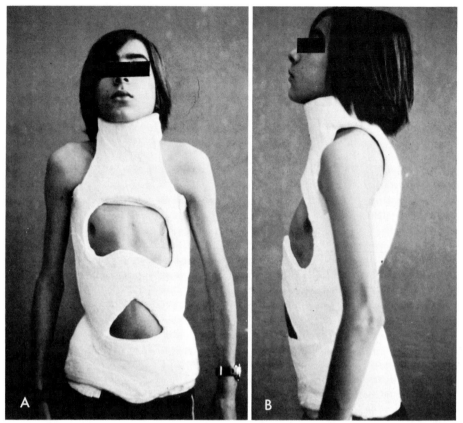

**Figure 19–4**  Postoperative cast as used by Dr. Stagnara. Note the head position with the cast causing head extension. The cast has a small chest window and also a small abdominal window. (Published with the permission of Dr. P. Stagnara.)

applied in one piece with a mandibular occipital section, using the distraction technique of Cotrel plus his derotation strap and a posterior thoracic window (Figs. 19–5 and 19–6).

## TECHNIQUES OF APPLICATION[5]

The commonest cast used is the postoperative Risser-Cotrel cast for scoliosis. This will be described first and the modifications in applying other casts will follow.

### Postoperative Risser-Cotrel Cast

The casting frame used is a modified Risser table (Fig. 19–7*A*). An overhead frame is added with pulleys for the derotation strap. The removable shoulder bar has been replaced by a flat bar, which allows application of a total contact cast. The sacral bar has been modified by the addition of a rectangular sacral seat, which allows for better application of the cast around the pelvis. There is a windlass at the head end and two at the foot end of the table for longitudinal traction.

The patient lies on a cart and is placed in two layers of tubular stockinet. The stockinet must be long enough to extend from mid-thighs to over the head. The outer layer is rolled up to around the lower abdomen. The patient is placed on the Risser table and positioned so that the removable cross bar lies at the level of the axilla (Fig. 19–7*B*). The cross bar is padded with a strip of felt. The sacral seat should comfortably support the pelvis with the sacral bar lying below the buttocks. The legs are supported on a wooden leg support which is not raised, maintaining a normal lumbar lordosis. A longitudinal canvas strap is *not* used in the postoperative cast.

Traction is applied with a disposable head halter, which is attached to the windlass at the head end of the frame. Muslin straps are

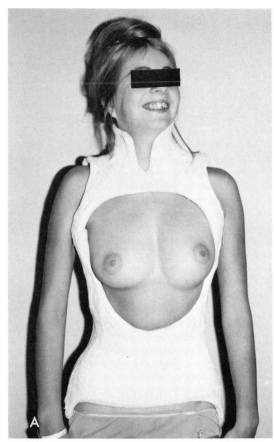
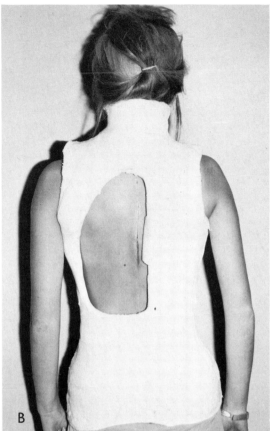

**Figure 19–5**  Risser-Cotrel cast. The cast is a combination of the principles of Risser and Cotrel. The cast extends from the mandible and occiput to the groin and buttocks. There is a large *thoracic* window anteriorly to allow full chest expansion. The cast is trimmed to allow full hip flexion and arm movement. Posteriorly the cast fits *under* the occiput and extends low over the buttocks to control pelvic tilt. A large window is removed over the concavity of the curve to allow expansion in this area with restriction over the rotational rib prominence.

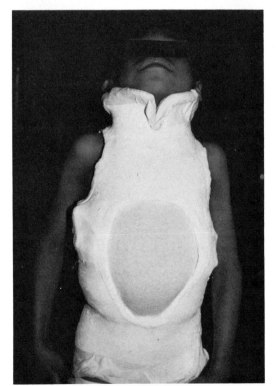

**Figure 19–6**  Example of a poorly fitted cast. The cast is poorly contoured to the patient. The anterior window is over the abdomen, and chest expansion is restricted. The neck applies distraction and extension, making normal functioning impossible.

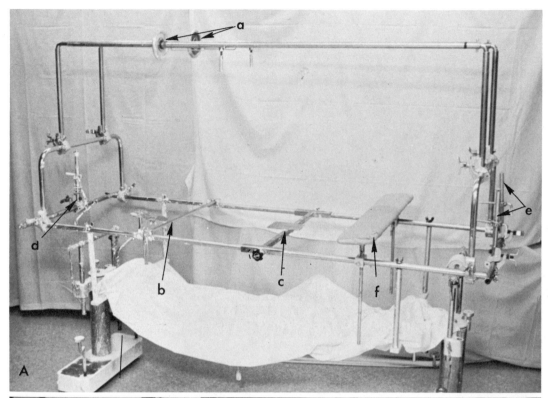

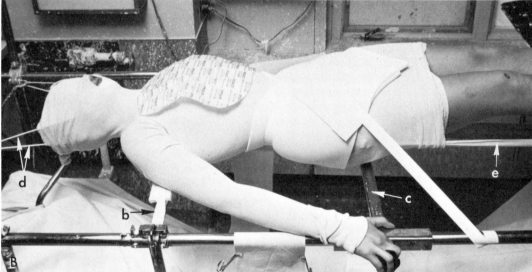

**Figure 19–7**   Technique of cast application. *A,* Casting frame. The frame is a modified Risser table with an overhead frame with pulleys (a) for the derotation strap. The patient lies on the shoulder bar (b) and sacral seat (c). Traction is applied via the windlass at the head of the table (d) and the two at the foot of the table (e). The feet are supported on the foot board (f), *no* hip flexion being used. *B,* The patient is placed in two layers of stockinet and positioned on the cast table. The shoulder bar (b) lies at the level of the axilla and the sacral bar and seat (c) lie just below the buttocks at the level of the greater trochanters. Longitudinal traction is applied via a disposable head halter (d), and muslin straps (e) are attached to windlasses. Note that the muslin straps pass around the pelvis between the two layers of stockinet and are tied at the level of the greater trochanter. The only padding used is ¼ ″ foam around the pelvis.

*Legend continued on opposite page*

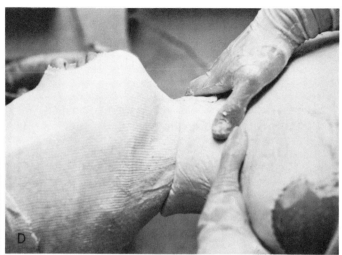

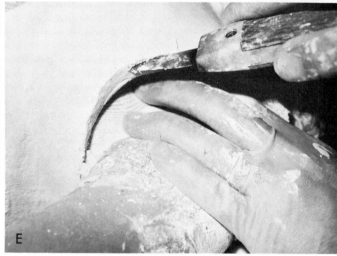

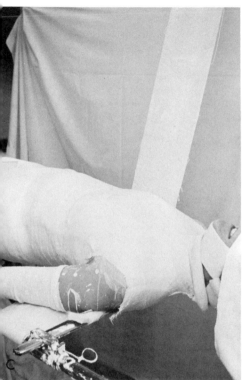

**Figure 19–7** *Continued. C,* Derotation strap. The Cotrel derotation strap passes from the side bar on the concavity of the curve, under the patient and to the pulley on the overhead bar on the side of the convexity of the curve. The strap is applied after the whole cast is applied and the plaster is setting. *D,* The neck is molded carefully to the contours of the patient. The plaster fits snugly around the neck and extends to below mandible and occiput with a fit the same as that of a well fitting Milwaukee-brace neck ring. *E,* The edges of the cast are finished by careful skiving. The cast is undercut to eliminate all sharp edges.

passed around the waist over one layer of stockinet, positioned just above the iliac crest, and tied on the opposite side at the level of the greater trochanter. Both straps are passed under the leg support to the foot of the table. They are attached to separate windlasses, and longitudinal traction is applied. The outer layer of stockinet is rolled over the muslin straps. These straps thus lie *between* the two layers of stockinet, allowing easy removal after the cast is applied. Maximal tolerated distraction is applied. The patient is awake and not sedated. Ketamine anesthesia is used in smaller children or in patients unable to cooperate. A four or six inch canvas strap is

attached to the frame so that it will pass under the patient and be applied to the convexity of the curve. Two straps are used for double curves.

The only padding used is $1/4$ inch foam rubber,* which is placed as a single sheet around the waist and hips and taped in place. No other padding is used. In very bony patients felt padding is added, being used as donuts *around* bony prominences. The stockinet must be free of wrinkles. The position of the patient is checked. The pelvis must be

---

*"Profex" brand, Airfoam Splint & Cast Padding—1/4", 1/2".

level with the torso and head in balance above it. The suprasternal notch lies over the pelvis. The head level is checked by elevating or lowering the head support, the head positioned so that the ears are over the middle of the shoulder.

Extra strong, resin-reinforced plaster is used, as it allows application of a thinner cast. Two six-inch rolls are applied, rolling from the pelvis upward, covering the torso evenly and going over the shoulders. Five by thirty-six inch splints (five to six layers thick) are applied posteriorly, starting over the buttocks and extending up, each splint overlapping the one previously applied. Splints are placed over the shoulders, running from the pelvis, over the shoulder, and then down the back. While the splints are incorporated using one or two plaster rolls, the neck is added. A four inch plaster roll is placed around the neck and mandible and reinforced using four by fifteen inch splints placed obliquely. The upper end of these splints is *below* the mandible and occiput, at the final level of the neck piece. These splints are incorporated with a four inch plaster roll. The application of plaster is rapid so that all the plaster still is wet, allowing molding and incorporation of the layers.

The Cotrel strap is placed under the patient *outside* the plaster and attached to the windlass on the overhead frame on the convexity, and a derotation force is applied to the convexity of the curve (Fig. 19–7C). The plaster is carefully rubbed to incorporate layers. The cast is molded to the contours of the body, care being taken especially posteriorly with molding under the occiput (Fig. 19–7D). Care is taken to mold over soft tissues with no pressure applied over bony prominences. In cases with a sharp "razor back" rib prominence, the Cotrel strap is not used, as localized pressure against the rib prominence can cause skin necrosis. Hand molding is used, ensuring that pressure on the apex of the kyphos is avoided, the molding being on the medial wall of the rib hump.

Once the plaster has set, the cast is trimmed. The neck is trimmed about half an inch below the mandible with an anterior notch for the trachea, the latter extending to the suprasternal notch. The pelvic section is trimmed above the pubis and laterally over the thighs to give enough room for 100 degrees of hip flexion. Note that the lower end of the cast is trimmed to resemble a Milwaukee brace pelvic section. The plaster is trimmed in the

area of the shoulders, allowing full arm motion. A large thoracic window is removed, extending to the epigastrium but leaving plaster covering the lower abdomen. Enough plaster is removed laterally to allow full chest expansion. Plaster should not compress the breasts.

The patient is removed from the Risser frame. The removable cross bar at the shoulder, once removed, allows the patient to be easily lifted onto a cart. The back of the cast is trimmed below the occiput and low over the buttocks. In patients with a very bony sacrum, extra felt padding is added at the sides of the sacrum to remove any pressure over the midline of the sacrum. A window is removed posteriorly on the side of the concavity of the thoracic curve, allowing the "thoracic valley" to be expanded with the use of breathing exercises. Sharp areas are removed by skiving the edges (Fig. 19–7E). The two layers of stockinet are pulled taut and fixed in place to the cast, using half-length three inch wide splints. No sharp edges or rough areas should remain.

The cast is usually applied five to seven days postoperatively. Absorbable intracuticular skin sutures are used so there is no need to delay cast application to remove skin sutures. After the cast is applied the patient is x-rayed supine and then is ambulated the same day. Constant attention to cast fit is necessary. Any area of pain is inspected for redness. The cast must be relieved in this area or, when necessary, padding added. The padding is applied around but never *over* bony prominences. If pain occurs under the cast, the area is windowed to inspect the skin. With this careful attention to cast application and fit, pressure sores are unusual.

With early ambulation, not more than five degrees should be lost between the supine and standing x-rays, the supine film being usually equal to or a few degrees better than the correction obtained on the day of surgery. If more than five degrees are lost the cause is usually a poor cast, and a new cast should be applied. The average cast time is eight to nine months, the cast being changed once. If the fusion extends above T4, a new Risser-Cotrel cast is usually applied. An underarm cast is used for the second cast if the fusion ends at T5 or below. With this technique, surgical correction is maintained, and five degrees loss between the day of surgery and one year postoperatively is average.[4]

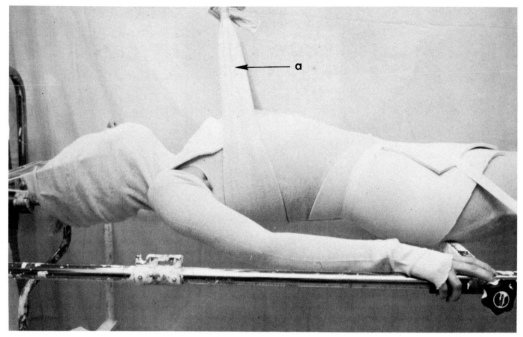

**Figure 19–8**  Position for hyperextension casting. The position is similar to that shown above in Fig. 19–7B for the Risser-Cotrel cast. The shoulder bar is removed after the patient is suspended by a hyperextension strap (a). This strap consists of a long piece of four inch tubular stockinet with a strip of ¼ " thick felt in the stockinet. The strap is attached to the pulleys on the overhead frame and is positioned at the apex of the kyphosis.

### Hyperextension Cast

The patient is placed in two layers of stockinet, positioned on the Risser frame as described above, and placed in traction (Fig. 19–8). In the patient with kyphosis the head is positioned more anteriorly as compared with a Risser cast. A hyperextension strap is placed around the patient and attached to the two pulleys on the overhead frame. This strap consists of a long piece of four inch tubular stockinet with a strip of one quarter inch felt placed *in* the stockinet. This strap is positioned over the apex of the kyphosis and is tightened until it lifts the patient off the shoulder bar. The two straps are tied together to allow adequate fit around the thorax. This causes restriction of breathing, and the patient must be reassured during cast application. The shoulder bar is removed, the patient being supported on the strap and sacral seat (Fig. 19–8). The position of the head is checked, as is the balance of the patient. Foam padding is placed around the pelvis.

The cast is applied as above, with care being taken to place reinforcing four inch splints vertically along the lateral aspect of the thorax. Once the plaster is set, it is trimmed.

The chest window is made large to allow full chest expansion. There is no posterior window, but the cast is windowed over the apex of the kyphosis, and the hyperextension strap is cut, the window being replaced. This prevents a ridge of pressure over the kyphosis and makes pressure sores over the kyphosis rare.

In cases with high thoracic kyphosis, the hyperextension strap is difficult to use. The patient is positioned with the apex of the kyphosis on the cross bar, and the latter is *not* removed. The bar then acts as the hyperextension force.

### Preoperative Cast

The preoperative cast is used to obtain preoperative correction. The cast is applied a day or two prior to surgery, surgery being performed through a large window in the cast. The basic technique of application is similar to the postoperative cast, with the following differences:

1. A longitudinal canvas strap is used, attached to a windlass at the foot of the frame

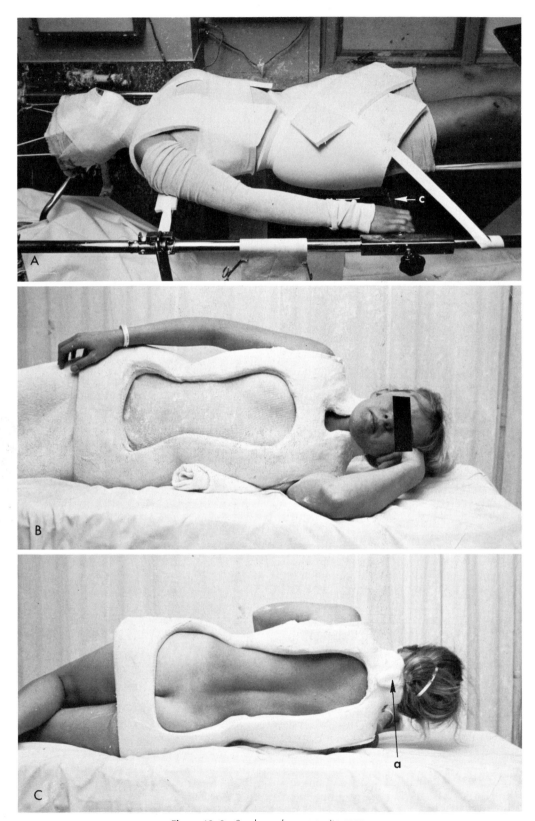

**Figure 19–9** *See legend on opposite page.*

and passing around the shoulder bar. This supports the patient and allows the cast to be applied low on the pelvis, allowing an adequate window to be removed for surgery. The patient is placed in two layers of stockinet and positioned on the Risser frame lying on the canvas strap. The sacral bar is positioned low on the buttocks or even in the upper thigh region, allowing the cast to be applied low anteriorly and posteriorly (Fig. 19–9A).

2. One-half inch foam padding is used over the pelvis, with additional foam padding over the shoulder, ribs, and sternal area.

3. The cast application technique is similar to the postoperative cast, except that the cast extends lower inferiorly. More splints are placed around the pelvic area and laterally along the thorax. The plaster is placed in areas that are not going to be removed when the cast is trimmed. This careful placement of splints assures the strength of the cast.

4. The anterior trimming of the neck is low to allow the neck of the cast to be bent out at the time of intubation. The cast is trimmed as shown in Figure 19–9B and C. Note that the neck is trimmed low posteriorly. This allows head and neck extension at the time of intubation. There is a four inch bar across the pubis with extensive cut over the abdomen and chest preventing pressure on the abdomen and chest in the prone position during surgery. Care must be taken not to remove the plaster on the lateral aspect of the thorax. If the cast is trimmed too widely in this area, the patient will fall out of the cast when positioned prone for surgery.

5. The occipital area is trimmed just below the occiput. A knob of plaster is placed in this area after the cast is trimmed. This knob is used during surgery to help support the wrapping around the head. This holds the head backward, preventing it from falling forward when the patient is positioned prone for surgery. If the head falls forward the

jugular veins are compressed against the cast resulting in venous obstruction and severe facial edema.

6. A large area is removed posteriorly, exposing an area for surgery and for taking the iliac bone. The cast extends over the buttocks.

7. The cast is skived and finished. The patient is kept supine after the cast is applied. A supine x-ray is taken to document the correction obtained in the cast.

## Underarm Cast (Fig. 19–10)

An underarm cast is used as the second cast for most spine fusions, the exception being high curves with the upper limit of the fusion above T5. This cast is also used for some cases of lumbar and all cases of lumbosacral fusions.

The technique of application is similar to the postoperative cast with the following exceptions:

1. The cast extends only to the sternum anteriorly and upper back posteriorly.

2. The patient is positioned low on the shoulder bar, which lies at the upper shoulders.

3. The arms are placed in a relaxed manner on the side bars and *not* pulled down.

4. Plaster is applied to under the arms with reinforcement anteriorly over the sternum and posteriorly as high as possible.

5. The cast is well molded around the pelvis and iliac crests. The cast is trimmed at the suprasternal notch and then to under the arms. A large thoracic window is removed leaving three to four inches (7 to 10 cm) above the window. This portion is cut wider than necessary, the final trim being performed with the patient sitting. No posterior window is removed.

---

Figure 19–9 Application of preoperative cast. A, Position for cast application. The position is similar to that shown above for the Risser-Cotrel cast in Fig. 19–7B. The patient is positioned on the longitudinal strap, and the sacral support (c) is positioned very low, behind the upper thighs. The padding consists of 1/2'' foam around the pelvis and over the shoulders and down the lateral thorax anteriorly and posteriorly. B and C, Completed cast. B, Anterior view shows the cast extending low anteriorly. There is a large chest and abdominal window but enough support is left laterally in the thoracic area to support the patient when prone. C, Posterior view shows that the cast extends very low over the buttocks. A large window is removed to allow an adequate area for prepping and draping, expecially in the area of the iliac donor site. A knob of plaster (a) is placed in the occipital area. This is used during surgery to help support the head wrapping.

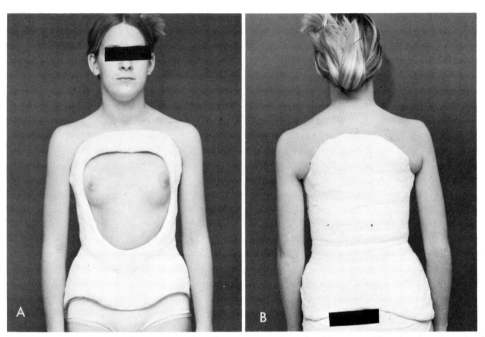

**Figure 19–10**   Underarm cast. This cast extends to the sternum with no shoulder straps. There is a large anterior thoracic window and *no* posterior window.

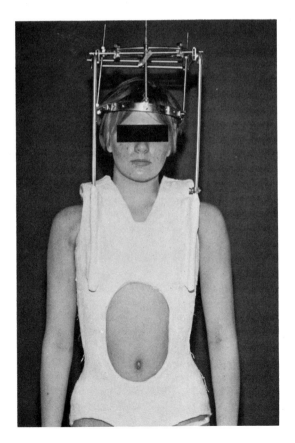

**Figure 19–11** "Old style" halo cast. The halo is supported by an overhead frame, which is attached to the cast anteriorly. A small anterior window was used. The halo cast was bulky and made it difficult for patients to get around, especially in cars.

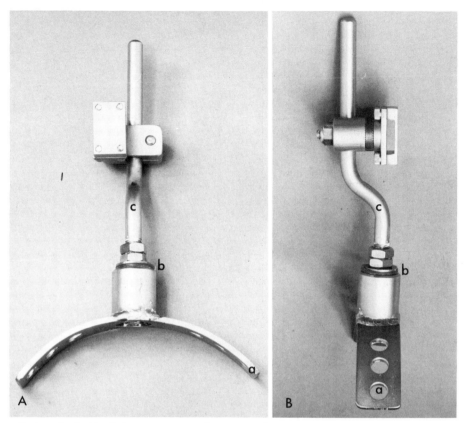

**Figure 19-12** "Lo-Profile" halo supports. Lateral view (*A*) and anterior view (*B*). The shoulder support (a) is malleable and is contoured to the shoulder straps of the cast. A silicone bushing (b) allows some motion of the upright (c). This upright is either straight or bent; the latter, which is illustrated, is necessary for children. The halo attachment allows control of halo height, tilt, and anteroposterior position.

**Halo Cast** (Figs. 19–11 to 19–15)

The halo cast is used for immobilization of cervical fractures and fusions, and fusion of cervicothoracic curves. This cast also aids in the postoperative immobilization of severe curves. The postoperative "old style" halo support consisted of two anterior uprights that extend to a frame to which the halo is attached (Fig. 19–11). The new "lo-profile" supports extend from the shoulder of the cast to the halo with silicone bushings at the junction of the uprights and shoulder supports (Fig. 19–12).[1] Both these supports allow a little motion, thus preventing the pin-skull interface from being the main site of motion. Both the halo supports allow for adjustments in head position.

The fit of the cast is as the postoperative cast, the differences being as follows:

1. The halo, having previously been applied, is suspended from the overhead frame and traction is applied to the halo. Counter-traction is supplied by the muslin straps as described previously (Fig. 19–16).

2. Felt padding is added over the shoulders and held in place with one or two turns of webril around the thorax.

3. The cast is applied extending over the shoulders, no neck being added.

4. The halo shoulder supports are contoured with bending irons to fit the shoulder sections of the cast. In children the uprights have a bend in them to allow the supports to be placed on the shoulders.

5. The connecting piece to the halo is applied, the uprights inserted and fitted to the shoulders. The head and uprights are positioned and the connecting pieces locked to the halo. The uprights are left loose while the shoulder portions are attached to the cast. Once this connection has completely set, the uprights are locked to the connecting pieces.

6. The cast is trimmed with anterior and posterior thoracic windows. A great deal of

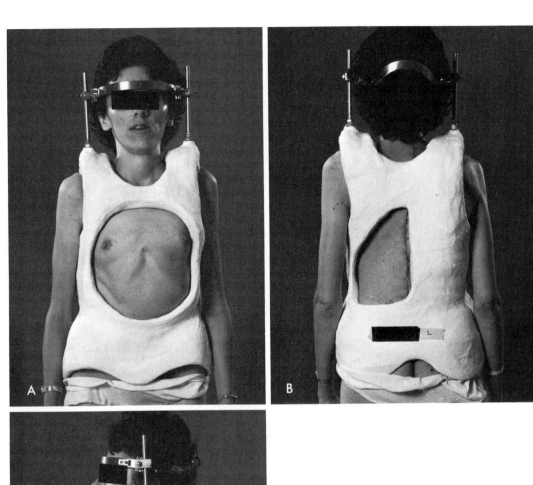

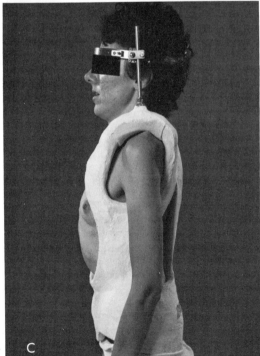

**Figure 19–13** Halo cast. The cast portion consists of a Risser-Cotrel cast with shoulder straps and large anterior and posterior windows. The halo is attached to the cast with "Lo-Profile" halo supports.

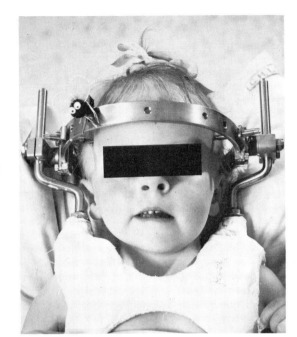

**Figure 19–14** A child in a halo cast needs contoured "Lo-Profile" supports to attach the halo to the cast.

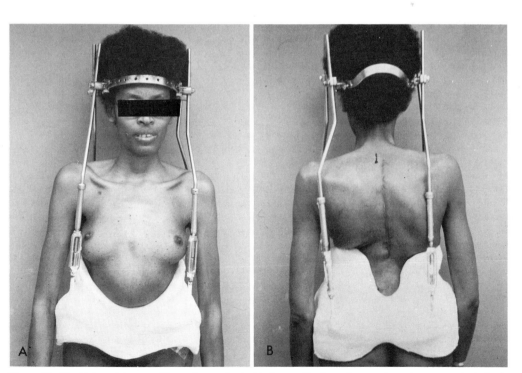

**Figure 19–15** Halo pelvic cast. Alternative method of halo cast fixation when no thoracic pressure is desired or as a form of ambulatory distraction. A well-molded pelvic section is attached to the halo via four contoured uprights, with turnbuckles for distraction.

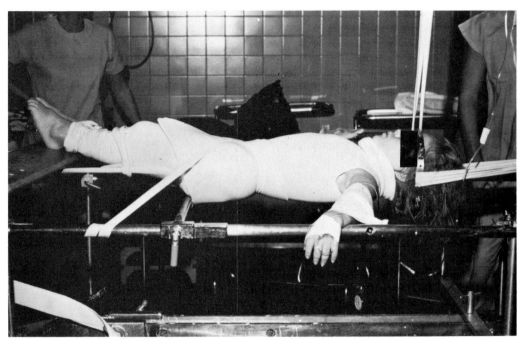

**Figure 19–16** Position for halo cast application. The patient is positioned on the Risser frame as for the application of a Risser-Cotrel cast. The halo is supported from the overhead frame, and traction is applied to the halo via muslin straps or rope.

care is necessary to trim and skive the cast sufficiently over the shoulders (Fig. 19–13).

7. Final adjustments in halo and head position are performed the following day once the patient stands and ambulates. This position is critical for position of fusion, plus the fact that in the halo cast the head position is fixed and thus must be as functional as possible.

### Cast With Leg Extension (Fig. 19–17*A*)

Any of the above casts may be extended down one or both legs to the knee or foot to aid in stabilizing the pelvis with certain lumbosacral fusions. The commonest use is with pelvic obliquity to allow the fusion to occur in a balanced position. In certain cases where traction in the cast is necessary, a femoral pin is incorporated in the cast to maintain this traction.

### Turnbuckle Cast (Fig. 19–17)

One of the commonest methods of obtaining correction prior to the use of Harrington instrumentation was with cast correction and fusion in the corrected position. A method

of obtaining cast correction was the turnbuckle cast. This is a cast that is wedged with the aid of turnbuckles incorporated in the cast. Guerin introduced the concept in 1842, and Risser modified it by moving the hinge from the side to over the spine.[7]

A cast is applied—either a Risser cast or halo cast with a leg extension to stabilize the pelvis where necessary. The cast is wedged opposite the apex with the hinges both in front and back over the spine. Initial correction is obtained using a cast spreader. A turnbuckle is attached on the side of the concavity, and by gradual distraction on this side the curve is corrected. Once maximal correction has been obtained, the cast is held in this position by plastering the two sides in and removing the turnbuckle.

While correction is being obtained, great care must be exercised to protect the skin. The skin should be watched for pressure and care taken not to pinch the skin during the period of correction.

It must be remembered that there are numerous methods of postoperative immobilization as described above. Each case must be carefully evaluated and the most appropriate method of immobilization used.

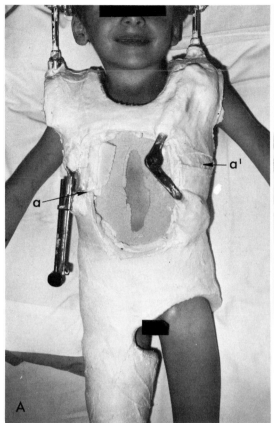

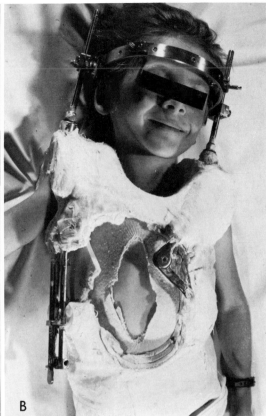

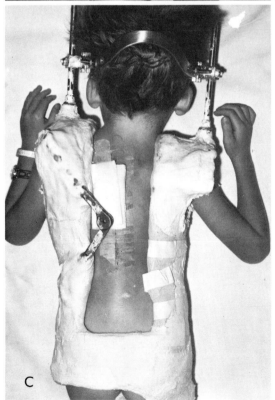

**Figure 19–17** Halo turnbuckle cast with leg extension. This cast is used to correct a curve with control of the head via the halo and the pelvis via the leg extension. *A,* The cast with the turnbuckle on the side of the concavity of the curve and anterior and posterior hinges over the spine. Note the plaster removed on the two sides a and a¹. *B,* The turnbuckle has been gradually lengthened with opening on the concavity of the curve. The wedge of plaster removed on the convexity of the curve has been closed, and the angle of the hinge is decreased. *C,* Posterior view after the area of the hinge has been sealed with plaster. The turnbuckle is removed and the cast filled in and reinforced, maintaining the correction.

## References

1. Anderson, S., and Bradford, D.S.: Lo-Profile halo. Clin. Orthop., *103*:72, 1974.
2. Cotrel, Y., and Morel, G.: Le technique de l' E.D.F. dans la correction des scolioses. Rev. Chir. Orthop., *50*:59, 1964.
3. Cotrel, Y.: Le corset de platre E.D.F. dans le traitement de la scoliose idiopathique. Med. Hyg., *28*:1032, 1970.
4. Leider, L. L., Jr., Moe, J. H., and Winter, R. B.: Early ambulation after the surgical treatment of idiopathic scoliosis. J. Bone Joint Surg., *55A*:1003, 1973.
5. Moe, J. H.: Methods of correction and surgical techniques in scoliosis. Orthop. Clin. North Am., *3*:17, 1972.
6. Ollier, M.: Techniques des platres et corsets des scolioses. Paris, Masson et Cie, 1971.
7. Risser, J. C., Lauder, C. H., Norquist, D. M., and Craig, W. A.: Three types of body casts. Am. Acad. Orthop. Surg. Instructional Course Lect., *10*:131, 1953.
8. Risser, J. C.: The appliction of body casts for the correction of scoliosis. Am. Acad. Orthop. Surg. Instr. Course Lect. *12*:255, 1955.
9. Sayre, L. A.: Spinal Disease and Spinal Curvature. London, Smith-Elder & Co., 1877.
10. Wullstein, L., and Schulthess, W.: Die Skoliose in inner Behandlung and Entschung Nach Klinishen und Experimentellen Studien. Z. Orthop. Clin., *10*:178, 1902.

# Chapter 20

# TECHNIQUES OF SURGERY

## POSTERIOR APPROACH[25]

### Spine Fusion[15]

The primary aim of surgical arthrodesis of the spine is to promote a physiologic state in skeletal tissue that will ultimately result in bone formation, maturation, and union. This is achieved by careful exposure, facet joint destruction, bony decortication, autogenous bone grafting, and adequate immobilization. One does not "fuse a spine"; rather, one produces conditions that are favorable for arthrodesis. This distinction should be obvious. Yet the failure to appreciate this point may result in failure to achieve an arthrodesis.

### POSITIONING THE PATIENT

For adequate exposure of the spine with minimal blood loss, the positioning of the patient is important. After intubation, the patient is placed prone on a four-poster or Hall frame (Fig. 20–1), which allows the abdomen to hang free. Intra-abdominal pressure will be minimized and venous bleeding appreciably decreased. A preoperative corrective cast with the abdominal chest window enlarged will likewise permit a freely dependent abdomen (see Chapter 19, p. 476).

The arms should be carefully supported, with the shoulders in no more than 90 to 100 degree abduction. The upper pads of the four-poster frame must rest not in the axillae but rather on the chest, and the elbows must be protected to prevent a pressure neuropathy.

The back is scrubbed with a surgical soap for 10 minutes and then painted with an iodine solution. The wound is draped. We have found an adhesive plastic drape to be useful in keeping the operative field and the cotton drapes dry.

### INCISION

A straight incision is made (see Fig. 20–1) through the dermis only. The incision should not follow the spinal curvature. The intradermal and superficial subcutaneous area is infiltrated with epinephrine solution (1 : 500,000). This reduces the capillary bleeding and helps to reveal fascial planes. The incision is deepened down to the fascia, and the skin margins are forcibly retracted, using multiple self-retaining retractors of the Adson or Weitlaner type. Small vessels are cauterized as they are encountered. The interspinous ligament overlying the spinous processes is identified. This identification is aided by maintaining strong distraction on the retractors as well as dissection with a sponge over the soft tissues. In curves of greater magnitude, it is important to remember that the dissection should proceed obliquely toward the apex of the curvature, in order to find the linea alba throughout the length of the area to be exposed. The exact centers of the spinous processes are then incised with a sharp scalpel through the cartilage cap and down to the bony tip (Fig. 20–2). Each half of the cartilaginous cap is pushed aside with the Cobb elevator, exposing the spinous process on all sides and initiating the subperiosteal stripping.

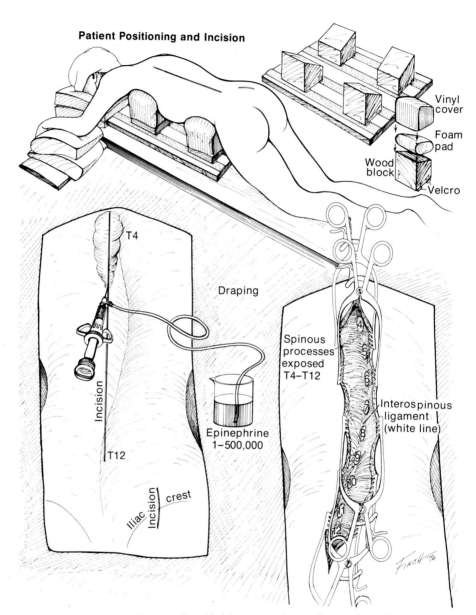

**Patient Positioning and Incision**

Vinyl cover

Foam pad

Wood block

Velcro

T4

Draping

Incision

Epinephrine 1-500,000

T12

Iliac crest

Incision

Spinous processes exposed T4–T12

Interospinous ligament (white line)

**Figure 20–1** Patient is positioned on a well-padded four-poster frame, allowing the abdomen to remain completely free. Following the skin preparation, a midline skin incision is made over the area of the spine to be fused. The incision is made just into the dermis, and the dermal and subcutaneous tissues are infiltrated with epinephrine 1:500,000 solution. The skin incision is then deepened down to the linea alba, dissection being facilitated by use of Weitlaner self-retaining retractors.

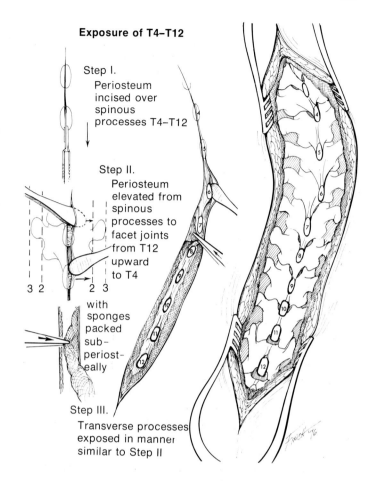

**Exposure of T4–T12**

Step I.
Periosteum incised over spinous processes T4–T12

Step II.
Periosteum elevated from spinous processes to facet joints from T12 upward to T4 with sponges packed sub-periost-eally

3 2 2 3

Step III.
Transverse processes exposed in manner similar to Step II

**Figure 20–2** After the spinous processes have been identified, the centers of the spinous processes are then incised with a sharp scalpel through the cartilage cap and down into the bony tip. A careful sharp subperiosteal dissection is then carried out, beginning at T12 and working proximally to the upper vertebra to be exposed. Hemostasis is facilitated by subperiosteal sponge packing. In general, it is preferable to expose the transverse processes only after all facet joints have been exposed throughout the area to be fused. Exposure too far laterally on the initial sweep often tears muscle, resulting in excessive blood loss. In the lumbar spine, the facet joint capsule is left intact. A sharp incision is made into the superior facet and the pars interarticularis, allowing the soft tissue with periosteum to then be dissected laterally out to the transverse process (see text).

After exposure of three or four spinous processes, the retractors are carefully introduced between the divided caps and spread slowly but firmly to put these tissues under tension. Excessive force will result in muscle tearing and unnecessary blood loss. Subperiosteal dissection is continued gently, exposing bare bone on all sides of each spinous process out to the facet joints. Continued retraction opens the soft tissues like a book. We find it most useful to begin distally and work proximally, since the oblique attachments of the short rotator muscles and ligaments are most easily detached from the lamina in this direction.

Liberal use of a scalpel to release tendinous and ligamentous attachments along the inferior margins of the lamina aids in the dissection. It is preferable to separate subperiosteally only to the facet joints on the first dissection with the Cobb elevator and to continue the dissection to the end of the transverse processes on the second dissec-

tion. Stripping far laterally on the initial sweep often tears muscle as well as the segmental vessel just lateral to the facet joint, resulting in excessive blood loss. The decision to dissect the concave and the convex sides singly or simultaneously is optional. All bleeding points are cauterized as they appear.

The success of clean subperiosteal stripping of spinous processes and laminae lies in gentle periosteal elevation, sharp division of resistant muscle insertions, and careful mechanical retraction with the self-retaining retractors. Gauze packing should be used to maintain hemostasis. The capsular covering of the facet joints is not removed until the exposure has been completed out to the ends of the transverse processes. Care should be taken not to damage the costotransverse articulation. A metallic marker is placed in the spinous process of the lowest vertebra exposed. An x-ray is then taken to confirm the correct level of exposure.

In the lumbar spine, if a transverse

process fusion is performed, exposure should proceed laterally to the tips of the transverse processes. A subperiosteal dissection should again be done, sweeping the periosteum and soft tissues just lateral to the facet joint. It is easiest to leave the joint capsule intact initially while this soft tissue dissection is being carried out. Retraction is maintained. A sharp incision is made along the superior facet and pars interarticularis, and the soft tissue with periosteum is swept laterally to the end of the transverse process. Great care should be taken not to forcefully dissect the transverse process; otherwise breakage will ensue. The bridge of intervening tissues between the transverse processes should be gently pushed laterally and the bleeders carefully cauterized.

Before facet fusion and decortication are begun, the joints should be cleared of all ligamentous and capsular attachments by using sharp curettes. In the thoracic spine (Fig. 20–3), the facet is uncovered by cutting and stripping the most inferior portion of the inferior facet with a clockwise and caudally directed force. With removal of this small inferior portion, the exposed cartilage of the superior facet is readily visualized. One may then sweep the curette medially, with the cutting edge directed downward, removing the ligamentous attachments to the lamina. The curette is then turned to face upward, and

curettement proceeds from a lateral to a medial direction on the inferior edge of the laminae above. In this fashion, ligamentous attachments and outer fibers of the ligamentum flavum are completely removed. Great care must be exercised in carrying out this manuever. One should always work toward the tip of the spinous processes rather than ventrally in order to avoid the inherent danger of slipping through the ligamentum flavum and into the dura. In the lumbar spine, the capsule overlying the joint is sharply curetted or rongeured away in preparation for the facet fusion.

### BONE GRAFT

Before decortication is carried out, a bone graft should be taken from the outer table of the ilium. The iliac crest is exposed through a separate incision, or, if the midline incision has extended down into the lumbar area, the original incision, slightly extended, will suffice. A vertical incision over the iliac crest is preferable, since this usually will give the best cosmetic scar. Subperiosteal dissection should expose approximately 50 per cent of the ilium. Care must be taken to avoid damaging the superior gluteal artery as it emerges from the sciatic notch. Cortical and cancellous strips of bone are taken and placed separately in a kidney basin, and the

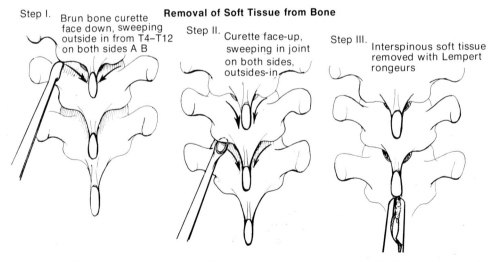

**Removal of Soft Tissue from Bone**

Step I. Brun bone curette face down, sweeping outside in from T4–T12 on both sides A B

Step II. Curette face-up, sweeping in joint on both sides, outsides-in

Step III. Interspinous soft tissue removed with Lempert rongeurs

**Figure 20–3** Before decortication is begun, the posterior elements are cleared of all ligamentous and capsular attachments, using sharp curettes. It is preferable to begin by cutting the capsular attachments off the lamina below, working from a lateral to a medial direction, and then cutting these attachments from the inferior edge of the lamina above by curetting again from a lateral to medial direction. Any remaining interspinous ligamentous or fatty tissue is then sharply rongeured away.

bone is covered with a blood-soaked sponge. Bleeding points may be packed with bone wax. A thrombin-soaked Gelfoam pack is placed over the graft site, and the area is packed off with sponge. By this maneuver, blood loss is minimized.

The success of the arthrodesis depends to a great degree on the adequacy of the bone graft. This portion of the surgery should not, therefore, be relegated to an inexperienced surgeon. A large amount of autogenous cancellous bone, harvested just before use and maintained in as biologic a state as possible, is essential to the success of arthrodesis. Bone grafts that are taken too early during the operative procedure, left exposed to operating room lights or laminar flow ventila-

tion, or placed in saline solutions will lose surface cell viability. They will thus offer little more than an inorganic scaffold for fibrous tissue ingrowth.

## FACET JOINT FUSION

Facet joint fusion is carried out by one of a variety of techniques, all of which are aimed at thoroughly destroying the articular facet and placing cancellous bone within the remaining space (Fig. 20–4). The Moe technique consists of elevating two hinged fragments of bone from adjacent transverse processes and moving them laterally to fill the intertransverse area. The joint surfaces are cleared of articular cartilage, and a block of

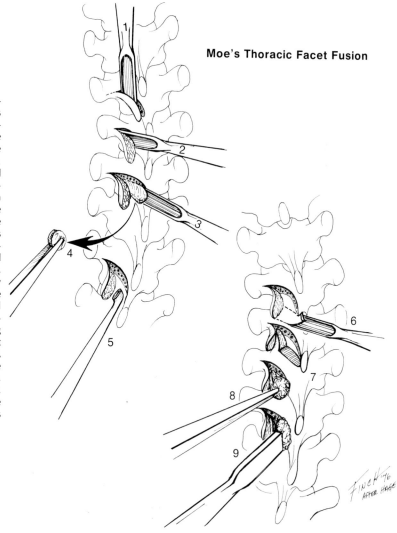

**Moe's Thoracic Facet Fusion**

**Figure 20–4** The Moe technique of facet joint fusion. A cut is first begun over the cephalad articular process at the base of the lamina. This is carried along the transverse process almost to its tip. This fragment is bent and levered laterally to lie between the transverse processes. It should remain hinged to the superior transverse process. The superior joint surface should not be included in this fragment. The joint surface is removed with a separate cut and discarded. The articular cartilage, which is now visible, is sharply curetted out. The cut is next made into the mid-portion of the caudal transverse process and curved inward and upward, decorticating the superior articular facet so that it creates another hinge fragment. A cancellous and/or cortical bone graft is now placed in the defect, which was previously the joint, and impacted in place, moving the two transverse process fragments more laterally.

cortical cancellous bone obtained from the laminae is placed in the defect. With a medium-size gouge, a cut is begun over the cephalad articular process at the base of the lamina. This cut is carried along the transverse process almost to its tip. This fragment is then bent and levered laterally to lie between the transverse processes. It should remain hinged to the superior transverse process. The cut that creates it should not be so deep that the superior joint surface is included in this fragment. The cephalad joint surface is then removed with the gouge and discarded.

The articular cartilage is now visible and is removed using a sharp curette. With the gouge held almost vertically, a cut is made into the midportion of the caudal transverse process and curved inward and upward, decorticating the superior articular facet so that it creates another hinged fragment. This will lie adjacent to the fragment cut from the cephalad transverse process. A good-sized fragment of cancellous and cortical bone is now cut free from the caudal lamina, and this is placed in the defect that was previously the joint. As it is gently impacted in place, it moves the two transverse process fragments laterally. This free graft spans the caudal and cephalad articular processes. For this free graft, cancellous bone with a little cortex, obtained from the lamina or the ilium, is the best.

The technique of Moe has the disadvantage of being more time-consuming than simpler methods described. Hall[12] uses a similar technique (Fig. 20–5), with the exception that he excises the joint surface totally and lays in it cancellous iliac bone at each facet joint level. Goldstein removes the joint by deep decortication and fills the area with cancellous bone. Risser, using the Hibbs technique, curettes the dorsal margin of cartilage from the joint, then interweaves flaps of bone into each other over the articulation. Decortication is complete, but iliac bone is seldom added, except sometimes in the lumbar spine.

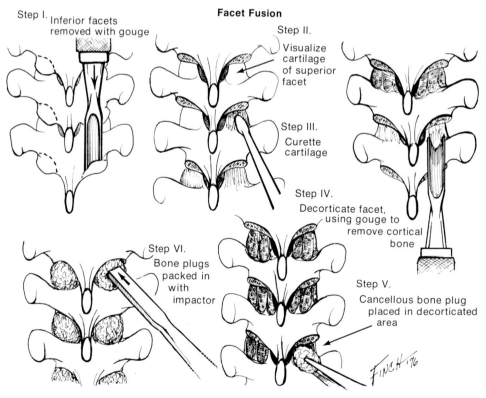

**Figure 20–5** An excellent facet joint fusion may be achieved by the method described by Hall. In the first step, the inferior facet joint is sharply cut with a semicircular gouge in the manner outlined. The bone fragment with underlying articular cartilage is removed in one piece. The superior facet cartilage is then easily visualized and is removed with a sharp curette. A trough is created by removing the outer cortex of the superior facet. Cancellous bone is then taken from the outer table of the ilium and snugly impacted into the decorticated area previously created.

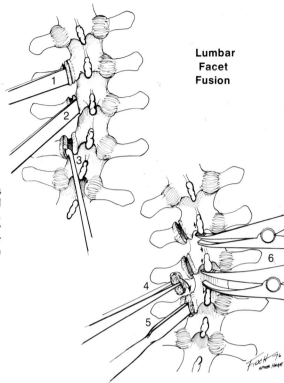

**Lumbar Facet Fusion**

**Figure 20–6** Lumbar facet fusion (Moe technique) is performed by cutting away the joint surfaces with a small thick osteotome. The floor of the joint is then curetted away. A block of the cancellous bone from the ilium is then firmly driven into the defect previously created. A Blount spreader applied between the spinous processes is helpful in visualizing the adequacy of facet joint removal.

As a transitional area is reached at T10–T11 and T11–T12, the articular processes become thin and predominantly cortical. The articulation does not provide an opportunity to construct a wide bridge of bone flaps. The best method of fusing these joints is to undercut the superior articular process with a gouge, creating a cavern. The cartilage is removed from its floor with a sharp curette. Cancellous bone is then carefully positioned and packed into the area thus created. Hard cortical bone should not be used.

In the lumbar spine, the facet joints are oriented in a sagittal direction. Facet fusion is best performed by cutting away the joint surfaces with a small thin osteotome (Fig. 23–6). The floor of the joint is curetted, and a block of cancellous bone from the ilium is firmly driven into the defect. Facet destruction and grafting are carried out on the convex and concave sides. A block facet fusion is unnecessary on the convex side above T10, provided the facet joints are destroyed during the decortication processes.

As a final step, the spinous processes are removed with a large bone cutter, and thorough decortication is performed over the entire exposed spine. Large amounts of cancellous iliac bone are placed over the whole

decorticated area out to the tips of the transverse processes. The remaining cortical bone is placed over this, and the spinous processes that were removed are cut into matchstick-sized fragments and then placed on the dorsum of the fusion mass. Before adding autogenous iliac bone, all joints should be inspected to be certain that the bone blocks remain in place.

***Rib Hump Deformities.*** If a rib hump elevation greater than 1.5 centimeters was present prior to surgery, the Cotrel transverse process osteotomy is carried out. This technique has been found to be a useful method of correcting rib hump deformity. The transverse processes are osteotomized as vertically as possible at their base with a sharp rib cutter and then hinged superiorly and laterally, allowing the rib to hinge forward at the costovertebral articulation (see Fig. 23–11). This procedure can be carried out safely provided the bone cutters are not placed further anteriorly than the inferior cortex of the transverse process (see Fig. 20–11).

## CLOSURE

The deep tissues are approximated with a running 0-chromic or Vicryl suture. A suction is placed in the subcutaneous tissues and put to wall suction. The subcutaneous tissues are approximated with 2–0 suture and the skin with a 3–0 subcuticular removable nylon suture or a self-absorbable type suture (Vicryl). A bulky pressure dressing is applied. Irrigation of the wound may be carried out during the surgical procedure with saline or an antibiotic type solution. However, once decortication has begun and bone grafts have been inserted, no further irrigation should be done. Suction drainage should not be instituted deeper than the subcutaneous tissues; otherwise, tamponading will not occur, and blood loss will be excessive.

## Harrington Instrumentation[7, 8, 9, 15]

The use of Harrington instrumentation in the treatment of idiopathic scoliosis has become such an accepted form of therapy that technical considerations may be over-

looked and success taken for granted. Such assumptions are inappropriate. The procedure itself will facilitate surgical correction of the deformity, maintenance of the correction, and successful arthrodesis of the spine. However, the use of the instruments as well as their limitations must be thoroughly understood.

## PLACEMENT OF THE HOOK

After the initial wide exposure and before facet fusion is begun, the site of Harrington hook placement must be selected and prepared. The upper hook is placed within the thoracic joint selected; the lower hook, under the lamina of the lower vertebra selected. The site for the upper hook is first prepared by removing all ligament and capsular tissues (Fig. 20–7). A small, 1/4 inch (0.6 cm.) osteotome is used to cut the inferior portion of the superior facet at a slightly oblique angle, the medial

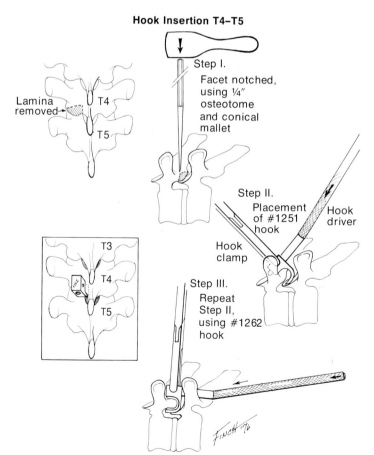

**Hook Insertion T4–T5**

Lamina removed

T4

T5

Step I.
Facet notched, using 1/4″ osteotome and conical mallet

Step II.
Placement of #1251 hook

Hook driver

Hook clamp

T3

T4

T5

Step III.
Repeat Step II, using #1262 hook

FINCH '96

**Figure 20–7** Preparation for the insertion of the upper hook of the Harrington assembly. A small (1/4 inch, 0.6 cm) osteotome is used to cut the inferior portion of the superior facet at a slightly oblique angle, as demonstrated. The facet joint is then easily identified and its most medial margin delineated. A #1251 hook is inserted into the facet interspace as demonstrated in Step II. The hooks should be tilted forward at least 45 degrees to assure proper placement and to prevent the tendency for the hook to improperly engage into the superior facet. Once the hook has engaged the pedicle, it may be impacted with a light mallet. This sharp hook is then removed and a flanged hook, #1262, is inserted and impacted into the pedicle, as demonstrated in Step III.

margin being more cranially directed. The facet joint is then easily identified and its most medial margin delineated. It is sometimes helpful to carefully insert a small Cobb elevator into the joint interspaces to further outline their cartilaginous surfaces. A #1251 hook is inserted into the facet interspace in the manner outlined. The hook should be tilted forward at least 45° to insure proper placement and contact with the inferior edge of the pedicle. When it has engaged the pedicle, it may be impacted with a light mallet. The hook is removed and a dull, flanged hook (#1262) or a dull unflanged hook (#1253) is similarly inserted and, likewise, firmly impacted into the pedicle. The flanged hook, if properly placed, will not damage the lamina but, on the contrary, will have a better grip into the bone and be less likely to dislocate.

The lower hook (#1254 dull hook) is inserted under the lamina of the vertebra selected (Fig. 20–8). If there is abundant room with a wide interspace, the ligamentum fla-

vum may be curetted out from its attachment to the lamina. Portions of the ligament may be removed. A sharp curette is very useful in exposing the dura and the superior margin of the laminar edge. The laminar edge is removed with a curette or with a Kerrison rongeur, giving a flat margin that extends to the pars interarticularis. On occasion, the lamina and the articular process of the adjacent cephalad vertebra will be thick and will interfere with rod insertion into the hook. If so, it should be carefully grooved with an osteotome or rongeurs, taking care to remove the articular surface. It is easiest to prepare the facet joint at the level of the lower hook and pack it with cancellous bone at this stage of the operation, prior to inserting the Harrington outrigger or the Harrington rod (Fig. 20–9).

### THE HARRINGTON OUTRIGGER

If a preoperative cast has not been used, the Harrington outrigger may be inserted be-

**Hook Insertion T11–T12**

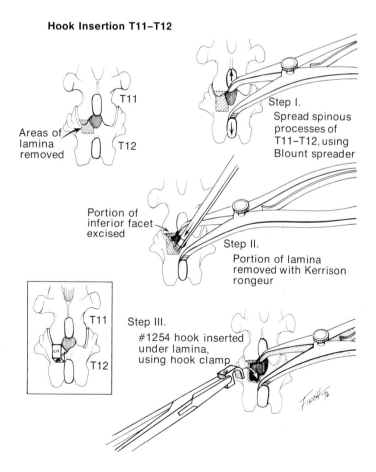

**Figure 20–8** Insertion of the lower hook assembly (#1254). It is best to curette out the ligamentum flavum from its attachment to the lamina. It is helpful to remove the most inferior portion of the inferior facet in order to better outline the limits of the ligamentum. A sharp curette or a knife may then be used to completely remove the ligamentum flavum and thus expose the dura. It is helpful to use a Blount spreader to obtain a wider exposure of this area. In Step II, portions of the lamina are removed with a Kerrison rongeur, giving a flat margin that extends to the pars interarticularis. It is easiest to prepare the facet joint at this level and pack it with cancellous bone prior to insertion of the Harrington outrigger or the Harrington rod. Insertion of the Harrington outrigger between the two hooks is demonstrated. Facet fusion is carried out as outlined in Figures 20–5 and 20–6.

Areas of lamina removed

T11
T12

Step I.
Spread spinous processes of T11–T12, using Blount spreader

Portion of inferior facet excised

Step II.
Portion of lamina removed with Kerrison rongeur

T11
T12

Step III.
#1254 hook inserted under lamina, using hook clamp

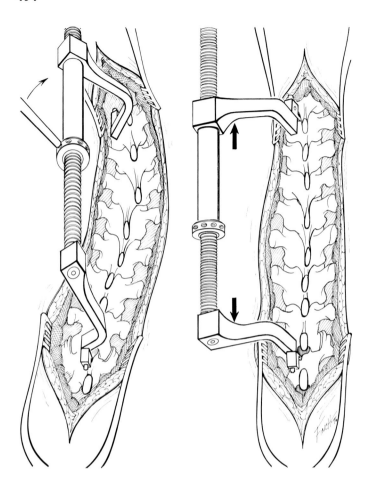

**Figure 20–9** The Harrington outrigger in place. Distraction is facilitated by having the assistant push over the apex of the curvature while the screw device is being tightened.

tween the two hooks prior to fusion of the facets and decortication. Careful, controlled distraction should be carried out. This may be facilitated by having the assistant put manual pressure over the convexity of the curvature. The outrigger has the advantage of facilitating correction, improving the exposure of the facet joints, and allowing fusion of the facet while the spine is in the corrected position. Current models of the Harrington outrigger do not permit calculation of the forces being generated in distraction. Therefore, only experience can indicate to the operating surgeon when the safe maximum distraction has been obtained. A preoperative cast, on the other hand, allows one to obtain good correction prior to surgery. However, its application is time-consuming for the flexible idiopathic curvature, and its use is not routinely recommended.

After the completion of the facet fusion and decortication (Fig. 20–10), the Harring-

ton outrigger is removed, the distraction strut bar is placed between the two hooks, and distraction is performed (Fig. 20–11). The Cotrel osteotomy at the base of the transverse processes on the convex side of the curvature will give additional correction and allow further distraction. Only experience can indicate to the operating surgeon the point at which the safe maximum distraction has been obtained. Distraction should not be carried out to the point of bony disruption, nor to the point of rod bending. Special hook holders are now available that can be inserted into the outrigger at its attachment to the Harrington hooks (Fig. 20–12). This modification allows the surgeon to insert the distracting rod assembly while the outrigger is still attached. It also facilitates insertion of the distraction rod.

At the completion of decortication, an 18-gauge wire is threaded around the upper end of the rod to prevent the rod from teles-

**Bony Decortication**

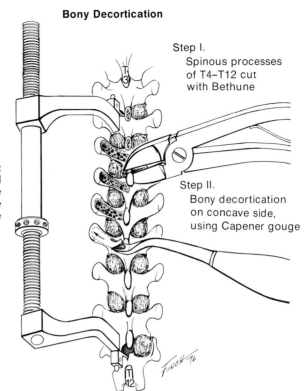

Step I.
Spinous processes
of T4–T12 cut
with Bethune

Step II.
Bony decortication
on concave side,
using Capener gouge

**Figure 20–10** Bony decortication is carried out after the facet joints have been prepared and packed with bone. Spinous processes are first cut with a Bethune bone cutter, and bony decortication on the concave side is carried out to the tips of the transverse processes. See Figure 20–11 for completion of method.

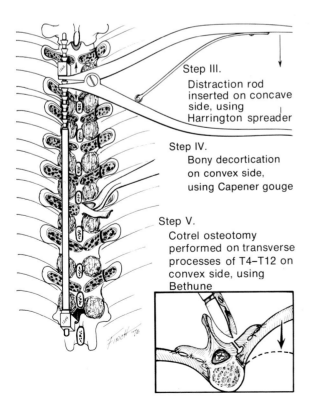

Step III.
Distraction rod
inserted on concave
side, using
Harrington spreader

Step IV.
Bony decortication
on convex side,
using Capener gouge

Step V.
Cotrel osteotomy
performed on transverse
processes of T4–T12 on
convex side, using
Bethune

**Figure 20–11** After the concave side of the curvature is completely decorticated (see Fig. 20–10), the Harrington outrigger is removed and a distracting rod inserted on the concave side, using the Harrington spreader. Bony decortication is then carried out on the convex side, and a Cotrel osteotomy completes the procedure. Cotrel transverse process osteotomy is performed if a rib hump elevation greater than $1\frac{1}{2}$ cm is present prior to surgery. The transverse processes are osteotomized as vertically as possible at their base with a sharp rib cutter and then hinged superiorly and laterally, allowing the rib to fall forward at the costovertebral articulation (Step V).

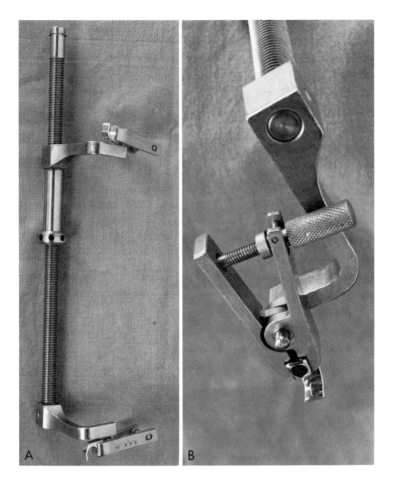

**Figure 20–12** A special hook bracket devised by Klaus Zielke of Tubingen, West Germany, is now available which may be inserted into the outrigger at its attachment to the Harrington hook. This modification allows the surgeon to insert the distracting rod assembly while the outrigger is still attached.

coping within the hook. (The Harrington rod collar may be used instead.)

The compression rod assembly should always be used with the distraction strut bar when there is an associated kyphosis, such as in the combination of scoliosis with Scheuermann's disease, or with compression alone, in the case of pure kyphosis. The insertion of the contraction assembly is more difficult (Figs. 20–13 and 20–14). There are two sizes of hooks (#1256 and #1259), which adapt to

two sizes of fully threaded rods: a larger rod ($\frac{1}{8}$ inch), and a smaller rod ($\frac{5}{11}$ inch). The smaller rod is more useful, since it is flexible and adapts readily to a kyphosis.

After thorough exposure of the spine as previously outlined, the hooks are first placed individually under the selected transverse processes, at the junction of the transverse process and the lamina. The sharp edge of the hook cuts the costotransverse ligaments. It is important to insert the hook several times so

**Figure 20–13** Procedure for insertion of the contracting assembly. The contracting assembly comes in two sizes, $\frac{1}{8}$ inch and $\frac{5}{11}$ inch. The smaller rod with the #1259 hook is generally more useful, since it is flexible and adapts readily to kyphosis. Insertion of this assembly is facilitated by careful and thorough preparation of the spine. The #1259 hooks should be placed individually under the selected transverse processes at the junction of the transverse process and the lamina. The sharp edge of the hook cuts the costotransverse ligament. Care should be taken to ensure that the hook does not cut into the transverse process and the seating is carried out easily in a horizontal fashion. If the hook must be tilted to slide under the transverse process, insertion will be extremely difficult once the rod is attached to the hook. Below T11 there are no suitable transverse processes, so the hooks must be placed under the lamina at this area. Appropriate amounts of bone are cut from the inferior lamina and inferior facet with an osteotome and Kerrison rongeur. A Blount spreader is then placed between the two spinous processes, and the #1259 hook is carefully inserted into place. Again, one should strive for placement of this hook in a horizontal fashion to facilitate its insertion once the rod is attached to the hook.

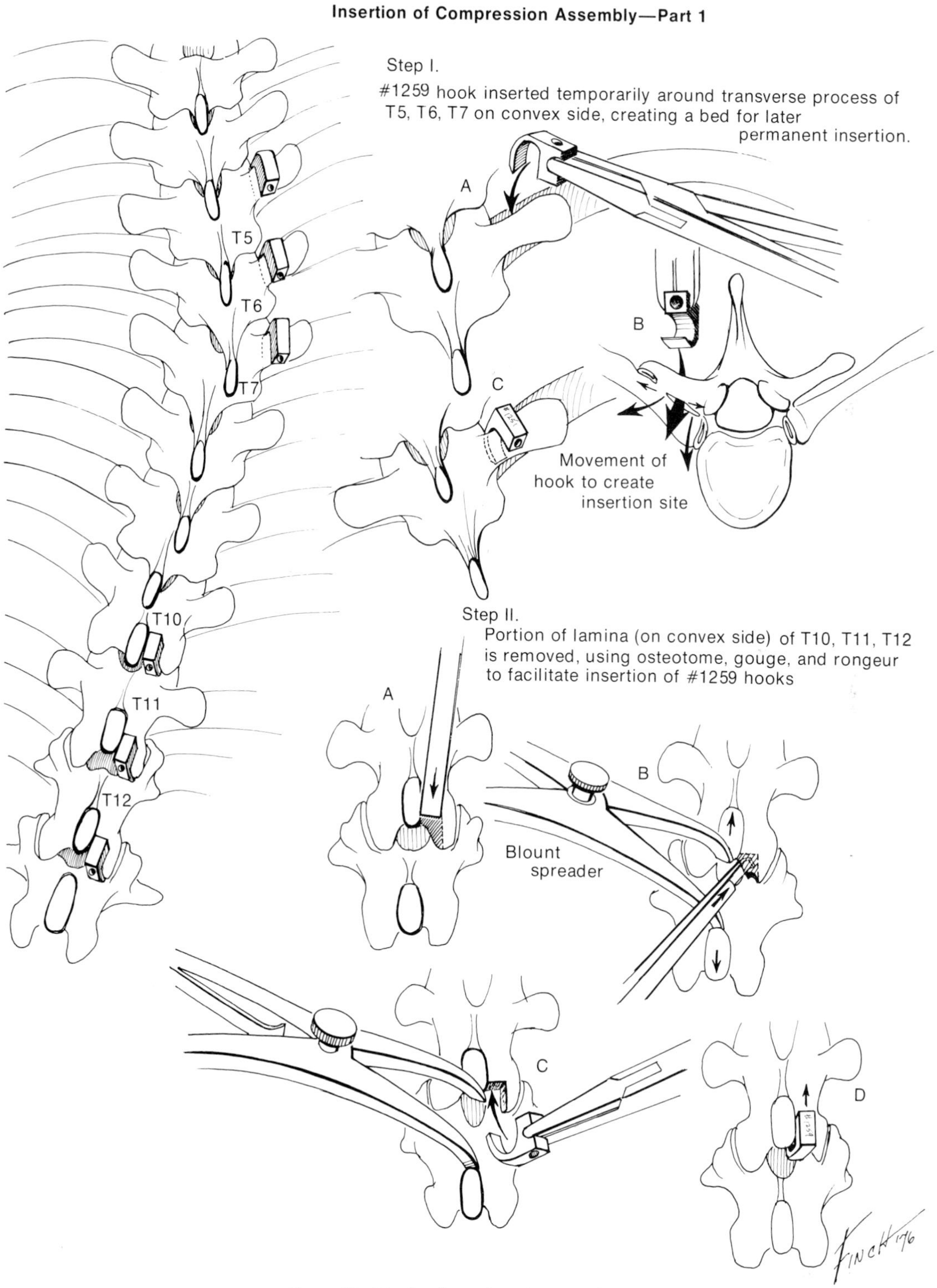
Insertion of Compression Assembly—Part 1
Step I.
#1259 hook inserted temporarily around transverse process of T5, T6, T7 on convex side, creating a bed for later permanent insertion.
A
B
C
Movement of hook to create insertion site
T5
T6
T7
T10
T11
T12
Step II.
Portion of lamina (on convex side) of T10, T11, T12 is removed, using osteotome, gouge, and rongeur to facilitate insertion of #1259 hooks
A
B
Blount spreader
C
D

**Figure 20–13** *See legend on the opposite page.*

Insertion of Compression Assembly—Part 2

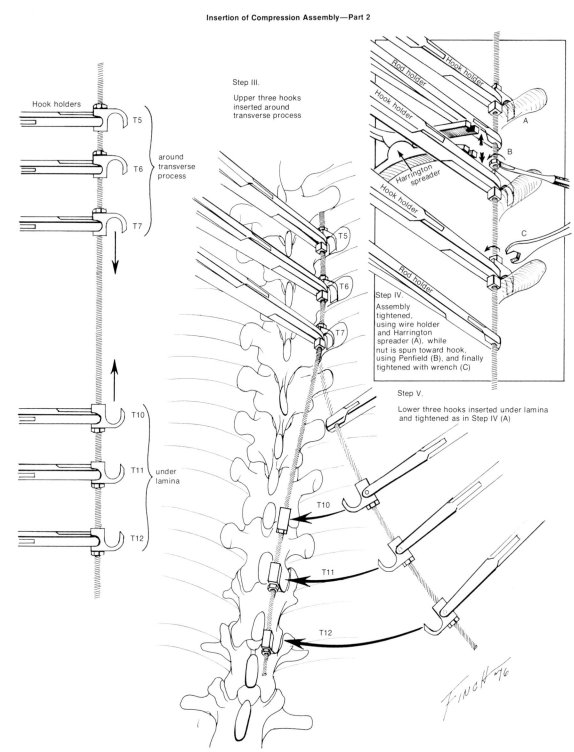

**Figure 20–14**  Insertion of the contraction assembly (continued from Fig. 20–13). After the transverse processes and laminae have been prepared as outlined, a threaded rod with the appropriate size hooks attached to it is then inserted. It is generally easier to insert the cranially directed hooks first, followed by insertion of the more caudally directed hooks in a single step. After the hooks are securely in place, they may be tightened with either a wrench or a spreader placed between a rod holder and a hook holder. The Moe elevator is used to tighten the nut between the hook holder and the rod holder after the distraction has taken place. After maximal contraction, the central threads adjacent to the nuts on the rod must be damaged with a clamp close to the nut to prevent them from unwinding and becoming loose.

that it will seat easily and slide horizontally under the transverse process when the rod assembly is finally attached to the hook. Care must be taken to ensure that the hook does not cut into the transverse process. If this does occur, the transverse process will be severely weakened and the hook will cut out. From T11 caudally there are no suitable transverse processes on which to seat the contraction hook. At these levels the hooks must be placed under the lamina, as close to the facet joint as possible.

*The Contraction Assembly.* After the transverse processes and laminae have been prepared to accept the contraction assembly, a threaded rod of the appropriate size, with the hooks attached along with the nuts, is inserted. Six hooks (three hooks cephalad and three caudad) have been found adequate. During the insertion, the more cranially directed hooks are placed first, followed by the insertion of the more caudally directed hooks. The compression assembly is then tightened by using the appropriate rod holders and Harrington spreader. The hooks can also be contracted by turning the nuts with a wrench. After maximal contraction, the central threads adjacent to the nuts on the rod must be damaged with a clamp close to the nut to prevent them from migrating.

The use of the contracting assembly for the scoliotic spine should be done only in those patients who have true kyphosis associated with scoliosis. The thoracic spines of most idiopathic curvatures are either flat or have some degree of thoracic lordosis. Under these circumstances, the use of the compression hook assembly may aggravate the thoracic lordosis. On the other hand, in patients with true kyphosis, the contracting assembly will facilitate correction of the scoliosis as well as the kyphosis.

In patients with true kyphosis without significant scoliosis, two compression assemblies are used. In these cases, it is very important that the head be elevated during the operation, since exposure and correction of the kyphosis are facilitated in this position. The upper hook assembly should be on the transverse process of the second, third, and fourth thoracic vertebra, whereas the three lower hooks are placed at the bottom of the kyphosis, under the lamina as previously described. The joints between the articular processes should not be prepared

with a dowel drill or blocked with bone, since this will prevent correction. They may, however, be curetted. The spinous processes are decorticated but not removed, since the fusion mass must be as thick as possible in the anterior-posterior plane to prevent loss of correction.

*Severe or Double Curvatures.* In those cases that demonstrate severe structural curvatures or double structural curvatures, two or more rods are occasionally necessary. In a severe structural curve in which x-rays demonstrate that the central area of the curve remains rigidly fixed, the best correction can often be obtained by using two distracting strut bars. One will span the inflexible central portion of the curve; the other will span the full extent of the curvature. A greater degree of fixation, and even correction, may thus be obtained.

Patients presenting with double structural thoracic curves or thoracic and lumbar curvatures may require the insertion either of a single rod in a "dollar-sign" fashion spanning both curves or of two parallel rods overlapping the junction of each curve by at least two segments. The preference is to use a single "dollar sign" rod in most cases, since kyphosis may develop at the junction of the two rods. In the thoracolumbar area particularly, though the two rods are overlapped by at least two segments, kyphosis may occur. If the fusion and rod placement must extend to T1 or T2, great care should be taken to assure that the excess portion of the rod does not protrude into the subcutaneous tissues of the neck. This can conveniently be prevented by reversing the rod and placing the #1254 hook at T1–T2 and the larger (#1253) hook below.

## SACRAL INSERTION OF ROD

For rod insertions into the sacrum, secure fixation may be provided by either the large alar hook or the sacral bar (Fig. 20–15). The ala of the sacrum provides excellent seating for the large sacral hook. Careful dissection must proceed out to the sacral ala, taking great care to avoid damaging the sacroiliac joint. The saddle of the hook is then inserted on the cortical surface of the ala. To seat the hook properly in this area requires complete removal of all soft tissues,

**Figure 20–15** Numerous types of hooks and rods allow one great flexibility in the internal fixation technique. *A,* The various hooks that we have found most useful. Beginning at the left and working clockwise are shown (1) the alar hook, (2) the sharp flanged #1253 hook, (3) the #1256 hook, (4) the #1253 hook, (5) the dull flanged #1262 hook, (6) the #1251 hook, (7) the André hook, and (8) the #1254 hook. The #1256 hook is generally used for the large threaded rod, while the #1259 hook, not shown, is used in conjunction with the smaller threaded rod. *B,* The types of rods available. From left to right— the standard distraction rod, the modified square-ended distraction rod, the larger contracting rod ($^5/_{16}$ in), and the smaller rod ($^1/_8$ in). The square ended distracting rod now is available in 1 cm increments, permitting more precise selection of proper size.

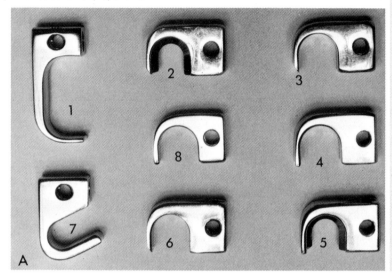
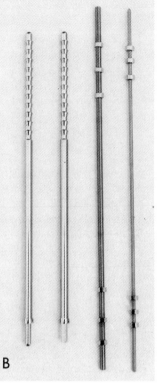

including those that overlie the alar surface. The bone itself, being cortical, should not be violated.

Certain circumstances may require the use of a transsacral bar for sacral fixation, particularly when there is severe lordosis of the lumbar spine. The bar can be inserted best with a slow-motor drill. It should pass through the posterior wing of the ilium and should cross the spine just posterior to the ligamentum flavum between the spinous processes of L5 and S1. After penetrating the opposite iliac wing through both cortices, its extra length is cut off with a heavy bolt cutter. The lower hook can then be placed into the sacral bar. Bone grafts can still be obtained from the cephalad portion of the ilium, but care must be taken not to weaken the firm seating of the bar.

In cases where the hook must be seated under the lamina of L5, a problem is sometimes encountered in which the lamina is vertical and wide, making placement of the hook too deep. The larger alar hook may be used to overcome this problem, or the lamina may be fenestrated more dorsally, permitting the hook to be inserted horizontally. Recently a special hook has been designed (André hook—Zimmer) that conforms to the vertical orientation of the laminae, assuring a secure fixation (see Fig. 20–15) when the hook is inserted into L5.

Occasionally, it is desirable to insert a short distraction bar from the sacral ala into the third or fourth lumbar vertebra to correct an "oblique take-off," or rather, a lumbosacral scoliosis. The insertion of the hook into the fourth lumbar vertebra must be as far anterior as possible, and this is achieved by placing a medium (#1256) sharp hook in a slot in the posterior portion of the pedicle, at the junction of the pedicle and the pars interarticularis and the transverse process. A portion of lamina must be removed to achieve this placement. A large threaded rod is then placed between a sacral hook at this point of fixation, and careful distraction is carried out. This provides an effective side thrust and realigns the vertebra with the sacrum.

*LOSS OF LUMBAR LORDOSIS*

Fusions to the sacrum or the fifth lumbar vertebra combined with instrumentation has often been associated with a loss or reversal of lumbar lordosis. This may frequently prove more disabling to the patient than the original problem for which surgery was undertaken.

Lumbar lordosis must be maintained. This is achieved by bending the rod in the lumbar area to conform to normal lordosis. After producing this bend in the rod, it may be necessary to place a second bend in the upper portion of the rod to conform to normal thoracic kyphosis. However, following the insertion of a bent rod, rotation of the assembly can occur, resulting in even greater loss of pelvic lordosis (Fig. 20–16). In order to overcome this problem, a square-ended rod inserted into a square hole in the hook has been devised (Fig. 20–17). This modification will prevent rod rotation after rod bending.

Rod bending does not seem to be associated with increased rod breakage. Rod breakage, on the other hand, is usually an indication of pseudarthrosis, but late breakage may occur even with a solid fusion. The limit to which a rod can be bent and still provide some corrective force is variable (Fig. 20–18). Generally, bending up to an angle of 35 to 40 degrees will not greatly compromise the effective distracting force. A rod that is bent more than this is difficult to insert and will continue to bend as distraction is applied. The rigidity of the deformity may necessitate bending the rod to greater than 50 degrees. If fixation does not appear secure, external fixa-

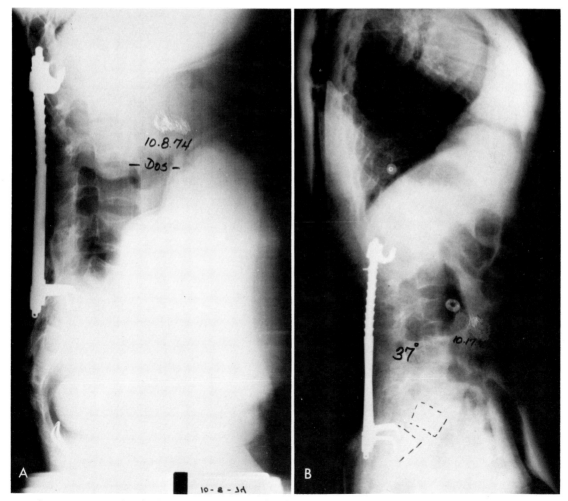

**Figure 20–16** Lumbar lordosis may be maintained in fusions carried to the sacrum by bending the Harrington rod assembly to conform to the lordosis. However, following the insertion of a bent rod, rotation of the assembly can occur, resulting in loss of lordosis. This can be avoided by use of the square-ended hook and rod.

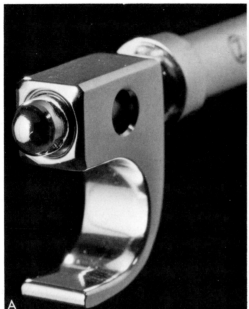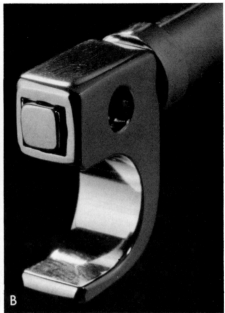

**Figure 20–17** *A,* Insertion of a Harrington distracting device into a #1254 hook. *B,* The junction of a modified rod with a modified hook. It can easily be seen that a bend placed into the customary rod may still rotate, but in the modified assembly, rotation of the rod is prevented.

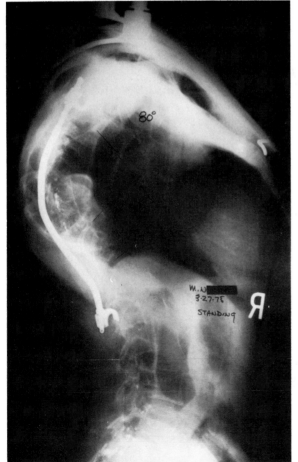

**Figure 20–18** Although bending of the rod is possible, as in this case, where a 65 degree bend was placed into the rod, the effective distracting force is greatly compromised. The fixation appeared secure, but external fixation in the form of a halo cast was supplemented for the postoperative immobilization. Note that not only is the rod bent in kyphosis to accommodate insertion into the upper hook but also that a bend is necessary in the lower end of the rod to achieve the lordosis essential for the rod to be inserted into the lower hook.

tion (Halo-cast) may be supplemental for postoperative immobilization. Bending should be carried out over the body of the rod and not at the ratcheted portion, lest weakening occur. For controlled and accurate bending, we have found the French bending device to be by far the most adaptable (Fig. 20–19).

## WAKE-UP TEST

We have found that the best technique for monitoring neurologic function following corrective spinal surgery, particularly after Harrington instrumentation insertion, is the "wake-up test" of Dr. Pierre Stagnara, Lyon, France. This provides, we feel, an effective method of allowing neurologic evaluation of the patient immediately after insertion of distracting rods or other manipulative spinal procedures. We have routinely adopted this technique, particularly in patients with congenital spine deformity where Harrington rods may occasionally be used. Following the insertion of the Harrington rod, the anesthesi-

ologist is instructed to begin waking the patient up while the patient is still intubated and the wound is open. With careful and controlled anesthesia technique, it is quite possible to ask the patient to move his hands and feet to command, immediately establishing the presence of cord function distal to the spinal surgery. Once this is elicited the anesthesia is deepened and the procedure is completed. If the patient can move his hands but is unable to move his feet, then one presumes that the possibility of neurologic damage is present, and the Harrington rod is removed. The patient is then instructed to move his feet again. We have had one such patient who was unable to move his feet after distraction had been carried out, but when the rod was taken down one or two notches, movement of the feet was possible. Patients rarely have any adverse reaction to this procedure, provided the anesthesia is properly and carefully carried out. Nor do they ever have any undesirable sequelae, and they rarely remember the procedure.

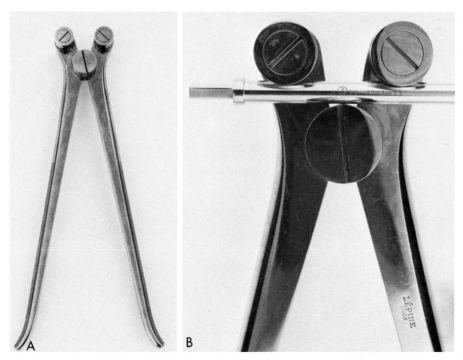

**Figure 20–19**   In order to achieve precise bending of the Harrington rods, we have found this bender, manufactured by Lépine (France) to be by far the most adaptable. (Also distributed by Du Puy.)

**Posterior Osteotomy for Ankylosed Facets.**

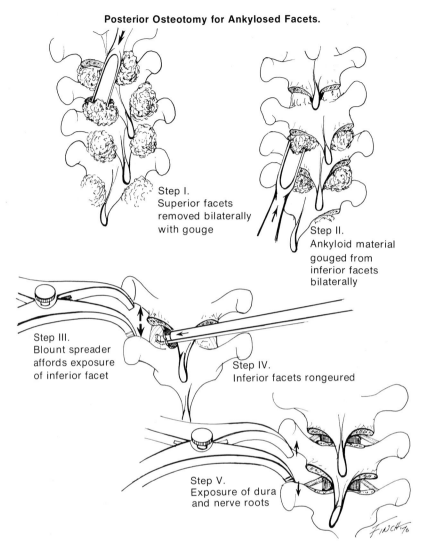

Step I.
Superior facets
removed bilaterally
with gouge

Step II.
Ankyloid material
gouged from
inferior facets
bilaterally

Step III.
Blount spreader
affords exposure
of inferior facet

Step IV.
Inferior facets rongeured

Step V.
Exposure of dura
and nerve roots

**Figure 20–20**   Facet osteotomy. Facet joints that have undergone spontaneous ankylosis must be osteotomized in order to achieve correction of the spinal deformity. The inferior articular process is excised sharply with a concave gouge, removing the osteophyte and the inferior facet. By orienting the gouge perpendicular to the bony surface, the facet is removed completely and safely, releasing the facet ankylosis. Osteophytes that remain on the superior facet may be likewise removed with a sharp gouge in the manner noted. A Blount spreader is then placed between the two transverse processes and spread gently in order to assure that the facet joint has been released completely. Release of the concave facet is usually all that is necessary. If little motion is demonstrated, even after releasing the convex side, careful laminotomy should be done over the ankylosed joint. The inferior as well as the superior facet should be removed laterally until the foramen is completely uncovered. Radical release in the facets bilaterally in the manner described will result in motion, provided a spontaneous anterior interbody fusion has not occurred. It is also possible, however, that the costotransverse joints have likewise become ankylosed, and a costransversectomy with removal of two centimeters of the apical four or five ribs on the concave side may be necessary.

## Posterior Osteotomy

Osteotomies through the posterior aspect of the spine may involve the facet joints alone or the posterior elements of the spine when they have been previously arthrodesed. Osteotomy through the facets alone may be carried out without difficulty, provided that the surgeon is cognisant of anatomical landmarks and variations associated with a malrotated spine (Fig. 20–20). Following exposure of the posterior elements as previously described, the facet joints that have undergone spontaneous ankylosis can be identified readily.

A sharp gouge may be placed at the junction of the transverse process with the inferior facet and oriented so that the concavity of the gouge covers the inferior articular facet. A cut should then be made perpendicular to the bony surface, cutting only deep enough to completely remove the inferior facet. By this careful maneuver, orienting the gouge properly, the inferior facet can be removed effectively and safely uncovering the superior facet and releasing the facet ankylosis.

In cases of severe ankylosis, the anatomical configuration of the facet may not be readily apparent. However, by placing the concavity of the gouge at the angle of the transverse process articulation with the lamina and cutting in a semicircular fashion through the outer shell of the inferior facet, the ankylosed joint is easily released. A Blount spreader should then be placed between the two transverse processes and spread gently in order to assure that the facet joint has been completely released. It may be necessary to extend this release to the convex side of the posterior element; however, this is rarely ankylosed. Release of the concave facet is usually all that is necessary. If the facet is completely fused and is not easily released by removing the inferior rim of the fact along with the ankylosed portion, a careful laminotomy should be done over the ankylosed joint.

Using angled Kerrison rongeurs, or gouge, osteotome, and curette, the inferior as well as as the superior facet is removed in a lateral direction until the foramen is reached. The pars interarticularis overlying the foramen is removed to completely release one half of the posterior element. A Blount spreader is then used between the transverse processes spanning this facet joint to determine whether the release has been complete and effective. If residual tightness is apparent, the release should be continued to the convex side of the curvature, releasing the facets in a similar fashion.

When the facets in the lumbar spine need to be released in order to free bony ankylosis, a similar cut is made in the inferior articular facet; however, the cut with the gouge should be made at a more sagittal plane to conform to the direction of the facet joint. Similarly, it is often useful to use an osteotome rather than a gouge, since this will conform best to the anatomical configuration of the facet joint in the lumbar area.

In the thoracic spine, after release of the ankylosed facet joint as described, one may find that little movement of the vertebral body is possible. On the concave side this may result from a "locking" effect of the costotransverse joints, which have likewise become ankylosed. The configuration of the ribs, which are held in place by the malrotated collapsing spinal deformity, may contribute to the fixation. One sees this particularly in cases of paralytic scoliosis with severe vertebral rotation. A costotransversectomy with removal of two centimeters of the apical four to five ribs is usually sufficient to allow complete release of the vertebral bodies.

## POSTERIOR OSTEOTOMY OF A PREVIOUSLY FUSED SPINE

Posterior osteotomies through previous posterior spine fusions, in either the presence or the absence of a pseudarthrosis, may prove a difficult surgical exercise (Fig. 20–21). However, careful attention to anatomical landmarks can make this a relatively safe procedure. Posterior osteotomies in the lumbar spine are somewhat easier to perform and allow a greater degree of correction, due to greater mobility of the lumbar spine.

Often in the case of very thick posterior fusions, it is difficult to determine where facet joints were located. The transverse processes provide a reliable anatomical landmark. One begins by outlining the osteotomy site just inferior to the transverse processes. A trough is cut into the fusion mass with osteotomes, gouges, and rongeurs of appropriate sizes. A thickened fusion mass will have characteristics similar to those to diaphyseal or metaphyseal bone. When the outer cortical shell is cut, cancellous bone of varying degrees of thickness will be found. By carefully removing this material, an inner cortex of bone is reached. An opening can be made with appropriate gouges or rongeurs, permitting entry of an angled Kerrison rongeur underneath this shell.

The dura at this point can be adequately visualized, and by progressively widening the opening, the dissection then proceeds in a lateral direction toward the intervertebral foramen. It is important to identify this area, since the osteotomy can be completed easily by making the cut directly through the pars interarticularis. If, on the other hand, one attempts to cut through the pedicle, the osteotomy will not be accomplished effectively. It

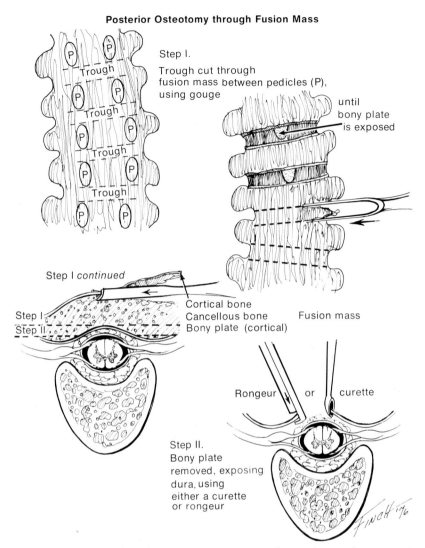

**Posterior Osteotomy through Fusion Mass**

Step I.

Trough cut through fusion mass between pedicles (P), using gouge

until bony plate is exposed

Step I continued

Step I

Step II

Cortical bone
Cancellous bone
Bony plate (cortical)

Fusion mass

Rongeur or curette

Step II.
Bony plate removed, exposing dura, using either a curette or rongeur

**Figure 20–21**  Posterior osteotomy through a previous posterior spine fusion. The site of osteotomy just inferior to the transverse processes is outlined. A trough is cut in the fusion mass with appropriate gouges. A thickened fusion mass will resemble metaphyseal bone. By cutting through the outer cortical shell, cancellous bone of varying degrees of thickness will be found. By carefully removing this, the inner cortex of bone is reached. An opening can be made in the mid-line, so that an angled Kerrison rongeur or angled curette can be inserted underneath this shell. The dura is adequately visualized, and by progressive widening of the opening, the section can proceed out laterally through the intervertebral foramen, completing the osteotomy. It is not necessary to osteotomize each level; in fact it is actually preferable to expose alternate levels, otherwise loosening will be too great and compromise of neural tissue can result.

is often helpful to use the Blount spreader to facilitate the correction and to crack through the last portion of cortical bone. Bleeding may become rather brisk at this point if epidural veins have been torn. However, hemostasis can be maintained with Gelfoam and cotton pledgets.

The manner in which posterior osteotomy wedges are made will be determined by the indication for the osteotomy. For example, if the osteotomy was done primarily for the purpose of loosening the posterior spine

and allowing further correction with the halo-femoral or halopelvic distraction, little planning is needed regarding the angle at which the osteotomy will be carried out. On the other hand, if the posterior osteotomy is being made in conjunction with 1) an anterior vertebral body excision or 2) a single-stage correction of an angular deformity, great attention must be directed toward planning and execution of the amount of bone to be removed and the area from which it is to be taken. In this situation it is preferable to leave the central midline broken cortex as a hinge and to make the osteotomy wide on the convex side and narrow on the concave side.

After the appropriate wedge or wedges are cut, one has the option of proceeding with skeletal traction, corrective casting, or internal instrumentation with wedge closure by use of the Harrington compression devices. The bony fusion mass provides excellent fixation for the compression as well as distraction hooks, and holes can be made in the fusion mass, with appropriate gouges to accept hooks of any size. For correction of an angular deformity in one stage, we have generally preferred to perform a single osteotomy in the thoracolumbar or lumbar spine and carry out immediate correction with the Harrington compression assembly, using two of the more narrow threaded rods, with four to six hooks on each rod. If the wedge of bone is carefully cut, bone-to-bone contact can be assured throughout the length of the osteotomy and strong fixation accomplished without undue difficulty. Occasionally, the distracting assembly may be necessary. However, one should realize that this device may serve to push the osteotomy apart on the side on which it is used, leading to a risk of delayed union or non-union. After the internal fixation is secure, the fusion mass is decorticated and bone is laid down over the osteotomy site. Additional iliac bone may be necessary if the local bone is insufficient.

## ANTERIOR SPINE FUSION*

### Transthoracic Approach

Transthoracic approach to the spine is preferable to the retropleural costotransversectomy approach, since far greater visibility is possible and the exposure is more extensive. The approach may be from the right or the left, depending primarily upon the discretion of the operating surgeon and the anatomy of the deformity. The great vessels lie anterior to the spine, and therefore, in either a right or left approach they will be out of the way, provided the exposure is carefully performed.

The level of the approach is determined by the procedure to be performed. The rib selected for removal should be the one above the upper level of the vertebral bodies to be exposed. If a lower rib is chosen, it will be

difficult to reach the upper portion of the deformity, since the downward inclination of the ribs will interfere with visualization. For example, if one removes the fifth rib, access from T5 to T11 can be accomplished without difficulty. Similarly, removal of the sixth rib gives access from T6 to T12, and removal of the seventh rib gives access from T7 to L1. There are exceptions to this rule. In some patients with horizontally oriented ribs, removal of the sixth rib gives access from T5 to T11. In other patients with very sloping ribs, removal of the fifth rib may give easy access from T6 through T11 only. Finally, in some patients with extreme rotation and collapsed chest walls, only two to three vertebrae may be approached with ease through one rib space. If, after rib removal, it is apparent that a higher exposure is necessary, one may divide the rib above at its posterior angle without removing it.

Proper positioning of the retractors will furnish greater exposure. It is possible to go as high as the third rib through this approach by careful mobilization and displacement of the scapula upward and forward. Approach to the first thoracic vertebra through the third is then possible, although difficult. If access from T1 to T4 is contemplated, it is also possible to reach this area by a sternal splitting incision from the suprasternal notch to the xiphoid. The thymus is retracted, the innominate vein is divided, and the trachea and esophagus are displaced to the left. This approach is a formidable one, and maneuverability is limited. Furthermore, the risk of complications would appear quite high. For these reasons, it is preferable to approach the highest thoracic vertebrae through a thoracotomy approach, removing the third or fourth rib.

After preparation of the skin (Fig. 20–22), the incision is made from the posterior angle of the rib to the tip of costal cartilage. The incision is carried down to the rib, and the rib is exposed subperiosteally and then detached anteriorly from the costochondral junction and as far posteriorly as possible (at least to the costotransverse articulation). The chest is entered by incising the pleura along the rib bed. The edges of the wound are covered with moist sponges, and rib retractors are inserted.

The parietal pleura is now incised along the vertebral bodies throughout the length of the spine to be exposed (Fig. 20–23). The discs will appear as prominences and the ver-

---

*See references 1, 2, 4, 5, 6, 10–14, 16.

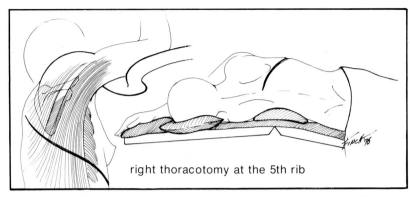

right thoracotomy at the 5th rib

**Figure 20–22**    The correct positioning for a patient undergoing a thoracotomy for exposure of the anterior spine at T5.

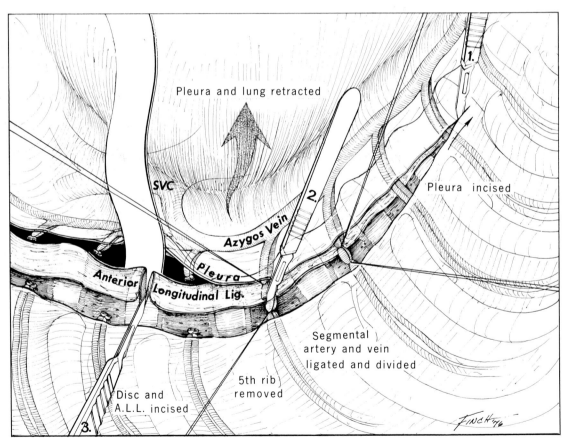

Pleura and lung retracted

SVC

Pleura incised

Azygos Vein

Anterior Longitudinal Lig.

Pleura

Segmental artery and vein ligated and divided

Disc and A.L.L. incised

5th rib removed

**Figure 20–23**    The exposure to the spine following removal of the fifth rib. First the parietal pleura is incised along the length of the spine to be exposed. The segmental vessels are identified overlying each vertebral body and are ligated and divided anterolaterally at least 1 cm away from the intervertebral foramen. By staying outside the periosteum, the areolar tissue with the divided vessels is pushed off the vertebral bodies and the anterior longitudinal ligament around to the opposite side and into the angle between the vertebral body and the transverse process. A malleable retractor provides excellent exposure. The disc and anterior longitudinal ligament may be incised and completely removed as necessary.

tebral bodies as depressions. The pleura may easily be dissected off the anterior longitudinal ligament. The segmental vessels will be visualized as they cross over the vertebral bodies. The vessels should be secured and ligated over the midportion of the spine anteriorly. It is possible, if the vessels are ligated too far laterally next to the intervertebral foramen, that the vascular anastomosis may be disrupted, and damage to the segmental feeder vessels to the spinal cord may result.

The dissection proceeds along either of two routes: 1) The areolar extraperiosteal plane or 2) the subperiosteal plane. Generally, the extraperiosteal plane is more common, but for inlay strut grafting the subperiosteal plane is preferable. If the extraperiosteal plane is chosen, the areolar tissue with the divided vessels is stripped off the vertebral bodies and anterior longitudinal ligament to the opposite side into the angle between the

vertebral body and the transverse process. Small bleeders will be encountered, and they should be cauterized. A sponge can be packed into the area and a malleable retractor then inserted to the opposite side of the vertebral bodies, providing excellent exposure and separating the great vessels from the operative field. No attempt is made to preserve the splanchnic nerves. Their division causes no problems.

## Thoracoabdominal Approach

Exposure of the thoracic and lumbar spines can be accomplished through a single incision by dividing the diaphragm from its costal attachments. For this approach, the tenth rib is generally removed (as described in the preceding section). The incision is extended from the costocartilage junction across the upper abdomen, to the lateral edge

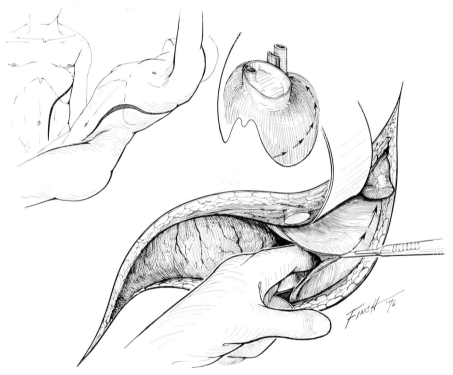

**Figure 20–24** The thoracoabdominal approach is carried out by an incision through the tenth rib. The incision is extended from the costocartilage junction across the upper diaphragm to the lateral edge of the sheath of the rectus abdominis muscle toward the symphysis pubis. The length of the incision depends upon the length of the lumbar spine to be exposed. After the tenth rib is removed from its costal attachment, a retroperitoneal entry into the abdominal cavity is accomplished. This is facilitated by blunt dissection with fingertips between the cut edges of the cartilage at the costochondral junction, peeling off the peritoneum from the underside of the diaphragm. The diaphragm is detached, leaving about 1 cm of its costal insertion as depicted in the figure. Stay sutures may be placed around the edge of the divided tissue where the diaphragm attaches to the spinal column in order to facilitate identification when surgical closure is carried out. Procedure continues in Figure 20–25.

of the rectus abdominis sheath and toward the symphysis pubis (Fig. 20–24). The length of the incision depends upon the length of the lumbar spine to be exposed. Through this incision, it is possible to expose all the way to the sacrum.

After the tenth rib is removed from its costal attachment, a retroperitoneal entry into the abdominal cavity is accomplished. This is facilitated by blunt dissection with fingertips between the cut edges of the cartilage, peeling off the peritoneum from the underside of the diaphragm. As this dissection proceeds laterally and posteriorly, the diaphragm will become free of its peritoneal attachment, and the viscerae will fall forward, away from the vertebral column. The diaphragm is then detached about one centimeter from its costal insertion. This leaves sufficient tissue on the rib to allow repair at the time of wound closure. The incision into the diaphragm extends posteriorly to the vertebrae. Sutures may be placed on the edge of the divided tissue where the diaphragm attaches to the spinal column in order to facilitate identification

when surgical closure is carried out. On the right side, the crus of the diaphragm is attached down to the body of the third lumbar vertebra, whereas on the left side it extends as far as the body of the second lumbar vertebra.

The exposure now proceeds cephalad and caudally, dividing the parietal pleura and identifying the vertebral bodies and the intervertebral discs (Fig. 20–25). The segmental vessels are identified and ligated as described previously. In the lumbar spine, the exposure is more difficult, since the psoas muscle overlies the anterolateral aspect of the vertebral body. Brisk bleeding may be encountered if the segmental vessels are not carefully identified and ligated. A surgical cautery is very helpful for this exposure. The sympathetic chain should be preserved if feasible. It is possible to retract this chain posteriorly toward the base of the transverse process of the vertebra. As one proceeds more distally, the iliac vessels will overlie the intervertebral disc at L4 and L5. By careful dissection, these vessels may be freed and displaced an-

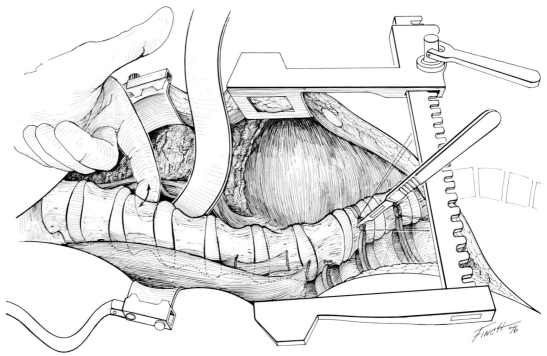

**Figure 20–25** Exposure (see Fig. 20–24) now proceeds proximally and distally along the spine from the areas to be visualized. The segmental vessels are identified and ligated in the manner previously described. In the lumbar spine the exposure is more difficult, since the psoas muscle overlies the anterior lateral aspect of the vertebral body. With careful dissection, however, more than adequate visualization is possible. As one proceeds distally, the iliac vessels will overlie the intervertebral disc at L4 and L5, but again by careful dissection, the vessels may be freed and displaced anteriorly, allowing exposure to the L5–S1 disc.

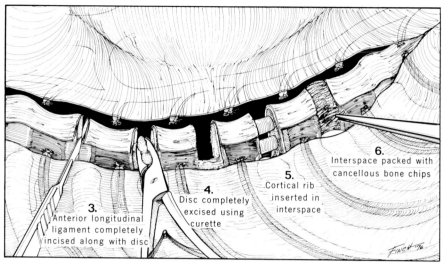

**Figure 20–26** Anterior interbody fusion is accomplished by complete excision of the anterior longitudinal ligament along with removal of the disc. The disc is removed to the posterior annulus, and the intervening cartilage is removed to the bony end-plates. If correction of the kyphosis is necessary, one should remove the posterior annulus along with the end-plates up to the posterior longitudinal ligament. Generally, however, this will not be essential, since removal of the disc material up to the posterior annulus will make it possible to hinge open the kyphosis and significantly correct the angular deformity. The rib bone that has been removed during the thoracotomy is cut into small pieces and wedged into each intervertebral space, hinging the vertebral bodies open and correcting the kyphosis. Remaining rib strips are then placed into the interspace, or, if desirable, cancellous bone from the iliac crest may be used to supplement the fusion mass.

teriorly, allowing exposure to the intervertebral disc between L5 and S1.

## Anterior Fusion

An interbody technique is best accomplished by complete removal of disc material and careful grafting with cancellous and cortical autogenous bone. Before the disc is removed, it is desirable to expose the annulus from the edge of one intervertebral foramen around anteriorly to the opposite foramen (Fig. 20–26).

Disc removal should be done in two stages. The annulus is first removed along with the nucleus, as completely as possible, at each interspace, leaving only the posterior portion of the annulus. Various sizes of rongeurs and curettes are helpful for this purpose (Fig. 20–27). The anterior longitudinal ligament and periosteum should not be re-

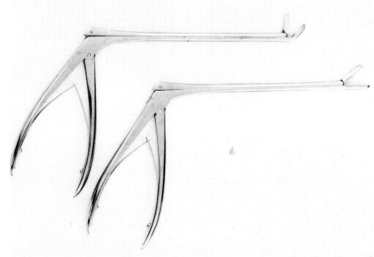

**Figure 20–27** These specially designed rongeurs have been extremely helpful in facilitating removal of disc and annulus material, especially in the lumbar spine. (Kindly furnished by Professor Hodgson, Hong Kong.)

moved from the vertebral body except where they overlie the annulus. After all of the involved disc spaces are exposed in this fashion, the cartilage end-plates are removed as completely as possible at each level. It is usually necessary to remove the end-plates up to the posterior annulus only, except in severe rigid kyphosis, where correction of deformity is necessary. In these cases, it will be necessary to remove the posterior annulus along with the end-plates up to the posterior longitudinal ligament. A long-handled angled curette and sharp, thin osteotomes are very useful for this portion of the procedure.

After each end-plate is removed, the disc space may be packed with Gelfoam or a sponge to minimize bleeding. The rib that has been removed in the thoracotomy exposure is now cut into small pieces, approximately one to two centimeters in length, and wedged into each intervertebral space. The remaining portions of the rib are cut into small matchstick-shaped grafts and carefully packed into the remaining open intervertebral spaces. If additional bone is necessary, cancellous and cortical bone can be taken from the iliac crest. The bone should be packed snugly in order to prevent fragments from dislodging. The parietal pleura can now be sutured over the anterior portions of the vertebral body, separating the dissection from the pleural cavity.

### Inlay Strut Fusion

When a major portion of a vertebral body has been removed, interbody bone grafting will not furnish sufficient support to achieve spine stability. In these cases, particularly where anterior decompression has been carried out, an inlay bone strut fusion will provide the necessary support.

Exposure proceeds as described, through the periosteal route. The intervertebral discs are removed and a trough is cut into the lateral portion of the vertebral bodies at the apex of the kyphosis (Fig. 20–28). The length depends on the area to be fused but usually extends two vertebrae above and two below the apical vertebra. The trough is deepened until the opposite cortex is approached. The vertebral bodies at the proximal and distal ends of the trough are then undercut, creating a cavity without violating either the lateral or the anterior cortex. This cavity should be at least one to two centimeters deep.

The rib previously removed is now prepared, cut to the proper length, and placed in the trough. One end is pushed into the undercut end vertebra. The surgical assistant forcefully pushes on the apex of the kyphosis, and the anesthetist pulls on the head, correcting the deformity while the surgeon maneuvers the free end of the rib strut into the opposite cavity in the end vertebra, "keying" the graft into place. Force is taken off the apex, allowing the graft to lock into position.

The remaining rib bone is cut into wedges and driven around each end of the strut as well as of the graft bed, further locking the graft into position. The interspaces are packed with rib bone as previously described. Iliac bone or fibula may be used in place of rib or to augment the rib strut as necessary. If an anterior cord decompression has been carried out, no loose fragments of bone should lie between the rib strut and the dura. A thin strip of Gelfoam should be placed on the dura and additional bone placed anterior to the strut.

### Anterior Strut Fusion

In the presence of an angular structural kyphosis, it may be necessary to place supportive bone grafts anterior to the vertebral bodies in order to achieve spinal stability and successful arthrodesis (Fig. 20–29). The length of the arthrodesis and strut graft depend on the severity of the kyphotic deformity. In general, the graft should extend from end vertebra to end vertebra of the structural part of the kyphosis and lie in the weight-bearing line of the spine if possible. The most common technical mistake is placement of the grafts between the apical two or three vertebrae only. Progression of the deformity, graft failure, and pseudarthrosis may result from an anterior fusion that is too short. If there is an associated scoliosis, it is desirable that the graft lie on the concave side of the curvature. If the scoliosis is significant (greater than 50 to 60 degrees), it may prove easier to approach the spine on the convexity of the scoliotic curvature, away from the great vessels, which will displace into the concavity. The graft may still be placed on the concave side of the curvature with little difficulty with this approach.

After the vertebral bodies are visualized, a subperiosteal rather than extraperiosteal

*Text continued on page 517*

**Inlay Graft Technique**

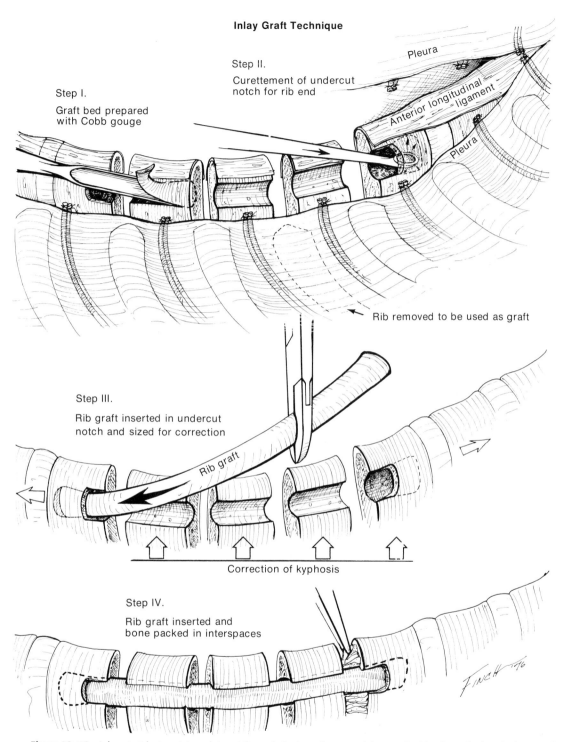

Step I.

Graft bed prepared with Cobb gouge

Step II.

Curettement of undercut notch for rib end

Pleura

Anterior longitudinal ligament

Pleura

Rib removed to be used as graft

Step III.

Rib graft inserted in undercut notch and sized for correction

Rib graft

Correction of kyphosis

Step IV.

Rib graft inserted and bone packed in interspaces

**Figure 20–28**  Inlay strut fusion. A trough is cut through the lateral cortex of the vertebral bodies to be fused. This trough is deepened for the appropriate length of the graft, at least to 1 to 2 centimeters. The opposite lateral cortex or the anterior cortex of the vertebral bodies should not be violated. A rib is prepared, cut to proper lengths, and placed in the trough as outlined. One end is pushed into the undercut end of the vertebra. The surgical assistant forcefully pushes on the apex of the kyphosis while the anesthetist pulls on the head, correcting the deformity, and the surgeon maneuvers the free end of the rib strut into the opposite cavity in the end vertebra, thus "keying" the graft into place. Force is taken off the apex, allowing the graft to lock in position. Remaining cut pieces of bone are then packed into each interspace, facilitating an adequate graft bed for bony fusion.

**Strut Graft Technique—Part 1**

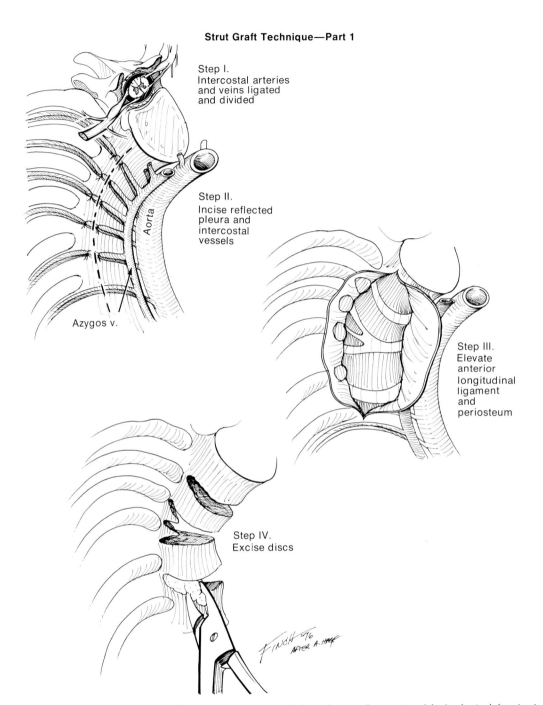

Step I.
Intercostal arteries
and veins ligated
and divided

Step II.
Incise reflected
pleura and
intercostal
vessels

Step III.
Elevate
anterior
longitudinal
ligament
and
periosteum

Step IV.
Excise discs

Aorta

Azygos v.

**Figure 20–29**   Anterior strut fusion. The length of the strut graft depends upon the severity of the kyphotic deformity. In general, the strut should extend from the end vertebra above to the end vertebra below the structural part of the kyphosis and lie in the weight-bearing line of the spine if possible. The most common error is placement·of grafts between the apical two or three vertebrae only. Progression of the deformity is then possible as a result of an anterior fusion that is too short. After the vessels are ligated as previously described, the periosteum with the anterior longitudinal ligament is elevated as a single flap of tissue.

*Legend continued on opposite page.*

**Strut Graft Technique—Part 2**

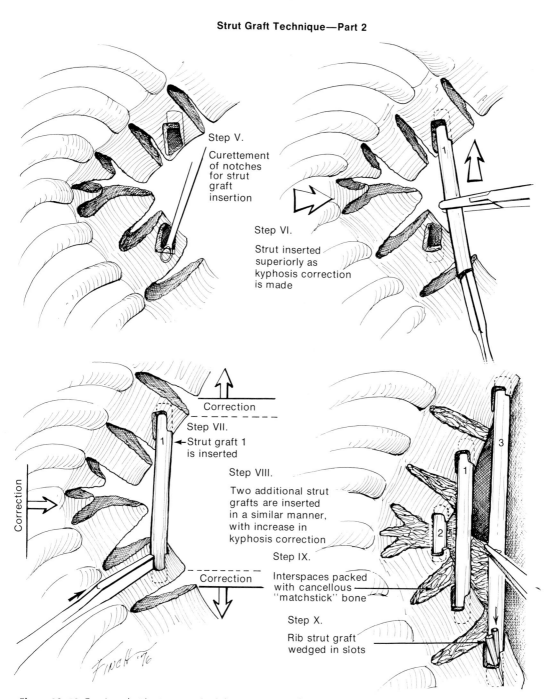

Step V.

Curettement
of notches
for strut
graft
insertion

Step VI.

Strut inserted
superiorly as
kyphosis correction
is made

Correction

Step VII.

Strut graft 1
is inserted

Step VIII.

Two additional strut
grafts are inserted
in a similar manner,
with increase in
kyphosis correction

Step IX.

Interspaces packed
with cancellous
"matchstick" bone

Step X.

Rib strut graft
wedged in slots

Correction

Correction

**Figure 20–29** *Continued*   The intervertebral discs are removed as previously described, and a tunnel is carved into the anterior body of the end vertebra below and above the apex of the curvature. Rib or fibula or even iliac strut is then cut to the appropriate length and wedged into place, applying a force over the apex of the curve as well as longitudinal traction on the head. Additional strut graft can then be inserted as outlined, and cancellous and remaining rib bone may then be inserted in each intervertebral disc space and on top of the periosteum between the strut graft and anterior cortex of the vertebral bodies. No attempt is made to reattach the periosteum.

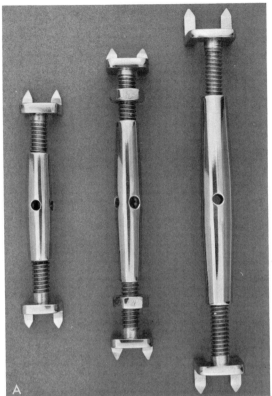

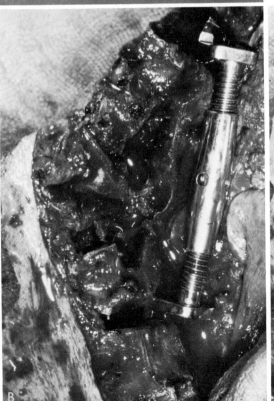

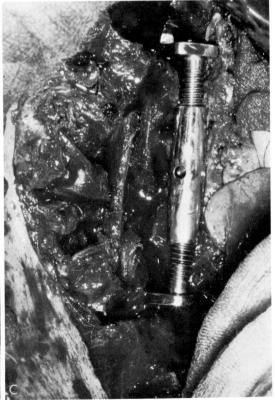

**Figure 20–30** To facilitate anterior strut graft insertion for severe kyphosis, the strut bar has proved to be of great help. This device may be locked into the vertebral body anteriorly and then carefully distracted, facilitating the anterior bone graft insertion. After the rib or fibula bone has been keyed into place, the device is removed. (Kindly furnished by Dr Waldemar Pinto, São Paulo, Brazil.)

dissection is preferable. After division of the segmental vessels, the anterior longitudinal ligament with the periosteum is elevated as a single flap to the opposite side of the vertebral bodies. The intervertebral discs are removed as described previously. A tunnel approximately one to two centimeters in length is then cut into the anterior body of the end vertebra above as well as the end vertebra below the apex. A rib, fibula, or iliac strut is then cut to the appropriate length. The fibula may provide greater strength than rib and may therefore be preferable, particularly in severe kyphosis. Iliac bone, on the other hand, offers the advantages of a cancellous component but will provide less support.

The strut graft is then keyed into the vertebral bodies in the fashion described in the preceding section (Fig. 20–30). By removing the periosteum, a bleeding bony surface on the anterior surface of the vertebral bodies faces the bone graft. This surface can be further curetted to cancellous bone, and the intervening space between the vertebral bodies and strut grafts can be packed with rib or iliac bone. The elevated periosteum lying deep to the strut graft acts as a protective wall, preventing the chips of additional bone from falling free into the thorax.

Usually two or more strut grafts may be inserted, depending on the severity and length of the kyphosis. No attempt is made to reattach the periosteum. It is actually impossible to do so. Gelfoam may be placed over the lateral surface of the graft area at the completion of the procedure to prevent small bone chips from dislodging. Provided the strut is well keyed into place, no problem results from the graft's lying against the lung tissue.

## Anterior Osteotomy

An osteotomy from the anterior approach may be carried out with a greater or lesser degree of difficulty, depending upon the deformity and the presence or absence of intervertebral disc tissue (Fig. 20–31). In a Type II congenital kyphosis, for example, a bony bar may be present in the most anterior portion of the vertebral body. Here disc material is absent anteriorly but is present laterally and posteriorly. It is relatively easy to

remove the bony bar anterior to the disc, completely excising the disc space using appropriately shaped gouges, rongeurs, and curettes. The anterior fusion as previously described is then performed. Occasionally, the bony ridge may be complete (to the posterior longitudinal ligament), and the osteotomy is, therefore, somewhat more difficult. In that case, one should begin with an anterior osteotomy, using a sharp osteotome and working carefully in a more posterior direction. The cancellous bone is removed with a sharp, angled curette.

Bleeding will become more brisk as one approaches the posterior cortical shell of the vertebral body, which is in juxtaposition to the posterior longitudinal ligament. As one approaches this cortical shell, the transition between cancellous and cortical bone is easily visualized. A Blount spreader is placed between the two vertebral bodies at the walls of the osteotomy and carefully spread. Usually this maneuver will serve to fracture the posterior cortex, allowing the vertebral bodies anteriorly to open like a clamshell. If it is not possible to fracture the posterior cortex of the bodies in this fashion, a gouge or osteotome can be carefully used to make a cut into this cortex at the posterior lateral limits. With the use of angled curettes and angled Kerrison rongeurs, the dissection can then be carried across to the opposite side of the vertebral body, completing the osteotomy and avoiding damage to the neural tissue.

## Anterior Cord Decompression

Decompression of the spinal cord anteriorly is not an unduly difficult procedure, provided that the exposure is adequate and the surgeon experienced (Fig. 20–32). The apex of the deformity at the site of cord compression should be adequately identified, and the chest entered at the rib or one rib higher than the point of this compression. The exposure of the vertebral bodies follows the same pattern as previously described. The anatomical landmarks of the costotransverse joint, pedicle, and costovertebral junction must be identified.

Anterior decompression is usually necessary for angular deformities in the lateral plane (kyphosis). Therefore, the chest cavity may be entered through either the right or the

*Text continued on page 520*

**Anterior Osteotomy**

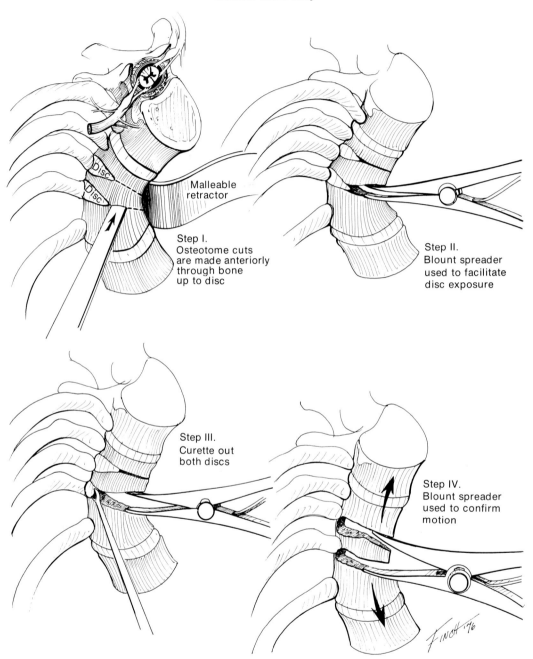

**Figure 20–31**  The technique for anterior osteotomy. In Type II congenital kyphosis, as noted, a bony bar may be present in the most anterior portion of the vertebral body. The bony bar is removed, using a sharp osteotome, beginning anteriorly and working posteriorly until the remaining disc material is entered. A Blount spreader may facilitate exposure, making it possible to completely remove the disc material back to the posterior longitudinal ligament. If the bony bridge is complete to the posterior longitudinal ligament, osteotomy must be complete through the posterior cortex. By the use of a Blount spreader, the posterior cortex remaining may be fractured, allowing the vertebral bodies to open anteriorly, like a clamshell.

**Anterior Cord Decompression**

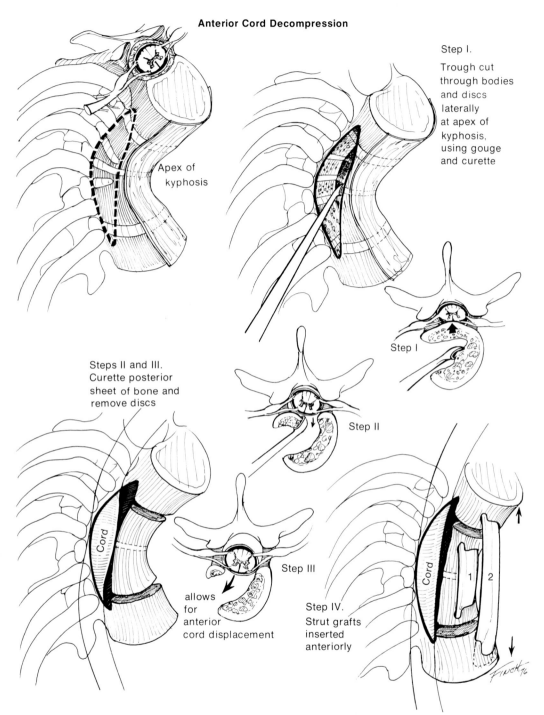

Step I.

Trough cut through bodies and discs laterally at apex of kyphosis, using gouge and curette

Apex of kyphosis

Step I

Steps II and III. Curette posterior sheet of bone and remove discs

Step II

Cord

Step III

allows for anterior cord displacement

Step IV. Strut grafts inserted anteriorly

Cord

**Figure 20–32** The technique of anterior cord decompression. Exposure should usually be on the concave side of the scoliosis, since the cord needs to be moved both forward and toward the concavity of the scoliosis for adequate decompression (see text). A trough is cut into the vertebral body and disc space at the apex of the curvature and deepened. Bleeding is controlled with bone wax. The posterior cortex of the vertebral body is identified. The posterior cortex is outlined all the way to the opposite posterior lateral surface of the vertebral body prior to removing this cortical shell. Angled curettes are essential for this dissection. The entire trough should be completed before the posterior cortex is removed. Starting away from the apex of the kyphosis, the posterior cortex is then removed, identifying the dura. Dissection then proceeds to the apex of the kyphosis. It will become apparent that the dura begins to move anteriorly into the space thus created. This may make exposure difficult and may be prevented by beginning the decompression on the far side (convex side of the lateral curvature) so that the cord will not move anteriorly into the created space until the last elements of bone and disc have been removed. A liberal use of bone wax is essential. The procedure is completed by anterior strut graft fusion (Fig. 20–29).

left side. Generally speaking, the left side is preferable, since the aorta is more easily managed than is the vena cava, should inadvertent tearing of the great vessels result. If, however, there is an associated scoliosis, the cord must be approached on the concave side of the scoliosis, since the cord needs to be moved both forward and toward the concavity of the scoliosis for adequate decompression.

If the scoliosis is greater than 50 to 60 degrees, it may prove technically difficult to proceed with a thoracotomy on the concave side. The aorta and vena cava are displaced into the concavity, and mobilization to achieve adequate exposure may be a problem. On the other hand, approaching on the convexity of the curvature, the vertebral bodies will lie just under the rib cage, and mobilization of the vessels is quite easy. Decompression may still be adequately performed on the concave side of the curvature.

After the thoracotomy is completed, a trough is cut into the vertebral body and the disc space at the apex of the curvature. The width of this trough should be approximately one third of the width of the vertebral body. As the trough is cut deeper and deeper, staying within cancellous bone, large venous bleeders may be encountered. This bleeding should be controlled with bone wax. The posterior cortex of the vertebral body can be identified by its cortical nature and outlined adequately with sharp, long-handled, angled curettes. It is essential to fully remove all the vertebral body bone to the opposite posterior lateral cortex before entering the spinal canal. Once the entire trough has been completed, then, and only then, should the posterior cortex be removed. Starting away from the apex of the kyphosis, the posterior cortex is removed and the dura can be identified. Dissection then proceeds to the apical vertebra until the apex of the kyphosis (and lateral curvature, if present) has been removed from the anterior portion of the spinal cord.

As bony and disc material are carefully removed with rongeurs and curettes, it will become readily apparent that the dura will begin to move anteriorly through the space thus created. This may serve to block the exposure, making it difficult to decompress the far side of the spinal canal. This situation is avoided by beginning the decompression on the far side (convex side of the lateral curvature) so the cord will not move anteriorly into

the created space until the last elements of bone and disc have been removed. Troublesome bone bleeding can be controlled by liberal use of bone wax. Epidural bleeding is controlled with Gelfoam and moist cotton or cotton pledgets. The posterior longitudinal ligament does not routinely need to be removed with the decompression, but it should be removed if there is any question of its interfering with the freedom of the dura and spinal cord.

If the kyphosis is extensive, it may be necessary to remove the majority of the apical vertebral body as well as sizable portions of the vertebral bodies above and below the apex. If, on the other hand, the kyphosis is moderate, only half or less than half of the vertebral body need be removed. In any event, after such a decompression, spine stabilization should be a routine element of the procedure, and a strong bicortical strut graft should be keyed into the vertebral bodies above and below the apex of the kyphosis. However, if it is a severe kyphosis, in the range of 150 degrees or more, it may be necessary to put the strut graft to four vertebrae above as well as below the apex of the kyphosis. In these cases of extreme degrees of angular deformity, two or more strut grafts are necessary.

After the decompression has been completed, the intervertebral discs over the area to be fused are carefully removed as previously outlined. Slots are then cut in the vertebral bodies into which the strut graft will be inserted. These strut grafts must be carefully keyed in place in order to prevent them from dislodging. After the slot has been cut and undermined approximately 0.75 to 1 centimeter, the graft is keyed in place. This maneuver is facilitated by having the assistant forcefully push over the apex of the kyphosis while the graft is toggled into the appropriate slot. Bicortical struts can then be wedged into the same slot to prevent the graft from displacing. A second strut is placed in a similar fashion, and the intervening disc spaces are packed with cancellous and cortical bone. No bone is placed deeply in the space where the decompression was carried out, even though the spinal cord may not completely fill that space. Gelfoam may be laid carefully over the dura, but all bone graft should be placed anterior and away from this cavity. No attempt is made to close the pleura over the defect; it is impossible to do so. The bone packed into the intervertebral disc spaces should be as firmly secured as possible, so that it will not dislodge and become loose in the pleural cavity. The chest cavity is then closed and drained in the customary fashion.

### Dwyer Instrumentation (Fig. 20–33)

The combined transthoracic retroperitoneal approach on the convex side of the curve provides a convenient exposure for the Dwyer instrumentation. It is best to select for removal the rib one level higher than the top vertebra to be instrumented. Since the Dwyer instrumentation has been most useful for thoracolumbar and lumbar curvatures, the tenth rib is usually selected for removal. Dissection is as outlined for the thoracoabdominal approach. The extraperiosteal exposure may be extended to the concave side of the vertebrae, far enough to enable a finger to be placed either to the head of the rib or to the transverse process in order to serve as a guide while passing the screw through the vertebral body.

When all the levels to be instrumented are exposed, the discs are excised. The disc is removed in two stages. The first stage is done by sharp dissection, removing approximately two thirds of the annulus fibrosis, followed by removal of the nucleus pulposus and the remnants of the annulus on the convex side of the curve. A sharp periosteal elevator is then slipped between the cartilage end-plate and the bony end-plate. This dissection is avascular, and bleeding is encountered only when the vertebral end-plates have been penetrated. Therefore, the end-plates are not removed until the discs at each vertebral level to be instrumented have been excised.

Attention is then directed to the upper vertebral body to be instrumented. One must select a staple of the proper size and drive it into place on the lateral side of the vertebral body, using the staple introducer. This also acts as a trocar for beginning the screw. The staple introducer is then removed, and the staple itself should fit snugly and tightly onto the vertebral body. An appropriately sized screw is picked by estimating the length required with a special gauge (Fig. 20–34). The screw is inserted through the hole in the staple and rotated firmly until it has just

engaged the opposite cortex, which is felt with the inserted finger. The next vertebral body is secured with a staple and a screw in a similar fashion, and the cable is introduced through the two screw heads (Fig. 20–35).

The end-plates are removed with a sharp chisel or angled curettes. Graft bone, which is obtained from the removed rib or the iliac crest, is placed in the disc space before the cable tensioner is applied to the cable, to close the space and to obtain close approximation. The actual corrective force is applied to the head of the screw by a special open-ended screwdriver, and the tensioner is used only to take out the slack of the cable. It is rarely necessary to exceed 10 to 20 kilogram-centimeters on the uppermost screw in order to close the interspace. If one uses more force, the upper screw may cut out. This is the weakest point of the fixation, and it is essential to avoid excessive tension.

Once the desired tension and correction have been obtained, the screw head is crimped with a special crimper. The next vertebral body is then prepared with a staple and screw. The end-plates are removed, the bone is packed in the interspace, the tensioner is introduced into the screw, and correction is similarly achieved. One then continues caudally along the lumbar spine, progressively correcting each level until the last vertebral body has been instrumented. A reinforcing collar is placed on the end of the cable at the last level (next to the last screw), so that a double crimp can be used to make the cable more secure. The cable is cut next to the reinforcing collar, which is moved distally approximately two to three millimeters and crimped. The cut end of the cable is thus inside the reinforcing collar and not exposed to the soft tissues surrounding this area. Exposed and frayed ends of the cable might otherwise lie disturbingly close to the iliac vessels (Fig. 20–36). One has the option as well of inserting all staples and screws into the vertebral bodies before starting the cable or proceeding as described.

With the Dwyer instrumentation device, L4 and usually L5 are conveniently reached once the iliac vessels have been mobilized. Reaching the sacrum, in our experience, is not practical or feasible with this technique but could be done under special circumstances and with modified instrumentation.

*Text continued on page 524*

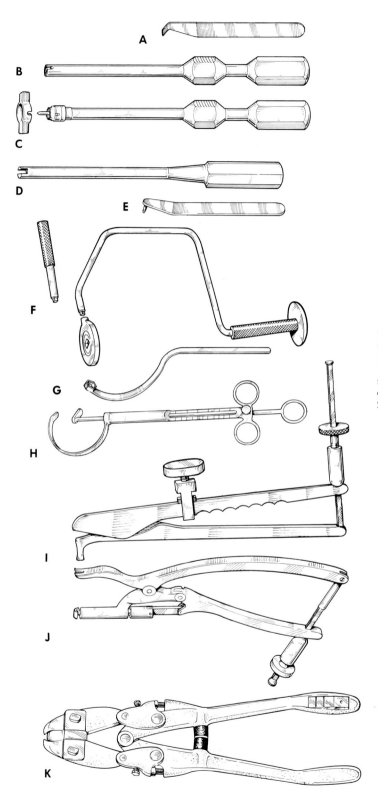

**Figure 20–33** Dwyer instrumentation. *A,* Staple starter. *B,* Hall self-holding screwdriver. *C,* Hall staple introducer. *D,* Hall open-ended screwdriver. *E,* Awl. *F,* Hall brace screwdriver. *G,* Hall box spanner. *H,* Hall calibrator. *I,* Dwyer cable tensioner. *J,* Hall cable tensioner. *K,* Simmons crimper.

*Figure continued on opposite page*

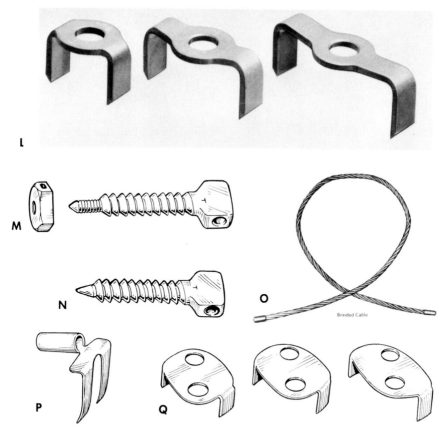

**Figure 20–33** *Continued* *L*, Dwyer staples. *M*, Hall screw with nut. *N*, Dwyer screw. *O*, Braided cable. *P*, Hall sacral anchor. *Q*, Hall double-hole staples. (Courtesy of Downs Surgical, Ltd.)

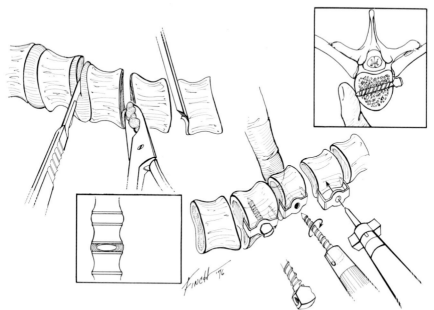

**Figure 20–34** Insertion of the Dwyer instrumentation device. The disc is removed in two stages. First, it is sharply dissected with a knife and rongeur, removing approximately two thirds of the annulus and the nucleus. A sharp periosteal elevator is placed between the cartilage end-plate and the bony end-plate, allowing complete removal of all cartilage. The proper size staple is introduced, using the staple introducer (this also acts as a trocar for beginning the screw hole). The staple should fit snugly and tightly into the vertebral body. The appropriate screw is then picked by estimating the length required with a special gauge. The screw is then inserted until it has engaged the opposite cortex, which is felt with the inserted finger. The next vertebral body is secured with a staple and a screw in a similar fashion. The cable may be introduced (see Fig. 20–35) through the two screw heads at this stage or after all vertebral bodies to be instrumented have been secured with a staple and a screw.

**523**

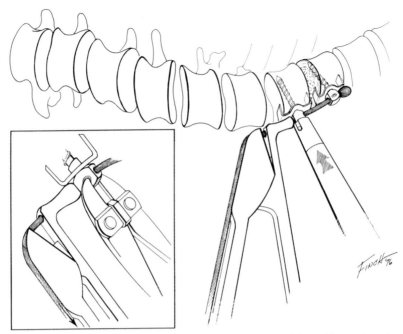

**Figure 20–35**   The cable is introduced through the two screw heads, and the cable tensioner is applied. Both the end-plates between the two vertebral bodies should be removed with a sharp chisel or an angle curette at this point and the interspace packed with cancellous iliac crest bone or with the rib bone that was removed previously. The cable tensioner is then tightened to obtain close approximation of the vertebral bodies. The actual corrective force is applied by a special open-ended screwdriver, and the tension is used only to take the slack out of the cable. The uppermost screw is the weakest point of the fixation, and excessive tension at this area must be avoided; otherwise, the screw will cut out. Once the desired tension and correction are obtained, the screw head is crimped with a special crimper.

## MODIFICATIONS

Various modifications have been made of the Dwyer instrumentation that provide a greater versatility for its use (Fig. 20–33). The upper screw has been designed to accept a nut on the opposite side of the vertebral body. This nut is introduced with the aid of a special S-shaped box spanner and is used to prevent the top screw from pulling out. This would appear to have some benefit, but the point of the screw, though dull, will protrude a few millimeters from the end of the nut, posing a possible source of future problems. Another modification, introduced by Dr.

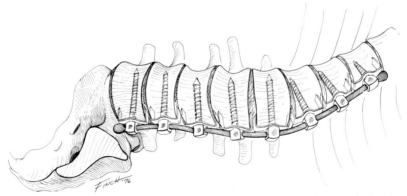

**Figure 20–36**   Instrumentation has proceeded to L5, and a reinforcing collar has been applied to the end of the cable. We prefer now to apply a second reinforcing collar and cut the cable and slide this second collar distally approximately 2 or 3 mm and then crimp it at that point. The cut end of the cable will then be inside the reinforcing collar and not exposed to the soft tissues surrounding the area.

John Hall, is the special brace screwdriver. The screwdriver's ratchet action has been designed to permit introduction of the screw without great difficulty under the upper rib margin.

A modification has been made in the instrumentation to permit fusion of the sacrum. A special anchor is inserted over the bodies of S1 and S2. The cable is threaded through the sacral anchor, and the technique of insertion is modified by beginning from S1 and working up to L3. One then starts at the top with another cable and works down to L2. With these two cables joined, a special double-holed staple is used in conjunction with two screws so the cables can overlap, thus enabling the final correction to be obtained at the apex of the curvature. We have

no experience with this technique, but Hall has found it occasionally of benefit.

Finally, a modification in the cable tensioner has been developed to permit threading of the cable through all the screw heads simultaneously and crimping of each screw at the same time. This may be helpful in cases where the spine is rather small, in order to avoid kinking the cable. Closure is begun by allowing the iliopsoas muscle to fall back over the implants in the retroperitoneal area, and the pleura and chest cavity are closed in a standard fashion.

## LIMITATIONS OF THE DWYER INSTRUMENTATION

It must be stressed that the Dwyer technique is primarily a method of instrumenta-

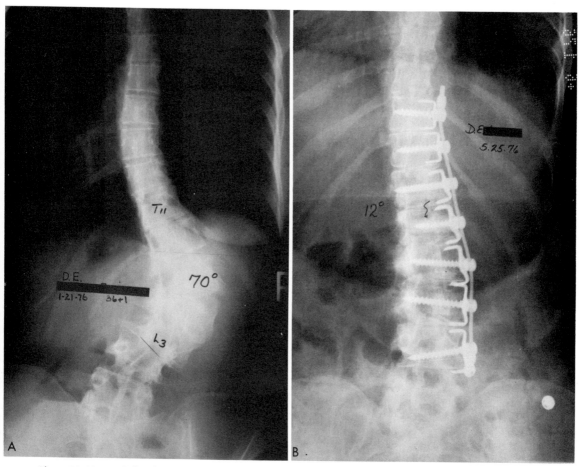

**Figure 20–37**  Methylmethacrylate is sometimes used in order to increase the strength and security of fixation. Although we do not recommend this as a routine procedure, it may prove of great help in salvaging a difficult situation where fixation is lost. A, An adult with a lumbar scoliotic curvature, treated by anterior Dwyer fixation. When the L1 vertebral body was being prepared, the screw cut out due to soft osteoporotic bone. Methylmethacrylate was then inserted and secure fixation achieved (B).

tion. It will not guarantee a solid anterior arthrodesis. We have found that in most cases the Dwyer procedure must be supplemented with a posterior spine fusion and Harrington rod instrumentation. Careful attention to details of anterior spine fusion is essential in order to avoid pseudarthrosis and cable failure. The end-plates must be removed and the area carefully packed with autogenous bone in order to prevent loss of correction. Some degree of kyphosis or reverse of lordosis will be produced in all patients if the screws are placed in the anterior half of the vertebral body. Dwyer instrumentation must not be performed in the presence of kyphosis, which will be increased by this procedure. In the immature spine, a complete disc excision is essential, because continued growth at the posterior portions of the remaining end-plate will lead to progressive kyphosis and possibly a pseudarthrosis. This operation is not recommended for patients under the age of 10 years because of the immaturity of the vertebral bodies and the size of the instrumentation. In elderly patients with osteoporosis, the bone is too weak to achieve secure fixation and loss of correction will occur. Methylmethacrylate can be used to increase the strength and security of fixation. Although we would not recommend this as a routine procedure, it may prove of great help in salvaging a difficult situation when fixation is lost while tightening the cable (Fig. 20–37).[3]

Finally, this technique should be reserved for the management of lumbar or thoracolumbar curvatures, as will be described in subsequent chapters. In the thoracic spine, this technique is not indicated, except perhaps in the case of severe lordoscoliosis, where the Dwyer instrumentation would offer the added advantage of correcting the lordosis as well.

## References

1. Burrington, J. D., Brown, C., Wayne, E. R., and Odom, J.: Anterior approach to the thoracolumbar spine. Arch. Surg., *111*:456, April, 1976.
2. Cook, W. A.: Transthoracic vertebral surgery. Ann. Thorac. Surg., *12*:54, 1971.
3. Dunn, H. K., and Bolstad, K. E.: Fixation of the Dwyer apparatus used in scoliosis. J. Bone Joint Surg., *56A*:1764, Dec., 1974.
4. Dwyer, A. F.: An anterior approach to scoliosis— a preliminary report. Clin. Orthop., *62*:192, 1969.
5. Dwyer, A. F.: Experience of anterior correction of scoliosis. Clin. Orthop., *93*:191, 1973.
6. Hall, J. E.: The anterior approach to spinal deformities. Orthop. Clin. North Am., *3*:81, 1972.
7. Harrington, P. R.: Correction and internal fixation by spine instrumentation. J. Bone Joint Surg., *44A*: 591, June, 1962.
8. Harrington, P. R.: Surgical instrumentation for management of scoliosis. J. Bone Joint Surg., *42H*:1448, 1960.
9. Harrington, P. R.: Technical details in relation to the successful use of instrumentation in scoliosis. Orthop. Clin. North Am., *3*:49, 1972.
10. Hodgson, A. R., and Stock, F. E.: Anterior spine fusion. Br. J. Surg., *44*:266, 1956.
11. Hodgson, A. R., Stock, F. E., Fang, H. S. Y., and Ong, G. B.: Anterior spine fusion. Br. J. Surg., *48*:172, 1960.
12. Hodgson, A. R.: Correction of fixed spinal curves. J. Bone Joint Surg., *47A*:1211, 1968.
13. Johnson, J. T. H.: Anterior strut grafts for severe kyphosis. Clin. Orthop., *56*:25, 1968.
14. Leathermann, K. C.: Resection of vertebral bodies. J. Bone Joint Surg., *51A*:206, 1969.
15. Moe, J. H.: Methods of correction and surgical technique in scoliosis. Orthop. Clin. North Am., *2*:17, 1972.
16. Riseborough, E. J.: The anterior approach to the spine for the correction of deformities of the axial skeleton. Clin. Orthop., *93*:207, 1973.

# Chapter 21

# TECHNIQUES OF TRACTION

## COTREL DISTRACTION

Cephalopelvic distraction by the method of Cotrel[3, 4] provides static as well as dynamic distraction to the spine (Fig. 21–1). The device as presently constructed has a pelvic and a cephalic portion. The pelvic component consists of two leather straps, overlaid with polyethylene foam, taking support from the iliac crest and crossing forward on the pelvis and backward on the sacrum. They then converge on each side toward a trochanteric pad and from there run to the foot of the bed, where they attach to pulleys and weights. Continuous traction is applied to the head by an occipital-chin device, designed so that most of the force is applied to the occiput and very little to the chin. The occipital and chin-piece straps are joined by means of an additional strap, which prevents the chinpiece from slipping under the chin.

The height of the pulley attached to the head halter must be carefully adjusted. The angle of traction from the horizontal plane should be approximately 40 degrees. If angled lower than this, most of the weight will be borne by the chin, which is exceedingly uncomfortable to the patient.

Distraction of the trunk by applying eight kilograms to the head and eight kilograms to the pelvic device is usually the maximum tolerated. This force may be achieved conveniently over a four-day period and continued for approximately two weeks. Because the forces are relatively small, they are easily borne by the patient, providing the device is properly applied. During the day,

patients are trained to do active stretching and respiratory exercises.

A complementary device can be fabricated that allows dynamic distraction of the spine (Fig. 21–2).[7] Active elongation against resistance is possible by fitting the patient with foot plates, adjusting a supplementary pulley to the occipital-chin strap, and securing the pelvic straps to the foot of the bed. By pressing down on the foot plate, the patient can stretch the trunk at will. We have had no personal experience with this dynamic modified traction.

Although the Cotrel device and technique of distraction continue to enjoy popularity in Europe, we have not found it a beneficial means of preoperative correction. The correction obtained is rarely more than that seen on preoperative side-bending x-rays. If preoperative distraction of a rigid curvature is considered necessary, we recommend halofemoral distraction.

## HALOFEMORAL DISTRACTION[1, 8, 10, 11, 12, 15, 16]

Since the first description of the halo skull traction method by Perry and Nickel in 1959, use of it in the treatment of scoliosis has become widespread. The advantages of this method lie in its complete yet comfortable control of the head and neck. The halo device coupled with femoral traction was first described by Moe in 1963, and results were presented in 1967. It has proved to be a valuable preoperative method of correcting spine deformity.

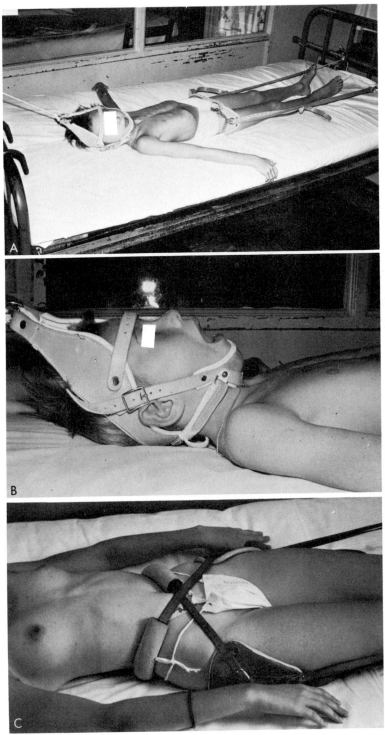

**Figure 21–1** The cephalopelvic distraction method of Cotrel. Traction is provided to the head by an occipital chin device and a pelvic component. *A,* The height of the pulley should be adjusted until it forms an angle of approximately 40 degrees with a horizontal. *B,* The occipital chin device is designed so that most of the force is supplied to the occiput and very little to the chin. *C,* The pelvic component consists of two leather straps overlaid with polyethylene foam, taking support from the iliac crest and crossing forward on the pelvis and backward on the sacrum. This component converges on the side toward a trochanteric pad and from there runs to the foot of the bed, attaching to pulley and weight.

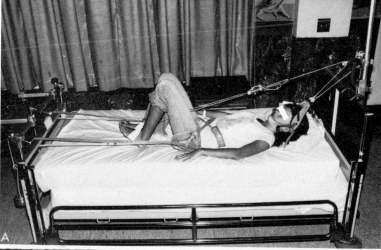

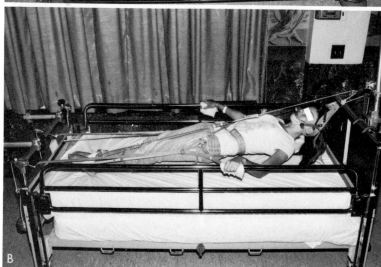

**Figure 21–2** A dynamic Cotrel distraction in use. See text for full description. (Kindly furnished by Dr. Dean McEwen, Alfred E. Dupont Institute, Wilmington, Delaware.)

## Insertion of the Halo Ring

In choosing the appropriate size halo, it is desirable to secure a ring size that allows a clearance of approximately one to three centimeters around the skull. For insertion of the halo ring, the head need not be shaved but the hair should be shampooed with a surgical soap scrub and left wet (Fig. 21–3). Local anesthesia alone is sufficient. A thin, narrow steel headrest is used to support the head. The assistant positions the halo below the maximum diameter of the skull, approximately 0.5 to 1 centimeter above the eyebrows and the pinnae of the ears. The skin is infiltrated over four sites with one per cent Xylocaine and epinephrine. Infiltration should be thorough and extended down to the periosteum.

The four pins are inserted, two posterolaterally and two anterolaterally. The anterolateral pins should be placed in the hairline in order to prevent unsightly scarring over the exposed forehead. The pins should be separated by an equal distance, if possible, to allow secure fixation. The assistant tightens one front pin and the diagonally opposite posterior pin simultaneously with the fingers to maximum finger tension. The other pair are tightened in a similar fashion. A final tension of 4 to 6 kilograms is achieved with a torque screwdriver. The pins should go through the periosteum into the outer table of the cranium but should not penetrate the inner surface.

If the torque screwdriver is not available, a short-handled screwdriver may be used, provided that care is taken to apply force with two or three fingertips only. It is impor-

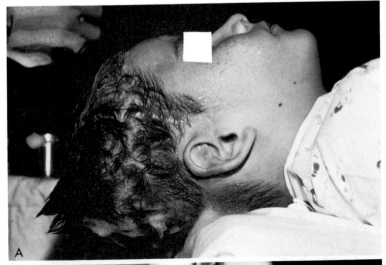

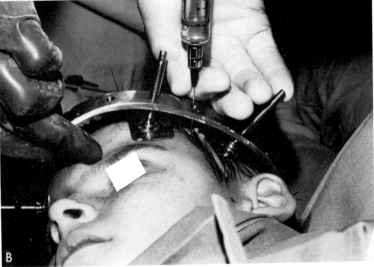

**Figure 21-3** *A,* For the application of the halo the hair need not be shaved but should be shampooed with a surgical soap scrub and left wet. Local anesthesia is generally sufficient, provided the individual is cooperative and well sedated. The assistant positions the halo below the maximum diameter of the skull, approximately 1 centimeter above the eyebrows and the ear lobes. The skin is infiltrated with Xylocaine, 1 per cent, with epinephrine *(B).*

*Illustration continued on the opposite page.*

tant to minimize the tendency to disturb the halo alignment as the pins are tightened, and it is best to alternate once or twice between the pairs of pins, applying tension in this serial fashion. When the maximum tension has been achieved, the pins are locked into position with special lock nuts and then fastened tightly to prevent the pins from working loose and inadvertently penetrating the skull. Plastic caps may be placed over the ends of the pins to prevent them from tearing sheets or bed garments.

General anesthesia (or ketamine in children) may also be used for halo application, and it is preferable in children. In summary, it is important that the halo lie below the maximum circumference of the skull. If the halo

lies further above the parietal eminence, it will have a tendency to migrate upward once distraction is instituted.

**Insertion of Femoral Pins**

For the insertion of the femoral pins, both knees are prepared with a sterile soap solution, and a local anesthetic is infiltrated over both sides of the femoral condyles at the metaphyseal-diaphyseal junction. Through a small stab incision a large unthreaded Steinmann pin is passed through the medial cortex of the distal femur at the metaphyseal-diaphyseal junction, through the cancellous bone, and emerges through the lateral cortex.

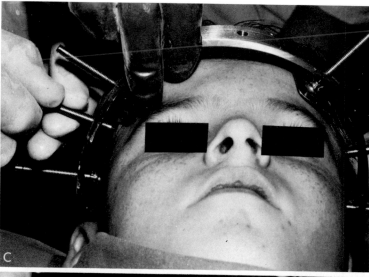

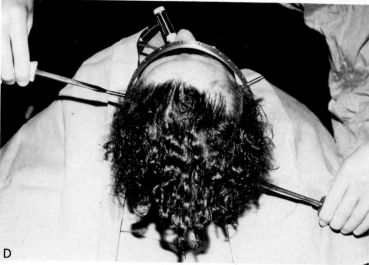

**Figure 21–3** *Continued* The four pins are then inserted, two posterolaterally and two anterolaterally *(C)*. The assistant tightens one front pin and the diagonally opposite posterior pin simultaneously with the fingers to maximum finger tension *(D)*. When maximum tension has been achieved, the pins are locked into position with special lock nuts *(E)*. The final tension of 4 to 6 kilogram centimeters is achieved with a torque screwdriver. If a torque screwdriver is not available, however, a short-handled screwdriver may be used, taking care to apply force with two or three fingertips only.

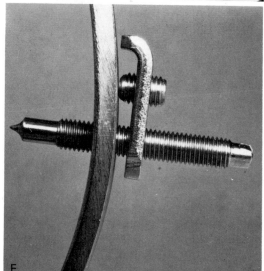

As it tenses the skin on the lateral surface, a small incision is made to allow the pin to pass through the subcutaneous and cutaneous tissues. A sterile dressing impregnated with an iodine solution is applied over the pins as they enter and exit through the skin, and the ends are secured in position with the use of a plaster of Paris bandage approximately 3 to 4 centimeters in width encircling the pins. When dried, the plaster is cut around the patella to prevent it from binding down and is split longitudinally to facilitate knee motion and prevent a possible tourniquet effect on the lower extremity. The plaster cuffs prevent medial-lateral migration of the pins and have vastly reduced pin tract infection.

A halo skid is then attached to the halo. This allows the patient free rotation without the pins' binding in the sheets. We have found a split mattress to be useful in positioning the patient, because it allows the body to rest at the same horizontal level as the halo with the attached skid. Likewise, a foam flotation pad provides comfort and may decrease skin pressure ulcerations (Fig. 21–4).

Halofemoral distraction is instituted, beginning with approximately 6 kilograms applied on the halo and 3 kilograms each on the femoral pins. The weights are steadily increased on a daily basis until a maximum of 12 kilograms on the halo and 12 kilograms on the femora equally divided between the two legs have been applied. Weights greater than 12 kilograms are no longer advised, and periods of traction longer than 2 to 3 weeks have not been beneficial in most cases. On

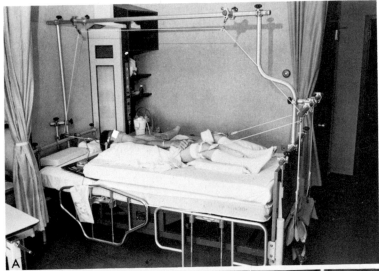

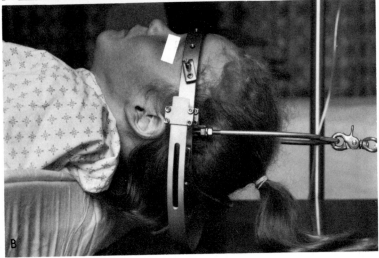

**Figure 21–4** *A,* A split mattress is useful for positioning the patient in halofemoral distraction, allowing the body to rest at the same horizontal level as the halo with the attached skid. *B,* A halo skid is attached to the halo, which allows the patient free rotation without the pins' catching in the bedclothes.

the other hand, Stagnara has found that distraction for 8 to 12 weeks may result in improved correction. If there is a fixed pelvic obliquity, greater weight may be applied on the high side of the pelvis to facilitate correction. With marked pelvic obliquity, traction can be performed only on the femur of the high side. Stagnara has modified halo skeletal traction by attaching the halo to an upright support on a wheelchair (Fig. 21–5). Progressive distraction is possible, with the patient's body providing the necessary counterweight. This technique would appear advantageous, since it allows the patient to be upright during the day. The patient can be placed back in halofemoral traction at night or can sleep in an inclined bed so that no femoral pins are needed.

The skull pins should be cleaned three to four times a day, using a hydrogen peroxide solution. Crusts, serum, and clots are removed around the pins, and the area is

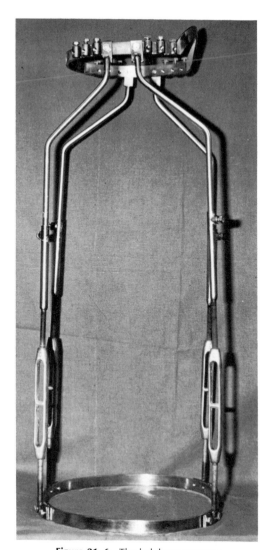

**Figure 21–6** The halohoop aparatus.

painted with Betadine. The halo should be tightened again in 24 to 48 hours, but continued tightening after this time may produce skull penetration. With frequent cleaning as noted, the pins will not become infected nor should they loosen in the skull. Antibiotics are not routinely necessary.

## HALOPELVIC DISTRACTION (HALOHOOP)[2, 5, 6, 13, 14, 15, 17]

The halohoop apparatus, originally designed by DeWald and Ray in 1970, has proved an excellent traction device for the management of severe rigid spinal deformities (Fig. 21–6). The advantages of this technique are gradual controlled correction of the

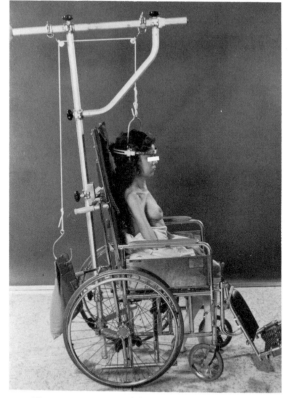

**Figure 21–5** A modified haloskeletal traction has been advocated by Stagnara (Lyon). Progressive distraction is possible as demonstrated with the patient's body providing the necessary counterweight. This technique is quite advantageous, since it allows the patient to be upright during the daytime. The patient can be placed back in halofemoral distraction at night.

deformity, unrestricted respiratory motion, easy access to the spine for surgery or wound care, and that the patient may be ambulatory in this device without loss of correction. The disadvantages of the technique include a diminished access to the iliac area for bone grafting, poor access to the L4–S1 area, and a high frequency of complications. Pin tract infections are common, and bowel perforation, nerve palsy, and paraplegia have been reported. The etiology of this paraplegia is unknown but appears to be on a vascular basis and is associated with excessive distraction forces. Finally, degenerative arthritis of the cervical spine is frequent and may be related to excessive forces across this area, especially when motion is prevented.

For application of the pelvic hoop, one must choose a hoop that allows a clearance of a minimum of 2.5 to 3.5 centimeters from the most bony prominences of the pelvis. It is important to plan the insertion and application of a hoop so that the pins will pass through the pelvis between the tables of the ilium and that the hoop, once attached to the iliac pins, will allow adequate clearance of the patient's legs on sitting. The rods should be placed across the pelvis so that they will be approximately perpendicular to the longitudinal axis of the spine when the patient is sitting. The important landmarks for rod replacement are the anterior superior iliac spine and the posterior iliac spine.

For hoop and rod insertion, the patient is placed under general anesthesia and is turned fully to one side to allow the abdominal contents to fall away from the iliac fossa. The hemipelvis is prepared and draped in a customary fashion (Fig. 21–7). An incision is made transversely below the anterior supe-

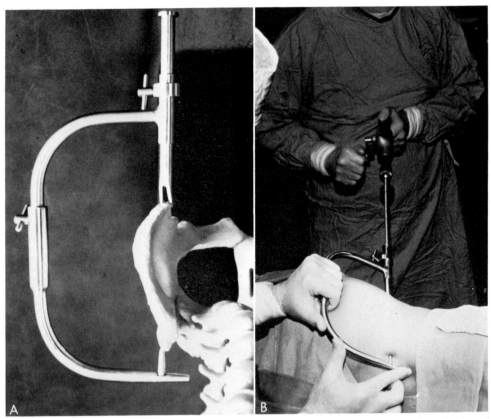

**Figure 21–7**   For insertion of the hoop and rod apparatus, the patient is prepared under general anesthesia and turned fully to one side to allow the abdominal contents to fall away from the iliac fossa. With the use of the special jig as noted (A), it is possible to insert the rod percutaneously from the anterior superior iliac spine to the posterior iliac spine without violating the pelvis and its contents (B). However, we have generally preferred to make an incision transversely below the anterior superior iliac spine as well as the posterior iliac spine and dissecting on the inner table of the pelvis beneath the iliacus muscle approximately 10 cm in each direction so that the inner table may be palpated and partially visualized as the rod is being inserted (C).

*Illustration continued on the opposite page.*

rior iliac spine and the posterior iliac spine. It is helpful to dissect on the inner table of the pelvis beneath the iliac muscle approximately 10 to 12 centimeters toward the posterior iliac spine so that the inner table may be palpated and partially visualized should any wandering or migration of the rods result. A deep Taylor retractor is placed subperiosteally to expose the entire iliac fossa. Iliac bone is then removed and stored in the bone bank for use in the subsequent spine arthrodesis. No bone should be removed at the posterior spine where the rod will exit.

The pelvic rod guide is firmly fixed against the ilium anteriorly and posteriorly against the posterior iliac spine. A drill hole is introduced in the direction of the anterior iliac spine, aiming toward the posterior iliac spine. The iliac rod, which is 1/4 inch thick, is driven across the pelvis. The rod has a self-tapping drill point and therefore should not migrate. However, the previous dissection as outlined allows the surgeon to determine quickly whether inner pelvic wall penetration is occurring. After the rod is penetrated through the posterior iliac spine, the rod guide fixture is removed. The rod should have equal portions protruding both anteriorly and posteriorly. Closure of the wounds is done in a usual manner.

The patient is now turned to the opposite side; the opposite hemipelvis is prepared and draped, and the same procedure is performed. It is helpful to be able to see the posterior portion of the first rod while inserting the second rod, in order to keep them in proper relationship.

With the patient still lying on his side, the hoop is brought up around the patient's legs and attached to the iliac rods. It is best

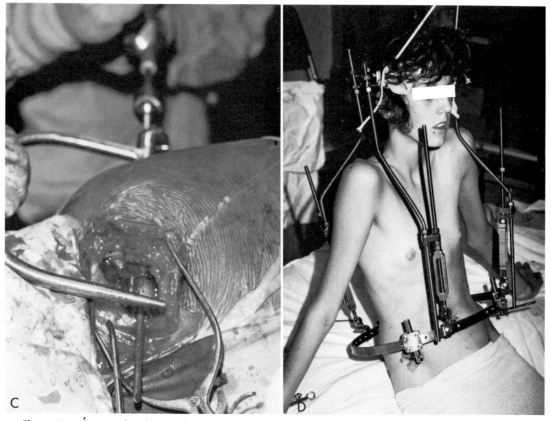

**Figure 21–7** *Continued*   Likewise, iliac bone may be removed at the same time and stored in the bone bank for use in the subsequent spine arthrodesis. After the rod is inserted, it should have equal portions protruding both anteriorly and posteriorly. Closure of the wound is done in a customary fashion. The patient is turned to the opposite side and the opposite hemipelvis is prepared and the rod inserted. The hoop is next attached to the rod and the uprights then attached from the halo to the loop, making certain that the head is correctly positioned over the pelvis and that pelvic obliquity, if possible, has been corrected (see text). We have generally preferred to apply the uprights at a second stage some two to three days later while the patient is awake and sitting (D).

to disassemble the rod holders, threading them over the iliac rods and then clamping them onto the hoop. If insufficient clearance occurs, preventing the patient from sitting, the rod holders may be inverted and the hoop placed above the rods.

After all the attachments are made, all portions of the system are loose and the patient is placed in a supine position with a pillow under the lumbar spine. At this time the hoop may be slid around the pelvis or moved in an anterior or posterior direction on the iliac rods. Further adjustment allows equal amounts of room between the patient's skin and the hoop. All nuts are then tightened securely.

The halohoop uprights are attached from the halo to the hoop. Make certain that the head is positioned directly over the pelvis and that the pelvis, if possible, has been corrected from any obliquity or forward tilt. Once the patient is in the halohoop apparatus, distraction is initiated slowly over a period of time, and the patient is observed carefully for neurologic dysfunction. We have found it preferable to apply the uprights while the patient is awake and sitting, two to three days later.

Distraction begins on the day after application and continues daily, usually one to three turns per day. All correction should be done while the patient is awake. If the discomfort is too much for the patient, the distraction can be lessened. Unfortunately the limits of distraction are not precisely defined. Once changes are seen in the cervical spine, such as overdistraction in the cervical spine intervertebral discs, distraction should be stopped until the neck becomes more supple. Strain gauges have been applied to the halohoop device and would appear to offer definite advantages. However, at the present time they are not commercially available. Cervical spine pain has frequently been the deciding factor, rather than the curve itself.

Pin wound tracts should be cleaned at least three times a day with hydrogen peroxide followed with Betadine ointment or topical antibiotics. The skin should not be allowed to "tent up" around the iliac pins. If this happens it is best to incise the skin so that it will not be tethered and to debride the area so as to prevent skin inflammation. Neurologic checks must be performed daily.

## References

1. Bonnett, C., Perry, J., Brown, J. C., and Greenberg, B. J.: Halo-femoral distraction and posterior spine fusion for paralytic scoliosis. J. Bone Joint Surg., 54A:202, 1972.
2. Clark, J. A., and Kesterton, L.: Halo pelvic traction appliance for spinal deformities. J. Biomech., 4:589, 1971. Pergamon Press. Printed in Great Britain.
3. Cotrel, Y.: The E.D.F. technique. In Keim, Hugo A. (ed.): Third Annual Post-Graduate Course on the Management and Care of the Scoliosis Patient, Dec. 2–4, 1971, New York Orthopedic Hospital, Columbia Presbyterian Medical Center.
4. Cotrel, Y.: Traction in the treatment of vertebral deformity. J. Bone Joint Surg., 57B:260, May, 1975.
5. Dewald, R. L.: Halo and halo hoop in scoliosis management. In Keim, Hugo A. (ed.): Third Annual Post-Graduate Course on the Management and Care of the Scoliosis Patient, Dec. 2–4, 1971, New York Orthopedic Hospital, Columbia Presbyterian Medical Center.
6. Dewald, R. L., and Ray, R. D.: Skeletal traction for the treatment of severe scoliosis. J. Bone Joint Surg., 52A:233, 1970.
7. Hensinger, R. N., and Macewen, G. D.: Evaluation of the Cotrel dynamic spine traction in the treatment of scoliosis. A preliminary report. Orthop. Rev., 3:27, 1974.
8. Kane, W. J., Moe, J. H., and Lai, C. C.: Halo-femoral pin distraction in the treatment of scoliosis. J. Bone Joint Surg., 49A:1018, 1967.
9. La Breche, B. G., Levangie, P. K., and Sharby, N. H.: A new approach to the pre-operative management of idiopathic scoliosis. J. Physical Therapy, 54:837, 1974.
10. Letts, R. M., and Bobechko, W. P.: Pre-operative skeletal traction in scoliosis. J. Bone Joint Surg., 57A:616, 1975.
11. Moe, J. H.: Methods of correction and surgical technique in scoliosis. Orthop. Clin. North Am., 2:17, 1972.
12. Nickel, V. L., Perry J., Garrett, A., and Heppenstall, M.: The halo. J. Bone Joint Surg., 50A:1400, 1968.
13. O'Brien, J. P.: The halo-pelvic apparatus. Acta Orthop. Scand. Suppl. 163. Copenhagen, Munksgaard, 1975.
14. O'Brien, J. P., Yau, A.C.M.C., and Hodgson, A. R.: Halo-pelvic traction: A technique for severe spinal deformities. Clin. Orthop., 93:179, 1973.
15. O'Brien, J. P., Yau, A. C. M. C., Smith, T., and Hodgson, A. R.: Halo-pelvic traction. J. Bone Joint Surg., 53B:217, 1971.
16. Perry, J.: The halo in spinal abnormalities: Practical factors and avoidance of complications. Orthop. Clin. North Am., 3:69, 1972.
17. Ransford, A. O., and Manning, C. W. S. F.: Complications of halo-pelvic distraction. J. Bone Joint Surg., 57B:131, 1975.

# Chapter 22

# SPONDYLOLYSIS AND SPONDYLOLISTHESIS

Spondylolisthesis is defined as a slipping forward of one vertebra on another. The origin of this word comes from Greek "spondylos," meaning vertebra, and "olisthesis," meaning to slip. The history of the recognition of this condition began with the work of Herbiniaux,[22] a Belgian obstetrician, who noted in 1782 that there were times when a bony prominence in front of the sacrum caused problems in delivery. He is generally credited with having first described the complete dislocation of the body of L5 over in front of the sacrum. The term spondylolisthesis was coined by Kilian in 1854,[26] who believed that the lesion was caused by slow subluxation of the lumbosacral facets. One year later, Robert[45] noted the location of the lesion to be in the pars interarticularis. Neugebauer, in 1881,[37] was the first to recognize that a slippage between L5 and sacrum can occur by elongation of the pars interarticularis, without a break in continuity. Lambl, in 1858,[27] was first credited with demonstrating the actual discontinuity of that portion of the neural arch known as the pars interarticularis, a defect in the neural arch, now referred to as spondylolysis.

## DESCRIPTION AND ETIOLOGY[29, 59, 61, 62]

The following classification represents the most recent one published and has been derived from previous classifications reported by Wiltse, Newman, and McNab. (Fig. 22–1).[61]

I. *Dysplastic*: In this type of spondylo-listhesis, congenital abnormalities in the upper sacrum and for the arch of L5 permit forward slippage of L5 to occur.

II. *Isthmic*: This is a lesion of the pars interarticularis in which three types can be identified: A: Lytic or fatigue fracture of the pars; B: Elongated but intact pars; C: Acute fracture.

III. *Degenerative*: Secondary to long-standing degenerative arthritis and intersegmental instability of the facet joints.

## Spondylolisthesis

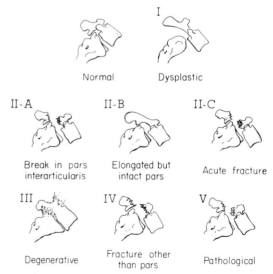

**Figure 22–1** Classification. (Reprinted from Bradford, D. S.: Spondylolysis and Spondylolisthesis. *In* Chou, S.: Spinal Deformity and Neurologic Dysfunction. New York, Raven Press, 1977.)

IV. *Traumatic*: Secondary to fractures in the areas of the bony hook other than the pars.

V. *Pathological*: In which there is generalized or localized bone disease (Paget's, etc.).

Dysplastic: In this type of spondylolisthesis, there is a congenital dysplasia of the upper sacrum and/or the neural arch of L5. This creates insufficient bony stock to withstand the forward thrust of the lumbar spine, and, therefore, the L5 lumbar vertebra gradually slips forward on the sacrum. The pars interarticularis may remain unchanged, but if it does, the slippage cannot exceed more than 25 per cent without cauda equina paralysis. Usually, however, the pars either elongates or fractures, making it difficult to tell this type from Type IIA or Type IIB (Fig. 22–2*A* and *B*). At surgery, the abnormal relationships are readily apparent. There is almost invariably a wide spina bifida of the sacrum and the L5 vertebra as well. This type usually goes on to a severe grade of slippage and, according to Wiltse, is about twice as common in girls as boys.[60]

Isthmic: In the isthmic type of spondylolisthesis, the basic defect is in the pars interarticularis. Subtype A is secondary to a stress or fatigue fracture. This is the most common type below age 50 and is rarely seen below age 5. It is never seen at birth and the youngest reported case is that by Borkow and Kleiger[4] in a child four months of age. The incidence of the defect in adult Caucasian males appears to be approximately 5 to 6 per cent, whereas in adult Caucasian females, it is 2 to 3 per cent.[3, 47] Stewart[42] found that Eskimos have by far the highest incidence, as high as 50 per cent in isolated communities north of the Yukon, whereas in blacks, it is appreciably less (less than 3 per cent).[47]

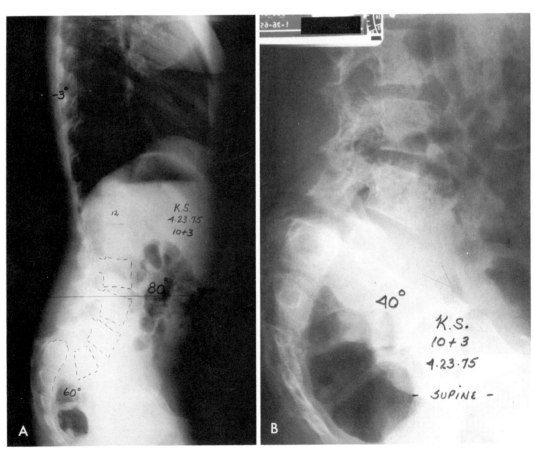

**Figure 22–2** Severity of the spondylolisthesis may be greater than appreciated when the supine x-ray is compared with the standing. In *B*, a dysplastic type, which has developed elongation of the pars with ultimate lysis, is apparent. (Reprinted from Bradford, D. S.: Spondylolysis and Spondylolisthesis. *In* Chou, S.: Spinal Deformity and Neurologic Dysfunction. New York, Raven Press, 1977.)

It should also be noted that there is approximately a 30 per cent incidence of spondylolisthesis in members of families of affected individuals.[59] Baker, in a study of 400 school children age 6, found 18 children with a defect (4.5 per cent). The parents of those positive were x-rayed, and 28 per cent were noted to have pars defects.[3] It is also of interest that spina bifida is thirteen times more frequent in patients with spondylolisthesis than in the general population. It is the opinion of many authors[12, 34, 39, 62] that the isthmic spondylolysis is a result of fatigue fractures from repeated trauma and stress, rather than any one acute traumatic episode. However, it differs from other fatigue fractures in the following respects: It tends to develop at an earlier age; there is a hereditary predisposition; callus formation is rarely seen; and the defect in the pars tends to persist, although occasionally healing may occur. In this regard, it is of interest that female gymnasts have a four times higher incidence of spondylolysis than their nonathletic female peers.[23] It is not known whether these stress fractures are due to flexion or extension stresses. It is known, however, that it never occurs in animals other than humans and that only humans have a true lumbar lordosis and a true upright posture.

Subtype B — elongation of the pars without separation. This is fundamentally the same lesion as in Subtype A. It is secondary to repeated stress fractures that heal with the pars assuming a more elongated position as the body of L5 slides forward. Eventually, it may separate as slippage continues to occur, making it difficult to differentiate from Subtype A. The fundamental disease as well as the presumed etiology is the same.

Subtype C — acute pars fractures. This is always secondary to severe trauma — usually, we feel, an extension type fracture. Slippage rarely occurs; heredity does not seem to play a role in the etiology of this type.

Degenerative: This is probably the most common type of spondylolisthesis. None of the affected patients are younger than age 40, and very few are younger than age 50. This type is four and five times more frequent in the female than in the male. Newman first gave this the descriptive title in 1963[39] although previous authors had referred to this and recognized its significance some 30 years before. There is no pars interarticularis defect in this type, and the slippage is never greater than 30 per cent, unless the patient has undergone a laminectomy. Advanced degenerative disease of the facet joints and disc is the exclusive finding that separates this condition from the other types of spondylolisthesis. The L4–L5 area is affected more commonly than other levels, and sacralization of L5 is four times more frequent.[48] The predisposing factor is thought to be a straight, stable lumbosacral joint, which puts increased stress on the intervertebral joint between L4 and L5, ultimately leading to hypermobility and degeneration of the articular processes and disc. Degenerative changes and the forward slipping combine to produce localized spinal stenosis, which may compress the nerve roots of the cauda equina.[48]

Traumatic: This type of spondylolisthesis is secondary to an acute injury that fractures some part of the bony "hook" other than the pars interarticularis and allows forward slippage of the vertebrae. This is always due to severe trauma and will usually heal with immobilization.

Pathologic: Generalized bone disease, such as Albers-Schonberg, osteogenesis imperfecta, and arthrogryposis, may lead to fractures or elongation of the pars interarticularis. Paget's disease also has been associated with elongation of the pars and spondylolisthesis. Local factors such as fractures of the pars at the upper end of a lumbar spinal fusion likewise have been reported. These are not common but are probably secondary to fatigue fractures from altered mechanics of the spine.

## SIGNS AND SYMPTOMS: CHILD AND ADOLESCENT

Spondylolisthesis in children behaves differently from that in adults. At least two types exist in children, producing pain in the back or legs or a combination of both. The types present as: 1) a defect in the pars with mild to moderate slip and backache predominating, with or without leg pain; and 2) a high grade of slip (Grade IV or V) with a typical spondylolisthesis build — a short type torso and heart-shaped buttocks. Pain in the back[1] is probably secondary to instability of the affected segment which produces strain on the intervertebral ligaments and joints. Herniation of the intervertebral disc is extremely uncommon. Pain also may rise from a defect in the pars, especially if there has been a fairly acute fracture. It should be emphasized that not every patient with spondylolysis or spondylolisthesis suffers from low back pain. We have seen patients with rather severe degrees of spondylolisthesis (75 to 100 per cent) who are totally asymptomatic! In fact, it is felt by some authors (Nachemson, personal communication) that spondylolysis with spondylolisthesis is not associated with back pain in any greater incidence than in the control population. The second type of pain is due to pressure on the roots of the cauda equina and is less common than backache. From the distorted anatomy created and the narrowing of the intervertebral foramen between the fifth lumbar and the first sacral vertebra, as well as the fibrocartilaginous callus of the fractured pars, pressure on the L5 root is produced. If the compression of the roots is severe, bilateral sciatica is evident. Compression can happen to other components of the cauda equina; that is, the sacral roots that pass over the top of the sacrum which are compressed at this site by the forward displacement of the lumbar vertebrae above. This latter type of compression is far less common than the foraminal compression at the fifth root.

The deformity of spondylolisthesis is very characteristic (Fig. 22–3). It is secondary to the forward slippage of the involved vertebra. When it becomes quite severe (75 to 100 per

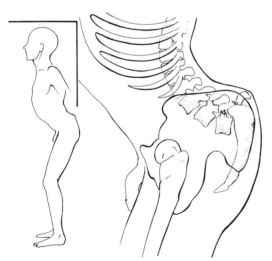

**Figure 22-3** The characteristic deformity of spondylolisthesis. Note that with severe deformity the sacrum becomes almost vertical, and the anterior superior iliac spine rides higher than the posterior superior iliac spine. The hips appear flexed even though they are fully extended in relation to the sacrum, while the knees become truly flexed if the patient attempts to stand straight.[20]

cent), compensating mechanisms are brought into play, and these must be recognized. As the vertebra slips forward, it leaves behind the lamina, spinous process, and the inferior articular facets. Consequently, there is a step-off palpable over the spinous processes from the one left behind to the ones slipped above. As the vertebrae above are carried further forward, the center of the body gravity, is displaced and to compensate for this, the lumbar spine above the lesion becomes hyperextended and the upper part of the trunk is thrown further backward. The pelvis becomes rotated about its transverse axis so that the sacrum actually becomes vertical.[20] One can clearly see this by noting that the anterior superior spine rises to the same level or even becomes higher than the posterior superior spine (Fig. 22–4). The buttocks appear "heart-shaped," secondary to the sacral prominence. The hip joint rotates with the tilted pelvis until the thigh, even in extreme degrees of full extension, fails to place itself vertically underneath the trunk. Consequently, when the patient tries to stand straight, his hips remain flexed beneath his torso and the knees must also remain flexed in order to place the feet beneath the body. If he attempts to stand with legs straight, the trunk must tilt forward at the hip, since the hips cannot hyperextend enough to compensate for this. As the slip becomes greater, the trunk is severely shortened, so there is an almost complete absence of the waistline, and the rib cage abuts on the iliac crest. It is useful also to think of this as a flexion deformity or a "kyphosis" of L5 on S1, for L5 not only is forward translated on S1 but also is forward tilted. The lumbar lordosis is compensatory for the kyphosis at L5–S1. This disturbed anatomy, along with the associated hamstring tightness, well described by Phalen and Dickson,[43] produces a peculiar yet characteristic gait.

These children often develop a functional scoliosis. This is also referred to as a "sciatic scoliosis" and is usually secondary to muscle spasm produced by the irritation of the nerve roots. If the scoliosis is a sciatic type scoliosis, it usually extends up from the sacrum. Idiopathic scoliosis may also be seen in association with spondylolisthesis as a coincident condition but is usually thoracic or thoracolumbar and is not secondary to muscle spasm or nerve root irritation.

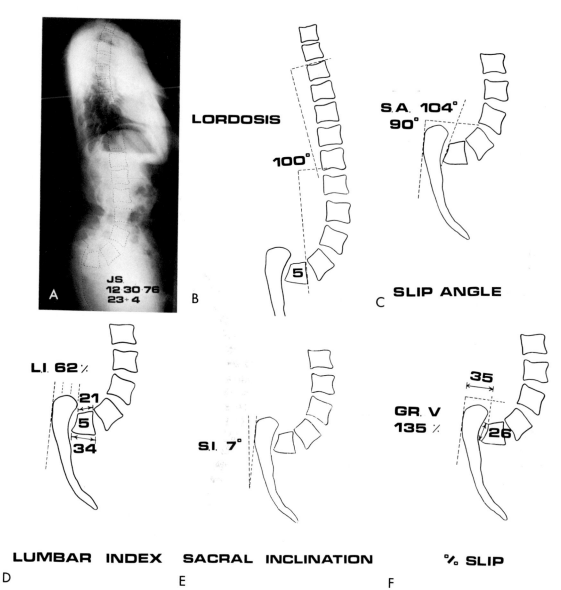

**Figure 22–4** Measurements concerning the degrees of slippage may be expressed in several ways. Transposing the vertebral outlines from *A*, the following angles may be constructed: *B*, Lordosis, Although we generally measure lordosis to the sacrum, this is not relevant in spondylolisthesis, since the sacrum frequently lies vertically. Therefore, the superior end-plate of L5 is used for the lower limit. The sacral angle *(C)* is a measure of L5–S1, kyphosis. The lumbar index *(D)* measures the trapezoidal shape of L5; the sacral inclination is measured by dropping a perpendicular to the floor and a line parallel to upper portion of the posterior half of S1. This gives one an impression as to the degree of vertical orientation of the sacrum. Calculation of the exact percentage slip *(F)* is often imprecise owing to the bony remodeling and formation that develops around the sacrum following a complete slip. The described technique, however, provides satisfactory accuracy.

Neurologic evaluation may reveal nerve root impairment, particularly involving the L5 nerve roots. With severe degrees of neurologic involvement, bowel or bladder signs or symptoms may develop, although this is uncommon.

The progression of spondylolisthesis may be slow or quite rapid. Progressive degrees of slip often occur during periods of rapid growth or just at the late juvenile or early adolescent period.

## SIGNS AND SYMPTOMS: ADULT

Pain in the adult from degenerative spondylolisthesis is either back or a combination of back and leg pain. The pain in the back is rarely severe and has often existed for several years with long periods of remission. Patients rarely associate their symptoms with activity, weather, or any other discernible factors.[48] Spinal stenosis type symptoms (spinal claudication) are uncommon, but when they occur, they usually are constant. These complaints are often relieved by sitting or lying down, in contrast to vascular claudication, which is usually relieved by standing in place. Radicular pain may be present. It is usually sensory in nature, but sometimes motor findings may be evident.

## DIAGNOSIS

With a well-marked deformity on physical examination, the diagnosis is rather simple. When the deformity is inconspicuous, adequate radiographic evaluation is essential. If there is a significant degree of slippage, a lateral x-ray will reveal the defect and the percentage of slip. Meyerding[25] has classified the percentage of slippage accordingly: Grade I, 0–25 per cent; Grade II, 25–50 per cent; Grade III, 50–75 per cent; and Grade IV, greater than 75 per cent (Fig. 22–4). If the gap at the defect is slight and there is no forward displacement, oblique radiographic projections are essential. Laminography is also helpful. In the anteroposterior projection, if the slip is severe, the body of L5 overlaps the upper sacrum, making a characteristic picture, referred to as "Napoleon's hat."

In cases of degenerative spondylolisthesis, the radiographic findings are characteristic: degenerative joint disease can be visualized, and a slippage of L4 on L5 is evident; without a defect in the pars interarticularis, disc space narrowing is usual. It should also be noted that standing x-rays in the lateral position are extremely valuable. Although supine x-rays may show a slippage, standing x-rays will often show the slippage to be much greater than would be appreciated on the supine film (Fig. 22–2). This has been noted by Lowe et al.,[30] and it has likewise been our experience. We would, therefore, recommend recumbent and standing lateral lumbosacral spine x-rays in order to compare the mobility of the slip, as well as its true magnitude. Hyperextension and hyperflexion x-rays are also useful to determine mobility. Preoperative evaluation may include a myelogram, since extrusion of an intervertebral disc may occur at or adjacent to the level of the spondylolisthe-

sis, thus impairing function of corresponding nerve roots. It is our experience that disc herniation in association with spondylolisthesis is extremely uncommon. From reports in the literature, it would certainly appear to be less than 5 per cent.[29] We have, therefore, not performed myelography as a routine procedure. In severe degrees of slippage (greater than 75 per cent), a complete "block" on the myelogram is characteristic but does not imply compression of neural tissues. In the adult, however, with degenerative spondylolisthesis unresponsive to conservative management, we would recommend myelography as a routine procedure prior to undertaking surgical intervention.

## TREATMENT

### Spondylolysis

*In the Child.* Although spondylolysis usually originates between 5 and 10 years of age with an incidence approaching 5 per cent, few of these patients are symptomatic. Those who do have symptoms respond for the most part to simple conservative measures. We do not feel that asymptomatic patients or those with minimal symptoms need to limit their activity. Repeated x-ray evaluation at six month intervals is advisable in those patients still growing. A small percentage of patients with persistent symptoms that do not respond to conservative measures may require surgical stabilization with a lateral process fusion from L5 to sacrum. Extension of the fusion to L4 is not necessary. There is no indication for a Gill procedure or a wide laminectomy. It should be stressed that symptomatic spondylolysis in the adolescent is most uncommon, and one should rule out other causes of back pain in children (e.g., infection, tumor, osteoid osteoma, herniated disc) before surgery is undertaken.

*In the Adult.* The conservative treatment for the adult with spondylolysis is the same as that for backache due to other causes. Heat, analgesics, exercises, anti-inflammatory medication, along with a corset or body jacket may be tried with some degree of success. For persistent pain, unresponsive to conservative management (at least 6 months), spine fusion should be performed. Myelography should be done and disc herniation surgically removed, if indicated. Generally, for patients under 50 years of age, we prefer spinal arthrodesis as the treatment of choice. Patients over 50 may usually be managed by laminectomy alone. Surgery is carried out primarily for the relief of pain. Although significant slippage rarely occurs as a result of the laminectomy, if it does develop and is felt to be a source of back pain, the patient may be managed by posterolateral spine fusion.

## Spondylolisthesis

*Dysplastic and Isthmic Type.* Treatment of the child with spondylolisthesis depends to a large part upon the severity of symptoms and the degree of slippage. If the symptoms are minimal and the slip is less than 25 per cent, conservative treatment consisting of routine back care, general abdominal strengthening exercises, and a temporary lumbosacral corset may prove helpful. Persistent symptoms, unresponsive to conservative management and interfering with normal childhood activities, necessitate surgical fusion. The necessity for operative intervention rests not only upon the severity of symptoms but also upon the degree of slippage. Further slipping may occur in the child, especially during the adolescent growth spurt.

If the L5 vertebral body is trapezoid in shape and the upper end of the sacrum has assumed a dome shape and somewhat vertical orientation, there is greater than 50 per cent likelihood that the patient will have progressive and severe slippage.[21, 54, 55] If the slippage continues to progress past 25 per cent or if the child is symptomatic, spine fusion is indicated. It is our feeling that the fusion should be performed in the growing child before the displacement exceeds one third the length of the vertebral body. Certainly, if the displacement is more than 50 per cent, even if the child has no symptoms, spine fusion is indicated.[21, 30, 36, 40, 60]

Any child in whom a defect is discovered early, especially below the age of 10, should have lateral standing roentgenograms taken of the lumbosacral area every six months until the completion of growth. This is particularly important in females because a high grade of slippage is twice as common in girls as in boys.[60]

Patients with the dysplastic (congenital) type defect are more likely to need surgical stabilization.[21] Surgery in the child consists of spine fusion with or without decompression by laminectomy (Fig. 22–5). Laminectomy (Gill procedure) as an isolated procedure in a growing child is contraindicated.[36] Further slippage with laminectomy alone will occur in a high percentage of cases.[29, 36] The most effective treatment is lumbosacral fusion, and we recommend extending the fusion from L4 to sacrum if slippage is greater than 50 per cent. The fusion should be done posterolaterally; it may be done through a midline incision, through a paraspinal approach, splitting the sacrospinalis muscle about two finger-breadths lateral to the midline, or an approach lateral to the paraspinal muscles. Fusion should extend out to the tips of the transverse processes from L4 down to the sacral alae, using autogenous iliac bone for grafting. It may be quite difficult to reach the L5 transverse process in extreme degrees of slippage, and therefore solidification of the fusion is assured by extending the fusion to the transverse process of L4. It is also helpful to countersink a cortical strut into a window made in the sacral alae and extend the strut to the transverse process of L4.[21] The articular facet joints of L4–L5 and L5–S1 should be cleaned of articular cartilage and cancellous bone packed into the facet joint.

Some doubt has been expressed as to whether a decompression with removal of loose posterior element of L5 should even be done in children, irrespective of the signs and symptoms of neurologic compromise. In fact, it is Wiltse's contention[60] that severely tight hamstrings, decreased Achilles reflexes, and even a foot drop will recover after a solid arthrodesis is effected. It is our feeling, however, that if the patient has severe hamstring tightness and/or a foot drop and bowel or bladder symptoms, a midline posterior approach with removal of the loose posterior element and fibrocartilaginous callus should be done. Removal of the posterior superior prominence of the sacrum has also been suggested, but we have not found this necessary. It should be stressed that, with all these decompressive procedures, spine stabilization by fusion, especially in children, must be undertaken.

Postoperatively, in the child with a slip of 50 per cent or more, we feel it is best to use a body cast extending to both thighs with the hips in hyperextension. Patients are kept in

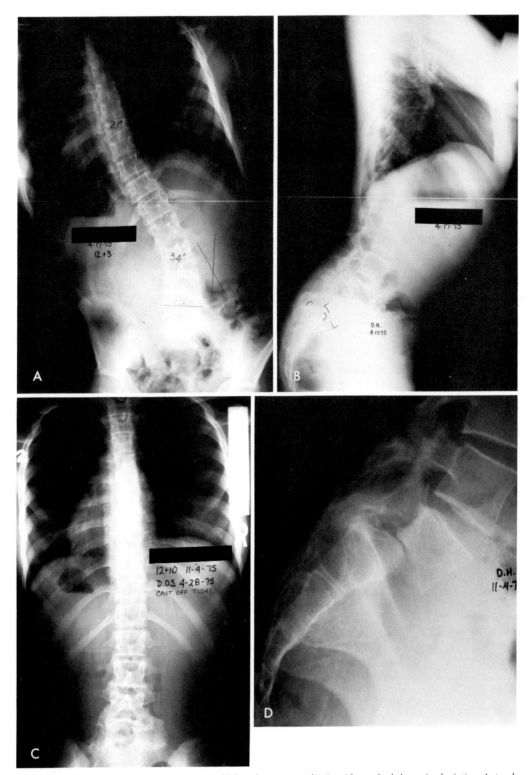

**Figure 22–5**  Spondylolisthesis in a 12 year old female. Note scoliosis with marked thoracic deviation. Lateral x-ray shows slippage greater than 50 per cent *(B)*. The patient underwent an L4–sacrum fusion and was kept in a double pantaloon cast and bed rest for four months, then placed in a body jacket and ambulated for two months. *C* and *D,* X-rays taken after the cast was removed. Note solid fusion and absence of scoliosis.

bed for four months, lessening the likelihood of further slippage. Then they may be ambulated with additional support (body cast) for two months. On the other hand, adult patients may be encouraged to begin ambulation one to two days after surgery. Routine abdominal isometric and gluteal sitting exercises are started two to four days after the operation. Sitting in straight backed chairs rather than on soft chairs is encouraged for the first two months after surgery, and patients are instructed to avoid excessive motion to the low back by rolling like a log instead of twisting and by bending at the knees when stooping to pick up objects from the floor. Corsets and braces may be used but do not appear to be essential for a solid arthrodesis. In the adult, if slippage is greater than 50 per cent, we prefer to apply a body spica cast with a single thigh extension after surgery, in order to facilitate greater immobilization of the lumbosacral spine and a more certain arthrodesis. The patient may then be ambulatory. The cast is continued for three to four months following discharge from the hospital.

Further slippage may occur after spine fusion, even if the patient is kept supine (Fig. 22–6). This has been noted by Newman,[38] Bosworth et al.,[5] Dandy and Shannon,[9] and Laurent and Osterman.[30] It is Wiltse's contention that the use of the midline posterior approach may increase the instability and permit further slippage. However, if a posterolateral approach is used, without removing the loose laminae, he feels that further slippage is less likely.[60]

## ALTERNATIVES IN MANAGEMENT

*Reduction of Spondylolisthesis.* In the past 25 years, increasing attention has been given to the possibility of reducing the spondylolisthesis and then performing surgical arthrodesis, either posteriorly or anteriorly or both. Jenkins in 1936 described the first successful attempt of reduction of spondylolisthesis.[25] In 1951, R. I. Harris further demonstrated that skeletal traction could indeed reduce spondylolisthesis.[20] Newman, in 1965,[38] described a method of reducing spondylolisthesis but felt that the reduction was never maintained during the period of consolidation of the posterior arthrodesis. Lance[28] reported successful reduction of the spondylolisthesis in 1966, and Harrington later proposed the technique of open reduction and internal fixation with distracting devices for severe degrees of slippage.[18, 19] Other authors since then have developed alternative procedures for reducing the spondylolisthesis that look quite promising.[11, 49, 50, 51] Particularly appealing is Scaglietti's technique for reduction of the spondylolisthesis with casting. In this technique, the patient is placed on a fracture table, and following longitudinal distraction the hips are hyperextended, actually reducing the spondylolisthesis and correcting the abnormal forward pelvic inclination. A plaster cast is then applied. The patient is kept in the plaster some four months before undergoing surgery, allowing reconstitution of the distorted anatomy. The second stage consists of a posterior spine fusion with internal instrumentation.

The Harrington technique consists of a spinal instrumentation from L3 to sacrum,[18] using a modified sacral bar with posterior interbody fusion and a lateral gutter fusion from L3 to sacrum. We have modified Harrington's technique and used it on five patients since 1972.[7] The technique consists of a posterior approach, instrumentation from T12 or L1 to sacrum, placing square-ended lower sacral hooks on the sacral alae, bending the rods to maintain a normal lumbar lordosis, removing the free-floating posterior element of L5, decompressing the L5 root, and then performing a lateral process fusion from L4 to sacrum, using iliac bone graft. The patients may be ambulated one week after surgery in a body cast, provided no loss of correction is demonstrated on x-ray. The rod is removed 12 to 24 months postoperatively, after the fusion is solid (Fig. 22–7). Complications have consisted of 1) facet subluxation at T12–L1, subsequently requiring open reduction and fusion of the facet between T12 and L1; and 2) a dislodged rod. However, no significant loss of correction occurred. Of concern is the loss of thoracic kyphosis and even the increase in pre-existing thoracic lordosis with this technique. Of great interest are the findings revealed at operation. After the posterior element is removed, the dura still remains tight and constricted without pulsations. Once distraction and partial reduction are carried out, pulsations appear, and the L5 root is visualized as it becomes decompressed from the pars adjoining the superior facet of L5 and the pedicle.[7] In fact, the visual decompression achieved by this distraction

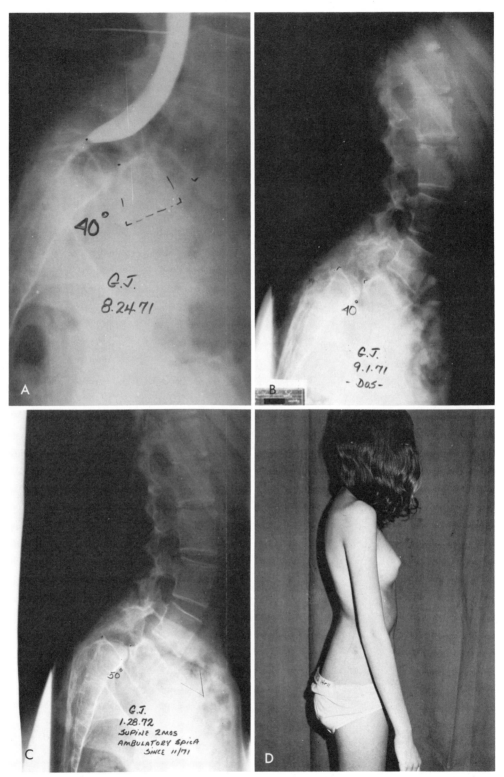

**Figure 22–6**   This patient with a severe slip (A) underwent a Gill procedure and L4–sacrum fusion on 9/1/71. (B) She was kept down for two months in a pantaloon spica and ambulated for two weeks in a walking spica. Fusion looked solid on 1/28/72 (C), and her clinical appearance was satisfactory (D). One can note, however, that on the x-ray's L–S angle has progressed to 50 degrees.

*Legend continued on opposite page*

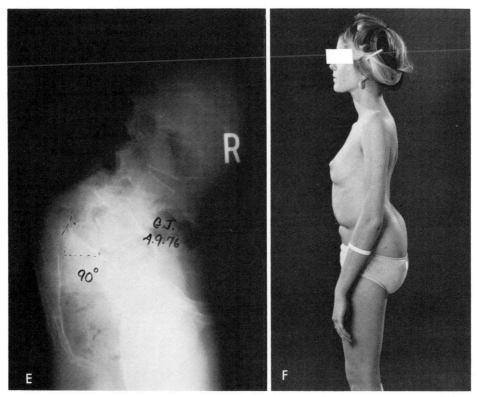

**Figure 22–6** *Continued* The slippage continued (*E*) and on last follow-up on 4/9/76 shows an unsatisfactory cosmetic result. The fusion is solid, however (*F*). (Reprinted from Bradford, D. S.: Spondylolysis and Spondylolisthesis. *In* Chou, S. N. (ed.): Spinal Deformity and Neurologic Dysfunction. New York, Raven Press, 1977.)

and reduction technique is far greater than that achieved by the Gill procedure.

The question, however, must be asked whether this technique is safe and worth the effort. Complications may be minimal if the technique is performed properly. The clinical and cosmetic results achieved are quite substantial, with a significant gain in height (1 to 2 inches) and a more normal appearing waistline. This would confirm the work of Ascani,[2] who has noted that with the reduction of the displacement by the hyperextension casting technique, cases of partial paralysis and existing bowel and bladder disturbances have disappeared. One must consider that even with a spine fusion (without a Gill decompression) further slippage may continue to develop while the fusion is solidifying (Fig. 22–8). This has been reported in 20 to 30 per cent of patients with more advanced degrees of slippage.[5, 9, 40] We have been impressed with the cast/traction technique of reduction of spondylolisthesis in children. For slips greater than 50 per cent, we feel that reduction

of the spondylolisthesis preoperatively, followed by surgical stabilization with or without Harrington rods, is an attractive alternative for the management of this severe deformity. For slips less than 50 per cent, the more standard techniques of fusion in situ remain the treatment of choice.

### Repair of the Defect

Techniques have also been described for direct repair of the defect in spondylolisthesis by either screw fixation across the fracture in the pars or fusion across the defect alone.[35] These techniques may be valid for slippage less than 25 per cent, but for greater slippage they would appear ineffective.

### ANTERIOR INTERBODY FUSION

Anterior interbody fusion for spondylolisthesis is seldom necessary in the child.

*Text continued on page 550*

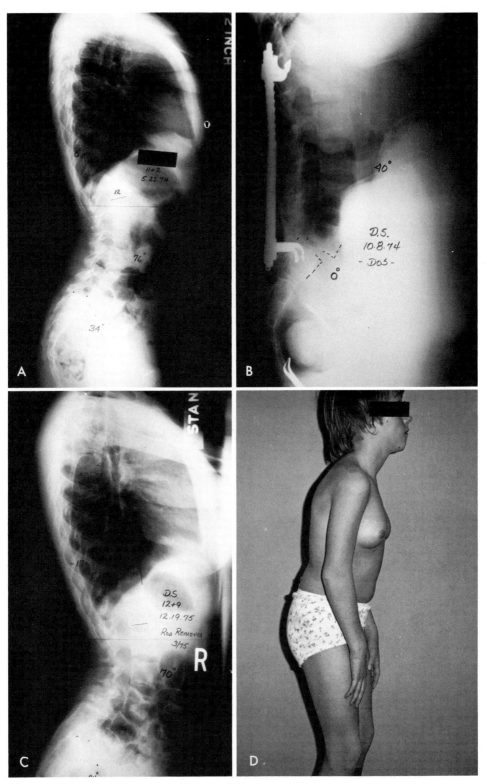

**Figure 22–7** *See legend on opposite page.*

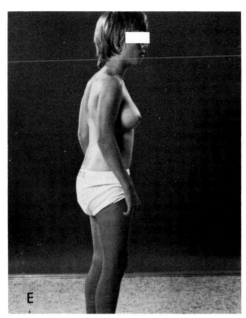

**Figure 22–7** *Continued* Reduction of the spondylolisthesis is possible and may be carried out by the Harrington device (*A* and *B*). The rod is placed from T12 to sacrum, but the fusion extends from L4 to sacrum. The rod is removed one year later (*C*). The L–S angle has been improved, as has been the degree of slippage. Some loss of correction has occurred. The initial appearance of the patient (*D*) and two years follow-up (*E*). (Reprinted from Bradford, D. S.: Spondylolysis and Spondylolisthesis. *In* Chou, S. N. (ed.): Spinal Deformity and Neurologic Dysfunction. New York, Raven Press, 1977.)

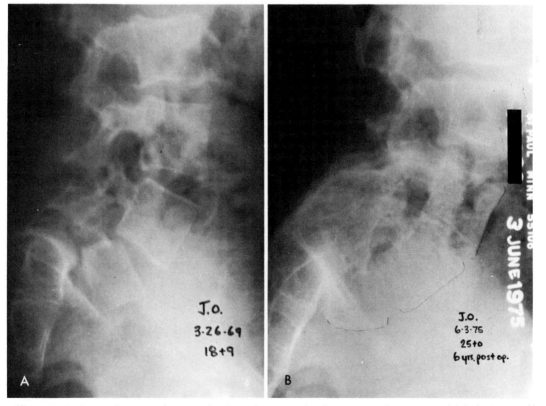

**Figure 22–8** Future slippage and increased L–S angulation noted in this patient with severe spondylolisthesis treated by fusion in situ without laminectomy.

Transperitoneal lumbar fusion was first performed by Capener in 1932[14, 23] and has recently received increased attention as a method to be used in conjunction with posterior reduction and fusion.[53] The reduction and the stability of reduction achieved by this technique appear greater than that achieved by posterior spine fusion with instrumentation by the Harrington technique. The exact indication for this method remains unclear, but it would appear physiologically to be the most certain method of achieving an adequate reduction, a solid fusion, and prevention of further slippage. With the exposure, damage to the sacral plexus is a risk with resultant retrograde ejaculation in the male.

## TRAUMATIC SPONDYLOLISTHESIS

Traumatic spondylolisthesis may generally be managed successfully with plaster cast immobilization.[46] Effect immobilization is best assured by the application of a cast that incorporates one thigh, facilitating increased immobilization of the lumbosacral articulation. It is of interest that some defects may heal without treatment while the patient continues vigorous athletic activities.[60] It is important to remember that acute fractures have medicolegal importance, if it can be proved that the lesion was caused by a given injury or accident. This is extremely difficult to do, however, since x-rays have rarely been taken prior to initial injury. Bone scans may help in determining whether active callus is present. If symptoms continue in spite of conservative management, operative intervention may be necessary, which consists of spinal stabilization by arthrodesis.

## DEGENERATIVE SPONDYLOLISTHESIS

The treatment of degenerative spondylolisthesis is basically that of the management of degenerative disc disease. Here, however, the situation is often complicated by spinal stenosis that develops secondary to forward slippage, centrally placed facet joints, and exuberant bone formation from osteoarthritic spurring around the facets. Most of these patients may be treated by conservative management, with analgesics, abdominal exercises, corsets, anti-arthritic drugs, and reassurance. Conservative therapy is adequate in

90 per cent of these patients.[46] Neurologic symptoms secondary to spinal stenosis are the conditions that usually bring the patient to the doctor and that ultimately make surgical treatment necessary. Decompression is the procedure of choice.[10] Myelography will show hourglass encroachment at the level of slipping and sometimes constriction sufficient enough to constitute a "block." A disc herniation at the level of slipping is also occasionally visualized. The disc herniation may be at a level actually lower than the slippage. Surgery consists of a laminectomy through a posterior approach.

The level at which the spinal canal is approached is sometimes difficult to identify because of transitional lumbosacral articulation or unsuspected fusion of the lumbosacral joints. Interoperative x-rays may be beneficial. The point of compression is where there is a slippage of L4 on L5 and the L5 nerve root becomes compressed as it passes between the upper edge of the body of L5 and the hypertrophic edge of the superior facet of the same vertebra.[41] It is best, therefore, to remove part of the laminae of the vertebrae above and below the level of the slippage. The lateral recesses must be well decompressed so that there is no question that the nerves are completely unroofed. If one confines the decompression to removing the lower half of the laminae and the spinous processes of the slipped vertebra and the upper half of the laminae in the spinous process of the subadjacent vertebra, adequate decompression can usually be achieved without producing greater instability.[48] The L5 root should be traced well out, taking off the corner of the superior articular process of L5, but usually not cutting through the pars of L5.

Even after adequate decompression has been achieved, mobility of the dura may be impaired because of tethering of a nerve root that has become adherent to the underlying annulus. This should be carefully dissected off and Gelfoam used to prevent adherence of the soft tissues to the dura following decompression. The step-off due to the malalignment of the vertebral bodies at the level of the slip should be identified to confirm that the proper level has been decompressed. If a herniated disc is found, it should be removed. Occasionally, the pars of L5 must be cut through in order to furnish adequate decompression, but this will lead to greater instability with the possibility of further slippage. It is interesting, however, that this does not appear to make these patients symptomatically worse, and Rosenberg has found that the increased slippage that may occur, which has been as much as 15 per cent in the year following surgery, has not subsequently progressed and seems to stabilize after that period.[48] The question of whether spine fusion should be done is still controversial. It is our opinion that spine fusion is not usually necessary in patients older than age 55.

## SCOLIOSIS DUE TO SPONDYLOLISTHESIS

There are two recognized patterns of curves caused by spondylolisthesis. First, and less common, is called "olisthetic" scoliosis. This condition was described by Tøjner[56] as a torsional scoliosis at the spondylitic vertebra. Instead of a symmetrical forward slipping of L5 on S1, one side slips farther forward than the other, thus producing a rotation or torsion of the spine. In this condition, there is relatively little lateral curvature, but the lumbar spine may show significant rotation (Fig. 22–9).

The second and more common pattern in our experience, is the "spasm" scoliosis. In this type, the curvature involves the whole spine, is not associated with rotation, and is quite similar to the scoliosis seen with a herniated intervertebal disc. The patient usually, *but not always*, has pain. This pattern is usually seen in growing children with Grade III or Grade IV slips. The curve disappears in the relaxed supine position and under anesthesia (Fig. 22–10). It spontaneously corrects following successful lumbosacral fusion.

On rare occasions, when a "spasm" curve has been present for many of the growing years, a lung structural curve may exist that does not disappear in the supine position, and the whole curve may require fusion.

### Diagnosis

Any patient with signs or symptoms pointing to the lumbosacral area should be

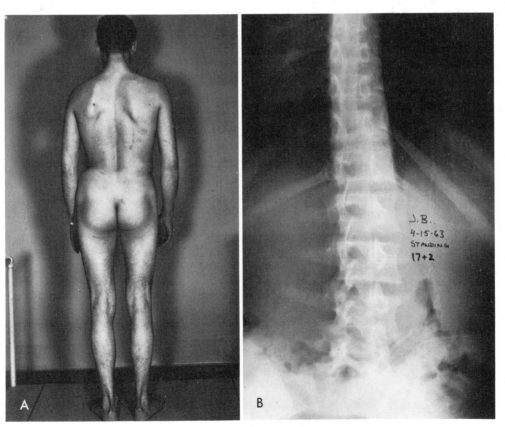

**Figure 22–9**  "Olisthetic scoliosis."

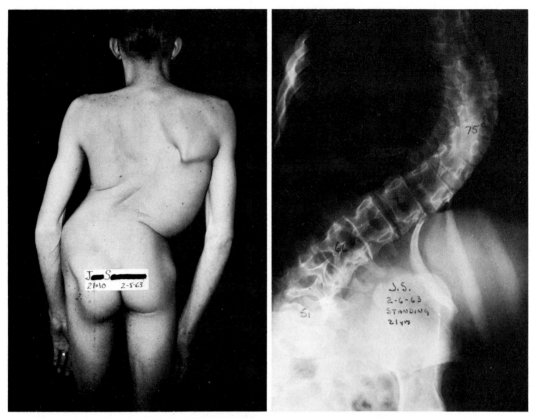

**Figure 22-10** "Spasm scoliosis."

suspected of having spondylolisthesis. Low back pain, leg pain, tight hamstrings, lumbosacral tenderness, a palpable "step-off" at the lumbosacral area, any curve emanating from the lumbosacral region, and any patient listing to one side on the forward bending test should be suspected of having spondylolisthesis.

For the definitive diagnosis, detail x-rays of the lumbosacral area are necessary. These should include a spot lateral of L5–S1, spot oblique views of L5–S1, and a "Ferguson" view (AP view of the sacrum and fifth lumbar vertebra. Because these views involve a significant amount of irradiation in the gonadal area, they should not be routinely ordered, but only when pathology is suspect in the lumbosacral region.

### Treatment

The treatment of scoliosis due to spondylolisthesis is lumbosacral fusion. The pro-

cedure of choice is a wide, transverse process fusion of L4 to S1. Theoretically, one could fuse only from the transverse process of L5 to S1, but patients presenting with these symptoms usually have a Grade II–IV slip, and the transverse process of L5 is both hypoplastic and displaced so far forward that an adequate fusion is difficult to achieve by fusion of L5 to sacrum only.

About one week postoperatively, the patient is placed on the Risser table or hip spica table, and a cast is applied from nipple line to just above both knees with the hips in full extension. Great care is taken to assure that the spine is straight above the pelvis. The patient *must not* be allowed to fuse in the scoliotic or deviated position. L4 must be directly above the center of the sacrum, and the top of L4 must be perfectly horizontal.

The patient is kept on bed rest in this cast for four to six months. A small lumbar cast or corset is used for an additional three to four months, ambulation beginning at four to six months. Immobilization is continued until the fusion is absolutely solid, as defined by vertical trabeculations in the fusion mass, extending from L4 to the alae of the sacrum.

## SCOLIOSIS ASSOCIATED WITH SPONDYLOLISTHESIS

Since both idiopathic scoliosis and spondylolisthesis are relatively common problems, it is quite possible for both to exist in the same person. In a study of 500 consecutive patients with idiopathic scoliosis who had routine oblique x-rays of the lumbosacral area, Fisk et al.[13] found an incidence of pars defects of 6.2 per cent. This corresponds closely to the incidence in the general population as reported by Roche and Rowe[47] of 5 per cent and Moreton[33] of 7.2 per cent.

The pattern of curvature in these patients is the typical curve of the idiopathic type and is not associated with tight hamstrings, deviation on forward bending, or marked decompensation as noted in patients with "spasm" scoliosis due to spondylolisthesis. It is not difficult to distinguish between the patient with scoliosis due to spondylolisthesis and the patient with idiopathic scoliosis coincident with spondylolisthesis.

In the patient with idiopathic scoliosis and spondylolisthesis, treatment is directed toward each problem.[17] If neither problem requires treatment, treat neither one. If the idiopathic scoliosis needs bracing, brace it. If the idiopathic scoliosis needs fusion, arthrodesis should be carried out. If the spondylolisthesis needs fusion, but the idiopathic curve needs bracing, fuse T5–L1 or L4–S1 and brace the curve. If the patient has a thoracic idiopathic scoliosis requiring fusion plus a spondylolisthesis requiring fusion (progressive slip and/or continuing pain), fuse both areas separately, e.g., T5–L1 and L4–S1.

It is only in the relatively rare circumstance of a lumbar idiopathic scoliosis of 50 degrees or more, coincident with a Grade III or Grade IV slip, that fusion would include both areas continuously, i.e., fusion from the top of the scoliosis curve to the sacrum.

Many physicians are afraid to fuse an idiopathic scoliosis down to L4, leaving a spondylolysis or Grade I spondylolisthesis at L5–S1. There appears to be no ground for such fears, as fusion of the idiopathic curve has not, in the authors' experience, increased either the degree of slip or the symptomatology of the slip.

## References

1. Adkins, E. W. O.: Spondylolisthesis. J. Bone Joint Surg., *37B*:48, 1955.
2. Ascani, C.: Personal communication.
3. Baker, D. R., and McHolick, W.: Spondylolysis and spondylolisthesis in children. Proceedings of the American Academy of Orthopaedic Surgeons, J. Bone Joint Surg., *38A*:933, 1956.
4. Borkow, S. E., and Kleiger, B.: Spondylolisthesis in the newborn. A case report. Clin. Orthop., *81*:73, 1971.
5. Bosworth, D. M., Fielding, J. W., Demarest, L., and Bonaquist, M.: Spondylolisthesis. J. Bone Joint Surg., *37A*:707, 1955.
6. Boxall, D. W., Winter, R. B., Bradford, D. S., and Moe, J. H.: Management of severe spondylolisthesis (Grade III and Grade IV) in children and adolescents. In press.
7. Bradford, D. S.: Spondylolysis and spondylolisthesis. *In* Chou, S. N. (ed.): Spinal Deformity and Neurologic Dysfunction. New York, Raven Press, 1977.
8. Buck, J. E.: Direct repair of the defect in spondylolisthesis, J. Bone Joint Surg., *52B*:432, 1970.
9. Dandy, D. J., and Shannon, M. J.: Lumbo-sacral subluxation. J. Bone Joint Surg., *53B*:578, 1971.
10. Davis, I. S., and Bailey, R. W.: Spondylolisthesis: Indications for lumbar nerve root decompression and operative technique. Clin. Orthop., *117*:129, 1976.
11. Del Torto, U.: Surgical reduction and stabilization of spondylolisthesis. Clin. Orthop. *75*:281, 1971.
12. Farfan, H. F., Osteria, V., and Lamy, C.: The mechanical etiology of spondylolysis and spondylolisthesis. Clin. Orthop., *117*:40, 1976.
13. Fisk, J., Winter, R. B., and Moe, J. H.: Scoliosis, spondylolysis, and spondylolisthesis: Their relationship as reviewed in 539 patients. In press.
14. Freebody, D., Bendall, R., and Taylor, R. D.: Anterior transperitoneal lumbar fusion. J. Bone Joint Surg., *53B*:617, 1971.
15. Friberg, S.: Studies on spondylolisthesis. Acta Chir. Scand. vol. LXXXII, suppl. LVI, 1939.
16. Gill, G. G., Manning, J. G., and White, H. L.: Surgical treatment of spondylolisthesis without spine fusion. J. Bone Joint Surg., *37A*:493, 1955.
17. Goldstein, L. A., Haake, P. W., DeVanny, J. R., and Chou, P. K.: Guidelines for the management of lumbosacral spondylolisthesis associated with scoliosis. Clin. Orthop., *117*:135, 1976.
18. Harrington, P. R., and Dickson, J. H.: Spinal instrumentation in the treatment of severe progressive spondylolisthesis. Clin. Orthop., *117*:157, 1976.
19. Harrington, P. R., and Tullos, H. S.: Spondylolisthesis in children. Observations and surgical treatment. Clin. Orthop., *79*:75, 1971.
20. Harris, R. I.: Spondylolisthesis. Ann. R. Coll. Surg. Engl., *8*:259, 1951.
21. Hensinger, R. N., Lang, J. R., and MacEwen, G. D.: Surgical management of spondylolisthesis in children and adolescents. Spine, *1*:207, 1976.

22. Herbiniaux, G.: Traite sur divers accouchments laborieux, et sur les polypes de la matrice. Bruxelles, J. L. DeBoubers, 1782.
23. Hodgson, A. R., and Wong, S. K.: A description of a technic and evaluation of results in anterior spinal fusion for deranged intervertebral disc and spondylolisthesis. Clin. Orthop., *56*:133, 1968.
24. Jackson, D. W., Wiltse, L. L., and Cirincione, R. J.: Spondylolysis in the female gymnast. Clin. Orthop., *117*:68, 1976.
25. Jenkins, J. A.: Spondylolisthesis. Br. J. Surg., *24*:80, 1936.
26. Kilian, H. F.: Schilderungen neuer Beckenformen und ihres Verhaltens in Leven. Mannheim, Verlag von Bassermann & Mathy, 1854.
27. Lambl, W.: Beitrage zur Geburtskunde un Dynackologie. von F. W. V. Scanzoni, 1858.
28. Lance, E. M.: Treatment of severe spondylolisthesis with neural involvement. A report of two cases. J. Bone Joint Surg., *48A*:883, 1966.
29. Laurent, L. E.: Spondylolisthesis. Acta Orthop. Scand., Suppl. 35, 1958.
30. Laurent, L. E., and Osterman, K.: Operative treatment of spondylolisthesis in young patients. Clin. Orthop., *117*:85, 1976.
31. Lowe, R. W., Hayes, T. D., Kaye, J., Bagg, R. J., and Leukens, C. A.: Standing roentgenograms in spondylolisthesis. Clin. Orthop., *117*:85, 1976.
32. Meyerding, H. W.: Spondylolisthesis. Surg. Gynecol. Obstet., *54*:371–377, 1932.
33. Moreton, R. D.: Spondylolisthesis. JAMA, *195*:671, 1966.
34. Mosimann, P.: Die Histologie der Spondylolyse. Archiv. Orthop. Unfallchir., *53*:264, 1961.
35. Nachemson, A.: Repair of the spondylolisthetic defect and intertransverse fusion for young patients. Clin. Orthop., *117*:101, 1976.
36. Nachemson, A., and Wiltse, L. L.: Editorial comment: Spondylolisthesis. Clin. Orthop., *117*:4, 1976.
37. Neugebauer, F. L.: The classic: A new contribution to the history and etiology of spondylolisthesis. Clin. Orthop., *117*:4, 1976.
38. Newman, P. H.: A clinical syndrome associated with severe lumbo-sacral subluxation. J. Bone Joint Surg., *47B*:472, 1965.
39. Newman, P. H., and Stone, K. H.: The etiology of spondylolisthesis, with a special investigation. J. Bone Joint Surg., *45B*:39, 1963.
40. Newman, P. H.: Surgical treatment for derangement of the lumbar spine. J. Bone Joint Surg., *55B*:7, 1973.
41. Newman, P. H.: Surgical treatment for spondylolisthesis in the adult. Clin. Orthop., *117*:106, 1976.
42. Osterman, K., Lindholm, T. S., and Laurent, L. E.: Late results of removal of the loose posterior element (Gill's operation) in the treatment of lytic lumbar spondylolisthesis. Clin. Orthop., *117*:121, 1976.
43. Phalen, G. S., and Dickson, J. A.: Spondylolisthesis and tight hamstrings, J. Bone Joint Surg., *43A*:505, 1961.
44. Risser, J. C., and Norquist, D. M.: Sciatic scoliosis in growing children. Clin. Orthop., *21*:137–154, 1961.
45. Robert: Monatsschrift, Fur Geburtskunde und Frauenkrankheiten, *5*:81.
46. Roche, M. B.: Healing of bilateral fracture of the pars interarticularis of a lumbar neural arch. J. Bone Joint Surg., *32A*:428, 1950.
47. Roche, M. B., and Rowe, G. G.: The incidence of separate neural arch and coincident bone variations. Anat. Rec., *109*:233, 1951.
48. Rosenberg, N. J.: Degenerative spondylolisthesis. Clin. Orthop., *117*:112, 1976.
49. Scaglietti, O., Frontino, G., and Bartolozzi, P.: Technique of anatomical reduction of lumbar spondylolisthesis and its surgical stabilization. Clin. Orthop., *117*:164, 1976.
50. Scaglietti, O., Frontino, G., and Bartolozzi, P.: Tecnica della ridozione de-la spondelolistesi lombare esua contenzione definitiva. Atti S.I.O.T., *292*:000, 1970.
51. Snijder, J. G. N., Seroo, J. M., Snijer, C. J., and Schijvens, A. W. M.: Therapy of spondylolisthesis by repositioning and fixation of the olisthetic vertebra. Clin. Orthop., *117*:149, 1976.
52. Stewart, T. D.: The age incidence of neural arch defects in Alaskan natives, considered from the standpoint of etiology. J. Bone Joint Surg., *35A*:937, 1953.
53. Taddonio, R. F., and DeWald, R. L.: Reduction and fusion of severe spondylolisthesis: 11th Annual Scoliosis Research Society Meeting, Ottawa, Ontario.
54. Taillard, W.: Le Spondylolisthesis chez l'enfant et l'adolescent. Acta Orthop. Scand., *24*:115, 1954.
55. Taillard, W. F.: Etiology of spondylolisthesis. Clin. Orthop., *117*:30, 1976.
56. Tøjner, H.: Olisthetic scoliosis. Acta Orthop. Scand., *33*:291, 1963.
57. Turner, R. H., and Bianco, A. J.: Spondylolysis and spondylolisthesis in children and teenagers. J. Bone Joint Surg., *53A*:1298, 1971.
58. Wiltse, L. L.: Spondylolisthesis in children. Clin. Orthop., *21*:156, 1961.
59. Wiltse, L. L.: The etiology of spondylolistheis. J. Bone Joint Surg., *44A*:539, 1962.
60. Wiltse, L. L., and Jackson, D. W.: Treatment of spondylolisthesis and spondylolysis in children. Clin. Orthop., *117*:92, 1976.
61. Wiltse, L. L., Newman, P. H., and Macnab, I.: Classification of spondylolysis and spondylolisthesis. Clin. Orthop. *117*:23, 1976.
62. Wiltse, L. L., Widell, E. H., and Jackson, D. W.: Fatigue fracture: The basic lesion in intrinsic spondylolisthesis. J. Bone Joint Surg., *57A*:17, 1975.

# Chapter 23

# MISCELLANEOUS PROBLEMS

## SCOLIOSIS SECONDARY TO OSTEOID OSTEOMA

The name osteoid osteoma was first proposed by Jaffe[15] in 1935 to designate a benign neoplastic lesion of bone characterized by a core of niduslike focus and reactive perifocal bony thickenings.[16-19] Several hundred cases have been described, with more than 50 involving the spine. The fact that these lesions may be the cause of painful scoliosis is not universally appreciated.

### CLINICAL FEATURES[11, 12, 13, 20, 23, 29, 32]

Osteoid osteoma of the spine affects males more frequently than females. The onset of symptoms is usually during the second decade, although cases have been reported in patients under 5 and over 40 years of age. The lesions are almost invariably located in the posterior elements of the vertebra; however, four cases have been reported in which the lesion involved the vertebral body.[7, 8, 13, 28] The lumbar spine is the most frequent area of involvement, followed by the cervical, then the thoracic area.

Pain is by far the most common symptom. It is usually described as a localized ache that increases with time. The pain may be aggravated by motion, but is not always relieved by rest or aspirin. Sometimes it is more severe at night and may be increased by coughing, sneezing, or defecation. Radi-

cular pain is common, particularly if the lesion involves the lumbar spine. We have had one patient who had no pain and was treated for scoliosis with a Milwaukee brace for two years until the correct diagnosis was made (Fig. 23–1).

Physical findings reveal tenderness and marked muscle spasm at the site of the lesion. Neurologic involvement may be present. This can present as weakness of the limb, cutaneous hypesthesia, positive straight leg raising, and deep tendon reflex changes. Atrophy has also been reported, but it is not clear whether this is from disuse secondary to radicular pain or whether it is due to neurologic involvement.

Scoliosis is common but may not be present if the lesion involves the spinous processes, sacrum, or vertebral body. The scoliosis is usually associated with torticollis in the cervical spine and pelvic obliquity in the lumbar spine. The magnitude of the scoliosis is variable. The curvature may be present as a "typical C-shaped curvature" but the so-called typical idiopathic curvature has also been seen in association with an osteoid osteoma. The lesion is located almost invariably on the concave side of the curvature and often in the apical posterior elements. The scoliosis usually demonstrates poor correctibility on side bending.

*Text continued on page 558*

**555**

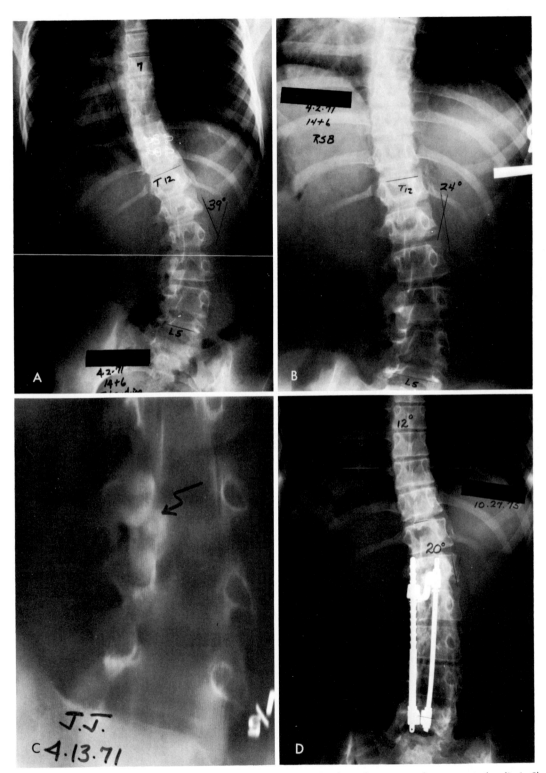

**Figure 23–1**    A, J.J., a 14 +6 year old female, had been in a Milwaukee brace for two years for treatment of scoliosis. She had no back complaints. B, Right side bending x-ray demonstrates poor correctability of the lumbar curvature. Sclerosis with bone formation in the left pedicle of L3 is noted. C, Tomography demonstrates the nidus and surrounding reactive sclerosis. D, Treatment consisting of removal of the pedicle, superor and inferior facets, was felt to render the spine unstable, so a spine fusion with instrumentation was carried out. Follow-up four years later demonstrates solid fusion with satisfactory spinal alignment.

*Illustration continued on the opposite page*

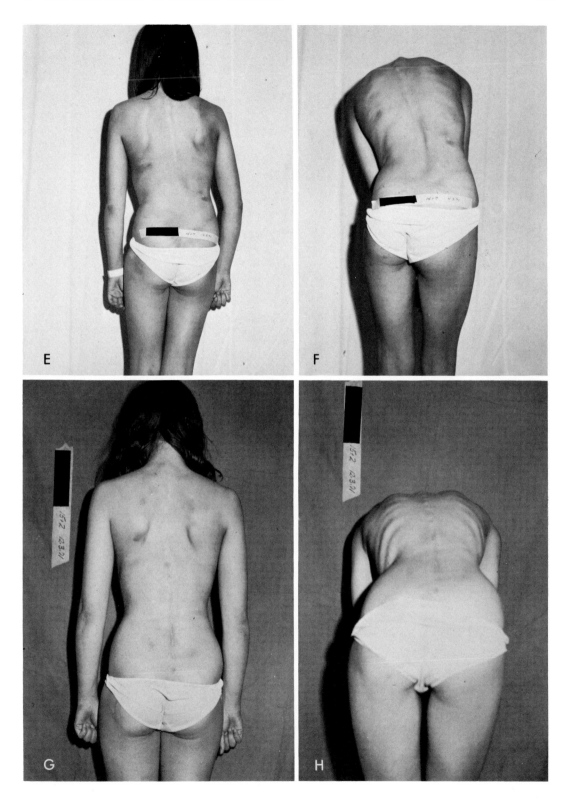

**Figure 23–1** *Continued E* and *F,* Preoperative photographs of patient, showing decompensated lumbar curve with restriction of forward bending. *G* and *H,* Clinical photographs taken eight months postoperatively show an excellent cosmetic appearance with no restriction on forward bending.

## RADIOGRAPHIC FINDINGS[1, 4, 9, 10, 20, 30, 34, 36, 37]

The roentgenographic appearance is that of a central radiolucent nidus with a surrounding sclerotic reaction but not as marked as that found elsewhere. In fact, the typical appearance is present in only one half of the cases. Initial x-rays may be negative, since the lesion may produce pain before it is radiographically detectable. Tomography of the spine is helpful, but even with multiple repeat projections, a central nidus may not be visualized. We have found the isotopic bone scan (technetium) to be of great value in identifying suspected osteoid osteomas (Fig. 23–2B). Osteomyelitis also gives a localized increased uptake of isotope, but the chronicity of the problem and a normal sedimentation rate allow one to rule out osteomyelitis. Angiography has been reported to be of help in the diagnosis of osteoid osteomas, but we have no experience with this technique.

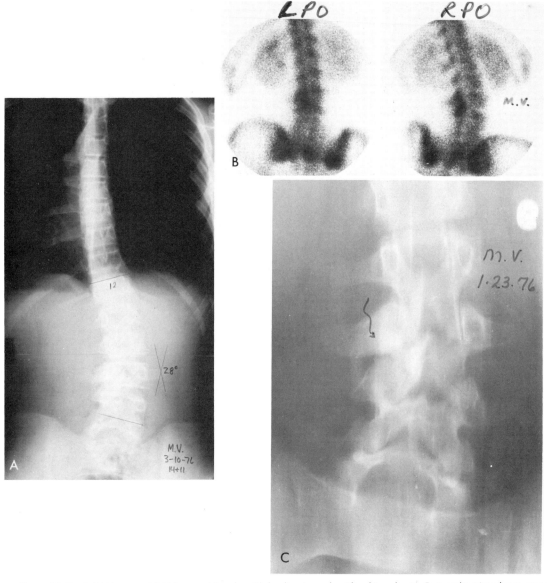

**Figure 23–2**  A, M.V. was a 14+11 year old male with back pain and a "fixed" scoliosis. B, A technetium bone scan revealed a "hot spot" in the lumbar spine coinciding with the area of bone formation at L3 on the left. C, Following removal of a portion of the laminae and inferior facet of L3 on the left side, his condition improved.

*Illustration continued on the opposite page*

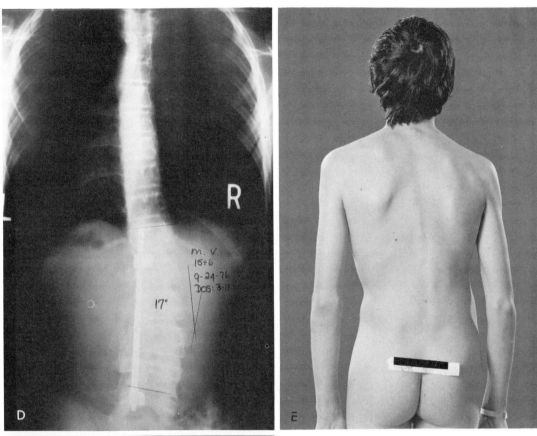

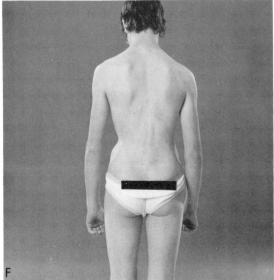

**Figure 23–2** *Continued D,* Two months later his symptoms recurred. No nidus was found at the original surgery; only sclerotic bone was present. In the area of the lesion additional reactive sclerosis was present. *E,* Removal of transverse process, pedicle, and remaining laminae on left was carried out. The nidus was identified underneath the transverse process at its junction with the pedicle. Spine fusion with instrumentation was carried out. Six months later the fusion appeared solid. He has remained asymptomatic since the second surgery. *F,* Clinical photograph one year following second operation.

## DIAGNOSIS[2, 3, 5, 7, 26, 32, 35, 41]

Most authors have commented on the length of time between the onset of symptoms and the diagnosis. It is most common to have one or more other diagnoses seriously entertained before the correct one is made. The diagnoses most frequently considered are lumbosacral strain, herniated nucleus pulposus, idiopathic scoliosis, arthritis, osteochondritis, hysteria, infection, and cord tumor.

## TREATMENT[20, 23, 31, 39]

Treatment consists of thorough surgical removal of the lesion in all patients. The findings at surgery include thickening of the cortex with an underlying small cavity containing cherry-red granulomatous tissue. There may be surrounding reaction in the soft tissues, but this is uncommon. There appears to be no reason or advantage to proceed with spine fusion at the time of surgical excision. Although the curvatures are relatively inflexible preoperatively, with removal of the nidus, the scoliosis will be expected to improve. If the curvature is moderately severe (less than 40 degrees), and the spine has been rendered unstable by removal of the articular facets and pedicle, consideration should be given to spine fusion. As a rule, however, we prefer to remove the lesion at a single stage and then brace the patient, particularly if the patient is skeletally immature. If the curvature is deforming and does not improve, consideration may be given to correction and fusion at a later stage.

It should be remembered that recurrences of this tumor[6] as well as multifocal lesions[35] have been reported. Similarly, spontaneous healing after the appearance of symptoms has been reported.[33, 39] Persistent pain and deformity after removal should lead one to suspect incomplete removal or recurrence[14, 25] (Fig. 23–2) or a multifocal lesion.[35]

## References

1. Caldicott, W. J. H.: Diagnosis of spinal osteoid osteoma. Radiology, 92:1192, 1969.
2. Coley, B. L., and Lenson, N.: Osteoid osteoma. Am. J. Surg., 77:3, 1949.
3. Dahlin, D. C., and Johnson, E. W., Jr.: Giant osteoid osteoma. J. Bone Joint Surg., 36A:559, 1954.
4. Dockerty, M. B., Ghormley, R. K., and Jackson, A. E.: Osteoid osteoma: A clinicopathologic study of 20 cases. Ann. Surg., 133:77, 1951.
5. Dubousset, J., Queneau, P., and Lacheretz, P.: Stiff and painful scoliosis in children. Rev. Chir. Orthop. 57:215, 1971.
6. Dunlop, J. A. Y., Morton, K. S., and Elliott, G. B.: Recurrent osteoid osteoma. Report of a case with a review of the literature. J. Bone Joint Surg., 52B:128, 1970.
7. Ferrer, T. M.: Osteoid osteoma of the vertebral column. Rev. Clin. Esp., 77:10, 1960.
8. Fett, H. C., Sr., and Russo, V. P.: Osteoid osteoma of a cervical vertebra. Report of a case. J. Bone Joint Surg., 41A:948, 1959.
9. Flaherty, R. A., Pugh, D. C., and Dockerty, M. B.: Osteoid osteoma. Am. J. Roentgenol., 76:1041, 1956.
10. Freiberger, R. H., Loitman, B. S., Helpern, M., and Thompson, T. C.: Osteoid osteoma. A report on 80 cases. Am. J. Roentgenol., 82:194, 1959.
11. Freiberger, R. H.: Osteoid osteoma of the spine. A cause of backache and scoliosis in children and young adults. Radiology, 75:232, 1960.
12. Golding, J. S. R.: The natural history of osteoid osteoma. With a report of twenty cases. J. Bone Joint Surg., 36B:218, 1954.
13. Heiman, M. L., Colley, C. J., and Bradford, D. S.: Osteoid osteoma of a vertebral body. Clin. Orthop., 118:159, 1976.
14. Hermann, R. M., and Blount, W. P.: Osteoid osteoma of the lumbar spine. J. Bone Joint Surg., 43A: 568, June, 1961.
15. Jaffe, H. L.: Osteoid osteoma. A benign osteoblastic tumor composed of osteoid and atypical bone. Arch. Surg., 31:709, 1935.
16. Jaffe, H. L.: Osteoid osteoma of bone. Radiology, 45:319, 1945.
17. Jaffe, H. L., and Lichtenstein, L.: Osteoid osteoma: Further experience with this benign tumor of bone. With special reference to cases showing the lesion in relation to shaft cortices and commonly misclassified as instances of sclerosing non-suppurative osteomyelitis or cortical bone abscess. J. Bone Joint Surg., 22:645, July, 1940.
18. Jaffe, H. L.: Osteoid osteoma. Proc. R. Soc. Med., 46:1007, 1953.
19. Jaffe, H. L.: Tumors and Tumorous Conditions of the Bones and Joints. Philadelphia, Lea and Febiger, 1958.
20. Keim, H. A., and Reina, E. G.: Osteoid osteoma as a cause of scoliosis. J. Bone Joint Surg., 57A:159, March, 1975.
21. Lichtenstein, L.: Bone Tumors, 2nd ed. St. Louis, C. V. Mosby, 1959.
22. Lindbom, A., Lindvall, N., Soderberg, G., and Spjut, H.: Angiography in osteoid osteoma. Acta Radiol., 54:327, 1960.
23. Maclellan, D. I., and Wilson, F. C., Jr.: Osteoid osteoma of the spine. A review of the literature and report of six new cases. J. Bone Joint Surg., 49A:111, Jan., 1967.
24. Moberg, E.: The natural course of osteoid osteoma. J. Bone Joint Surg., 33A:166, Jan., 1951.
25. Morrison, G. M., Hawes, L. E., and Sacco, J. J.: Incomplete removal of osteoid osteoma. Am. J. Surg., 80:476, 1950.
26. Morton, K. S., and Barlett, L. H.: Benign osteoblastic change resembling osteoid osteoma. Three cases

with unusual radiological features. J. Bone Joint Surg., 48B:478, Aug., 1966.

27. Mustard, W. T., and Duval, F. W.: Osteoid osteoma of vertebrae. J. Bone Joint Surg., 41B:132, Feb., 1959.

28. Paus, B. C., and Kim, T. K.: Osteoid osteoma of the spine. Acta Orthop. Scand., 33:24, 1963.

29. Ponseti, I., and Barta, C. K.: Osteoid osteoma. J. Bone Joint Surg., 29:767, July, 1947.

30. Prabhakar, B., Reddy, D. R., Dayananda, B., and Rao, G. R.: Osteoid osteoma of the skull. J. Bone Joint Surg., 54B:146, Feb., 1972.

31. Pritchard, J. E., and McKay, J. W.: Osteoid osteoma. Can. Med. Assoc. J., 58:567, 1948.

32. Rushton, J. G., Mulder, D. W., and Libscomb, P. R.: Neurologic symptoms with osteoid osteoma. Neurology, 5:794, 1955.

33. Sabanas, A. O., Bickel, W. H., and Moe, J. H.: Natural history of osteoid osteoma of the spine. Review of the literature and report of three cases. Am. J. Surg., 91:880, 1956.

34. Sankaran, B.: Osteoid osteoma. Surg. Gynecol. Obstet., 99:193, 1954.

35. Schajowicz, F., and Lemos, C.: Osteoid osteoma and osteoblastoma. Closely related entities of osteoblastic derivation. Acta Orthop. Scand., 41:272, 1970.

36. Sherman, M. S.: Osteoid osteoma associated with changes in adjacent joint. Report of two cases. J. Bone Joint Surg., 29:483, April, 1947.

37. Sherman, M. S.: Osteoid osteoma. Review of the literature and report of thirty cases. J. Bone Joint Surg., 29:918, Oct., 1947.

38. Sim, F. H., Dahlin, D. C., and Beabout, J. W.: Osteoid-osteoma: Diagnostic problems. J. Bone Joint Surg., 57A:154, March, 1975.

39. Vickers, C. W., Pugh, C. D., and Ivins, J. C.: Osteoid osteoma. A fifteen-year follow-up of an untreated patient. J. Bone Joint Surg., 41A:357–358, March, 1959.

40. Wallace, G. T.: Some surgical aspects of osteoid osteoma. J. Bone Joint Surg., 20:777, July, 1947.

41. Young, H. H.: Non-neurological lesions simulating protruded intervertebral disk. JAMA, 148:1101, 1952.

# SPINAL CORD TUMORS

Tumors of the brain and spinal cord are uncommon, comprising less than two per cent of total tumors seen.[27] Spinal cord tumors are only one-quarter to one-fifth as common as intracranial tumors.[5, 18] All reports of spinal cord tumors in children note the large delay in the diagnosis.[1, 5, 11, 12, 14, 20] A high index of suspicion must exist to allow for early diagnosis and treatment. Currently with the aggressive therapy used, the mortality rate is low, and the prognosis is improving.[1, 7, 17, 21, 24, 25, 32]

Spinal cord tumors have been divided into the intradural and extradural groups.[1, 18, 19, 28] Extradural tumors are usually malignant, being metastases from primary carcinomas and sarcomas as well as reticuloendothelial malignancies. Occasionally an extradural tumor can be part of a dumb-bell neurofibroma. Intradural tumors can be divided into the extramedullary group, comprising neurofibromas and meningiomas, and the intramedullary group of gliomas and ependymomas. These tumors are commonest in the third to the seventh decades. Schott found the incidence of the tumors in adults to be 25 to 40 per cent extradural, 60 per cent extramedullary, and 5 to 10 per cent intramedullary.[28] The relative incidence in children is 20 per cent gliomas, 20 per cent sarcomas, 17 per cent developmental tumors and dermoids, and only 10 per cent neurofibromas.[28] Haft et al. in their small series found that one third of their cases of spinal cord tumors in children were intramedullary and one half extradural.[15]

The delay in diagnosis of these tumors in children is due to a failure to fully appreciate the early signs and symptoms of cord compression. The early symptoms are glossed over, or an incorrect diagnosis is made. The features that should alert the clinician include back pain, motor disturbances, sensory phenomena, sphincter disturbances, and musculoskeletal abnormalities.[1, 20]

## PAIN

Low back pain, often associated with spinal rigidity, is the most frequent presenting symptom in spinal tumors.[1, 18, 20, 23, 35] Persistent low back pain in a child should be evaluated with care, and if no obvious cause of the pain is found, the possibility of a spinal cord tumor should be considered. A valuable sign at this stage is spinal rigidity.[3, 20, 26] When the child is examined and asked to bend foward, restriction of forward bending and/or deviation on forward bending is seen. This abnormality is often painless and may be subtle, so any deviation of forward bending should be viewed with suspicion (Fig. 23–3).

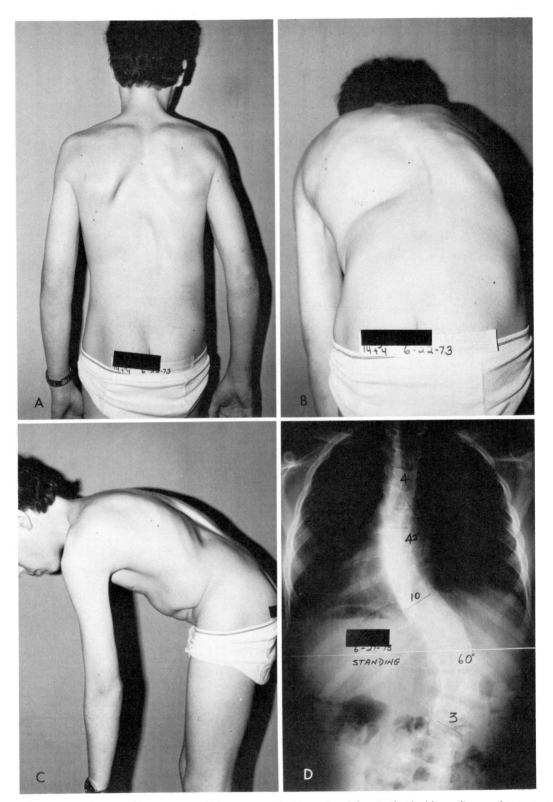

**Figure 23–3** *A,* D.W. This 14+4 year old boy presented with a spine deformity that had been diagnosed two years earlier and treated with exercises. This posterior view of his back showed decompensation to the left and a rigid lumbar scoliosis with lumbar muscle spasm. *B,* Forward bending showed the marked lumbar muscle spasm with deviation of the trunk to the left. *C,* Side view of forward bending shows the spinal rigidity with restriction of forward bending. Neurologic examination showed minor sensory and proprioceptive loss in one leg. *D,* Anterosposterior standing x-ray shows a left thoracic curve of 42 degrees and a right lumbar curve of 60 degrees. The marked decompensation to the right is noted. The presence of a left thoracic curve is very suspicious, as it is rare in "idiopathic" scoliosis.

*Illustration continued on the opposite page*

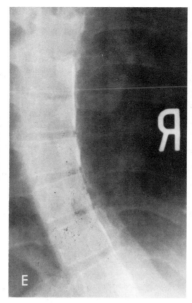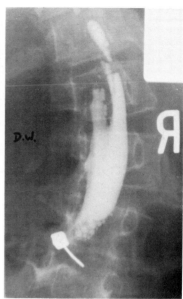

**Figure 23–3** *Continued E*, Myelogram shows widening of the whole spinal cord with only a trickle of dye alongside the cord. At surgery an ependymoma of the whole cord was found which was partially resected in a two-stage procedure.

## MOTOR FUNCTION

Weakness is one of the most common early presentations of spinal neoplasms in children. When the onset of the weakness is rapid, with paraparesis or paraplegia, diagnosis is easy. An insidious onset of weakness is difficult to detect. The family often notes a change in posture or gait. A child tends to spare a limb while at play or shows a change in his gait pattern. Careful evaluation with muscle testing is essential, but some early changes are subtle and may be missed even when the index of suspicion is high (Fig. 23–4).

## SENSORY CHANGES

The child seldom complains of sensory symptoms apart from pain. Objective assessment of sensory loss is difficult and unreliable due to the unwillingness or inability of the child to cooperate.

## SPHINCTER DISTURBANCE

Sphincter disturbance in the infant and toddler is impossible to evaluate. In an older child, regression of sphincter control may be the first manifestation of a cauda equina lesion. The presence of constipation, urinary incontinence, or nocturia should not be overlooked.

## MUSCULOSKELETAL ANOMALIES

Scoliosis, foot deformity, and pain are important presenting features (Figs. 23–3 and 23–5).[4, 6, 8, 33] A high index of suspicion is necessary to enable an early diagnosis to be made. Cases of scoliosis should be considered idiopathic only if no other cause is found. Subtle neurologic changes should be sought. With the forward bending test any sign of spinal rigidity, with inability to bend forward or persistent deviation to one side, should alert the physician. Any case of scoliosis associated with pain is a spinal cord tumor until proved otherwise. Any abnormal curve pattern on x-ray must be viewed with suspicion, especially left thoracic curves in adolescents or markedly decompensated curves (Figs. 23–3*D*, 23–4*A*, 23–5, 23–6).

A subtle presenting feature of intraspinal lesions is foot deformity. A cavus foot is often the presenting feature of spinal dysraphism or a spinal cord tumor. All children with foot deformities should have their backs examined and have a full neurologic evaluation, with a consultation by a neurologist or neurosurgeon where necessary.

## X-RAYS[1, 7, 9, 15, 18, 21, 25, 29, 31, 33, 34]

The plain anteroposterior and lateral x-rays often reveal signs of intraspinal pathology. Erosion or deformity of vertebral

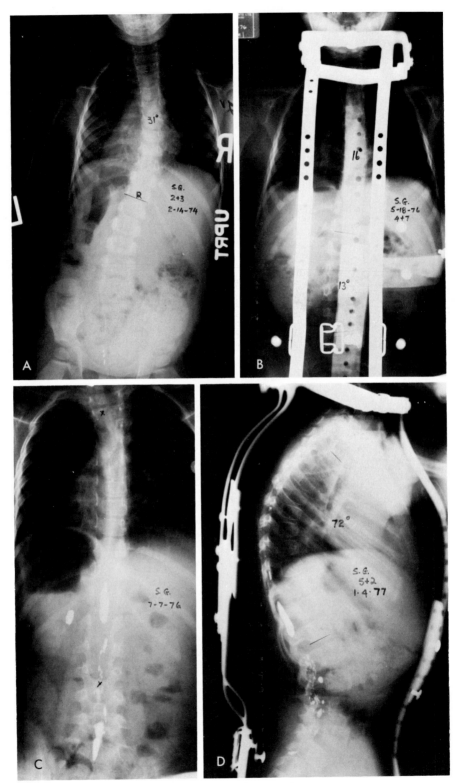

**Figure 23–4** *See legend on opposite page.*

bodies, asymmetry or erosion of pedicles, or an increase in the interpediculate distance should be sought. A spinal tap will reveal a block in the flow of cerebrospinal fluid on the Queckenstedt test and an elevated CSF protein level. A myelogram is essential for diagnosis and should be performed when the index of suspicion is high. A number of negative myelograms on a few children is far better than missing the diagnosis because of reluctance to perform a myelogram on a child.

Commonly the diagnosis is missed. The most common diagnoses made include poliomyelitis, trauma with back pain, and idiopathic scoliosis.[2, 5, 6, 16, 22] In any case where the natural history or response to treatment is different from that expected with that diagnosis, the patient should be re-evaluated.[1, 2, 5, 6, 14, 15, 16, 22, 33, 35]

## TREATMENT

The first extramedullary intradural tumor excision was by Sir Victor Horsley in 1887. Current neurosurgical treatment of spinal cord tumors is surgical excision and irradiation for radiosensitive lesions.[1, 7, 10, 13, 14, 17, 18, 21, 24, 29, 30, 32] Intraspinal lesions are approached using microsurgical techniques with myelotomy and reoperation after two weeks with excision of the tumor. Symmetrical irradiation is used with portals chosen to minimize the effects on vertebral growth. In certain types of tumors adjunctive chemotherapy is added. Constant orthopedic supervision is necessary in these children to detect the onset of postlaminectomy

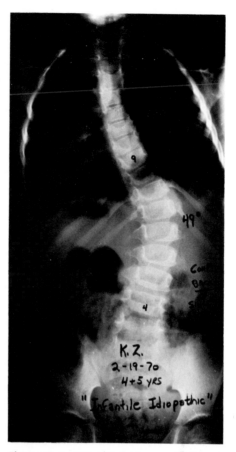

**Figure 23–5** K.Z. This 4+5 year old girl presented with a decompensated right thoracolumbar curve of 49 degrees. Neurologic examination was normal except that the patient had a vague complaint of back pain and a burning sensation passing around the chest. She was diagnosed as an infantile idiopathic scoliosis and placed in a Milwaukee brace. Two years later she was correctly diagnosed as having spinal cord tumor, and the astrocytoma was partially excised and irradiated. The presence of the vague neurologic symptoms plus the unusual curve pattern should have raised the index of suspicion.

kyphosis (see page 595). In some cases surgical treatment of the co-existing scoliosis is necessary.

---

**Figure 23–4** *A*, S.G. This 2+3 year old child presented with a right thoracic scoliosis of 31 degrees. Because of the unusual appearance of the curve, neurologic consultation was obtained, but no abnormality was found. The curve was flexible on side bending. A Milwaukee brace was fitted. *B*, Correction in the brace was excellent. Six months after brace fitting the mother had noted limping but this could not be verified, and the neurologic examination was normal.

Just after two years of brace wearing the correction was excellent, with the right thoracic curve corrected to 16 degrees. The patient had an abnormal gait for two weeks. She walked with a crouched gait. There was weakness of her quadriceps and anterior tibial muscles on the right. Referral to a neurologist was made. *C*, A myelogram showed a total block at the level of the conus with a raised spinal fluid protein of 1200. A laminectomy and myelotomy showed an intramedullary cyst, but no tumor. Postoperatively the gait was normal. Two weeks later she gradually became paraplegic and the myelogram showed a block at L1 and T8. The laminectomy was extended from T3 to L3. A Grade II astrocytoma was found, and subtotal resection was performed. The x-ray shows the extent of the laminectomy. *D*, Postoperatively the tumor was irradiated. Neurological return was gradual over the next nine months, with return of sphincter control and only residual minor foot weakness. Because of the extent of the laminectomy, a long kyphosis has resulted. The x-ray shows the kyphosis controlled in a Milwaukee brace. If the control is not maintained, an anterior fusion is planned.

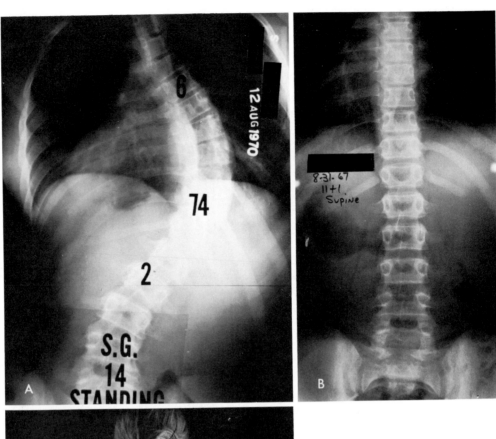

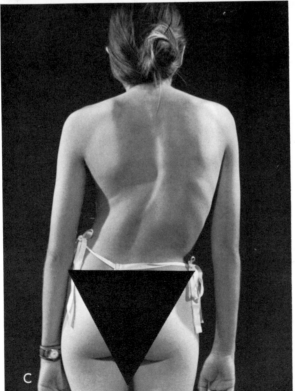

**Figure 23–6**   *A,* S.G. This 14+1 year old girl presented with a 74 degree curve. Neurologic examination was normal. *B,* This supine x-ray was taken three years previously and showed a minimal curve. *C,* This clinical photograph showed deformity and decompensation. No spinal rigidity was present on forward bending.

A spine fusion and Harrington instrumentation was carried out with no complication and an excellent result. Six years later, following the birth of her first child, there was a sudden onset of leg weakness. A myelogram showed a spinal cord tumor, which on exploration was diagnosed as a very low grade astrocytoma. In retrospect this tumor was probably present on initial presentation, but there were no clues to its presence other than the rapid progression of the scoliosis

# References

1. Austin, G.: The Spinal Cord. Springfield, Ill., Charles C Thomas, 1972.
2. Bailey, A. A., and Craig, W. McK.: Intraspinal meningiomas simulating degenerative diseases of the spinal cord. Proc. Staff Meet. Mayo Clin., 24: 233–238, 1950.
3. Bennett, G. E.: Tumors of cauda equina and spinal cord. Report of four cases in which marked spasm of erector spinal and hamstring muscles was outstanding sign. JAMA, 89:1480–1483, 1927.
4. Boldrey, E., Adams, J. E., and Brown, H. A.: Scoliosis as a manifestation of disease of the cervicothoracic portion of the spinal cord. Arch. Neurol. Psychiatry, 61:528, 1949.
5. Craig, W. McK.: Need for consideration of intraspinal tumors as a cause of pain and disability. JAMA, 164:436–437, 1957.
6. Curtiss, P. H., and Collins, W. F.: Spinal-cord tumor—a cause of progressive neurological changes in children with scoliosis. A report of three cases. J. Bone Joint Surg., 43A:517–522, 1961.
7. Cushing, H.: Meningiomas; Their Classification, Regional Behavior, Life History, and Surgical End Results. Springfield, Ill., Charles C Thomas, 1938.
8. Dalloz, J. C., Queneau, P., Canlorbe, R., and Rubin, S.: Modifications de la statique rachidienne au cours des compressions medullaires pour tumeur chez l'enfant. Arch. Franc. Pediatr., 20:309, 1963.
9. Ekelund, L., and Cronquist, S.: Roentgenological changes in spinal malformations and spinal tumors in children. Radiology, 13:541, 1973.
10. Elsberg, C. A., and Beer, E.: The operability of intramedullary tumors of the spinal cord. A report of two operations with remarks upon the extrusion of intraspinal tumors. Am. J. Med. Sci., 142:636–647, 1911.
11. Grant, F. C.: Notes on series of spinal cord tumors. Am. J. Surg., 23:89–95, 1934.
12. Grant, F. C.: Spinal Cord Tumors. Penn. Med. J. 39: 591–593, 1936.
13. Grant, F. C.: Surgical experiences with extramedullary tumors of the spinal cord. Ann. Surg., 128: 679–684, 1936.
14. Grant, F. C., and Austin, G. M.: The diagnosis, treatment, and prognosis of tumors affecting the spinal cord in children. J. Neurosurg., 13:535, 1956.
15. Haft, H., Ransohoff, J., and Carter, S.: Spinal cord tumors in children. Pediatrics, 23:1152, 1959.
16. Haslam, R.: "Progressive cerebral palsy" or spinal cord tumor? Two cases of mistaken identity. Dev. Med. Child Neurol., 17:232, 1975.
17. Horrax, G., and Henderson, D. G.: Encapsulated intramedullary tumor involving the whole spinal cord from medulla to conus: Complete enucleation with recovery. Surg. Gynecol. Obstet., 68: 814–819, 1939.
18. Ingraham, F. D., and Matson, D. D.: Neurosurgery of Infancy and Childhood. Springfield, Ill., Charles C Thomas, 1954.
19. Iyengar, B., and Chandra, K.: The pattern of distribution of tumors of brain and spinal cord. Indian J. Cancer, 11:134, 1974.
20. Melvill, R. L.: The pitfalls in early diagnosis of childhood spinal compression. S. Afr. Med. J., 50:621, 1976.
21. Naffziger, H. C., and Stone, R. S.: Treatment of tumors of the spinal cord. In Treatment of Cancer and Allied Diseases. New York, Hoeber, 1940.
22. Oberhill, H. R., Smith, R. A., and Bucy, B. C.: Neoplasms of central nervous system simulating degenerative disease of spinal cord. JAMA, 151: 612, 1953.
23. Paillas, J. E., Vigouroux, R., Serratrice, G., and Courson, B.: Compressions medullaires d'origire tumorale chez l'enfant. Sem. Hop., 39:2663, 1963.
24. Pool, J. L.: The surgery of spinal cord tumors. Proc. Congress Neuro. Surg., 17:310, 1970.
25. Rand, R. W., and Rand, C. W.: Intraspinal Tumors of Childhood. Springfield, Ill., Charles C Thomas, 1960.
26. Richardson, F. L.: A report of 16 tumors of the spinal cord in children; the importance of spinal rigidity as an early sign of disease. J. Pediatr., 57:42, 1960.
27. Sanyal, S., Biswas, S. K., Sengupta, K. P., and Pal, N. C.: Primary spinal cord tumors—a review of 98 cases. Indian J. Cancer, 12:389, 1975.
28. Schott, G. D.: Spinal tumors 1, Classification. Nursing Times, 71:2055, 1975.
29. Schott, G. D.: Spinal tumors 3, Investigation, treatment, and prognosis. Nursing Times, 72:57, 1976.
30. Shuman, R. M., Ellsworth, C. A., and Leech, R. W.: The biology of childhood ependymomas. Arch. Neurol., 32:731, 1975.
31. Simril, W. A., and Thurston, D.: The normal interpedicular space in the spine of infants and children. Radiology, 64:340–347, 1955.
32. Svien, H. J., Thelen, E. P., and Keith, H. M.: Intraspinal tumors in children. JAMA, 155:959–961, 1954.
33. Tachdjian, M. O., and Matson, D. D.: Orthopaedic aspects of intraspinal tumors in infants and children. J. Bone Joint Surg., 47A:223, 1965.
34. Till, K.: Observations on spinal tumors in childhood. Proc. R. Soc. Med., 52:333–336, 1959.
35. Toumey, J. W., Poppen, J. L., and Hurley, M. T.: Cauda equina tumors as cause of the low back syndrome. J. Bone Joint Surg., 32:246–256, 1950.

# HYSTERICAL (CONVERSION) SCOLIOSIS

Although unusual, scoliosis as a psychosomatic manifestation can occur, and the astute physician should be aware of this possibility (Fig. 23–7).

Three cases were reported by Gillette,[2] one a boy age 7, one a girl age 6, and the third a female age 20 with both a hysterical lateral curve and a hysterical club foot. Schulthess[4] shows an example of an adolescent female also with a hysterical lateral curve and hysterical club foot.

Blount et al. reported 8 cases in 1974.[1] The curve patterns were not characteristic of any structural or other functional curves. They looked like children bending voluntarily in unusual positions.

Perves[3] reported 5 cases in 1976. All were female, with the ages ranging from 9 to 25. He felt all the patients had a "disturbed or unfavorable social milieu."

The peculiar position may be held throughout the examination. It may be present standing and disappear while prone or supine. It may persist while prone but with distraction may then vanish. A few may disappear only while asleep or under an anesthetic.

There is no true structural rotation. Shoulder elevation is usually quite pronounced but out of proportion for the curve. The patient may have other psychosomatic manifestations that give clues to the diagnosis. One of Blount's patients, a male aged 16, had a collection of 23 lawn sprinklers.

A high index of suspicion and astute clinical diagnosis are the keys to this problem. A thorough neurologic exam is essential. Treatment is psychiatric. Orthopedic treatment by exercises, braces, or surgery is contraindicated.

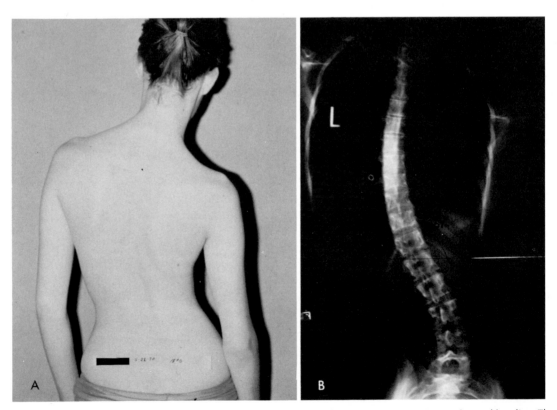

**Figure 23–7**  *A,* An 18 year old female with a long left curvature. There was no true rotation on forward bending. The curve persisted in the prone position but disappeared when supine. The curve also disappeared during sleep or anesthesia. *B,* The x-ray, which shows a long, sweeping curve extending into the cervical spine but without rotation, is highly suspicious for hysteria just by its pattern. This girl required extensive psychiatric treatment.

## References

1. Blount, W. P., Waldram, D. W., and Dicus, W. T.: The diagnosis of "hysterical" (conversion) scoliosis. Presented to Scoliosis Research Society, 1974. J. Bone Joint Surg., 56A:1766, 1974.

2. Gillette, A. J.: Quotation from Am. Orthop. Assoc. News, VI:11, Jan., 1974.
3. Perves, A.: Scolioses psychogeniques. Paper presented at the French Scoliosis Society, 1976.
4. Schulthess, W., In Jaochimstal: Handbuch der Orthop. Chirurgie, vol. II, p. 1012. Jena, Verlag Von Gustav Fisher, 1905–1907.

# DWARFS

By definition, dwarfs have a disproportionate short stature, as compared to midgets, whose body proportions are normal. In dwarfs, the disorder of bone growth and maturation often affects some part of the skeleton with greater intensity, creating disproportionate growth between the axial and appendicular skeleton and between different parts of the extremities.

Dwarfs have been described from earliest times. In Egypt they were held as gods or art figures. In the middle ages they lived with royalty and served as counselors and were the subjects of painters (Fig. 23–8). It is only recently that they have been recognized for what they are—intelligent contributing members of society.

The most significant problem of dwarfs is not so much their shortness of stature but the medical problems complicating their underlying condition. Most of these affect the musculoskeletal system, with the spine usually being involved. The more common types of dwarfism will be discussed in relation to the spine problems and their treatment.

## ACHONDROPLASIA[6, 27, 44, 57]

Achondroplasia is the most common form of shortness of stature. It was first described by Parrot[46] in 1878 and Kauffman[25] in 1892. It is transmitted as an autosomal dominant inheritance and is obvious at birth. About 90 per cent are due to a new mutation, the parents being unaffected. The picture is of short stature with the adult reaching a height of 127 cm. (four feet, two inches). The classical appearance of these patients is a short-limbed rhizomelic (proximal segment shortening) dwarf with a slightly enlarged head and depressed base of the nose. The characteristic clini-

cal[4, 6, 13, 33, 34, 41, 51, 57] and radiographic features are well described.

The spine shows typical changes. The most diagnostic finding is narrowing of the lumbar interpediculate distance. Normally, the interpediculate distance gradually increases as one progresses from the first to the fifth lumbar vertebrae. In the achondroplast, in infancy, this distance is the same throughout the lumbar area or narrows (Fig. 23–9). This interpediculate distance becomes narrower as the child develops, giving marked lumbar constriction noted in adult-

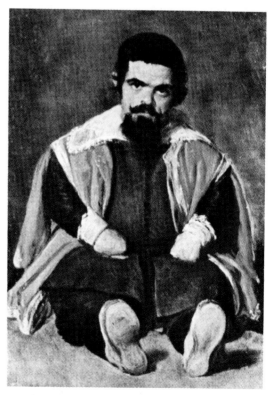

**Figure 23–8** Portrait of Sebastian de Morra, a dwarf in the court of Prince Baltasar Carlos of Spain, painted by Diego Velázquez in 1643.

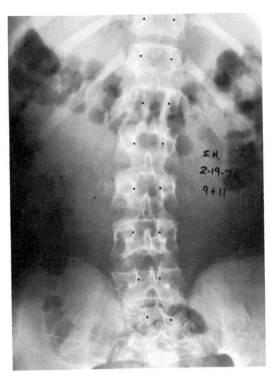

**Figure 23–9**  S.H. This anteroposterior spine x-ray of a 9+11 year old achondroplast shows the narrowing of the interpediculate distance. In the lower thoracic area the distance between the pedicles is widest, and in the lumbar area this distance gradually decreases.

The interpediculate distance is one-half to one-third that of a nonachondroplastic control. Much of this decreased interpediculate distance is related to pedicle hypertrophy, which encroaches on the spinal cord. In addition, the inferior articular facets are hypertrophic, further decreasing the available space. If the entire cross section of the spinal canal is examined, the area is one-third to one-half smaller in the achondroplast than in the control. In addition, the nerve root foramen is narrower in the achondroplast, adding foraminal stenosis to the canal stenosis. The canal in the achondroplast has just enough space for the spinal cord or cauda equina, with no extra space being present. There is thus no safety factor, and *any* further loss of space will produce neurologic symptoms.

Other factors may decrease the area of the borderline spinal canal. These have been called extrinsic factors by Lutter and Langer.[37] Multiple disc herniations in the achondroplast are a known cause of neurologic deficits.[10, 49, 52] The herniations cause acute signs of nerve root compression but have been erroneously blamed for the other neurologic presentations. Because of the concave posterior border of the vertebral body, the spinal canal is narrowest in the area of the end-plates and discs, and thus any myelogram in an achondroplast will show indentations in this area. The myelogram can easily be misinterpreted as multiple disc herniations, instead of the classic spinal stenosis of the achondroplastic spine.

In the adult achondroplast, degenerative spondylosis and arthrosis are common. These result in further reduction of the space available for the neural elements.[1, 17, 22, 61] With aging, symptoms of spinal stenosis with claudication symptoms are common and occur in over 40 per cent of adult individuals, according to Nelson.[46]

All newborn achondroplasts have mild kyphosis in the thoracolumbar area. This may be associated with anterior wedging of the vertebral body in this area—the so-called bullet type vertebra (see Fig. 23–12*A*). Once the infant stands, the kyphosis usually regresses, resulting in lordosis in this area. In a small percentage of cases, the kyphosis persists and progresses during the period of growth.[45, 46] This kyphosis can result in pressure on the neural contents of the spinal canal and paraplegia.

hood. Another radiographic finding in the lumbar spine is a concave posterior border of the lumbar vertebral bodies.

Due to the cartilage growth abnormality, there is a relative increase in the cartilage versus bone. This gives a disc space that is widened as compared to the normal. In the nonachondroplast spine, the ratio of vertebral body to disc is approximately three to one. In the anchodroplast, this ratio approaches one to one. In addition, the abnormal bone growth gives pointed vertebral bodies. This is especially prominent in the thoracolumbar area.

The problems seen in the achondroplastic spine are: 1) neurological symptoms, 2) kyphosis, 3) cervical root compression, 4) scoliosis, and 5) low back pain. There are intrinsic and extrinsic anatomical factors that form the basis of these complications.

When the normal spine is compared to that of the achondroplast, certain intrinsic differences are found (Fig. 23–10).[1, 9, 21, 37, 38]

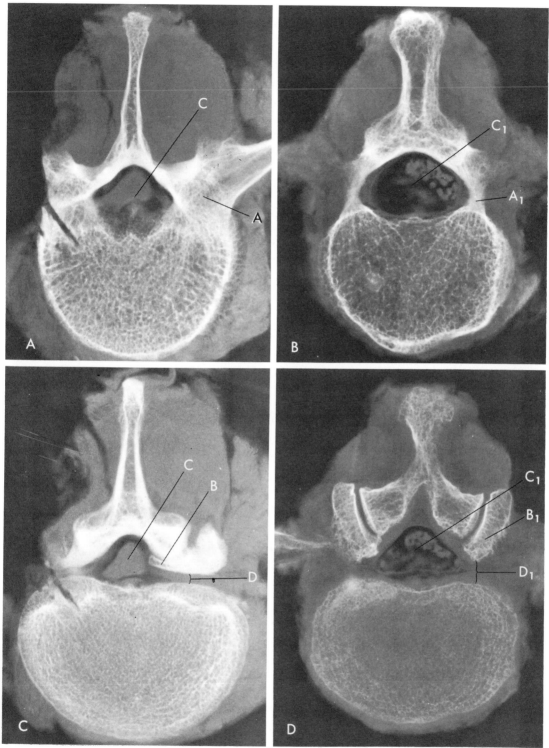

**Figure 23–10**   Cross sections of the lumbar spine of an achondroplast (*A* and *C*) are compared to a matched nonachondroplast (*B* and *D*). In the achondroplast the pedicles are broader and shorter (A) when compared to the normal (A₁). The facet joints are hypertrophied encroaching on the spinal canal (B), no encroachment being present in the nonachondroplast (B₁). The total cross-sectional area of the spinal canal in the achondroplast is decreased (C) when compared to the non-achondroplast (C₁), leaving just enough space for the spinal cord. The nerve root foramen in the achondroplast is markedly narrowed (D) when compared to the nonachondroplast (D₁).

These anatomical intrinsic and extrinsic factors in the spine of the achondroplast form the basis of the spine problems that occur.

## Neurologic Syndromes

Four types of neurologic deficits have been described by Lutter and Langer in a review of 14 cases and an additional 20 cases reported in the literature.[15, 26, 37, 48, 59, 61, 62] These deficits are listed in the probable order of frequency.

a) *Type I:* There is a progressive insidious onset of paresthesia, sciatic pain, and back pain, usually followed by an inability to walk and urinary incontinence. There is a high correlation of this deficit with kyphosis,[37] with mechanical compression being the cause of the neurologic symptoms. The symptoms are continuous and progressive and have commonly led to paraparesis or paraplegia. Surgical decompression by laminectomy is generally unsuccessful, and anterior decompression in one case showed some return of function. Anterior decompression and anterior fusion to remove the bone at the apex of the kyphosis and stabilize the deformity is the operation of choice. It is technically difficult owing to the small spinal canal.

b) *Type II:* Intermittent claudication occurs in relation to activity and is relieved by rest. Neurologic examination at this stage is normal or may show hyperreflexia. With progression, posterior column symptoms and paresthesia are marked. With progression, paraparesis or paraplegia may occur. The kyphosis in these cases is not striking. The symptoms are due to vascular causes rather than mechanical compression. With the small subarachnoid space there is compression of the spinal veins with physiological activity. This results in venous engorgement, decreased blood flow, and neural tissue anoxia. With rest, the engorgement decreases. If operated before permanent long tract signs occur, a laminectomy will result in improvement in symptoms. The laminectomy must be extensive, including inferior facet removal and nerve root foramen decompression.

c) *Type III:* Herniated nucleus pulposus. The onset and presentation are those of a herniated nucleus pulposus with leg pain, positive straight leg raising, and specific root sensory and motor loss. A large laminectomy for excision of the involved disc is necessary, and good results are expected.

d) *Type IV:* Acute onset. This rare presentation is of acute severe back pain associated with physical activity or trauma. These patients usually present with Type I progressive symptoms with sudden onset of paraparesis or paraplegia. The results of surgery in this group are poor.

In summary, it can be seen that knowledge of the different neurologic syndromes in the achondroplast is important, as the prognosis of treatment of the different syndromes varies. Early recognition and early appropriate surgery are important. When a laminectomy is indicated, it must include removal of the inferior facets along with nerve root foraminal decompression (Fig. 23–11). The surgery is difficult and time-consuming and may need to be performed in two stages. If concern about spinal stability is present after the laminectomy, stabilization using an anterior fusion is necessary.

## Kyphosis

As has already been mentioned, kyphosis is common in the newborn achondroplast and is often associated with "bullet shaped" vertebrae in the thoracolumbar area (Fig. 23–12*A*). This kyphosis usually regresses once the infant stands. Occasionally this kyphosis persists and progresses during growth. The Type II neurologic syndrome is associated with kyphosis, and thus early treatment of the kyphosis will prevent this complication.

Patients with kyphosis should be followed carefully. If, after standing in infancy, the kyphosis does not decrease, a Milwaukee brace should be fitted to control it. If there is progression in the brace, or the patient presents with a marked kyphosis, fusion anteriorly and posteriorly is necessary (Fig. 23–12). This should be done before paralysis begins.

## Cervical Root Compression

The anatomical changes in the spine in the achondroplast involve the cervical as

*Text continued on page 576*

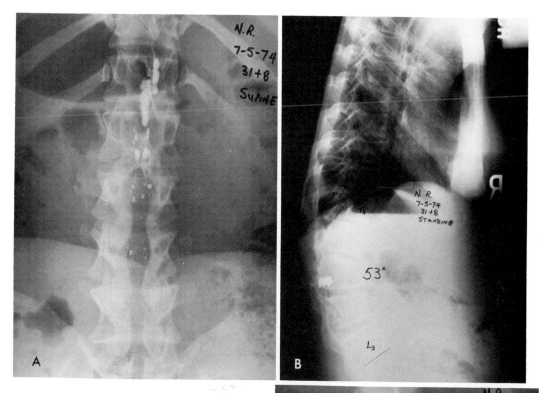

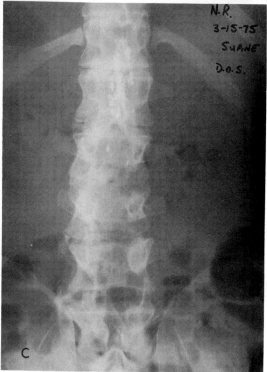

**Figure 23–11**  *A,* N.R. This 31+8 year old female achondroplast presented with Type II neurologic symptoms. A laminectomy had been previously performed. Anteroposterior x-ray of the lumbar spine demonstrating the laminectomy. The laminectomy is narrow and if compared with the anatomical x-rays in Fig. 23–10 there will be seen a simple unroofing has been performed without increasing the size of the spinal canal. *B,* Lateral x-ray on admission shows a 53 degree lumbar kyphosis, which had increased following the laminectomy. *C,* Treatment consisted of an anterior interbody fusion to stabilize the spine followed five months later by decompressive laminectomy. The laminectomy removed all bone encroaching on the spinal canal, and the nerve root foramina were all enlarged. Primary nerve root compression was by the facet joints. She was held in a brace for two years postoperatively as interbody fusion progressed slowly. There was marked improvement in the claudication symptoms.

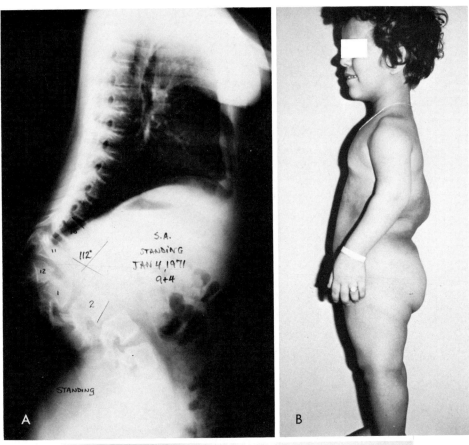

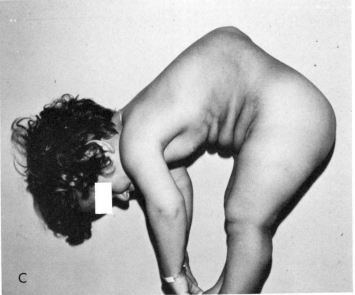

**Figure 23–12**  *A,* S.A. This 9+4 year old female achondroplast presented with a 112 degree thoracolumbar kyphosis. The "bullet shaped" wedge vertebra is seen at T12, with wedging of the vertebrae above and below it. *B,* Initial clinical photographs show the short limbs with marked proximal shortening, enlarged head, and depressed base of nose. The thoracolumbar kyphosis is well seen on forward bending *(C).*

*Illustration continued on the opposite page.*

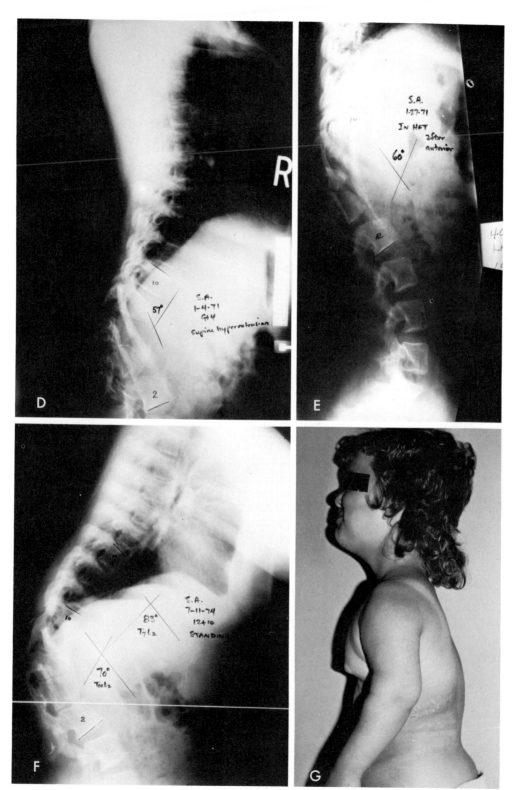

**Figure 23–12** *Continued D,* A hyperextension x-ray shows that the kyphosis is flexible, correcting to 57 degrees. *E,* Treatment consisted of halofemoral traction followed by an anterior fusion from T10 to L2 using a rib graft. This lateral x-ray in traction after the anterior fusion shows correction of the kyphosis to 60 degrees and the rib strut is seen. A posterior fusion was performed two weeks later. Patient was kept supine for five months in a halo cast and then ambulated, total cast time being 10 months. She was then placed in a Milwaukee brace. *F,* Lateral x-ray 3½ years postoperatively shows control of the original area of kyphosis. The area of kyphosis has lengthened, and additional surgery may be necessary. Bracing is continued. *G,* Lateral clinical photograph 2½ years postoperatively shows the markedly improved kyphosis.

*Illustration continued on the following page.*

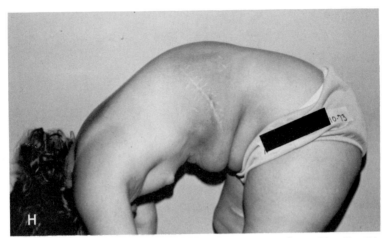

**Figure 23–12** *Continued*    The improvement is well seen on forward bending (*H*).

well as the lumbar spine. Odontoid hypoplasia is not present, but there is failure of posterior atlanto-occipital segmentation, with absence of motion and instability at this level, according to Dorst.[16] A significant number of achondroplasts develop cervical root compression because of the narrow canal and intervertebral foramina as they grow older. Treatment is initially nonoperative, but if symptoms progress and there is cervical instability, fusion is indicated. Decompression may be considered, but there

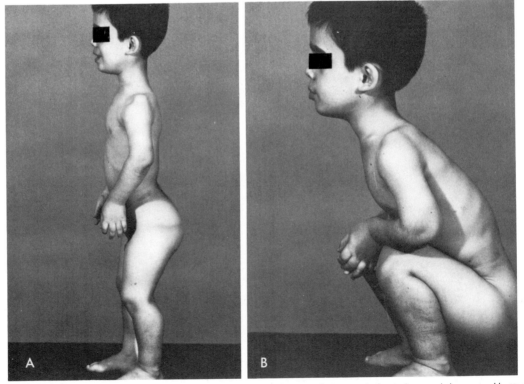

**Figure 23–13**    *A,* W.E. This 10 year old achondroplast shows the typical picture of of protuberant abdomen and buttocks with increased lumbar lordosis. *B,* W. E. When sitting on the haunches, or "hunkering," the lumbar lordosis decreases with increase in the lumbar spinal canal and less stress on the facet joints.

*Illustration continued on the opposite page.*

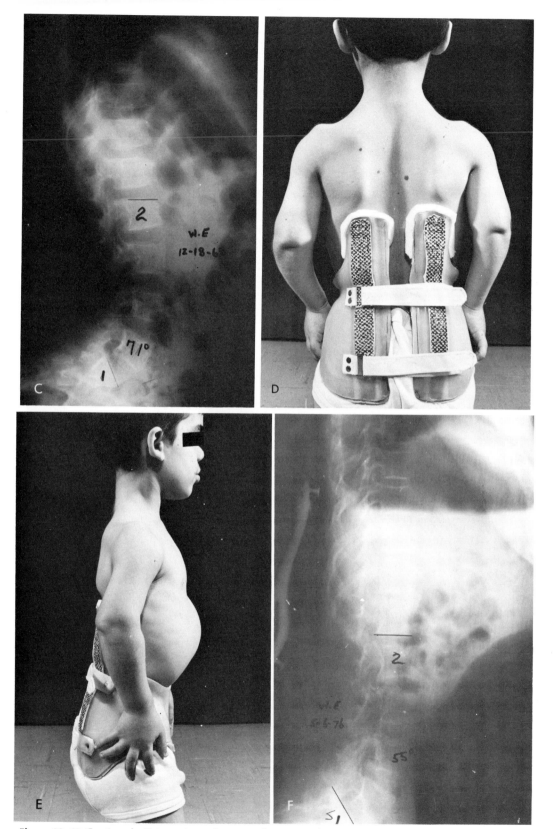

**Figure 23–13** *Continued   C,* Lateral standing x-ray shows a 71 degree lumbar lordosis with most of the angulation occurring at L5 and S1. *D,* A TLSO was fitted to control the lordosis. *D* shows the posterior view and *E* the side view. *F,* A lateral standing x-ray in the brace shows control of the lordosis with reduction to 55 degrees.

are no reports in the literature of this approach The narrow spinal canal with no excess space makes this procedure very hazardous.

### Scoliosis

Scoliosis is more common in the achondroplast than has been appreciated. Seventy-five per cent of Langer's series had some mild degree of scoliosis.[34] The curves tend to be short and in the thoracolumbar area. Progression occurs in the adolescent as in idiopathic scoliosis. The treatment principles follow those of idiopathic scoliosis, with the use of the Milwaukee brace or surgery, with one exception. Treatment is more aggressive in the achondroplast because the spinal cord in these patients with the narrow spinal canal does not tolerate changes as safely as does a normal cord.

### Low Back Pain

Low back pain is common in almost all achondroplasts and may even begin in childhood. It appears to be associated with the mechanical disadvantage placed on the lumbar facets due to the increased lumbar lordosis and the protuberant abdomen and buttocks. The narrowed lumbar spinal canal may also be a factor in this pain (Fig. 23–13A). This pain occurs with standing, and achondroplasts prefer to sit on their haunches or "hunker" (Fig. 23–13B). This compensatory mechanism of hunkering is interesting. In standing, the hips extend and the lumbar lordosis increases, the canal size decreases, and there is increased stress on the lumbar facet joints. The lordosis is associated with a large lumbosacral angle. With hip flexion, as in "hunkering," the lordosis and lumbosacral angle · decrease, the canal size increases, and there is less stress on the lumbar facet joints.

If the lumbar lordosis can be controlled, this back pain is decreased. A TLSO controlling the lordosis will adequately control the back pain (Fig. 23–13).

An understanding of the spine problems in the achondroplast is helpful in discussing the spine problems of the other types of disproportionate short stature.

### HYPOCHONDROPLASIA[6, 8, 27, 28, 36]

Hypochondroplasia is a form of short-limbed rhizomelic dwarfism with an autosomal dominant mode of inheritance. It is important to distinguish this entity, for the clinical appearance closely resembles achondroplasia. It is also important to differentiate this condition from achondroplasia, as spine problems are rare. Neurologic symptoms do not occur, and scoliosis is not reported.

Radiographically, the hypochondroplast shows minimal interpediculate narrowing with minimal reduction in spinal canal area. The pelvis is normal, and the long bones show a slight flaring of the metaphyseal-epiphyseal junction. With these features, a correct diagnosis and an excellent prognosis for spine problems can be made.

### DIASTROPHIC DWARFISM[2, 5, 6, 27, 31, 44, 57, 58, 60]

The word diastrophic is based on a Greek word meaning twisted, tortuous, or crooked and was used by Lamy and Maroteaux to describe this type of severe dwarfism.[29] The condition is severe dwarfing of the rhizomelic type with severe joint contractures and club feet, "hitchhiker's" thumbs, ear deformities, and cleft palate. It is inherited as an autosomal recessive. The spine problems in this condition are severe.

Radiographically, the interpediculate distance increases to L4 and then narrows slightly. The vertebral bodies are slightly flattened (platyspondyly), and the vertebral body height/disc ratio is approximately normal. The epiphyseal ossification abnormalities seen in extremities are not seen in the spine.

There are three problems seen in the spine of the diastrophic dwarf: 1) Spinal stenosis, 2) scoliosis and kyphosis, and 3) cervical kyphosis.

### Spinal Stenosis

The canal size in the diastrophic is only slightly decreased, and thus spinal stenosis is rare. The signs and treatment are the same as those mentioned under achondroplasia.

## Scoliosis and Kyphosis

Some degree of spinal curvature is present in more than 80 per cent of patients with diastrophic dwarfism. The scoliosis and kyphosis in the diastrophic develop in early childhood. The curves are both progressive, tend to become severe, and are usually fairly rigid (Fig. 23–14). With the known tendency to progression, Milwaukee bracing should be instituted early. If the curve is severe on initial presentation or does not respond to the brace, spinal fusion is indicated (Fig. 23–14). The treatment is thus preventive, as the correction obtained is poor. With progression, the deformity affects both the ability to ambulate and the pulmonary capacity.

## Cervical Kyphosis

The odontoid process is normal in diastrophics, and subluxation does not occur. Cervical kyphosis may occur and tends to be progressive. The progression can be severe, resulting in cord compression and quadriplegia (Fig. 23–15). If cervical kyphosis is present and progressive, Milwaukee brace treatment is instituted (Fig. 23–16). If control of the curve is not possible in the brace, a spinal fusion is performed. If the kyphosis is flexible, a posterior fusion is sufficient, but with severe or rigid kyphosis anterior fusion is necessary. In both cases the spine is immobilized using a halo cast.

## SPONDYLOEPIPHYSEAL DYSPLASIA

The spondyloepiphyseal dysplasias are a heterogenous group of conditions in which bony abnormalities are more or less confined to the vertebrae, the epiphyses of long bones, and the carpal and tarsal bones. There are many terms used for these conditions, and various classifications have been proposed by Maroteaux[39, 42, 43] and Rubin.[47] Bailey divides the spondyloepiphyseal dysplasias (SED) as follows: a) SED congenita, b) pseudoachondroplasias, c) pseudo-Morqui syndromes, and d) SED tarda syndromes.[6] The first and last of these are common and will be discussed.

## SED Congenita[6, 20, 27, 44, 47, 56, 57]

Spranger and Weidemann first described this entity in 1966.[53, 54] This condition of short-trunked dwarfism must be differentiated from Morquio syndrome. It is transmitted by autosomal dominant inheritance. The diagnosis is difficult at birth, as the limbs appear shorter than the trunk, and the frontal bossing makes confusion with achondroplasia possible.

The characteristic stance is one of lumbar lordosis with a large protuberant abdomen. This is more obvious owing to the hip flexion contractures and the coxa vara due to the proximal femoral epiphyseal dysplasia. This lordosis tends to throw the center of gravity forward, and affected individuals tend to walk with their heads hyperextended. Radiographically, the vertebrae show a decrease in height of the vertebral body with occasional marked hypoplasia at the thoracolumbar junction. The upper vertebral bodies often appear oval or pear shaped.

The spine problems in SED congenita are odontoid hypoplasia, kyphosis, and scoliosis.

Odontoid hypoplasia with atlantoaxial instability is common in SED congenita. This has resulted in cord compression in one third of Kopit's cases.[27] The instability is due to the odontoid hypoplasia aided by the lax ligaments and hypotonia. Flexion extension cervical spine views are necessary, and if instability is present, early fusion is indicated.

Kyphosis is a frequent finding in SED congenita in the thoracic or thoracolumbar area. In the latter area, it is due to the vertebral hypoplasia. With this kyphosis, active early bracing is necessary, and with progression, fusion is indicated.

Scoliosis may develop in later childhood. The curves are progressive and thus, when noted, should be braced. If there is progression in the brace, spinal fusion is necessary (Fig. 23–17).

## SED Tarda[6, 23, 27, 57]

This condition is of late onset, from mid-childhood onward. The spine and proximal joints are mainly involved. The most common type of SED tarda is the "X" linked type, being inherited as an "X" linked reces-

*Text continued on page 586*

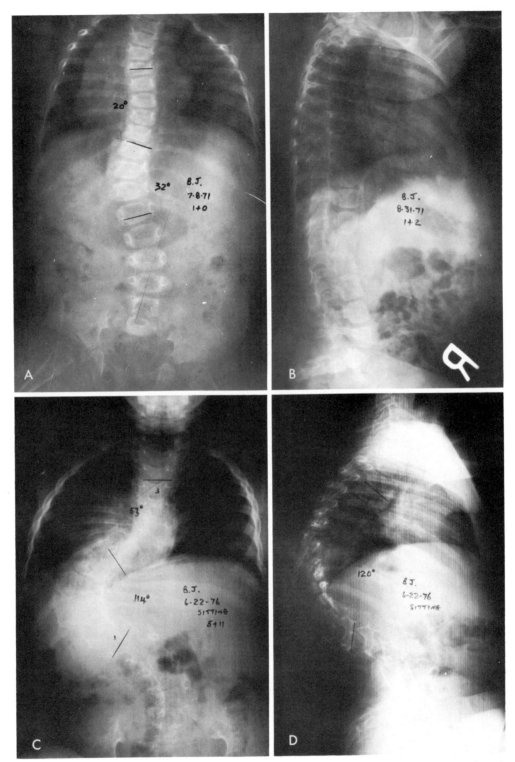

**Figure 23-14**  *A,* B.J. Anteroposterior x-ray of a one year old diastrophic dwarf showing a T5–T10 right thoracic curve of 20 degrees and a T10–L1 left thoracic curve of 32 degrees. *B,* A lateral x-ray two months later shows minimal lumbar kyphosis. *C,* No treatment was instituted. She presented at age 5+11 with marked progression and a T3–T8 right thoracic curve of 53 degrees and a T8–L1 left thoracic curve of 114 degrees. *D,* The sitting lateral x-ray shows 120 degrees of kyphosis.

*Illustration continued on the opposite page*

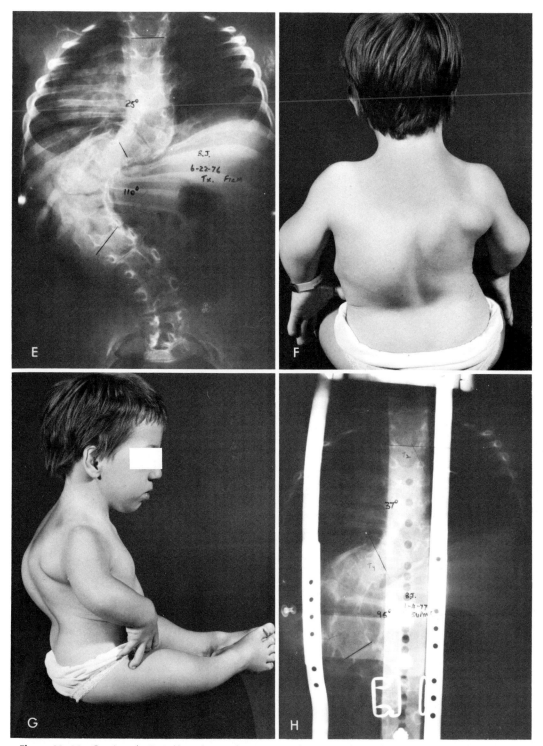

**Figure 23–14** *Continued* *E,* A film taken with maximum distraction shows the rigid nature of the deformity with scoliosis correcting to 25 degrees and 110 degrees. *F* and *G,* Clinical back and side views show typical short-limbed dwarfism with marked spinal deformity. *H,* A posterior spinal fusion was performed from T3 to L4. The anteroposterior supine x-ray in the postoperative holding Milwaukee brace shows the correction to 37 degrees and 95 degrees.

*Illustration continued on the following page*

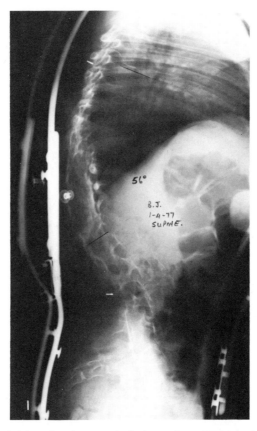

**Figure 23-14** *Continued    I,* A lateral supine x-ray in the brace shows the kyphosis corrected to 56 degrees.

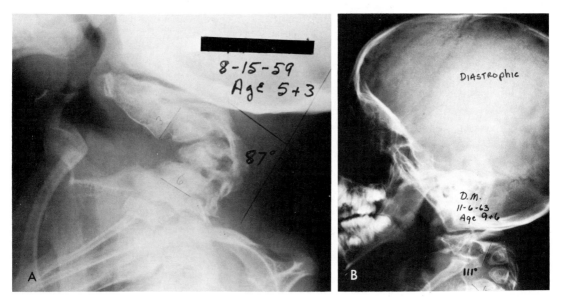

**Figure 23-15**   *A,* D.M. This 5+3 year old boy first presented with a cervical kyphosis of 87 degrees. This progressed, and he became partially paraplegic at age 6+11. The paraplegia cleared in halofemoral traction, and a Milawaukee brace was fitted. The family refused surgical therapy. *B,* By 1963 the kyphosis had increased further, and the patient became quadraparetic. This lateral x-ray, nine months later, shows the C3–C6 kyphosis of 111 degrees. Treatment was refused by the family. The boy remained quadriplegic and died suddenly at age 18.

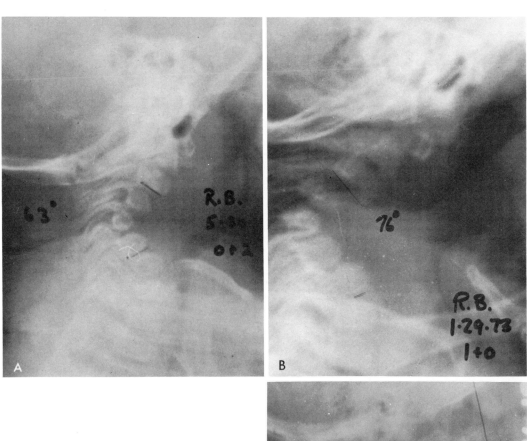

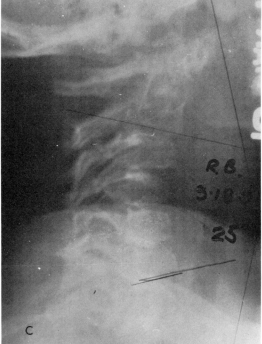

**Figure 23–16** *A,* R.B. This lateral cervical spine x-ray of a 2 month old diastrophic dwarf shows a 63 degree cervical kyphosis. *B,* By the age of one year the kyphosis had increased to 76 degrees. A Milwaukee brace was fitted to try to control the curve. *C,* Three years later the kyphosis was well corrected to 25 degrees with the use of the brace.

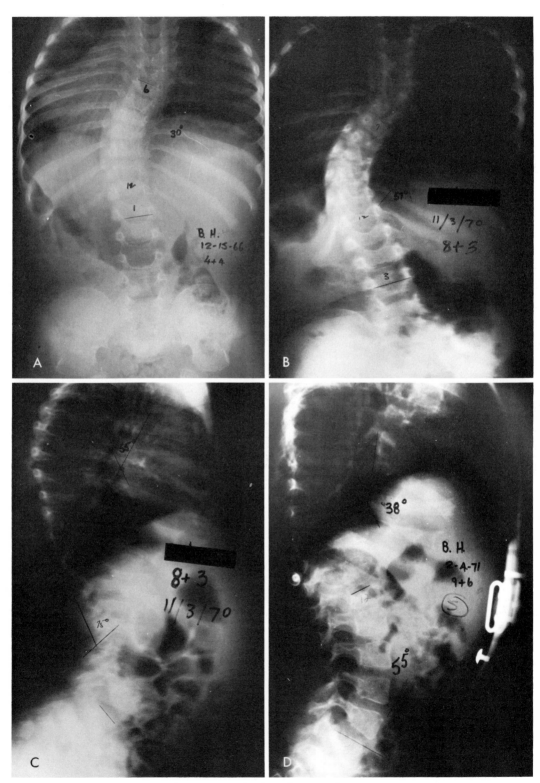

**Figure 23–17** *See legend on opposite page.*

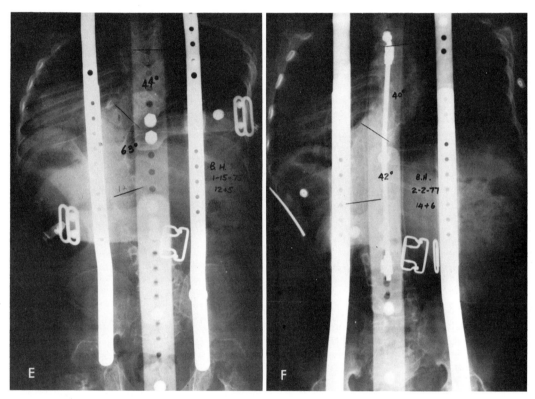

**Figure 23–17** *A,* B.H. This 4+4 year old boy with SED congenita presented with a T6–L1 left thoracic scoliosis of 30 degrees. *B,* In the next four years the curve progressed to 57 degrees. A Milwaukee brace was fitted to control the curve. *C,* A lateral x-ray at this time showed a kyphosis of 55 degrees. *D,* The kyphosis responded well to brace therapy, correcting to 38 degrees. *E,* The scoliosis was initially controlled but by age 12+5 had progressed to 44 degrees and 63 degrees. *F,* A posterior spinal fusion and Harrington instrumentation was performed from T2 to L2. The patient was immobilized post-operatively in his Milwaukee brace. This anteroposterior x-ray 2 years postoperatively in the brace shows a solid fusion with correction maintained at 40 degrees and 42 degrees.

sive. The individual is a short-trunked dwarf. The spine x-ray is diagnostic, as described by Langer.[30] The lumbar vertebral bodies on a lateral view are deformed, with a build-up of bone in the central and posterior portions of the superior and inferior vertebral plates. There is also a lack of visible bone in the distribution of the ring apophysis.

The most characteristic problem in both the spine and hips is early degenerative changes with pain. The back pain may have its onset in adolescence. Treatment of the spine is essentially nonoperative.

Scoliosis can occur, being slightly more common than in the general population. Early bracing is necessary but is difficult owing to the short neck and barrel chest.

## MULTIPLE EPIPHYSEAL DYSPLASIA[6, 7, 14, 18, 19, 27, 47, 50, 57]

This is a group of entities defined by Maroteaux as conditions in which the changes in the long bones are limited to the epiphyses, and the spinal lesions are limited to the vertebral plates without notably affecting the height of the vertebrae.[42] The multiple epiphyseal dysplasias have been classified by Bailey into the congenital group ("stippled epiphysis") and tarda groups, each being subdivided according to the specific epiphyseal involvement.[6]

Clinically, they are short-trunk dwarfs with mild to moderate shortness, reaching an adult height of 135 cm. (five feet, two inches). The age of onset varies from age two to early childhood, depending on the specific syndrome. The x-ray changes are restricted to the epiphyses of the named specific subgroups. The vertebrae show irregularity of the vertebral end-plates with some flattening. These changes are more marked in the thoracic spine.

The spine problems encountered are back pain and kyphosis. Back pain starts in the adolescent years and usually increases with age. The pain is related to the early degenerative changes.

Kyphosis occurs in the thoracic area and may be progressive. Radiographically, it appears as severe Scheuermann's disease and can be effectively treated with a Milwaukee brace. Principles of bracing are similar to those followed with Scheuermann's disease (see Chapter 14 page 331).

## MORQUIO'S DISEASE

Morquio or Morquio-Brailsford disease is the most common type of mucopolysaccharidosis.[12, 43] It is inherited as an autosomal recessive. It is the prototype of the short-trunked dwarfism group, and the general features are well known.[6, 27, 40, 44, 57]

Radiographically, the spine is normal at birth, changes appearing at about two years of age. All the vertebrae are flat (platyspondyly), and the anterior aspects of the body are "flame" or "tongue" shaped. These changes are usually most marked in the thoracolumbar area (Fig. 23–18). The odontoid process is hypoplastic or missing, and instability is common.

Clinically, the problems are related to the odontoid hypoplasia and the kyphosis.

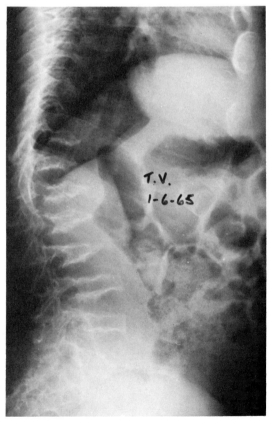

**Figure 23–18**  T.V. Lateral x-ray of the spine of a boy with Morquio's disease showing the markedly flattened vertebrae with an anterior "tongue."

## Odontoid Hypoplasia

The odontoid is hypoplastic, and the transverse ligament of the axis is lax. This allows anterior subluxation of the axis on the atlas with compression of the upper cervical spinal cord. Blaw and Langer found that all eight patients in their series of Morquio's disease had a hypoplastic odontoid with five of the eight demonstrating neurologic symptoms.[11] In addition, these patients fatigue easily.[32] Minimal trauma or induction of anesthesia may cause sudden death. Early detection of the instability is essential. Routine periodic flexion and extension views of the cervical spine are essential, and when instability is demonstrated, posterior atlantoaxial fusion is necessary (Fig. 23–19). Some surgeons advocate prophylactic fusion in these cases.

## Kyphosis

The kyphosis in the thoracolumbar area must be treated vigorously. Early bracing is necessary, as progression occurs. With increasing kyphosis, fusion both anteriorly and posteriorly is necessary. Rarely, the kyphosis can cause spinal cord compression. In these cases, anterior spinal cord decompression and spinal fusion is the treatment of choice.

## METATROPHIC DWARFISM[3, 6, 27, 35, 44, 51, 57]

Metatropos is a Greek word meaning changing pattern and was the term chosen by Maroteaux et al. to describe this syndrome.[41a] These individuals resemble achondroplasts during infancy and in later life resemble individuals with Morquio's disease. In addition, they show, radiographically, a supra-acetabular notch, dumb-bell shaped ends of long bones, and a coccygeal tail. The disease appears to have an autosomal recessive mode of inheritance.

Radiographically, the spine in the newborn shows a delay in ossification of the vertebral bodies, which appear as small tonguelike bony islands in front of well-developed spinous processes. These bony islands are widely separated from one another so that it appears as if there are two ossification centers per vertebral body (one posterior, one anterior). Platyspondyly persists, especially in the thoracic area, while occasionally the

lumbar vertebrae become wedge-shaped (Fig. 23–20*A*). The lumbar interpediculate distance narrows slightly but not as much as in achondroplasts. The most clinically important radiographic finding is odontoid hypoplasia.

Clinically, two problems exist: 1) Odontoid hypoplasia and 2) kyphoscoliosis.

## Odontoid Hypoplasia

Odontoid hypoplasia is a common finding in metatrophic dwarfism. All patients with this diagnosis should have lateral flexion and extension x-rays of the cervical spine to rule out atlantoaxial instability. High cervical cord compression with generalized weakness contributes significantly to the problems in these individuals. Even if no clinical or radiographic evidence of instability is present, these children are more susceptible to minor trauma about the head region. When instability is present, surgical stabilization is necessary (Fig. 23–20). Prophylactic fusion should be considered when no instability exists but where the odontoid hypoplasia is marked.

## Scoliosis

Scoliosis usually presents at an early age with marked progression occurring. Some degree of kyphosis commonly accompanies the scoliosis. Early bracing is necessary, and where bracing fails, fusion is indicated (Fig. 23–21). Often the curve is controlled until adolescence, when a rapid increase occurs.

### SUMMARY

Individuals with disproportionate short stature have many musculoskeletal problems. It is important to classify these patients correctly, as the potential problems vary depending on the specific diagnosis.

In general, the scoliosis that develops has an early onset, tends to be rigid, and is progressive. Because of the high incidence of progression, bracing is commenced at a smaller degree of curvature compared to idiopathic scoliosis. For larger curves or curves that do not respond to a brace, early posterior fusion is performed. The individual is short, and any curvature makes him shorter. The disability (cardiopulmonary and ambulation) from an untreated scoliosis is severe.

Kyphosis is a common problem occurring

*Text continued on page 593*

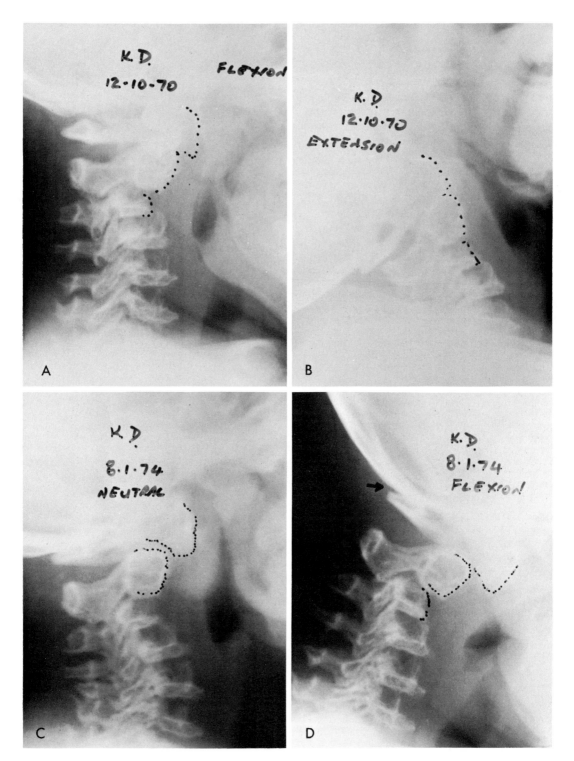

**Figure 23–19**  K.D. Initial flexion *(A)* and extension *(B)* views of a girl with Morquio's disease and odontoid hypoplasia show minimal instability. *C,* Repeat x-rays were taken routinely. Three years and eight months later the lateral cervical spine film in neutral shows anterior subluxation of C1 on C2. This subluxation is increased in flexion and reduced with extension.

*Illustration continued on the opposite page*

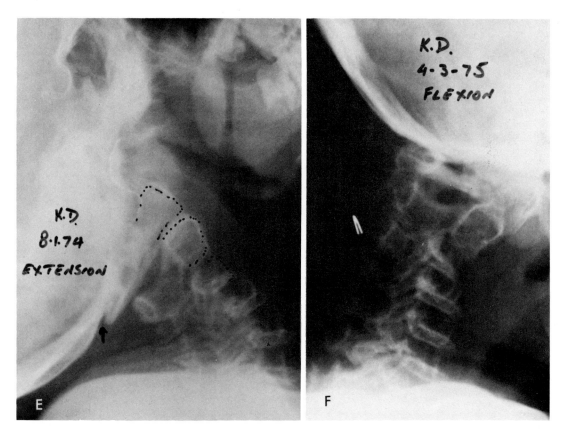

**Figure 23–19** *Continued*  *E,* The occiput is fused to C1, no motion being present: *F,* A posterior spinal fusion was performed from occiput to C3. This lateral flexion view when the halocast was removed shows a solid fusion with no subluxation.

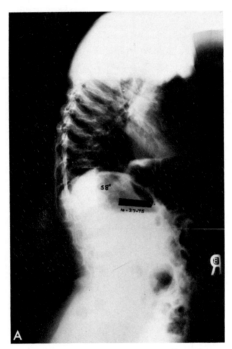

**Figure 23–20**   *A,* D.B. Lateral spine x-ray shows platyspondyly throughout the spine, with a 58 degree kyphosis. Lateral x-ray of the cervical spine demonstrated odontoid hypoplasia. X-rays in flexion *(B)* and extension *(C)* show instability with C1–C2 subluxation. A posterior C1–C2 fusion was performed. When the Halo-cast was removed five months later, lateral x-rays show a solid fusion with no instability or flexion *(D)* and extension *(E)*.

*Illustration continued on the opposite page*

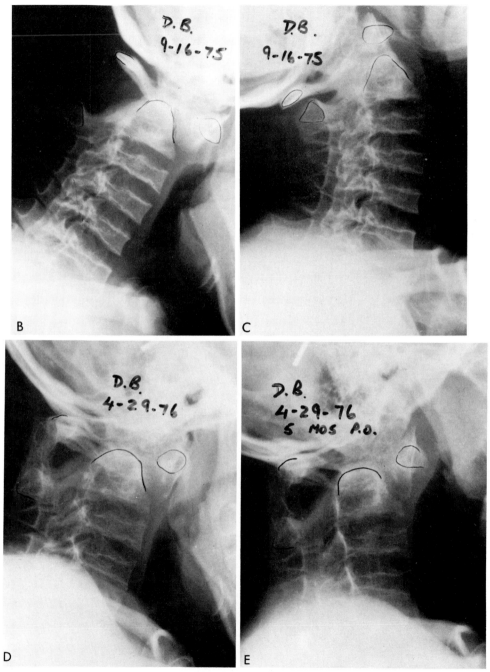

**Figure 23–20** *Continued*

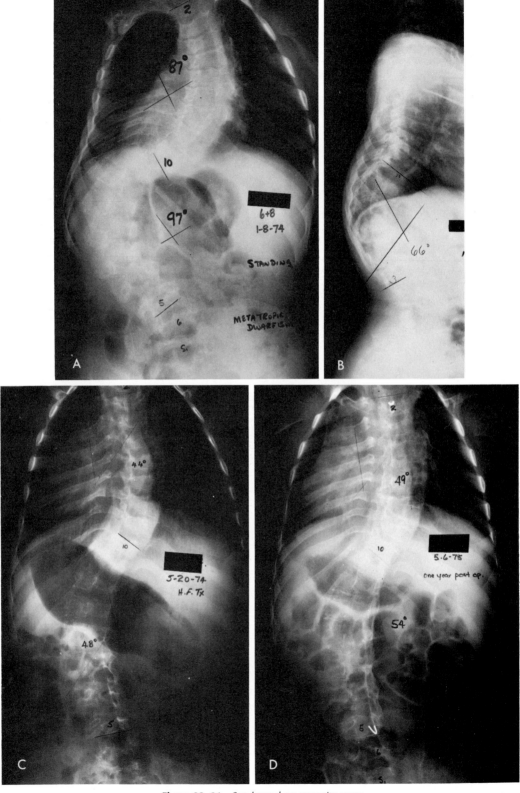

**Figure 23–21**  *See legend on opposite page.*

**TABLE 23-1  Frequency and Severity of Spine Problems in Dwarfs**

| Name | Cervical Spine | Scoliosis | Kyphosis | Interpediculate Distance |
|------|----------------|-----------|----------|--------------------------|
| Achondroplasia | Occasional foraminal stenosis | Occasional | Thoracolumbar | Decreased |
| Hypochondroplasia | Normal | No | No | Slightly decreased |
| Diastrophic dwarfism | Cervical kyphosis | Frequent-progressive | Frequent-progressive | Decreased below L5 |
| SED congenita | Odontoid hypoplasia frequent | Early onset progressive | Thoracolumbar progressive | Normal |
| SED tarda | Normal | Minimal | Minimal | Normal |
| Multiple epiphyseal dysplasia | Normal | Minimal | Minor problem | Normal |
| Morquio's disease | Odontoid hypoplasia | Minor problem | Thoracolumbar | Normal |
| Metatrophic dwarfism | Odontoid hypoplasia | Frequent severe-progressive | Frequent progressive | Slight narrowing |

at the thoracolumbar area. It is usually associated with dysplastic vertebral bodies. The kyphosis is often progressive, and thus bracing should be started early; otherwise it will be unsuccessful. There is a high incidence of spinal cord compression associated with this progressive kyphosis. Surgical treatment of the kyphosis is indicated. Atlantoaxial subluxation and instability are common. The ligamentous laxity and general hypotonia add to this instability. Patients with these problems are often tired, and their activity level is decreased. After stabilization, these symptoms disappear. In the diseases where odontoid hypoplasia is common, routine lateral flexion and extension x-rays of the cervical spine are necessary. Where hypoplasia plus subluxation is present, posterior atlantoaxial fusion is performed. If hypoplasia without subluxation is present, periodic x-rays are necessary to detect subluxation. Some authors suggest prophylactic fusion since the chance of subluxation is high.

The commonest problem in the treatment of spine deformities in these patients is the reluctance to perform a spinal fusion. The patient is short, and with a fusion, "growth will be stunted." This is a fallacy, as all that occurs is curve progression and decreased patient function. This reluctance denies the patient the adequate treatment that is indicated.

**Figure 23-21**  A, M.G. This 6+8 year old girl with metatrophic dwarfism presented with a severe scoliosis. The anteroposterior spine x-ray shows an 87 degree T2–T10 right thoracic curve and a T10–L5 97 degree left lumbar curve. B, A lateral x-ray shows a T10–L3 kyphosis of 66 degrees. C, Treatment consisted of halo-femoral distraction, which corrected the right thoracic curve to 44 degrees and the left lumbar curve to 48 degrees. D, A posterior spinal fusion was performed from T2 to L5. The patient also had a C1–C2 fusion for cervical spine instability. She was immobilized in a halo-cast supine for five months. A Milwaukee brace was fitted. This anteroposterior x-ray one year postoperatively shows maintenance of correction and an apparently solid fusion. She was kept in the brace. One year later there was a definite pseudarthrosis at the apex of the kyphosis, which was successfully repaired. She will be maintained in the brace for a prolonged time.

## References

1. Alexander, E.: Significance of the small lumbar spinal canal: Cauda equina compression syndromes due to spondylosis. Part 5: Achondroplasia. J. Neurosurg., *31*:513–519, 1969.
2. Amuso, S. T.: Diastrophic dwarfism. J. Bone Joint Surg., *50A*:113, 1963.
3. Bailey, J. A., II, Dorst, J. P., and Saunderson, R. W., Jr.: Metatrophic dwarfism recognized retrospectively from the roentgenographic features. Birth Defects: Original Article Series, *5*:376–381, 1969.
4. Bailey, J. A., II: Orthopaedic aspects of achondroplasia. J. Bone Joint Surg., *52A*:1285–1301, 1970.
5. Bailey, J. A., II: Forms of dwarfism recognizable at birth. Clin. Orthop., *76*:150–159, 1971.
6. Bailey, J. A.: Disproportionate Short Stature. Philadelphia, W. B. Saunders Co., 1973.
7. Bateman, D.: Two cases and specimens from third case of punctate epiphyseal dysplasia. Proc. R. Soc. Med., *29*:745, 1936.
8. Beals, R. K.: Hypochondroplasia. J. Bone Joint Surg., *51A*:728–736, 1969.
9. Bergstrom, K., Laurent, U., and Lundberg, P. O.: Neurological symptoms in achondroplasia. Acta Neurol. Scand., *47*:59–70, 1971.
10. Blau, J. N., and Logue, V.: Intermittent claudication of the cauda equina. An unusual syndrome resulting from central protrusion of a lumbar intervertebral disc. Lancet, *1*:1081–1086, 1961.
11. Blaw, M. E., and Langer, L. O.: Spinal cord compression in Morquio-Brailsford's disease. J. Pediatr., *74*:593–600, 1969.
12. Brailsford, J. F.: Chondro-osteodystrophy. Am. J. Surg., *7*:404, 1929.
13. Caffey, J.: Achondroplasia of pelvis and lumbosacral spine. Am. J. Roentgenol., *80*:449–457, 1958.
14. Conradi, E.: Vorzeitiges Auftreten von Kochen und eigenartigen Verkalkungskernen bei Chondrodystrophia fetalis Hypoplastica: Histologische und Rontgenuntersuchungen. J. Kinderheilkd., *80*:86, 1914.
15. de Gispert, C. I.: Complicaciones neurologicas de la acondroplasiz. Rev. Clin. Esp., *53*:127–131, 1954.
16. Dorst, J. P.: Unpublished observation, 1972. Quoted by Kopits, 1976.
17. Duvoisin, R. C., and Yahr, M. D.: Compressive spinal cord and root syndromes in achondroplastic dwarfs. Neurology, *12*:202–207, 1962.
18. Fairbank, H. A. T.: Generalized diseases of skeleton. Proc. R. Soc. Med., *28*:1611, 1935.
19. Fairbank, H. A. T.: Dysplasia epiphysealis punctata. Synonyms: stippled epiphyses, chondrodystrophia calcificans congenita. (Hunermann). J. Bone Joint Surg., *31B*:114–122, 1949.
20. Fraser, G. R., Friedmann, A. I., Maroteaux, P., Glen-Bott, A. M., and Mittwoch, U.: Dysplasia spondyloepiphysaria congenita and related generalized skeletal dysplasia among children with severe visual handicaps. Arch. Dis. Child., *44*:490–498, 1969.
21. Grossiord, A., Guiot, G., Held, J. P., Tournilhac, M., and Besson, J.: Lesions medullaires dans l'achondroplasie: Role des anomalies vertebrales. Rev. Neurol., *94*:329–334, 1946.
22. Hancock, D. W., and Phillips, D. G.: Spinal compression in achondroplasia. Paraplegia, *3*:23–33, 1965.
23. Jacobsen, A. W.: Hereditary osteochondro-dystrophia deformans. A family of 20 members affected in five generations. JAMA, *113*:121–124, 1939.
24. Kash, I. J., Sane, S. M., Samaha, F. J., and Briner, J.: Cervical cord compression in diastrophic dwarfism. J. Pediatr., *84*:862, 1974.
25. Kaufmann, E.: Untersuchungen uber die Sogenannte foetale Rachitis (Chondro-dystrophia faetalis). Berlin, Georg Reimer, 1892.
26. Kissel, P., Hartemann, P., Barrucand, D., and Montaut, J.: Compression medullaire et achondroplasie. Rev. Neurol., *109*:489–498, 1963.
27. Kopits, S. E.: Orthopaedic complications of dwarfism. Clin. Orthop., *114*:153–179, 1976.
28. Kozlowski, K.: Hypochondroplasia. Polish Rev. Radiol. Nucl. Med., *29*:450–459, 1965.
29. Lamy, M., and Maroteaux, P.: L'anisme diastrophique. Presse Med., *68*:1977, 1960.
30. Langer, L. O., Jr.: Spondyloepiphyseal dysplasia tarda. Hereditary chondrodysplasia with characteristic vertebral configuration in the adult. Radiology, *82*:833–839, 1964.
31. Langer, L. O., Jr.: Diastrophic dwarfism in early infancy. Am. J. Roentgenol., *93*:399–404, 1965.
32. Langer, L. O., Jr., and Carey, L. S.: The roentgenographic features of the KS mucopolysaccharidosis of Morquio (Morquio-Brailsford's disease). Am. J. Roentgenol., *97*:1–20, 1966.
33. Langer, L. O., Jr., Bauman, P. A., and Gorlin, R. J.: Achondroplasia. Am. J. Roentgenol., *100*:12–26, 1967.
34. Langer, L. O., Jr., Bauman, P. A., and Gorlin, R. J.: Achondroplasia: Clinical radiologic features with comment on genetic implications. Clin. Pediatr., *7*:474–485, 1968.
35. Larose, J. H., and Gay, B. B., Jr.: Metatropic dwarfism. Am. J. Roentgenol., *106*:156–161, 1969.
36. Leri, A., and Linossier, M.: Hypochondroplasia hereditaire. Bull. Soc. Med. Hop. (Paris), *48*:1780, 1924.
37. Lutter, L. D., and Langer, L. O.: Neurological symptoms in achondroplastic dwarfs—surgical treatment. J. Bone Joint Surg., *59A/1*:87–91, Jan., 1977.
38. Lutter, L. D., Lonstein, J. E., Winter, R. B., and Langer, L. O.: Anatomy of achondroplastic lumbar canal. Clin. Orthop. *126*:139–142, 1977.
39. Maroteaux, P., Lamy, M., and Bernard, J.: La dysplasie spondylo-epiphysaire tarde: description clinique et radiologique. Presse Med., *65*:1205–1208, 1947.
40. Maroteaux, P., Lamy, M., and Foucher, M.: Maladie de Morquio: etude clinique, radiologique et biologique. Presse Med., *71*:2091–2094, 1963.
41. Maroteaux, P., Lamy, M.: Achondroplasia in man and animals. Clin. Orthop., *33*:91, 1964.
41a. Maroteaux, P., Spranger, J., and Wiedemann, H. R.: Der Metatrophische Zwergwuchs. Arch. Kinderheilkd., *173*:211, 1966.
42. Maroteaux, P.: Spondyloepiphyseal dysplasias and metatrophic dwarfism. Birth Defects: Original Article Series, *5*:35, 1969.
43. Morquio, L.: Sur une forme de dystrophie osseuse familiale. Arch. Med. Enf., *32*:129–140, 1929; and *38*:5–24, 1935.

44. Nelson, M. A.: Orthopaedic aspects of the chondrodystrophies. The dwarf and his orthopaedic problems. Ann. R. Coll. Surg., *47*:185–210, 1970.

45. Nelson, M. A.: Spinal stenosis in achondroplasia. Proc. R. Soc. Med., *65*:1028–1029, 1972.

46. Parrot, J. M. J.: Sur les malformations achondro-plastiques et le dieu. Path. Bull. Soc. Antropol. (Paris), *1 (3rd Series):* 296, 1878.

47. Rubin, P.: Dynamic Classification of Bone Dysplasias. Chicago, Year Book Medical Publishers, Inc., 1964.

48. Schatzker, J., and Pennel, G. F.: Spinal stenosis as a cause of cauda equina compression. J. Bone Joint Surg., *50B*:606–618, Aug., 1968.

49. Schreiber, F., and Rosenthal, H.: Paraplegia from ruptured discs in achondroplastic dwarfs. J. Neurosurg., *9*:648–651, 1952.

50. Silverman, F. N.: Dysplasies epiphysaires: Entite proteiforme. Ann. Radiol., *4*:833–867, 1961.

51. Silverman, F. N.: A differential diagnosis of achondroplasia. Radiol. Clin. North Am., *6*:223–237, 1968.

52. Spillane, J. D.: Three cases of achondroplasia with neurological compressions. J. Neurol. Neurosurg. Psychiat., *15*:246–252, 1952.

53. Spranger, J., and Wiedemann, H. R.: Dysplasia spondyloepiphysaria congenita. Lancet, *2*:642, 1966.

54. Spranger, J. W., and Wiedemann, H. R.: Dysplasia spondyloepiphysaria congenita. Helv. Paediat. Acta, *21*:598–611, 1966.

55. Spranger, J. W., and Gerken, H.: Diastrophischer zwergwuchs. Z. Kinderheilkd., *98*:227, 1967.

56. Spranger, J. W., and Langer, L. O., Jr.: Spondyloepiphyseal dysplasia congenita. Radiology, *94*:313–322, 1970.

57. Spranger, J. W., Langer, L. O., and Wiedemann, H. R.: Bone dysplasias: An atlas of constitutional disorders of skeletal development. Philadelphia, W. B. Saunders Co., 1974.

58. Stover, C., Hayes, J. Y., and Holt, J. F.: Diastrophic dwarfism. Am. J. Roentgenol., *89*:914, 1963.

59. Stroobandt, G., Laterre, E. C., Vincent, A., and Cornelis, G.: Compression radiculo-medullaire d'origine rachidienne chez une achondroplase. Neurochirugie, *16*:295–306, 1970.

60. Taybi, H.: Diastrophic dwarfism. Radiology, *80*:1, 1963.

61. Vogel, A., and Osborne, R. L.: Lesions of the spinal cord (transverse myelopathy) in achondroplasia. Arch. Neurol. Psychiatr., *61*:644–662, 1949.

62. Weber, G.: Ruckenmarkskompression bei chondrodystropie. Schweizer Arch. Neurol. Psychiatr., *71*: 291–308, 1953.

# POST LAMINECTOMY SPINE DEFORMITY

A large number of laminectomies are performed every year for excision of ruptured intervertebral discs and for the treatment of spinal stenosis. Deformities following these laminectomies are rare, and the authors have seen only two cases of progressive kyphosis in adults following such laminectomies. Increase in an existing kyphosis occurs with treatment of cord compression by laminectomy (see Chapter 23, page 600). The most common occurrence of deformity following laminectomies in children are those associated with the treatment of a spinal cord tumor. With the recent aggressive treatment of these tumors by laminectomy and excision, radiotherapy and chemotherapy, a large number of children are surviving and presenting to the orthopedic surgeon late with severe post laminectomy spine deformity.

## INCIDENCE

The occurrence of post laminectomy spine deformities is rare except in children treated for spinal cord tumors.[4,7] Haft in 1959 reported 30 children who had laminectomies for spinal cord tumors, and, of 17 with adequate follow-up, 10 developed spine deformities (33 per cent).[6] In Tachdjian and Matson's series of 115 children with spinal cord tumors, 46 developed spine deformity (40 per cent).[9] Boersma reported that half of the 51 children in his series developed spine deformity after laminectomy for spinal cord tumors.[1] Dubousset et al. in 1970 reported 55 children, 78 per cent of whom developed late post-laminectomy spine deformity.[5] Taking all these series together, the incidence of this deformity is 49 per cent. This figure is misleading, as a large number of children die from the tumor, making the incidence of deformity greater in those that survive.

## TYPES OF DEFORMITIES

The majority of deformities following a laminectomy occur in the thoracic spine. Kyphosis and scoliosis can develop, kyphosis being the more common and more severe deformity. The kyphoses are of two types—a

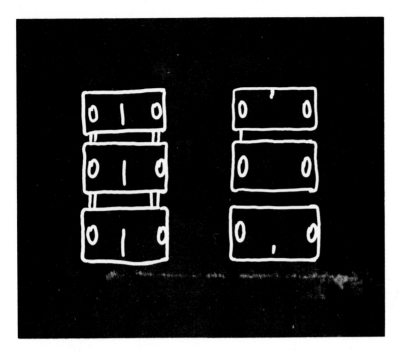

**Figure 23–22** Diagrammatic representation of the spine using the technique of Dubousset et al.[3] On the left the normal spine is represented with vertebral bodies, pedicles, and intact spinous processes. The facet joints are represented by two parallel lines joining the vertebral bodies on each side. On the right a laminectomy is shown. The spinous processes are removed. On the left the facet is partially removed, and a single line is drawn, while on the right the facet removal is complete, and no line is drawn.

short angular kyphos or a gradual rounded kyphos. The configuration depends on the character of the laminectomy, as discussed below. The kyphoses are progressive and in the authors' series led to cord compression in five cases.[8]

Scoliosis occurs less commonly than kyphosis, but usually occurs in the area of the laminectomy and is associated with kyphosis. Less commonly scoliosis occurs below the area of laminectomy and is related to paralysis resulting from the cord tumor or its treatment. In rare cases the scoliosis is the first sign of a cord tumor (see Chapter 23, page 561), and progression occurs after the laminectomy.

## PATHOGENESIS

The most important factor in the development of the deformity is mechanical. The posterior ligament complex plays an important stabilizing role, which is complemented by normal muscle tone. Gravity normally exerts a flexion bending movement on the thoracic spine, which is resisted by the posterior ligament complex and spine extensors. After laminectomy there is disruption of the posterior ligament complex with removal of the interspinous ligaments, spinous processes, and laminae and partial or complete removal of the facet joints. With this loss of posterior stability the normal flexion forces produce kyphosis.

The most important factor in development of deformity is the integrity of the facet joints. If the laminectomy is diagrammatically represented using the technique of Dubousset et al.,[5] a correlation between the facet integrity and deformity is found (Fig. 23–22). If the facets are completely removed at one level, a sharp angular kyphos results with the apex at this level. The intervertebral foramen is enlarged in this area, and the disc space opens posteriorly (Fig. 23–23). In addition, if the facet is partially removed on one side, a sharp angular scoliosis develops

**Figure 23–23**  *A,* This girl had a laminectomy from T3 to T6 at age 20 months for excision of a neuroblastoma of the spinal cord with postoperative irradiation. A lateral x-ray at the age of three years and four months shows a 45 degree kyphosis. An anteroposterior x-ray at this age shows a minimal right thoracic scoliosis. The absent facet joints bilaterally at T5–T6 junction are well seen. *B,* The laminectomy is diagrammatically shown. There is a T2–T6 laminectomy with no facets between T4 and T5 on the right and bilaterally between T5 and T6. In addition, the facets were partially removed between T4 and T5 on the left. *C,* Standing lateral x-ray at age 9 years and 10 months shows a sharp angular kyphosis measuring 137 degrees. Note that the maximal deformity is between T5 and T6, the site of complete facet removal. The disc space is open posteriorly with an enlarged foramen at this level. *D,* A standing anteroposterior x-ray at age 9 years and 10 months shows a 78 degree right thoracic scoliosis. This angulation is due to the decreased stability on the right side, as the facets are removed at two levels on this side.

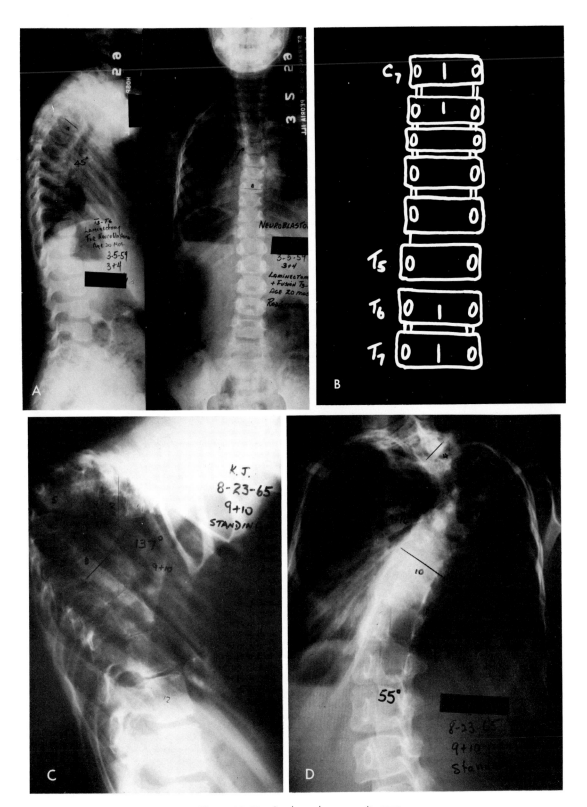

**Figure 23-23** *See legend on opposite page.*

in addition to the kyphosis. If the facets are preserved in part, a gradual rounding kyphosis develops (Fig. 23–24). By careful evaluation of the post laminectomy x-rays with examination of the facet joints, an accurate prediction of the potential deformity can be made.

In the pathogenesis of the spine deformity, factors other than the mechanical ones mentioned are important. Radiotherapy damages the growth plates, adding to the deformity (see Chapter 11, page 303). The tumor can destroy local tissue, the obvious example being an eosinophilic granuloma with collapse of the vertebral body. A spinal cord tumor can cause extensive paralysis of the paraspinal muscles; this adds to the increasing deformity. It is well known that of children with a high paralysis occurring under the age of ten, 100 per cent develop a collapsing paralytic deformity.[2, 3]

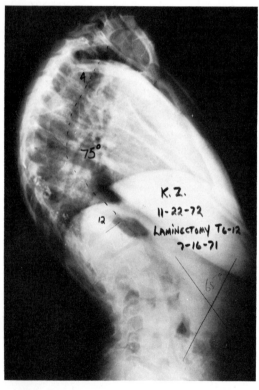

**Figure 23–24** K.Z. This girl had a spinal cord astrocytoma biopsied at age 5 years and 10 months with postoperative irradiation. The laminectomy extended from T6 to T12, and the facets were removed partially from T7 to T10. This lateral x-ray, 14 months postlaminectomy, shows a gradual rounding kyphosis of 75 degrees.

## TREATMENT

The first rule must be *prevention* of these progressive post laminectomy deformities. Consultation between neurosurgeon and orthopedic surgeon is desirable at the time the tumor is treated. The ideal is for the orthopedic surgeon to visualize the extent of the laminectomy intraoperatively. The facet joints do *not* have to be removed for adequate treatment of most cord tumors. The facets should be preserved whenever possible.

Postoperatively the child is carefully followed by the orthopedic surgeon, and at the first sign of progressive deformity a cast or brace is fitted to control the deformity. In the authors' experience this nonoperative control is possible but is only temporary.

If the deformity progresses in the brace, a spine fusion should be performed. The only exception is the case with an extremely poor prognosis related to a very malignant tumor. This is rare today, as with more aggressive care of these tumors more children are surviving. A more aggressive surgical approach is perhaps warranted.

Posterior fusion alone is difficult, and the pseudarthrosis rate is high. A small amount of bone surface is available after the wide laminectomy, and kyphotic problems have a tendency to pseudarthroses with a posterior fusion alone. The anterior approach is thus mandatory with an inlay strut graft technique (Fig. 23–25). With very extensive laminectomies and an excellent prognosis the approach should be more aggressive with an early anterior fusion *before* the deformity occurs.

Cases presenting late with kyphosis and scoliosis require preoperative correction using halofemoral or halo-Cotrel traction with hyperextension for the kyphosis. The presence of kyphosis and the absence of posterior elements are prime indications for an anterior fusion. In these cases a strut graft anterior fusion is necessary (see page 512), the spine being approached via the concavity of the scoliosis, when it is mild. With marked scoliosis and marked vertebral rotation the approach via the convexity of the scoliosis often gives a better exposure of the spine. Placement of the graft in the weight-bearing line of the spine is essential.

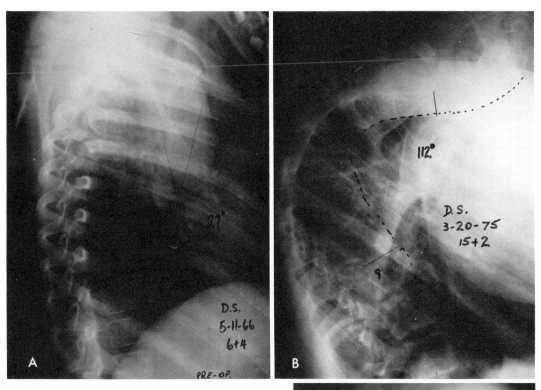

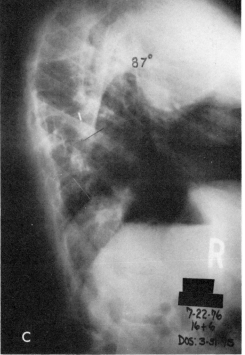

**Figure 23–25** *A,* D.S. This 6 year and 4 month old boy underwent a laminectomy with partial excision of a spinal cord neuroblastoma and a thoracotomy 10 days later for excision of an intrathoracic extension. This preoperative lateral x-ray shows a 27 degree thoracic kyphosis. *B,* Nearly nine years later, at age 15 years and 2 months, the kyphosis had increased to 112 degrees. There was a rapid increase during the rapid growth spurt. *C,* Treatment consisted of halofemoral traction for seven days followed by a transthoracic anterior spine fusion with intervertebral disc excision and insertion of multiple rib grafts. Postoperatively he was placed in a halocast for six months, a Risser cast for four months, and a Milwaukee brace for eight months. This lateral x-ray, 16 months postoperatively, shows a solid fusion and an 87 degree kyphosis.

## References

1. Boersma, G.: Curvatures of the Spine Following Laminectomies in Children. Amsterdam, Born, p. 257, 1969.
2. Brown, H. P.: Spine deformity subsequent to spinal cord injury. Ortho. Sem. Rancho Los Amigos Hosp., 5:41, 1972.
3. Brown, H. P., and Bonnett, C. C.: Spine deformity subsequent to spinal cord injury. Proc. Scoliosis Research Society Meeting, Wilmington, Delaware, 1972. J. Bone Joint Surg., 55A:441, 1973.
4. Cattell, H. E., and Clark, L. G.: Cervical kyphosis and instability following multiple laminectomies in children. J. Bone Joint Surg., 49A:713, 1967.
5. Dubousset, J., Guillaumat, M., and Mechin, J. F.: Paper presented to Neurosurgical Congress of Infants, Versailles, 1970, Chapter XI, p. 185. In Rougerie, J. (ed.): Les Compressions Medullaires non Traumatiques de l'Enfant. Publ. Paris, Masson et Cie, 1973.
6. Haft, H., Ransohoff, J., and Carter, S.: Spinal cord tumors in children. Pediatrics, 23:1152, 1959.
7. Haritonova, K. I., Tziuian, J. L., and Ekshtadt, N. K.: Orthopaedic sequelae of laminectomy. Orthop. Traumatol. Protez., 11:32, 1974.
8. Lonstein, J. E., Winter, R. B., Bradford, D. S., Moe, J. H., and Bianco, A. J.: Post laminectomy spine deformity. Presented to Annual Meeting of American Academy of Orthopaedic Surgeons. J. Bone Joint Surg., 58A:727, 1976.
9. Tachdjian, M. O., and Matson, D. D.: Orthopaedic aspects of intraspinal tumors in infants and children. J. Bone Joint Surg., 47A:223, 1965.

# CORD COMPRESSION

## DEFINITION

Neurologic deficits can be associated with scoliosis and kyphosis. They can be due to spinal cord tumors (see Chapter 23, page 561), extramedullary tumors, bone lesions, or compression of the spinal cord by the spine deformity. Compression of the spinal cord by the deformity is discussed in this section.

## INCIDENCE

Numerous reports of this rare complication are in the world literature,[7, 8, 9, 11, 12, 13] the majority being single case reports. The first report is by MacEwen in 1888 of a case successfully treated by laminectomy.[9] Two large series are those of Marchetti et al.[10] and Roaf.[11] Thirty-eight patients with this complication have been seen by the authors at the Twin Cities Scoliosis Center. As with the other reported cases, the commonest cause of the spine deformity in this series is congenital kyphosis. Other causes of deformity include neurofibromatosis, inactive tuberculosis with increasing kyphosis, post laminectomy kyphosis, achondroplasia kyphosis, and a miscellaneous group. In *all* the cases seen, kyphosis was the main spine deformity. The kyphosis is severe and averages 94 degrees, with many cases over 120 degrees.[8]

In all the congenital kyphoses, the kyphosis was due to failure of vertebral body formation—a posterior hemivertebra classified as Type I kyphosis by Winter et al.[13] Scoliosis was usually minor and was present in association with the kyphosis. Only in neurofibromatosis was the scoliosis a major component of the deformity.

The exact incidence of this complication is unknown, but it is preventable. In analyzing the cases seen by the authors, a common feature was early detection of the spine deformity but *no* treatment, with steady progression of the kyphosis. With this progression the neurologic loss occurred on an average of *10 years* from the diagnosis of the deformity. Early and adequate treatment would have prevented progression of the kyphosis and cord compression.

## PATHOGENESIS

In analyzing the reported cases, certain common features were found. This complication is commonest in severe kyphotic deformities (usually congenital), in the upper thoracic spine, in males, in the second decade of life.

The pathogenesis of the cord compression depends on the differential "growth" of the vertebral column and spinal cord. In severe kyphoses there is angulation of the spinal cord over the anterior bone, the cord taking the shortest route across the concavity of the curve. The dura is tethered to the skull at the foramen magnum and to the sacrum. With the kyphosis and growth the dura tends to pull the spinal cord against the anterior bone (Fig. 23–26). This differential growth is more obvious during the rapid growth spurt in the second decade, the time when neurologic complications most often become manifest. In addition, the kyphosis rapidly increases during the phase of growth, increasing the compression of the spinal cord.

A similar effect is seen when placing this deformity in traction. Traction lengthens the vertebral column by correcting the small flexible curves on either side of the rigid kyphosis. There is traction on the spinal cord, which is pulled against the anterior bone, with resultant cord compression and neurologic loss. Traction is therefore dangerous in the treatment of rigid kyphosis. Any correction of the kyphosis, performed surgically, involves straightening the curve and actually reduces the anterior pressure on the spinal cord.

A common site for cord compression by kyphosis is the upper thoracic spine. The spinal cord in the area of T4 to T9 has been shown to have the poorest blood supply from both feeder and perforating arteries.[3, 4] In addition, the spinal canal is narrowest in the upper thoracic area, and in this area the spinal cord is the least elastic and thus more sensitive to stretch.[1]

## PRESENTATION

The neurologic loss is usually of sudden onset with rapid progression. Rarely the onset follows trauma to the back; e.g., a fall, direct trauma to the back in playing or wrestling, or even turning on a Stryker frame.

Numerous classifications of the neurologic loss are available. The most practical and useful has been to divide the lesions into minor neurologic deficit, paraparesis, and paraplegia. A minor deficit is one that does not affect the patient's activities, and usually the patient is not aware of the deficit; this includes hyperreflexia, mild clonus or minor spasticity, and a positive Babinski sign. The paraparesis can range from mild to severe with marked functional restriction. Paraplegia is complete motor and sensory loss.

## TREATMENT

With the presentation of a spine deformity and neurologic deficit an accurate evaluation is essential to establish the diagnosis.

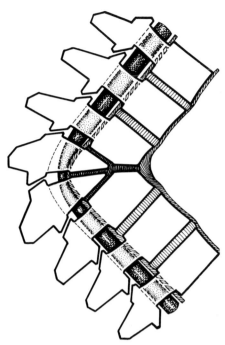

**Figure 23–26** Diagram to show cord compression due to a congenital Type I kyphosis. The spinal cord is compressed at the apex of the deformity by the anterior bone. The cord is narrowed at this site with obstruction in the subarachnoid space as shown by myelography.

A full history of the deformity is necessary. In addition, a history of the onset and progression of the neurologic loss should be included. The physical examination should be complete with emphasis on the spine deformity and neurologic examination.

After full radiologic evaluation of the spine deformity, the etiology of the deformity is diagnosed. When kyphosis is absent the occurrence of scoliosis alone plus cord signs should be viewed with suspicion. Three patients have been seen with this combination, and full evaluation showed a separate cause for the neurologic loss; an arteriovenous malformation, a demyelinating disease of the spinal cord, and a case of aorto-iliac occlusive disease with leg weakness due to ischemia. The authors have knowledge of only one case of scoliosis causing cord compression. This was a child with a congenital scoliosis due to a unilateral failure of vertebral body segmentation. A part of the unsegmented bar was a large fibrocartilaginous mass that compressed the spinal cord.

A myelogram is necessary for two reasons. First, it will reveal other causes of

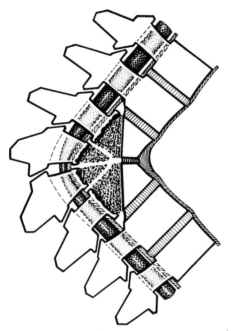

**Figure 23-27** Diagrammatic representation of anterior spinal cord decompression. The spine at the apex of the kyphosis is visualized via a transthoracic approach. The bone at the apex of the kyphosis is removed, leaving the posterior cortex and far cortex intact. The posterior cortex is carefully removed starting away from the apex and working toward the apex and toward the surgeon.

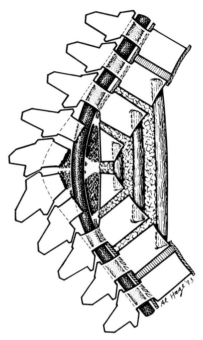

**Figure 23-28** The decompression has been completed, and the spinal cord has moved forward into the area of excised bone. No bone remains compressing the cord, and spinal cord pulsations return. The intervertebral discs are excised, and an anterior strut graft fusion is performed. This is reinforced with a posterior fusion with Harrington instrumentation where possible.

neurologic deficit such as cord tumors, neurofibromas, etc. In addition, it will confirm the presence of spinal cord compression at the apex of the kyphosis. In these cases there is narrowing of the dye column with a partial or complete obstruction at the apex of the kyphosis. To visualize this area adequately, a modification of the myelographic technique is necessary. The technique preferred is that described by Gold and Leach,[5] in which a large volume of Pantopaque (up to 90 ml) is used. This fills the subarachnoid space and allows excellent visualization of any pathology. Smaller volumes can be used, but it is necessary to remove the needle and

turn the patient supine. Unless this is done it is impossible for the dye to pool at the apex of the kyphosis to allow visualization of this area.

When the diagnosis has been made and confirmed by myelography, treatment is instituted. The treatment of minor deficits differs from that of severe neurologic loss. In the latter group removal of the bone anterior to the spinal cord is necessary. With minor deficits, the patient can be treated with correction of the deformity and stabilization. The minor neurologic signs will usually resolve. With flexible deformities, the correction is performed using preoperative hyperextension

**Figure 23-29** *A*, R.C. This boy contracted tuberculosis of the spine at age 3 years and 8 months. He was hospitalized from 1948 to 1951 and was discharged with a progressive thoracic kyphosis. This lateral x-ray on admission in 1948 shows destruction of T7 and T8 with paravertebral calcification: *B*, At the age of 9 years and 7 months he had the sudden onset of a T7 spastic paraparesis. This was due to a paravertebral tuberculous abscess which was drained via a costotransversectomy. There was complete neurologic recovery, and a year later he underwent a posterior spinal fusion (8/1/55). The kyphosis continued to progress, and this lateral x-ray (4/21/64) at the age of 19 years and 4 months shows a 135 degree kyphosis. He was neurologically normal and doing heavy farm work. *C*, At age 21 there was the sudden onset of a T10 spastic paraparesis. A myelogram was not performed. He underwent an anterior transthoracic spinal cord decompression from T8 to T10. The operative bleeding was excessive, and an anterior spinal fusion was not performed. He had many postoperative respiratory problems. Neurologic recovery was complete, and the family refused an anterior arthrodesis.

Eighteen months later he had a recurrence of the spastic paraparesis, and a myelogram showed narrowing at the area of kyphosis. This lateral x-ray shows the kyphosis of 135 degrees on admission with this third episode of paraparesis. Gentle traction and hyperextension were used, and there was gradual neurologic return over the next two months. An anterior strut graft fusion was performed with a halocast used for six months and a Risser cast for a further six months. *D*, This lateral x-ray six years postoperatively shows a solid anterior fusion with the strut grafts well seen. He is neurologically normal.

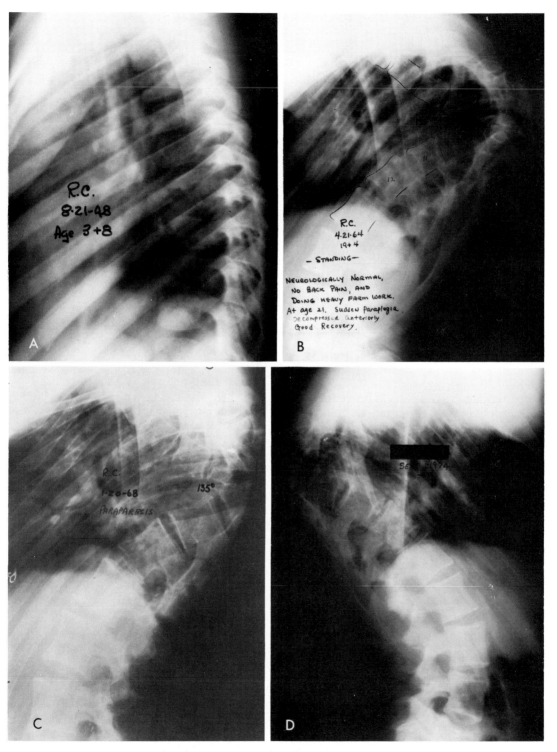

**Figure 23–29** *See legend on opposite page.*

traction and serial hyperextension casts or occurs at the time of stabilization. The stabilization is achieved with a spinal fusion performed posteriorly, when the kyphosis is slight, or with anterior fusion supplemented by a posterior fusion with Harrington compression instrumentation, for kyphoses over 60 degrees. A strut graft anterior fusion is performed (see Chapter 20, page 512) using fibula when necessary for the most anterior strut. Multiple struts of rib are used, filling the concavity of the kyphosis with bone.

When paralysis or paraparesis is present, a hyperextension x-ray is of utmost importance. If the kyphosis is flexible on hyperextension, correction of the deformity alone may relieve the anterior compression of the spinal cord and make surgical decompression unnecessary. Thus all cases with a *flexible kyphosis* are placed in hyperextension to correct the deformity as much as possible. The correction is obtained by using either a Bradford frame or placing a rolled towel under the mattress in the area of the kyphosis to give a hyperextension force. Correction may also be achieved using serial hyperextension casts. With improvement of the neurologic deficit to normal, or a residual minor deficit, the correction of the kyphosis is maintained using a two-stage anterior and posterior spinal fusion. It is usual when scoliosis as well as kyphosis is present to approach the spine via the concavity of the scoliosis. With severe scoliosis and kyphosis an exposure via the convexity of the scoliosis is possible. The strut graft must be placed to stabilize both the kyphosis and the scoliosis.

If the kyphosis is rigid, or there is no improvement in the neurologic loss using traction, cord decompression is necessary. The most effective approaches are posterior decompression using the Hyndman and Schneider radical posterior decompression,[7, 12] a lateral approach via the Capener method,[2] and a direct transthoracic or anterior approach. Laminectomy does *not* decompress the spinal cord, because the compressing bone is anterior. All the laminectomy achieves is loss of posterior stability with increase in the kyphosis and deterioration in the neurologic picture. An extension of the laminectomy was described by Hyndman and Schneider for removal of

anterior bone. This is most effective with significant scoliosis and involves the removal of a large amount of bone—laminae, pedicles, transverse process, and ribs—to adequately visualize and remove the anterior bone. This leaves a very unstable spine with insufficient bone anteriorly for a fusion base. With significant kyphosis a Capener decompression can remove anterior bone, the approach being posterolateral. This was first described for decompression of tuberculous spinal abscesses.[2]

As the compressing bone is anterior, the anterior route for decompression is the most effective. This was pioneered by Hodgson and Stock[6] for the treatment of spinal tuberculosis. The spine is approached anteriorly using the transthoracic approach in the thoracic spine and a combined transthoracic retroperitonial approach in the thoracolumbar area. A wedge of bone is removed from in front of the spinal cord, allowing the cord to move forward into the space created (Fig. 23-27). The technique is described fully in Chapter 20, page 517. Following the decompression, an anterior strut graft fusion is performed, and two weeks later a posterior fusion is necessary to maintain any correction achieved and ensure stabilization (Fig. 23-28). This combined anterior and posterior approach has been shown to be the most effective method of stabilizing severe kyphoses.[8] Patients are placed in a halo cast and kept supine for four to six months. They are then ambulated in a cast, total cast time being nine to twelve months (Fig. 23-29).

In rare cases where decompression is necessary but the pulmonary functions are so poor that a transthoracic approach is contraindicated, decompression is performed via the Capener approach. The drawback of this approach is that anterior stabilization is not possible at the same time.

In our experience, the anterior route for spinal cord decompression is the most effective and gives the best results in alleviation of the cord compression. A laminectomy proved useless for correction of the neurologic deficit. Most commonly this procedure gave an increased deficit owing to the manipulation of the tight spinal cord and removal of the stabilizing posterior bone with increasing kyphosis and increasing cord compression.[8]

## References

1. Breig, A.: Biomechanics of the Central Nervous System. Stockholm, Almquist and Wiksell, 1966.
2. Capener, N.: The evolution of lateral rachotomy. J. Bone Joint Surg., 36:173, 1954.
3. Dommisse, G. G.: The Arteries and Veins of the Human Spinal Cord from Birth. New York, Longman, Inc., 1975.
4. Dommisse, G. G.: The blood supply of the spinal cord. J. Bone Joint Surg., 56B:225, 1974.
5. Gold, L., Leach, C., Kieffer, S. A., Chou, S. N., and Peterson, H. O.: Large volume myelography. Radiology, 97:531, 1970.
6. Hodgson, A. R., and Stock, F. E.: Anterior spine fusion. Br. J. Surg., 44:266, 1956.
7. Hyndman, D. R.: Transplantation of the spinal cord. Surg. Gynecol. Obstet., 84:460, 1947.
8. Lonstein, J. E., Moe, J. H., Winter, R. B., Bradford, D. S., Chou, S. N., and Pinto, W. C.: Cord compression due to untreated spinal deformity. (In preparation.)
9. MacEwen, W.: Case report in surgery of the brain and spinal cord. Br. Med. J., 2:302, 1888.
10. Marchetti, P. G., Faldini, A., and Ponte, A.: Il Trattamento Chirurgico delle Scoliosi. Report of 53rd Congress of the Italian Society for Orthopedics and Traumatology. Pisa, October, 1968, p. 265.
11. Roaf, R.: Spinal deformity and paraplegia. Paraplegia, 2:112, 1964.
12. Schneider, R. S.: Transposition of the compressed spinal cord in kyphoscoliotic patients with neurological deficits. J. Bone Joint Surg., 42A:1027, 1960.
13. Winter, R. B., Moe, J. H., and Wang, J. F.: Congenital kyphosis. J. Bone Joint Surg., 55A:223, 1973.

# ARTHROGRYPOSIS SCOLIOSIS

Arthrogryposis was first described in 1841 by Otto.[6] Stern, in 1923, is generally credited with originating the name arthrogryposis multiplex congenita.[8] Scoliosis has been mentioned in numerous articles concerning arthrogryposis, but the incidence has varied from a low of 0 per cent to a high of 42 per cent.[2, 3, 4, 5] The cause of arthrogryposis is as yet unknown. The diagnosis of arthrogryposis multiplex congenita may be quite difficult, since there is no histologic, laboratory, or clinical test specific for the condition. Many extraneous conditions are thus often included within this diagnosis. The widely accepted diagnostic criteria include: multiple flexion or extension contractures present at birth; marked limitation of active and passive motion of the involved joints but motion relatively free over the small range of motion remaining; the joints appear cylindrical and fusiform; sensation is intact; the tendon reflexes are diminished or absent; and the muscular atropy is not progressive, although the joint contractures may worsen with time. Skin creases over joints are generally absent. Flexion contractures are usually associated with skin webbing across the joint.

Drummond and McKenzie reported 50 patients with arthrogryposis of the neuropathic type.[1] All the patients had rigid contractures present at birth involving at least two extremities. Scoliosis occurred in 14 of the 50 patients reviewed, an incidence of 28 per cent. There were 8 girls and 6 boys.

Eight of the 14 patients had curves of at least 40 degrees by age 10. Only 2 of the 50

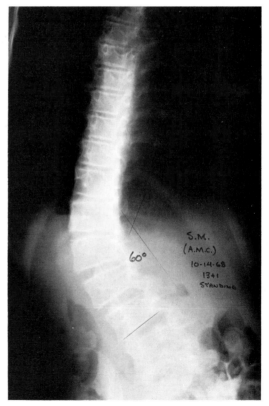

**Figure 23–30** Arthrogryposis scoliosis in a 13 year old male. The lumbosacral curve was more rigid than the thoracolumbar curve. A Milwaukee brace was prescribed at this time.

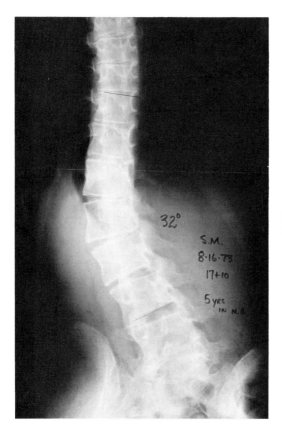

**Figure 23–31** Same patient as in Fig. 23–30. After five years in the Milwaukee brace, there has been improvement of the thoracolumbar curve but not the lumbosacral curve.

children died in childhood, both having severe scoliosis. Seven of the patients had congenital scoliosis associated with their arthrogryposis. Four children had long curves typical of paralytic scoliosis, and these occurred either in infancy or in early childhood. These progressed to become long, rigid, decompensated curves. The authors recommended prompt treatment of the curve before it became severe (Figs. 23–30 and 23–31).

The spinal problems are not easy to manage. Brace treatment is appropriate for small curves of 50 degrees or less, particularly in growing children. Exercises have no beneficial effect. Quite often the patient is denied adequate spinal treatment because of multiple other handicapping conditions that distract the treating physician's eye from the scoliosis problem.

Surgical treatment in these patients has not been easy. The connective tissue is tough and tight, and the bones are osteoporotic. In our personal experience, blood losses have been larger than those of similar idiopathic curves. Following correction and

fusion, loss of correction has been minimal, partly owing to the stiff nature of the curvatures. The bones heal well, and pseudarthrosis has not been a problem. Halofemoral traction has been successful in correcting some of the more severe curvatures. Harrington rods have been well tolerated, although the soft bone leads to a higher incidence of hook dislocation.

## References

1. Drummond, D. S., and McKenzie, D. A.: Scoliosis and arthrogryposis. Scoliosis Research Society, San Francisco, 1974. J. Bone Joint Surg., *56A*:1763, 1974.
2. Friedlander, H. L., Westin, G. W., and Wood, W. L.: Surg., *50A*:89, 1968.
3. Gibson, D. A., and Urs, N. D. K.: Arthrogryposis multiplex congenita, J. Bone Joint Surg., *52B*:483, 1970.
4. Lloyd-Roberts, G. C., and Lettin, A. W. F.: Arthrogryposis multiplex congenita. J. Bone Joint Surg., *52B*:494, 1970.
5. Mead, N. G., Lithgow, W. C., and Sweeney, H. J.:

Arthrogryposis multiplex congenita. J. Bone Surg., 40A:1285, 1958.
6. Otto, A. G.: Monstorum Sexentorum Descriptio Anatomica. Vratislavial Museum Anatomica Pathologicum 323, 1847.

7. Siebold, R. M., Winter, R. B., and Moe, J. H.: The treatment of scoliosis in arthrogryposis multiplex congenita. Clin. Orthop. 103:191, 1974.
8. Stearn, W. G., Arthrogryposis multiplex congenita. JAMA, 81:1507, 1923.

# OSTEOGENESIS IMPERFECTA

Osteogenesis imperfecta is one of the most common hereditary disorders of connective tissue.[10] Although it may present a wide variety of clinical and surgical problems to the orthopedic surgeon, reports of the incidence, natural history, and treatment of spine deformities have received scant attention in the literature.[1, 2, 6, 8, 9, 11]

## INCIDENCE AND NATURAL HISTORY

The classification of osteogenesis imperfecta has varied considerably from one reported series to the other. Looser, in 1906, classified the condition as either "congenita" or "tarda" and stated that both types were expressions of the same disease.[10] In the "congenita" form, the child has multiple fractures that have occurred sometime before birth, micromelia, and caput membranacum.[9] This type may be caused by new autosomal dominant mutation or may develop secondary to autosomal recessive inheritance.[7] In the "tarda" form, fractures occur at the time of birth or later. This type is inherited as an autosomal dominant with incomplete penetrance and variable expressivity. The "tarda" form has been subdivided again into the "gravis" (occurring from one year onward) depending upon the age at which fractures occur.[10] Falvo et al.[6] have divided the "tarda" group into a type I and type II, depending on whether bowing of long bones is present or not (Type I demonstrating bowing of the lower extremity long bones, while Type II patients do not).

Since the classification of disease types has varied so much among different authors writing about osteogenesis imperfecta, an accurate portrayal of the incidence of scoliosis is difficult to establish. King and Bobechko,[9] using the classification described above, found that 43 per cent of patients with osteogenesis imperfecta "congenita" had scoliosis, whereas 70 per cent of "tarda gravis" and 28 per cent of "tarda levis" demonstrated scoliosis. Thoracic curvatures were the most common. On the other hand, Falvo and co-workers, using their classification, found scoliosis in 92 per cent of the patients with osteogenesis imperfecta congenita, 44 per cent in the "tarda" I type and 11 per cent in the "tarda" II type.[5] Hoek, in his series of 46 patients, found 70 per cent with scoliosis.[8] He stated that the severity of the disease correlated with the prevalence of scoliosis and the degree of curvature.

The most definitive and complete review has recently been presented by Benson et al., who reviewed a series of 143 patients with osteogenesis imperfecta.[4] They found that of the 123 spines evaluated, 68 per cent had some degree of curvature. Curvatures were mild in young children and became more severe with advancing age. Curvatures over 80 degrees were seen only in patients over 12 years of age. The factors that directly correlated with the incidence and severity of the curvature were the thin bones in the "congenita" type of osteogenesis imperfecta. In these cases, a progressive and significant curvature could invariably be predicted (Fig. 23–32).

The etiology of these spinal deformities is unknown. It may well be due to a combination of several factors related to the softness or brittleness of the bone, which leads to compression fractures and vertebral collapse. Multiple fractures with alterations of vertebral growth plates,[10] laxity of ligaments with loss of intrinsic support to the spine, and abnormalities of the biochemistry and physiology of the intervertebral disc could all be associated with pathogenesis of scoliotic and kyphotic curvatures.

*Text continued on page 611*

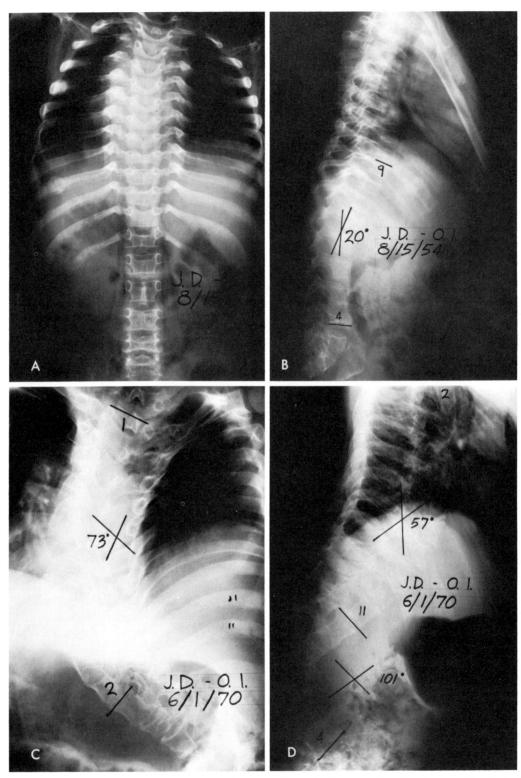

**Figure 23-32**    *A* and *B*, Minimal thoracolumbar kyphosis with no significant scoliosis in a six year old patient with a congenital type of osteogenesis imperfecta. *C* and *D*, The marked progression of these curvatures, which were untreated. At this time, the patient was age 22 and presented with early cardiopulmonary failure secondary to the scoliosis as well as the thoracic lordosis. He expired shortly thereafter from cardiopulmonary failure.

*Illustration continued on the opposite page*

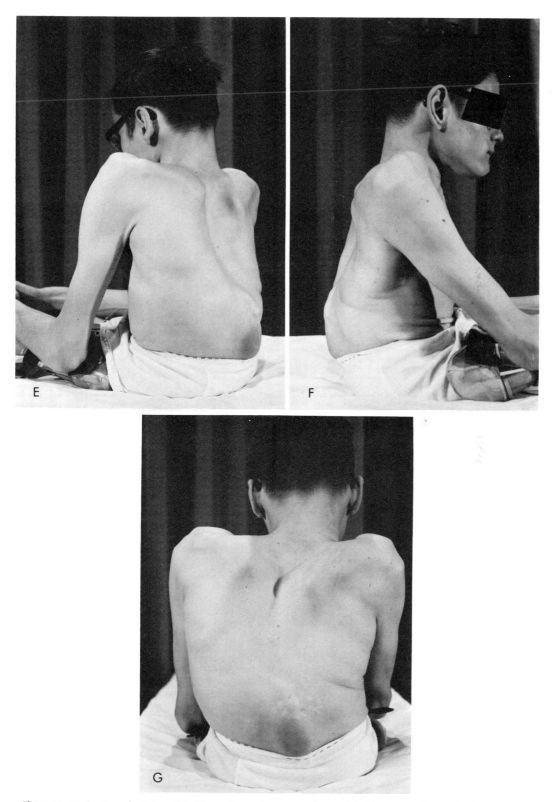

**Figure 23–32** *Continued* *E, F,* and *G,* The patient as he appeared at age 21 with a severe thoracic lordosis and thoraco-lumbar kyphosis.

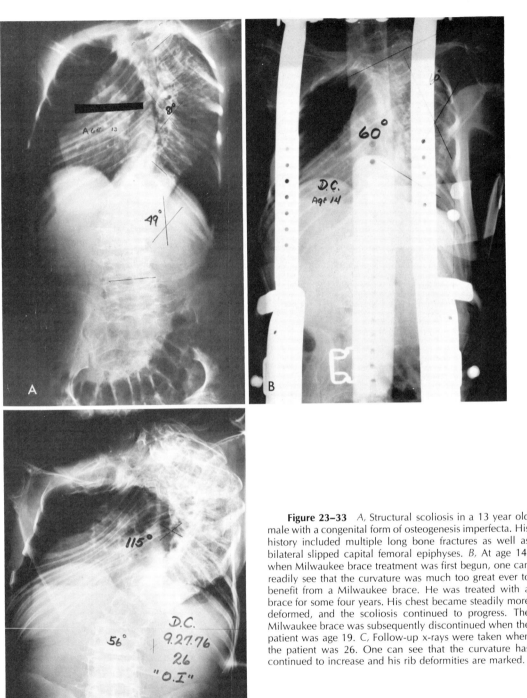

**Figure 23–33** *A,* Structural scoliosis in a 13 year old male with a congenital form of osteogenesis imperfecta. His history included multiple long bone fractures as well as bilateral slipped capital femoral epiphyses. *B,* At age 14, when Milwaukee brace treatment was first begun, one can readily see that the curvature was much too great ever to benefit from a Milwaukee brace. He was treated with a brace for some four years. His chest became steadily more deformed, and the scoliosis continued to progress. The Milwaukee brace was subsequently discontinued when the patient was age 19. *C,* Follow-up x-rays were taken when the patient was 26. One can see that the curvature has continued to increase and his rib deformities are marked.

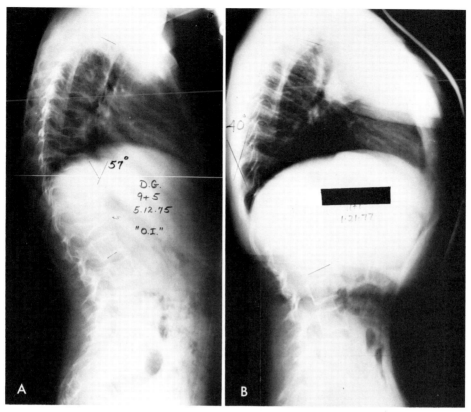

**Figure 23–34**  *A,* Patient with osteogenesis imperfecta and kyphosis. Because of increasing back pain and progressive deformity, the patient was treated in a Milwaukee brace. *B,* One can see a marked improvement in the kyphosis and a decrease in the vertebral wedging and a restoration of bone height. Although this is only a preliminary result, the patient's symptoms have been greatly relieved.

## TREATMENT

The treatment of spine deformities in isolated cases has been described,[1, 3, 8, 9] but no large series has been reported. The treatment has been either nonoperative, using the Milwaukee brace, or surgical correction by spine fusion with or without Harrington instrumentation. The greatest experience was recently reported by Benson et al.[4] and consists of 9 of 143 patients treated with a Milwaukee brace. These authors showed rather conclusively that the Milwaukee brace is not only ineffective but also detrimental, since it deformed the rib cage and did not improve the scoliosis.

Our own experience, although limited, would support their findings and conclusions (Fig. 23–33). Spinal bracing to control progressive scoliosis in these patients would appear ill advised and without benefit. We have, however, found the Milwaukee brace of some benefit in controlling or at least reliev-ing the symptoms associated with kyphosis (<60 degrees) and compression fractures (Fig. 23–34).

For progressive spinal curvatures, spine fusion with Harrington instrumentation would appear to be the preferred form of treatment. Although the experience with this form of surgical treatment for the deformed spine in a patient with osteogenesis imperfecta is not widespread, the results from scattered reports appear to be sufficiently encouraging to justify its continued use. The presence of soft osteoporotic bone might cause some concern about the integrity of internal fixation. Waugh has reported satisfactory fixation in osteoporotic bone with the use of Harrington rods secured with methylmethacrylate around the upper hook.[13] It is our feeling that should any treatment appear indicated, surgical correction with fusion would be preferred to the Milwaukee brace or any other type of spinal orthosis. Since the correction of the curve is difficult if not impossible, the prevention of increase by arthrodesis is the most important concept.

Curves progressing beyond 50 degrees should be fused, even without correction if such be the situation.

### References

1. Albright, J. A., and Grunt, J. A.: Studies of patients with osteogenesis imperfecta. J. Bone Joint Surg., *53A*:1415, 1971.
2. Aufdermaur, M: Die Wirbelsaule bei der Osteogenesis Imperfecta. Orthop. 103 bd.
3. Bauze, R. J. Smith, R., and Frances, M. J. O.: A new look at osteogenesis imperfecta. J. Bone Joint Surg., *57B*:1–12, 1975.
4. Benson, D. R., Donaldson, D. H., and Millar, E. A.: Natural history of the spine and osteogenesis imperfecta. Review of 143 cases. Scoliosis Research Society—proceedings, 1976, Ottawa.
5. Falvo, K. A., Klain, D. B., and Krauss, A. N.: Pulmonary function studies in osteogenesis imperfecta. Am. Rev. Resp., Dis., *108*:258, 1973.
6. Falvo, K. A., Root, L., and Bullough, P. G.: Osteogenesis imperfecta. Clinical evaluation and management. J. Bone Joint Surg., *56A*:783, 1974.
7. Herndon, C. N.: Osteogenesis imperfecta; Some clinical and genetic considerations. Clin. Orthop., *8*:132, 1956.
8. Hoek, K. J.: Scoliosis in osteogenesis imperfecta. Proceedings of the Western Orthopedics Assoc. J. Bone Joint Surg., *57A*:136, 1975.
9. King, J. D., and Bobechko, W. P.: Osteogenesis imperfecta. J. Bone Joint Surg., *53B*:72–89, 1971.
10. McKusick, V. A.: Heritable Disorders of Connective Tissues, 4th ed. St. Louis, C. V. Mosby, 1972.
11. Rothman, R. H., and Simeone, F. A.: The Spine. Philadelphia, W.B. Saunders Co., 1975.
12. Smith, R., Francis, M. J. O., and Bauze, R. J.: Osteogenesis imperfecta. Quart. J. Med., New Series, XLIV, *176*:555–573, 1975.
13. Waugh, T.: Application of methylmethacrylate to scoliosis—the biomechanical basis. Presented at the Scoliosis Research Society Annual Meeting of 1970.

# SPINAL INJURY

Deformities to the axial skeleton following trauma have only recently begun to receive the attention they rightfully deserve. In the past decade alone, a greater awareness and appreciation by the orthopedic surgeon of the acute and chronic complications associated with spinal injuries has resulted in a more rational basis for early and long term management. It has become increasingly apparent that proper, expeditious, and intelligent treatment of acute injuries will tend to eliminate the late development of spinal deformity.

Spinal deformity developing acutely or chronically following spinal injury is related to four factors: 1) the type of injury—stable versus unstable, 2) the age of the patient at the time of injury, 3) the degree and level of neurologic deficit, and 4) type of acute surgery performed.

## STABILITY OF THE VERTEBRAL COLUMN

The stability of the vertebral column is dependent to a great degree on the soft tissue support. Posteriorly the supraspinous and interspinous ligaments along with the capsules of the posterior lateral joints and ligamentum flava provide what has become known as the posterior ligament complex. The integrity of this ligament complex is felt to be essential for spinal stability. Anteriorly, the intervertebral disc, the periosteum, and the anterior and posterior longitudinal ligaments provide additional functional support to the vertebral column. One can consider the spine as two connected structural columns; an anterior column consisting of vertebral bodies, discs, and ligaments and a posterior column consisting of the neural arch, facet joints, and interconnecting ligaments.

Injuries to the spine may damage one or both of these structural columns and in the process may produce varying degrees of spinal instability. It is important to determine whether this instability is acute or chronic. Acute instability implies a fracture that is capable of further displacement soon after injury with immediate neurologic damage. Chronic instability implies an injury that may further angulate, producing greater deformity months or even years after injury.

Slow and progressive neurologic damage may result from chronic instability but only as a late consequence of marked angulation. Disruption of both anterior and posterior columns results in acute instability. Chronic instability is less common but may result from damage to the anterior column alone over multiple levels (i.e., multiple compression fractures) or traumatic injuries and surgical procedures that jeopardize the integrity of the posterior column.

## PATHOMECHANICS AND CLASSIFICATION OF SPINAL INJURY

Classifications of spinal injuries have developed that have taken into consideration forces which may result in damage to either the anterior or posterior column or a combination of both structural columns. In considering mechanisms involved in injuries, it is useful to describe the relationship of one vertebral segment to another in the conventional X, Y, and Z axis of three dimensional space (Fig. 23–35). Angular motion around the three axes would include flexion, extension, rotation, and lateral bending, while nonangular motion (translation) would include distraction, compression, anterior-pos-

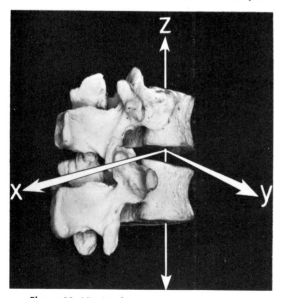

**Figure 23–35** Mechanisms involved in spinal injury, described as a relationship of one vertebral segment to another in the conventional X, Y, and Z axis. Angular motion is a normal component of the intact spine, whereas nonangular (translational) motion is not. (Used by permission of Minn. Med., 59:711, 1976.)

terior shear, and lateral shear. For translational displacement to occur, both structural columns of necessity would be disrupted, and acute instability would result. For instance, the flexion (slice) fracture described by Holdsworth would ultimately result in lateral translational displacement and be indicative of acute spinal instability. Such injuries with marked displacement of both structural columns usually result in neurologic deficit at the time of injury. Acutely unstable injuries that have not been properly reduced and held in position, either by external support or by internal fixation until adequately healed, may further angulate weeks, months, or years after the original injury, producing severe degrees of spinal deformity. It must also be remembered that even so-called stable injuries as classified by Holdsworth may lead to chronic instability. For instance, multiple compression fractures over contiguous segments of the spine or severe bursting injuries may lead to progressive kyphosis with delayed neurologic sequelae secondary to cord angulation.

## LEVEL OF NEUROLOGIC INJURY AND OF PATIENT

Stable vertebral fractures in children, in contradistinction to those in the adult, rarely if ever result in progressive or delayed angulatory deformity. This is particularly true in stable fractures that occur before the age of 10. Multiple compression fractures in children have a remarkable tendency for spontaneous healing and ultimately result in complete restoration of vertebral height. Rarely are changes suggestive of Scheuermann's disease present over the vertebrae initially injured.[17, 18] Lateral wedge fractures in children may result in minimal scoliosis, but progressive spine deformity is rarely if ever observed. This favorable prognosis might best be explained by the absence of severe damage to the growth zone of the vertebral bodies at the time of initial injury.[1] This is in contradistinction to the unstable fracture dislocations that may occur in children or those lesions to the spine associated with paraplegia or quadraplegia. The classical report of Kilfoyle et al.[21] and the experience developed at Rancho Los Amigos Hospital over the past 15 years demonstrates conclusively that approximately 85 per cent of patients who sustain a spinal cord injury prior to the adolescent growth spurt will develop a spinal deformity.[6] This deformity may be lordosis, scoliosis, or kyphosis, or a combination of each. We also have found this a predictable pattern, one which unfortunately continues to be poorly appreciated.

## ROLE OF SURGERY IN ACUTE SPINAL INJURIES

The role of emergency surgery (i.e., within 24 hours) following acute spinal injury associated with neurologic deficit is controversial. Although open reduction and fusion have been advocated for some 30 years, postural reduction as stressed by Guttman[13] continues to receive substantial support, particularly in Europe. Poor fixation devices were a primary factor leading many workers to this nonoperative approach. Recent experience, however, as reported by Harrington and others, has shown that the technique of open reduction and Harrington rod fixation

of unstable fractures is a safe technique, which improves nursing care, shortens rehabilitation, and is effective in maintaining fracture reduction and promoting bony healing.[2, 3, 4, 9, 10, 14, 15, 19] Furthermore, nonoperative measures often fail to reduce the fracture and may lead to greater pain and deformity.[10, 22, 24]

We now feel that, except in those cases with a progressive neurologic deficit or an open fracture, immediate decompression or stabilizing procedures are probably ill-advised. When the patient's condition becomes stable, we recommend that unstable thoracic and lumbar spinal injuries with or without a neurologic deficit be managed by open reduction of the fracture, internal fixation, and spine fusion. We feel the unstable fracture should be stabilized in order to prevent late deformity, skin ulceration, and pain. Furthermore, anatomic realignment of the fracture and spinal canal remains the most certain method of decompressing the neural elements, a consideration that is relevant only in the neurologically incomplete situation.

Complete absence of neurologic func-

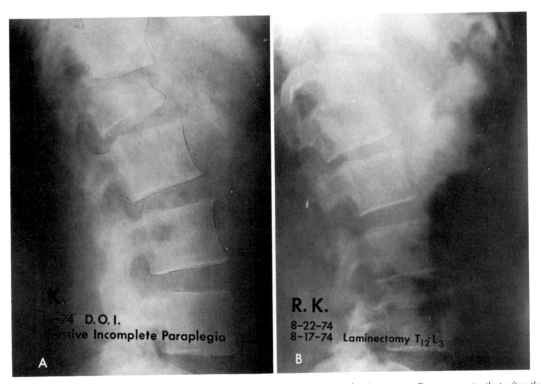

**Figure 23–36**  *A*, This patient with an incomplete lesion underwent a laminectomy. One can note that after the laminectomy, the anterior step-off has not been relieved. If anything, it has actually increased as the spine has gone into greater kyphosis (*B*).

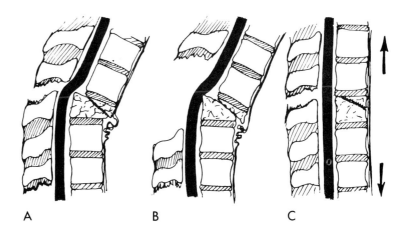

**Figure 23–37** *A,* Unstable injuries with or without neurologic deficit must be stabilized to prevent late deformity and pain. Laminectomy alone does not decompress but will lead to greater deformity *(B).* Anatomical realignment is the preferred method for decompressing the neural elements *(C).* (Reprinted by permission of J. Bone Joint Surg.[10])

A     B     C

tion for 24 hours below the level of injury indicates an irreversible neurologic deficit. Treatment in these cases should be directed toward the patient's rehabilitation as a paraplegic. No longer is it justified to perform a laminectomy to "assure the family and patient that everything possible was done." This approach is without documented benefit, and furthermore the laminectomy may produce greater spinal instability and will convert a stable injury into an unstable one. It is our feeling that maximal neurologic damage occurs at the time of injury and heroic measures such as cord cooling and myelotomy offer little benefit. Furthermore, laminectomy as an isolated procedure will not decompress the neural elements (Fig. 23–36). The compression that exists in these injuries is anterior, and therefore posterior unroofing procedures do little more than produce spinal instability. It must also be stressed that patients who have a sustained spinal cord injury at the age of 18 years or younger and undergo a laminectomy as initial treatment are much more likely to develop kyphosis than those who do not undergo a laminectomy. It is readily apparent that this problem may develop in the cervical as well as the thoracic and lumbar spine.[6, 7, 23] We have not seen or heard of a documented case of complete traumatic paraplegia that was improved neurologically by a laminectomy.

## MANAGEMENT OF THORACIC–LUMBAR FRACTURES

In our experience, spinal deformity following spine fractures with or without neurologic deficit is a preventable problem.

Unstable injuries should be stabilized, unnecessary ill-advised laminectomies should be avoided, and children sustaining a traumatic paraplegia prior to the adolescent growth spurt should be braced until the completion of growth.

Stable or unstable injuries with neurologic deficit require a careful but realistic approach. Those lesions associated with complete and persistent interruption of spinal cord function over 24 hours will not be benefited by surgery directed at reversing the neurologic deficit. Treatment, rather, should be directed toward the patient's rehabilitation as a paraplegic.[6] On the other hand, incomplete cord lesions or lesions involving the cauda equina carry a favorable prognosis for some degree of significant functional neurologic improvement. We do feel that greater improvement is possible when adequate decompression is carried out. Anatomical reduction of the fracture is, in our minds, the most efficacious and beneficial method of achieving decompression (Fig. 23–37).

## PLAN OF MANAGEMENT: UNSTABLE INJURIES WITH OR WITHOUT NEUROLOGIC DEFICIT

Following injury, the patient is managed on a Foster or horizontal Stryker turning frame. A vertical turning circle-electric bed should be avoided, since axial loading of the spine may result in severe displacement of the bony fragments. Following stabilization of the patient, usually during the first week following injury, the patient is taken to surgery. The patient is anesthetized, intubated, and then carefully turned on to a four poster frame. After skin preparation, the fracture is

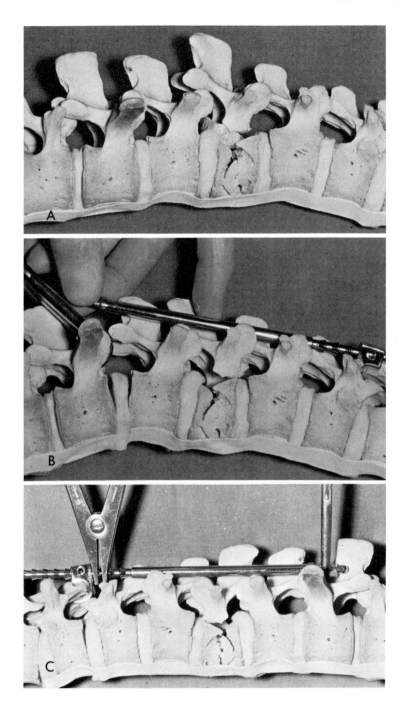

**Figure 23–38**   The method of fracture reduction using the Harrington device. Usually the anterior longitudinal ligament is intact and can act as a tether to prevent overdistraction. However, it may be disrupted, so one can not count on this, and overdistraction must be prevented at all cost. Actually, the technique is one of anatomic realignment using the three-point principle. Hooks are placed two levels above and two levels below the fracture site (B), and by levering the lower end of the rod into the lower hook, fracture reduction is achieved (C). If the kyphosis is very structural, it may be beneficial to use an outrigger on one side of the spine while the distracting rod is being placed in position, or one may have to bend the first Harrington rod to conform to the kyphosis and then put a second Harrington rod in on the opposite side, not bent, then cut out the first bent rod and place a straight one in its place. By using this technique, reduction can be achieved. It must be stressed that overdistraction must be avoided.

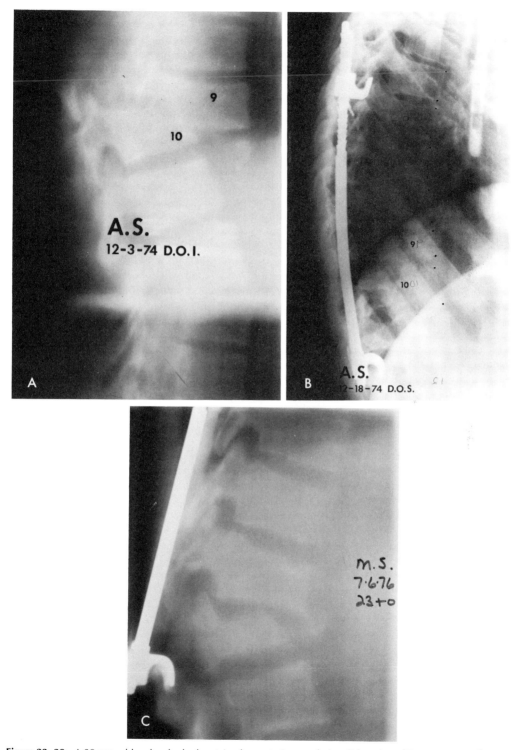

**Figure 23–39** A 20 year old male who had sustained an anterior translation dislocation of T10 on T11. By the use of the Harrington distraction device, anatomical reduction of the fracture was achieved. *C,* Improper positioning of the Harrington rods will not reduce the fracture but rather will allow the fracture to go into greater kyphosis and displacement. (*A* and *B* used by permission of Raven Press, New York.[3])

exposed through a midline incision. If the patient has a complete neurologic deficit, Harrington hooks are placed two levels above and two levels below the fracture. Using the outrigger the fracture may be reduced and a distraction rod levered in position between the two hooks on the opposite side of the outrigger. The distraction rod actually acts by a three-point principle, anatomically realigning the spine (Fig. 23–38). Overdistraction is to be avoided, and the spinous processes should be wired together if there is any tendency for this to occur. Decortication by using a rongeur is carried out, and iliac crest bone is added. One week after surgery, the patient is mobilized after application of a body cast. If sensation is absent, the patient is immobilized in a bivalved plastic body jacket rather than plaster. Rehabilitation is then begun. External immobilization is continued for four to six months (Fig. 23–39).

If the patient is neurologically intact or has an incomplete neurologic deficit, a limited laminectomy over a single level at the time of fracture reduction has proved to be a useful procedure in identifying and removing loose bony fragments and disc material within the canal. Although this material is quite uncommon, we have seen it, and its removal would certainly appear indicated, especially in incomplete lesions. A limited laminectomy is also helpful in visualizing the dura as the fracture is being reduced and realigned by the Harrington device. Through this opening, one may palpate the anterior "step-off" prior to fracture reduction and after spinal realignment to assure that decompression is complete and thorough.[10] If the reduction has not been complete and anterior impingement remains, one may remove the articular process and pedicle on one side to provide lateral exposure in the region of the deformity. The vertebral body is then entered, and with appropriate rongeurs and angled curettes the cancellous bone under the posterior cortical shell is removed. Once this undermining is complete, the thick cortical shell can be fractured anteriorly away from the anterior aspect of the dural sac. This decompression is accomplished without retraction of the dura, and when it is complete, one can see the dural sac move anteriorly, and dural pulsations appear distal to the area of the previous compression. This technique has greatest applicability at the thoracolumbar junction and in the lumbar spine (Fig. 23–40). In the thoracic spine, if anterior decompression is still necessary after fracture reduction and alignment has been done, it is preferable, we feel, to accomplish this through a transthoracic approach.

If treatment has been delayed more than three to four weeks, anatomic reduction of the fracture is more difficult and sometimes impossible. If the patient has an incomplete neurologic deficit that is felt to require decompression, a combined anterior and posterior approach will be necessary, the posterior procedure to provide more stability and the anterior procedure to provide decompression and fusion. We do not recommend doing this at one sitting (although it is technically possible to do so), but rather we advise proceeding first with the anterior decompression and fusion, followed one to two weeks later with a posterior spine fusion with Harrington rod instrumentation (Fig. 23–41). If the patient presents months later with kyphosis secondary to the injury and laminectomy and is totally paraplegic, anterior and posterior fusion will be necessary, since the deformity is relatively fixed, and adequate correction and fusion cannot be obtained by posterior fusion alone (Fig. 23–42).

*Stable injuries with no neurologic deficit* require little treatment. This group of injuries would include anterior wedge, lateral wedge, and burst (compression) fractures, where injury to the posterior elements has not resulted. Analgesics for pain along with bed rest for several days is usually sufficient. Transient ileus is common and should be treated when present. These comments must be tempered, however, by the evidence – that severe degrees of bursting (>50 per cent of the body) and multiple compression fractures over several contiguous segments may demonstrate a tendency to cause progressive angulation and deformity (chronic instability) and require surgical stabilization as a secondary procedure.

As a general rule, the use of a brace or body jacket for one to two months for most of these stable fractures that have not been operated on may offer some benefit. We favor the Williams chair back brace for lower lumbar spine injuries and the Jewett brace for injuries involving T8 to L2. Injuries higher than T8 require an over-the-

*Text continued on page 622*

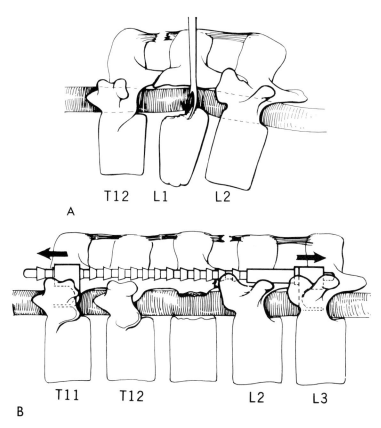

T12   L1      L2

A

T11      T12           L2      L3

B

**Figure 23–40**   Technique for a limited laminotomy at the time of anatomical reduction of a fracture. Although partial reduction may be achieved with a Harrington device, comminuted bony elements may still be protruding posteriorly against the anterior aspect of the dural sac. If this is still palpated after reduction of the fracture is achieved, as best as can be with the Harrington device, removal of the most posterior portion of the body with sharp curettes and rongeurs is possible through this lateral approach *(A)*. The procedure is then completed *(B)* and autogenous iliac bone graft added to furnish a solid arthrodesis. Usually it is necessary to approach the spine on one side only in order to carry out this decompression. This technique works best at the thoracolumbar junction or the lumbar spine and only in cases of incomplete neurologic deficit. (Used by permission of J. Bone Joint Surg.[10])

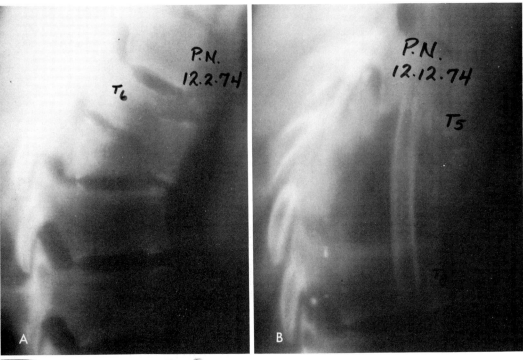

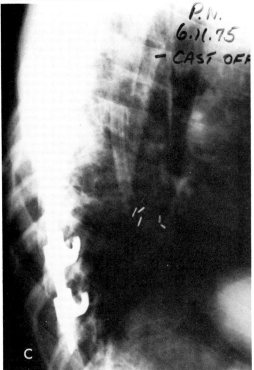

**Figure 23–41** (*A*) This 22-year-old male sustained a flexion compression injury to T6–T7 with an incomplete paraplegia (sensory sparing and useless motor activity in one foot). After 3 to 4 weeks of bed rest, this neurologic deficit showed no significant improvement. Following anterior cord decompression and fusion (*B*) and posterior spine fusion with Harrington rod instrumentation (*C*), his deficit rapidly improved. Some three months later he was ambulatory with assistive devices, and when last seen two years after surgery he had only residual unsustained clonus with minimal spasticity in one leg. His bowel and bladder functions are normal, and he is walking without assists. (Used by permission of Raven Press, New York.[3])

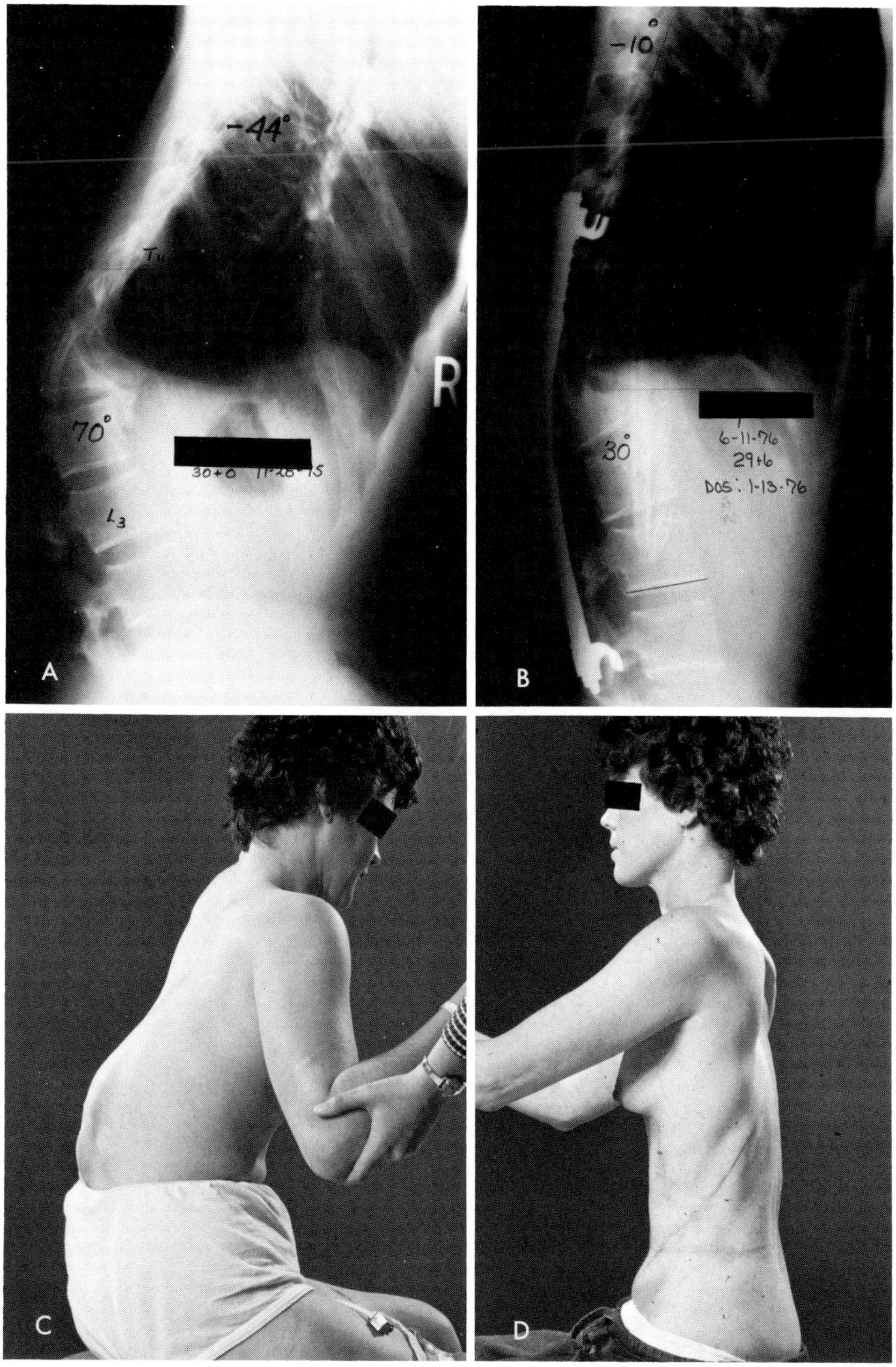

**Figure 23–42** A 30-year-old woman who sustained a complete paraplegia in 1970. Three days after injury a laminectomy from T12 to L2 was carried out. Her paraplegia remained complete. Progressive kyphosis with loss of sitting balance and back pain was the ultimate result *(A)*. Following anterior spine fusion, using fibula strut bone graft, and a posterior spine fusion with Harrington instrumentation, an excellent correction of her kyphosis was achieved and a solid fusion resulted *(B)*. C, The patient preoperatively; *D,* the patient postoperatively. She has remained asymptomatic. (Used by permission of Raven Press, New York.[3])

shoulder plaster body jacket. There is little evidence that these supports appreciably affect the end result; however, they do little harm, and patients often seem more comfortable with their use. The follow-up from such injuries demonstrated that 25 per cent have enough symptoms to produce some disability.[20]

*Stable lesions with a neurologic deficit* should be managed along the guidelines outlined. If the lesion is a complete one, surgery is contraindicated. If the lesion is incomplete and decompression is felt to be indicated, it should be carried out at the site of compression which is anterior.

These indications for surgery as outlined should provide a helpful guideline for the management of the patient with acute spinal injury secondary to a fracture. The question may logically arise as to whether all patients with unstable fractures truly need surgery. Granted that some patients with fractures and complete paraplegia with minimal degrees of translational displacement in the thoracic spine (involving, for instance, a 10 per cent step-off of one vertebral body on another) may do quite satisfactorily with a polypropylene body jacket after three to four weeks of bed rest. In these borderline situations and if the patient is completely paraplegic, we would try early mobilization without surgery. Any tendency of the spine to displace or angulate would then be an indication for surgery. Likewise, the question of whether to use distracting rods or compression rods is not easily resolved. As a general rule, distraction rods are best in situations of translational displacement, while contracting rods work best in those deformities presenting as distraction injuries (chance fractures or late kyphosis with chronic instability). In these cases, Weiss springs could be used in preference to the Harrington compression rod. However, we personally feel that the fixation is inferior and that the possibility of producing a lateral curvature through unequal tension is increased.

Finally, the indication for spine fusion is relative. Good results have been reported with instrumentation alone, but the rods must be removed 6 to 12 months post insertion. We would favor spine fusion because it obviates the need for rod removal as a secondary procedure.

## MANAGEMENT OF PARAPLEGIA IN CHILDREN

Based on the preceding discussion, it is apparent that spinal deformity following spinal injuries with or without paraplegia is for the most part a preventable problem: unstable injuries should be stabilized, unnecessary ill-advised laminectomies should be avoided, and children sustaining a traumatic paraplegia prior to the adolescent growth spurt should be braced until the completion of growth. In this regard, we have found that the bivalved polypropylene body jacket is an excellent orthosis. It serves to stabilize an unstable collapsing spine, allowing easy removal and easy application and avoiding the skin complications associated with plaster of Paris. Not all deformities will necessarily be prevented by early bracing, but it is our experience that the incidence of those requiring surgical stabilization will be greatly lessened by bracing from injury through the completion of the adolescent growth period.

Surgery is indicated for those patients with progressive spinal deformity uncontrolled by bracing during the growth periods or those patients presenting with significant spine deformity (greater than 40 degrees) after growth was complete. Spine fusion with Harrington rod instrumentation is the procedure of choice, and the fusion with instrumentation for the collapsing spine in children and adolescents must extend to sacrum. Failure to include the sacrum in the fusion will result in progressive pelvic obliquity, loss of sitting balance, and pressure ulceration over unequal weight distribution applied to the ischium. Postoperative immobilization is best carried out with a plastic polypropylene bivalved body jacket well-molded over the ilium, allowing easy and frequent removal while the patient is in the supine position in order to inspect the skin for possible skin ulcerations. Dwyer instrumentation may occasionally be useful for the paralytic posttraumatic spine deformity associated with severe structural pelvic obliquity. The posterior arthrodesis with Harrington instrumentation must always be carried out with extension of the fusion to the sacrum; otherwise the pelvic obliquity will recur, and correction will be lost (Fig. 23–43). For further details, see Chapter 8.

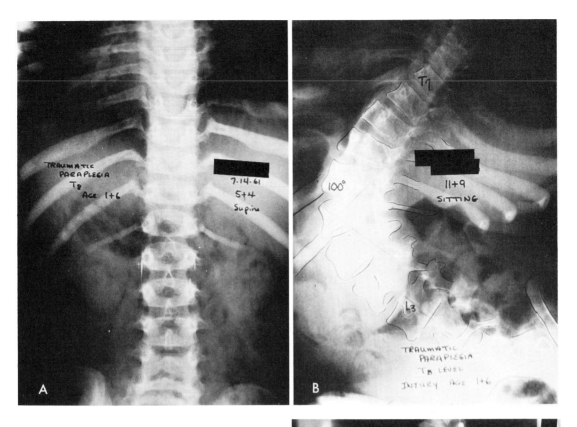

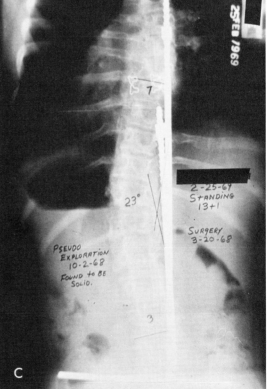

**Figure 23–43** This 5-year-old patient sustained a traumatic paraplegia at age 1+6. Untreated at age 11, a severe structural scoliosis is evident. Extensive spine fusion with Harrington rod instrumentation was necessary (C). (Used by permission of Raven Press, New York.[3])

## References

1. Aufdermaur, M.: Spinal injuries in juveniles: Necropsy findings in twelve cases. J. Bone Joint Surg., 56B:513, 1974.
2. Bedbrook, G. M.: Use and disuse of surgery in lumbo-dorsal fractures. J. West. Pacific Orthop. Assoc., 6:26, 1969.
3. Bradford, D. S.: The role of internal fixation and spine fusion in thoracic and lumbar spine fractures. In Chou, Shell N. (ed.). New York Raven Press, 1977 (in press).
4. Bradford, D. S. Akbarnia, B., Winter, R. B., and Seljeskog, E.: Surgical stabilization of fracture and fracture dislocations of the thoracic spine. The Spine, 2:185, 1977.
5. Bradford, D. S., and Thompson, R. C.: Fractures and dislocations of the spine—indications for surgical intervention. Minn. Med., 59:711, 1976.
6. Burke, D. C.: Traumatic spinal paralysis in children. Paraplegia, II:268, 1974.
7. Cattell, H. S., and Clark, G. H.: Cervical kyphosis and instability following multiple laminectomies in children. J. Bone Joint Surg., 49A:713, 1967.
8. Cullen, J. C.: Spinal lesions in battered babies. J. Bone Joint Surg., 57B:364, 1975.
9. Dickson, J. H., Harrington, P. R., and Erwin, W. D.: Harrington instrumentation in the fractured, unstable thoracic and lumbar spine. Texas Med., 69:91, 1973.
10. Flesch, J. R., Leider, L. L., Erickson, D. L., Chou, S. N., and Bradford, D. S.: Harrington instrumentation and spine fusion for thoracic and lumbar spine fractures. J. Bone Joint Surg., 59A:143, 1977.
11. Frankel, H. L., Hancock, D. O., Hyslop, G., Melzak, J., Michaelis, L. S., Ungar, G. H., Vernon, J. D. S., and Walsh, J. J.: The value of postural reduction in the initial management of closed injuries of the spine with paraplegia and tetraplegia. Paraplegia, 7:179, 1969.
12. Gillespie, R., and Wedge, J. H.: The problems of scoliosis in paraplegic children. J. Bone Joint Surg., 56A:1767, 1974.
13. Guttmann, L.: Surgical aspects of the treatment of traumatic paraplegia. J. Bone Joint Surg., 31B:339, 1949.
14. Harrington, P. R.: Instrumentation in spine instability other than scoliosis. S. Afr. J. Surg., 5:7, 1967.
15. Harrington, P. R.: Technical details in relation to the successful use of instrumentation in scoliosis. Orthop. Clin. North Am., 3:49, 1972.
16. Holdsworth, F. W.: Fractures, dislocations and fracture-dislocations of the spine. J. Bone Joint Surg., 52A:1534, 1970.
17. Horal, J., Nachemson, A., and Scheller, S.: Clinical and radiological long term follow-up of vertebral fractures in children. Acta Orthop. Scand., 43:491, 1972.
18. Hubbard, D. D.: Injuries of the spine in children and adolescents. Clin. Orthop., 100:56, 1974.
19. Katznelson, A. M.: Stablilization of the spine in traumatic paraplegia. Paraplegia, 7:33, 1969.
20. Kaufer, H.: The thoracolumbar spine. In Rockwood, Charles A., Jr., and Green, David P. (eds.): Fractures. Philadelphia, J. B. Lippincott, 1972.
21. Kilfoyle, R. M., Foley, J. J., and Norton, P. L.: Spine and pelvic deformity in childhood and adolescent paraplegia. J. Bone Joint Surg., 47A:659, 1965.
22. Lewis, J., and McKibben, B.: The treatment of unstable fracture-dislocations of the thoracolumbar spine accompanied by paraplegia. J. Bone Joint Surg., 56B:603, 1974.
23. Morgan, R., Brown, J. C., and Bonnett, C.: The effect of laminectomy on the pediatric spinal cord injured patient. J. Bone Joint Surg., 56A:1767, 1974.
24. Roberts, J. B., and Curtiss, P. H.: Stability of the thoracic and lumbar spine in traumatic paraplegia following fracture or fracture dislocation. J. Bone Joint Surg., 52A:115, 1970.

# TUBERCULOSIS OF THE SPINE

### HISTORY

Tuberculosis of the spine has been reported in Egyptian mummies[15] dating from 3000 B.C. The earliest example shows thoracic spine involvement with pronounced kyphosis and a psoas abscess.[10] The first written description of this disease was given by Hippocrates (450 B.C.).[29] It was Sir Percival Pott who first accurately described the disease that bears his name, and his description included autopsy findings.[61]

### INCIDENCE

Tuberculosis is still prevalent in densely populated parts of the world: Africa, Asia, Mexico, and parts of South America. It is much rarer in countries with adequate housing, nutrition, and public health preventive measures. In the United States there are an average of 31,000 cases reported annually, the number of cases remaining approximately constant since 1970. The number of extrapulmonary cases has also been static at 3500 to 4000 per year.[8]

### SITE

The spine is the site of involvement in over half the cases of bone and joint tuberculosis. Hodgson reports that in 1000 consecutive cases of bone and joint tuberculosis, the spine is involved in 58.7 per cent.[40] This contrasts to nontuberculous bone infection, in which the spine is involved in only two to five per cent of cases.[51] All areas of the spine do not have the same predilection for this disease. In 587 consecutive cases of spinal tuberculosis, Hodgson found a peak incidence at L1, with a rapid fall-off above and below this level.

The sex incidence of spinal tuberculosis is equal. The age of involvement depends on many factors. In areas with marked overcrowding with an undernourished population and no preventive measures, the child is exposed to the infection early in life and develops the disease in childhood. With improvement in housing and nutrition the child is not exposed to infection till school age, or even into adulthood. With improvement in antituberculosis measures there is a gradual upward shift in age of infection.

## ETIOLOGY

Henriques pointed to the first clue in reviewing osteomyelitis complicating urologic procedures. He found a high incidence of spine involvement.[25] He postulated that the pathway for the infection was via the venous plexus of Batson.[4] Attempts by Blocklock to produce spinal tuberculosis by injection of tubercle bacilli either into the vertebrae directly or into the left ventricle, both combined with a spinal injury, were unsuccessful.[5] Hodgson performed experiments on monkeys, rabbits, and rats, injecting tubercle bacilli directly into kidney, ovary, prostate, and other abdominal and pelvic organs. The animals were sacrificed at intervals after infection. A primary lesion was found in the injected organ, with a secondary focus in the spine.[35, 40] The infection was traced from the primary focus in the kidney to the spine via the venous plexus of Batson. There was, in addition, a spine focus in vertebrae at higher levels. By latex injection of the plexus in animals and humans, an understanding of this venous system was obtained. In quadrupeds the plexus is poorly formed and consists mainly of two lateral veins with few interconnections. In the biped the plexus is larger with many communications. The plexus is an important bypass for venous blood from the lower limbs, pelvis, and abdomen when the pathway via the inferior vena cava is obstructed as in coughing,

sneezing, Valsalva maneuver, and any physical stress involving breath holding.[4] The role of this plexus physiologically and as an avenue for spread of metastases has been well described by Batson,[4] Eckenhoff,[13] and Herlihy.[26, 27]

## PATHOGENESIS[23, 32,35]

Once the tubercle bacilli reach the vertebral body metaphysis, the infection is established and follows a definite pattern. This pathology has been well described by Hodgson and co-workers from their experience with operative treatment.

The first stage is a prepurulent phase of granulation tissue. This consists of an inflammatory reaction with Langhan's giant cells, epithelioid cells, and small inflammatory cells. The inflammation initially is closely related to the vessels but spreads rapidly with thrombosis of vessels, cellular edema, and death. In addition, there is a hypersensitivity immunologic reaction, which adds to the inflammatory process. With the spread of the infection and tissue necrosis a paraspinal abscess is formed (Fig. 23–44A).

The paraspinal abscess is the hallmark of active spinal tuberculosis as pointed out by Swett et al. in 1940.[69] The abscess is initially small and is surrounded by edema of the paraspinal tissues. With increased tissue destruction the abscess increases in size. Initially the pus is fluid and greenish-yellow, but later in the disease process it becomes thicker and whiter with the consistency of toothpaste. After many years it becomes still thicker and even solid as calcification occurs. In the pus are small necrotic fragments of bone, cartilage, and granulation tissue.

As the abscess spreads it strips the periosteum off the vertebrae. This renders the vertebrae avascular, and with minor trauma or the spread of the infection, pathologic fracture occurs, forming a sequestrum of dead bone in the pus. The sequestrum may be small or large, and if large may be forced backward into the spinal canal, causing paraplegia. The intervertebral disc is an avascular structure and is not involved in the disease. With the destruction of the bone above and below the disc, it becomes detached and lies free in the pus.

The abscess cavity is surrounded by a

wall of granulation tissue with edema of the surrounding tissue. When the abscess is in contact with the dura an inflammatory reaction results with pachymeningitis. With healing of the lesion the granulation tissue may turn into fibrous tissue and may "strangulate" the cord, causing late-onset paraplegia.

The process of spread of the infection with superficial destruction of the vertebral body was termed the "aneurysmal syndrome" by Ghormley and Bradley in 1928.[22] With increased pressure in the abscess cavity the body attempts to discharge the pus to the exterior. Numerous organs can be penetrated in the process, including trachea, esophagus, lung, vena cava, heart, mediastinum, liver, kidney, intestine, and urinary system. The most frequently involved organ is the lung. Another common site is the paravertebral muscles with formation of a sinus posteriorly or a cold psoas abscess with the pus presenting in the groin.

With the vertebral body destruction the spine collapses into kyphosis (Fig. 23–44B). If the loss is greater on one side than on the other, scoliosis results. Kyphosis is the more marked deformity, the scoliosis usually being minor.

With control of the infection by the body, revascularization of some of the surrounding bone occurs. The granulation tissue becomes fibrous and in parts osseous. Calcification also occurs in the pus as it becomes less liquid and more caseous in nature. A fibrous or bony bridging occurs between the vertebrae above and below the abscess. The bony bridging appears to be caused by ossification of the paravertebral ligaments and is more common in the lumbar spine.[62] Compensatory lordosis occurs above and below the kyphosis, and this is accompanied by changes in the vertebrae and discs in this area. There is a reversal of the height-width ratio of the vertebrae, especially in the lumbar area. The normal lumbar vertebra is wider than it is tall. With the lordosis this ratio is reversed, the vertebra in the area of lordosis being taller. In addition, the intervertebral disc in the area of lordosis becomes wedged.

## X-RAY CHANGES[30–32, 34–38]

In summary, the x-ray changes seen with spinal tuberculosis can be divided into soft tissue changes and bony changes.

### Soft Tissue Changes

The early changes occur in the paravertebral tissues, with a paravertebral shadow due to edema and abscess formation. Depending on the extent of the involvement and exact site in the vertebra the paravertebral shadow may be globular, fusiform, or unilateral. With destruction of the vertebrae the abscess will contain sequestra or areas of calcification.

### Bony Changes

The earliest bony change is osteopenia of the vertebral body, followed by erosion and loss of bone. In the early phase this is best seen on tomography. With spread of the infection, vertebral loss and collapse occur leading to kyphosis (Fig. 23–49B and C). With healing, bony and fibrous bridging is seen with changes in the height-width ratio of the adjacent vertebrae and wedging of the intervertebral disc.

## DIFFERENTIAL DIAGNOSIS

In the classic case, no difficulty exists in the diagnosis of spinal tuberculosis. When the presentation and x-ray appearance are less typical, difficulty in diagnosis can exist. The common differential diagnosis includes atypical pyogenic osteomyelitis, eosinophilic granuloma, metastatic disease to the vertebrae, congenital kyphosis, and brucellosis.

## TREATMENT

### Historical

The treatment for tuberculosis has varied since its first description by Hippocrates. Treatment has been both operative and nonoperative. Pott, in his monograph in 1779, wrote, "The remedy for this dreadful disease consists merely in procuring a large discharge of matter."[61] Pott and later Charcot applied a red-hot iron to the abscess in cases of paraplegia, to drain the abscess and reduce the pressure on the spinal cord.

With the introduction of antiseptics and aseptic surgery, direct operative attacks on the disease were performed in the United

States, United Kingdom, France, and Germany. In 1891, Hadra performed the first stabilization of spinal tuberculosis using wires wrapped around the spinous processes.[24] The stabilization was more widely used after Hibbs described his fusion procedure in 1911.[28]

At the turn of the century a change occurred in the treatment of tuberculosis. With the use of sanitaria, patients were moved to special centers remote from the cities and treated with "fresh air and sunshine." The nonoperative approach was strengthened by the discovery of chemotherapeutic agents effective against *M. tuberculosis*. Streptomycin was the first effective drug and was introduced in 1945. PAS was developed in 1946 and INH introduced in 1951. These agents have recently been shown to be very effective in entering the abscess cavity of the spinal lesion.

Many surgeons were dissatisfied with the results of nonoperative therapy and developed and used techniques for drainage of the tuberculous abscess. Capener developed the lateral rachotomy approach,[7] which was extended by Dott and Alexander to a costotransversectomy approach.[12] Griffiths et al. extended the approach to anterolateral approach.[23] In 1955 Hodgson and Stock[30] revived the anterior approach to the spine first devised by Ito et al. in 1934[43] for treatment of spinal tuberculosis. This approach removed all the contents of the abscess and stabilized the spine using an anterior fusion.

Today three philosophies in the treatment of spinal tuberculosis exist, all using 18 months of chemotherapy for control of the disease. One approach is the use of nonoperative therapy with the addition of bed rest, hospitalization, or a plaster jacket in some cases.[20, 47, 49, 50, 68] A number of surgeons routinely drain the abscess, some using debridement alone and others adding anterior fusion.[3, 8.4, 18, 32, 48, 59, 77, 78] Tuli from Varanasi, India, practices a "middle path" regimen with a basic nonoperative therapy and selective surgical intervention.[70, 72]

In order to try to establish scientifically an effective treatment program for spinal tuberculosis, the Medical Research Council of Britain established a Working Party on Tuberculosis of the Spine. Using different centers the variables in treatment were compared. A series of controlled clinical trials were planned, the study being restricted to thoracic and lumbar portions of the spine in nonparalytic patients (mainly children). The details of the trial in each center were determined by the resources available there, the incidence of the disease being high in all cases. In Masan, Korea, ambulatory outpatient treatment was compared to an initial period of six months' bed rest in hospital. In Pusan, Korea, ambulatory outpatient therapy was used comparing cases with and without splintage in a plaster jacket. In Bulawayo, Rhodesia, ambulant outpatient therapy was compared to simple debridement. In Johannesburg and Pretoria, South Africa, a comparison as in Hong Kong was established. In all the centers chemotherapy was administered for 18 months using double or triple drug therapy. An initial evaluation at a minimum of three years after the start of treatment has been made in all centers,[53-56] with Korea reporting in addition after five years.[57]

A favorable result in the study was defined as radiologically healed disease with all abscesses and sinuses healed, full physical activity, and no central nervous system involvement. In Masan, Pusan, and Bulawayo, the ambulant outpatient treatment groups showed 88 per cent, 82 per cent, and 86 per cent favorable results. The addition of six months' bed rest, nine months' splintage in a plaster jacket, open debridement, or the use of streptomycin did not significantly affect the result. There was however, an increase in the kyphosis of an average of 15 degrees, and 43 patients had central nervous system involvement on admission or developed it under treatment.[53-55, 57]

In Hong Kong, debridement and grafting gave 87 per cent favorable results compared with 86 per cent in the debridement alone group — figures very similar to those in the ambulatory studies. There was, however, a significant difference when considering bony union and stability of the kyphosis, factors that Hodgson says are essential when considering a good result of treatment. Debridement plus fusion gave 93 per cent healing with bony fusion compared with 69 per cent in the debridement series and 46 per cent in the nonoperative series in Korea. In addition, only 1 patient in Hong Kong presented with or developed central nervous system involvement compared with 43 patients in the other three centers, a large number of these developing during the course of treatment.[56] As all these reports are of a short term follow-up, the long term results will be valuable for a true comparison of the treatment modalities available.

### Principles of Treatment[2, 2A, 14, 16, 21, 30–32, 36, 37, 41, 42, 44, 45, 52, 60, 63, 64, 66, 73–76, 79]

The problems in spinal tuberculosis that require treatment are the acute disease with or without paraplegia and the late problems accompanying a healed lesion. These are a severe kyphotic deformity, mechanical back pain secondary to the compensatory lordosis, and late-onset paraplegia. The disease is in the vertebral bodies with destruction of bone and anterior growth potential giving an unstable kyphosis (Fig. 23–44). In addition, culture permits rational chemotherapy.

### ACUTE DISEASE

As seen in the above comparison of the various treatment modalities, a favorable result is achieved in the same percentage of all groups, irrespective of what is added to chemotherapy. The object of treatment is to achieve a stable spine with the least chance of central nervous system involvement.

In a classic presentation with back pain, mild kyphosis, and an ill patient, the diagnosis is easy. With unusual presentations either clinically or radiologically, spinal tuberculosis must be considered. The diagnosis of tuberculosis in another site is important, and intravenous pyelography and urine culture are important. To aid in the diagnosis of the spinal lesion laminography can be very helpful.

In the acute phase the exact treatment will depend on the stage of the disease and the extent of the vertebral destruction. The longer the period between the onset of the disease and the presentation, the more vertebral bodies are involved in the infection.

### EARLY MILD DISEASE, NO KYPHOSIS

Diagnosis of spinal tuberculosis in this early stage is very unusual. If the diagnosis is made, chemotherapy is started. With this early diagnosis and early chemotherapy, treatment without surgery is possible (Fig. 23–45). If there is no response to chemother-

apy and the vertebral destruction increases, debridement as described under Destruction of Several Vertebral Bodies (below) is performed.

### DESTRUCTION OF ONE VERTEBRAL BODY

If the diagnosis is made with only one vertebral body destroyed, treatment is initially nonoperative with chemotherapy. If the vertebral destruction extends to involve more than one body and the kyphosis increases, debridement is necessary.

One disadvantage of this nonoperative approach in areas where tuberculosis is not common is confirmation of diagnosis. A needle biopsy to obtain a culture is possible but very dangerous. Hemorrhage can accompany the needle biopsy, and paraplegia has been described as a result of the biopsy.[67] A costotransversectomy can be used, but this is better for drainage than exicision and grafting.

### DESTRUCTION OF SEVERAL VERTEBRAL BODIES

With a more extensive disease and destruction of two or more vertebral bodies, the anterior approach of Hodgson is the treatment of choice where facilities are available. This is also used in the above cases where nonoperative treatment is unsuccessful. The debridement will confirm the diagnosis and allow culture and sensitivity of the organism. The abscess will be evacuated, eliminating all necrotic tissue. The fusion will correct existing deformity and prevent future deformity (Fig. 23–46).

After a short course of chemotherapy, surgery is performed. Using the anterior exposure (see page 507) the spine and abscess are visualized. A "T" or "I" shaped incision is made in the abscess wall once the segmental vessels have been coagulated or ligated. The contents of the abscess—pus, bony sequestra, intervertebral disc, and granulation tissue—are all removed. The remaining cavity should have bleeding walls with raw bone at the two ends. An inlay strut rib graft is placed in the cavity with the ends recessed in the vertebral bone. As many struts as possible are used, increasing the amount of bone graft and the stability. In adults consideration should be given to using iliac bone in

*Text continued on page 633*

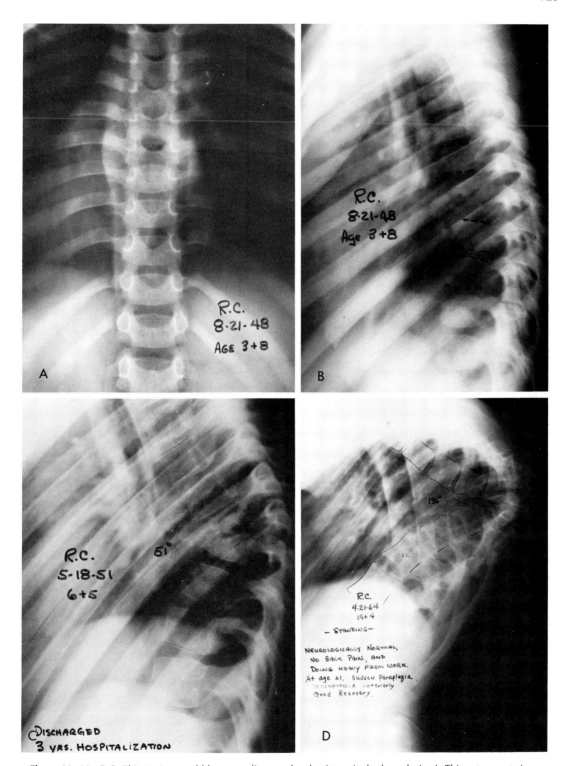

**Figure 23–44** R.C. This 3+8 year old boy was diagnosed as having spinal tuberculosis. *A,* This anteroposterior x-ray shows a paravertebral soft tissue mass. *B,* The lateral x-ray on admission shows vertebral destruction and kyphosis due to the vertebral collapse. *C,* Treatment consisted of bed rest for 2½ years with "diet, vitamins, and sunshine." This lateral x-ray on discharge shows destruction of three vertebral bodies with a 51 degree kyphosis. *D,* At age 9+7 there was the sudden onset of spastic paraparesis treated with a costotransversectomy with full return of function. A posterior fusion was performed a year later. At age 19+4 the lateral x-ray shows that the kyphosis had increased to 135 degrees. He was neurologically normal with no back pain and was doing heavy farm work. Two years later there was the onset of paraplegia.

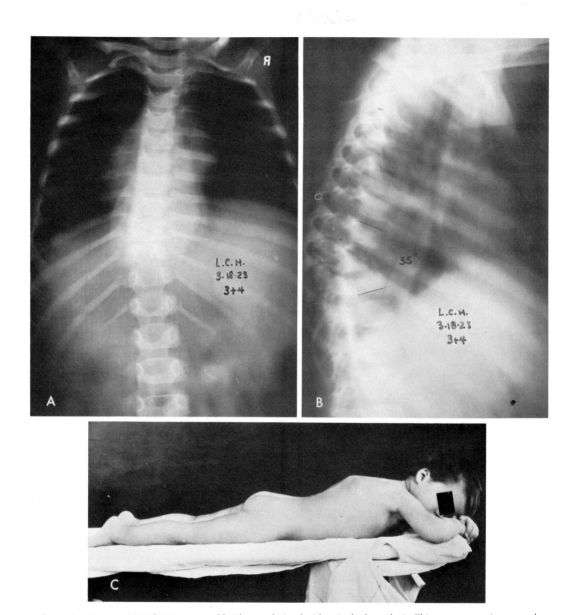

**Figure 23–45** *A,* L.C.H. This 3+4 year old girl was admitted with spinal tuberculosis. This anteroposterior x-ray shows a large paravertebral abscess. *B,* The lateral x-ray on admission shows involvement of one vertebral body and a 35 degree kyphosis. *C,* Clinical photograph on admission shows the thoracic kyphosis. *D,* Treatment consisted of bed rest for 10 months. A body jacket was worn for 7 months and a Taylor brace thereafter. This lateral x-ray at age 10+9 shows that the infection has destroyed two vertebral bodies and the kyphosis has increased to 65 degrees. *E,* Clinical photograph at age 10+9 shows the increased kyphosis. *F,* A posterior fusion was performed at age 14. Forty-one years later the kyphosis is stable at 60 degrees. She is asymptomatic and works full-time as a medical secretary.

*Illustration continued on the opposite page*

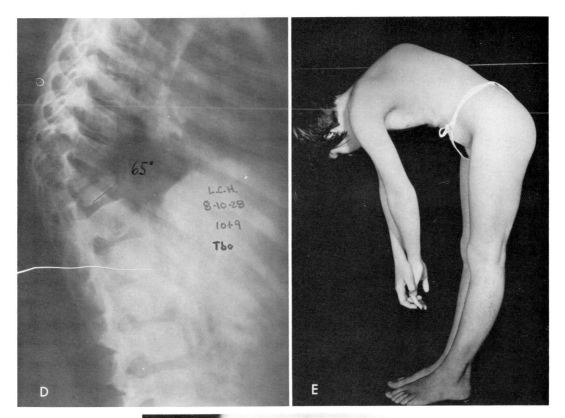

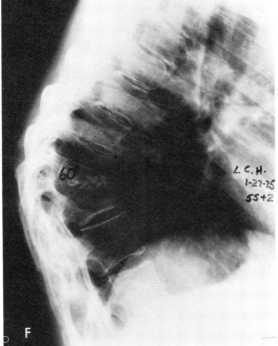

**Figure 23–45** *Continued    See legend on opposite page.*

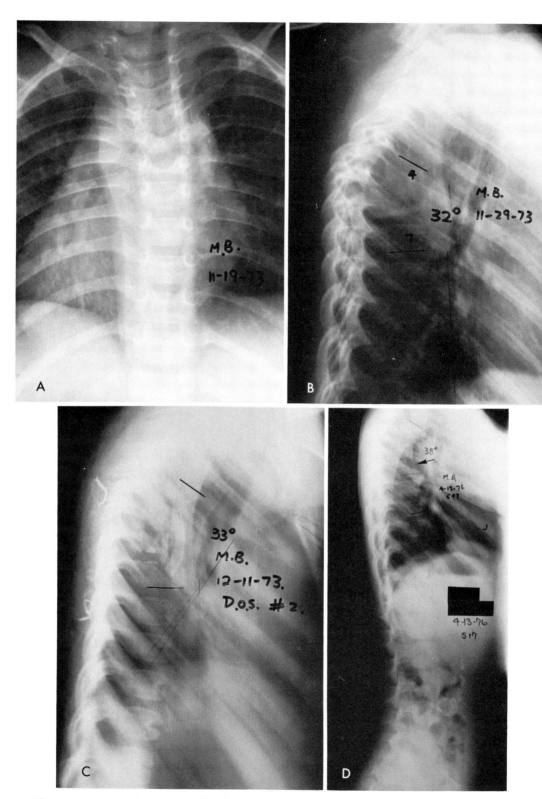

**Figure 23–46**   M.B. This 2+9 year old girl presented with spinal tuberculosis with marked systemic symptoms of two months' duration. *A,* This anteroposterior x-ray shows the marked paravertebral abscess. *B,* The lateral x-ray shows destruction involving three vertebral bodies with collapse and a 32 degree kyphosis. *C,* After two weeks of chemotherapy, an anterior exposure was undertaken with debridement and anterior fusion using rib struts. Two weeks later a posterior fusion was performed. This lateral x-ray on the day of the posterior fusion shows the anterior fusion. *D,* The fusion was held in a cast for six months, four months being supine. Two years later the lateral x-ray shows a solid fusion with a well-visualized anterior strut.

**632**

*Illustration continued on opposite page*

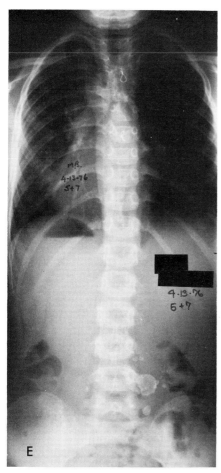

**Figure 23–46** *Continued* E, Anteroposterior x-ray shows no evidence of scoliosis.

children to 6 months in adults, total immobilization varying from 4 to 12 months, until a solid fusion is present. Using spot lateral and oblique x-rays, the fusion is assessed. In difficult cases laminography is valuable to determine the state of the anterior fusion and incorporation of the strut grafts.

## ACUTE DISEASE PLUS CORD INVOLVEMENT[1, 17, 40, 61, 65, 71]

In acute spinal tuberculosis the spinal cord can be involved in two ways: 1) pressure of the abscess with sequestra can compress the spinal cord; 2) the disease process extending through the meninges can involve the cord directly When present in the acute phase, the paraplegia or paraparesis is an indication for immediate operation. After starting chemotherapy, immediate operative decompression of the abscess is performed. The dura is carefully exposed and any granulation tissue carefully removed from its surface. If the dura does not pulsate, consideration should be given to incising the dura and inspecting the cord for a tuberculoma or tuberculous involvement.

After decompression an anterior fusion is performed, the treatment being the same as that described above. Usually after evacuation of the abscess and relief of external pressure on the cord, neurologic return is rapid and complete. If there is direct involvement of the spinal cord, recovery is rare.

## LATE KYPHOTIC DEFORMITY

Spinal tuberculosis with healing results in a kyphotic deformity. The greater the number of vertebrae destroyed by the infection, the greater is the anterior instability and the greater will be the kyphosis. The most severe deformities are found at the thoracolumbar junction, followed by midthoracic and cervicothoracic kyphosis. Midthoracic kyphosis is associated with impairment of pulmonary function. Thus patients with kyphosis present with complaints of pain in the area of the kyphos or pain secondary to the compensatory lordosis and rarely with pain due to pulmonary decompensation. The kyphosis can also result in spinal cord compression and paraplegia.

***Kyphosis Alone.***[33, 39] Surgical treatment of the kyphosis can be either stabilization of the kyphosis to prevent increase or correc-

addition to rib bone, owing to its greater osteogenic potential. Postoperatively the patient is nursed on a regular bed with gentle regular turning.

In young children there is the possibility of posterior growth resulting in increasing kyphosis. In addition, in these cases, because of the very soft rib bone, graft fracture, displacement, and fibrous union can occur. To minimize these complications, a posterior fusion of the involved area of the spine should be added two weeks later using autologous iliac bone graft (Fig. 23–46). In adults, where anterior stability is in jeopardy because of extensive bony loss, the addition of a posterior fusion with Harrington instrument will improve the stability.[19, 40]

All patients are placed in a cast 7 to 10 days postoperatively. A period of bed rest is used varying from 2 to 3 months in young

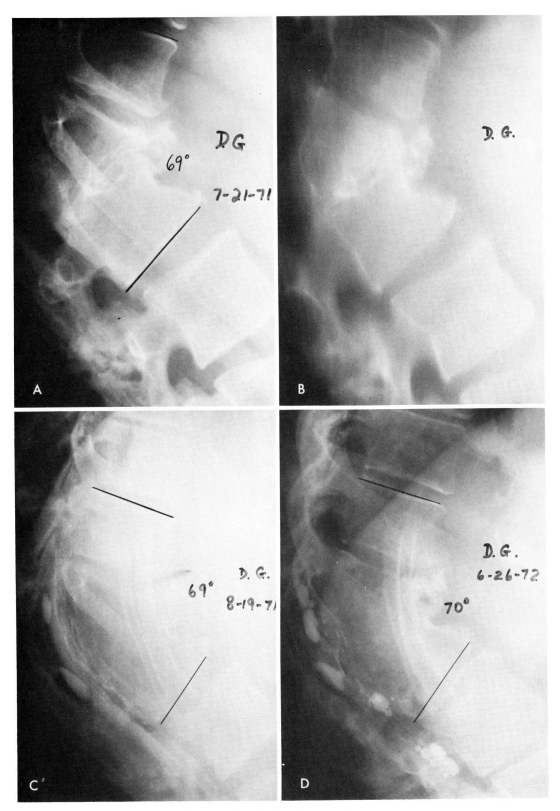

**Figure 23–47** *See legend on opposite page.*

tion and stabilization of the deformity. Stabilization requires an anterior exposure with debridement of any caseous material and chronic fibrosis with insertion of multiple anterior strut grafts. The most anterior strut needs to be strong, and fibula is often used for this.

Surgical correction of the deformity is difficult, as the kyphosis is rigid. After preoperative evaluation, including pulmonary function tests and laminography of the area of kyphosis, a staged surgical procedure is carried out, as pioneered by Yau et al.[80]

   i) Application of the halopelvic apparatus.
  ii) Anterior spinal osteotomy and decompression of the spinal canal.
 iii) Posterior osteotomy where spontaneous fusion is present—this is either seen on laminography or discovered after an initial period of distraction.
  iv) Distraction in the halopelvic apparatus with a special pad fitted to apply pressure to the kyphosis.
   v) Anterior fusion, after maximal correction obtained.
  vi) Posterior spinal fusion two weeks later, fusion extending into the compensatory curves above and below the kyphosis.
 vii) Postoperative immobilization in the halopelvic apparatus for six to eight weeks, followed by a cast till the fusion is solid.

The average correction after this series of procedures is very meager and perhaps not worth the halopelvic distraction and prolonged treatment. With the use of the Pinto distractor anteriorly, similar correction is obtainable, making the halopelvic distraction unnecessary.

***Kyphosis Plus Paraplegia.***[6, 40, 46] In a case of healed inactive tuberculosis, late-onset paraplegia occurs owing to one of two causes.[40] With increasing kyphosis the spinal cord is stretched over the bone anteriorly with compression and resulting neurologic loss. This is the commonest cause of late-onset paraplegia. More rarely the healing granulation and fibrous tissue constrict the cord.

Evaluation of the late-onset paraplegia includes laminography and myelography (see page 37). In the past, laminectomy was the approach used for operative decompression, but this gave very poor results. Menard, in 1900, pointed out the fact that the compression occurs from the *front* of the spinal cord and that in most cases the neural arch, which is removed at laminectomy, is not in contact with the compressed spinal cord.[58] He pioneered an anterior decompression via a costotransversectomy approach with rapid improvement of nerve function. This approach fell into disfavor following a series of fatal complications. Seddon, in his classic on Pott's paraplegia in 1935,[65] pointed out the role of anterior compression and the futility of laminectomy. Since the anterior approach of Hodgson and Stock[40] anterior decompression has become a safe and effective method to remove this bone.

Using an anterior transthoracic approach the apex of the kyphos is visualized, and all residual caseous material removed. The bone compressing the spinal cord is removed, and the spine is stabilized using an anterior fusion (see page 518) (Fig. 23–47). When there is a significant amount of fibrosis on the surface of the dura, this is carefully removed until dural pulsations return. In the attempts to remove this fibrous tissue a dural leak and cerebrospinal fluid fistula can result.

With the application of these treatment principles, the acute disease, chronic disease, and cases with spinal cord compression can be appropriately treated.

---

**Figure 23–47** *A,* D.G. This 37-year-old male was treated for spinal tuberculosis and tuberculous meningitis at age 14. He presented with progressive spastic paraparesis of three weeks' duration. The lateral x-ray shows a T11–L1 69 degree kyphosis. *B,* A laminogram showed a knuckle of bone protruding posteriorly into the spinal canal. A myelogram showed a partial obstruction at this level with anterior compression of the dye column. *C,* An anterior transthoracic spinal cord decompression was performed, and the spine was stabilized using an anterior fusion with rib strut grafts. This lateral x-ray two weeks postoperatively shows the kyphosis of 69 degrees and the strut grafts. *D,* The patient was uncooperative postoperatively and would not remain supine. He did not tolerate the holding casts and was held in a Milwaukee brace. Ten months later evaluation showed full return of function, and this x-ray shows the kyphosis stabilized at 70 degrees with a solid anterior fusion.

## References

1. Ahn, B. H.: Treatment for Pott's paraplegia. Acta Orthop. Scand., *39*:145, 1968.
2. Alexander, G. L.: On neurological complications of spinal tuberculosis. Proc. R. Soc. Med., *39*:730, 1946.
2A. Arct, W.: Operative treatment of tuberculosis of the spine in old people. J. Bone Surg., *50A*:255–267, 1968.
3. Bailey, H. L., Gabriel, M., Hodgson, A. R., and Shin, J. S.: Tuberculosis of the spine in children. Operative findings and results in one hundred consecutive patients treated by removal of the lesion and anterior grafting. J. Bone Joint Surg., *54A*: 1633–1657, 1972.
4. Batson, O. V.: The vertebral vein system. Caldwell Lecture 1956. Am. J. Roentgenol. Radium. Ther. Nucl. Med., *78(2)*:194–212, 1957.
5. Blocklock, J. W. S.: Injury as an etiological factor in tuberculosis. Proc. R. Soc. Med., *50*:61–68, 1956.
6. Bouvier, H.: Leçons Cliniques sur les Maladies Chroniques de l'Appareil Locomoteur. Paris, Bailliere, 1858.
7. Capener, N.: The evolution of lateral rachotomy. J. Bone Joint Surg., *36B*:173, 1954.
8. Center for Disease Control: Atlanta, Personal communication, 1977.
8A. Chu, C. B.: Treatment of spinal tuberculosis in Korea using focal debridement and interbody fusion. Clin. Orthop., *50*:235–253, 1967.
9. Clemns, H. J.: Die Venensysteme der menschlichen Wirbelsäule. Berlin, Gruyther, 1961.
10. Derry, O. G.: Pott's disease in ancient Egypt. Med. Press Circ., July, 1938, pp. 196–200.
11. Dickson, J. A. S.: Spinal tuberculosis in Nigerian children. J. Bone Joint Surg., *49B*:682–694, 1967.
12. Dott, N. M.: Skeletal traction and anterior decompression in the management of Pott's paraplegia. Edinb. Med. J., *54*:62, 1947.
13. Eckenhoff, J. E.: Circulatory control in the surgical patient. Ann. R. Coll., Surg. Engl., *39*:67, 1966.
14. Editorial: Tuberculosis of the Spine. Br. Med. J., *4(5945)*:613, 1974.
15. Elliot, Smith, G., and Dawson, W. R.: Egyptian Mummies. London, 1924, p. 157.
16. Fang, H. S. Y., Ong, G. B., and Hodgson, A. R.: Anterior spinal fusion. The operative approaches. Clin. Orthop., *35*:16–33, 1964.
17. Felländer, M.: Paraplegia in spondylitis—results of operative treatment. Paraplegia, *13*:75, 1975.
18. Felländer, M.: Radical operation in tuberculosis of the spine. Acta Orthop. Scand., Suppl. 19, 1955.
19. Fountain, S. S., Hsu, L. C. S., Yau, A. C. M. C., and Hodgson, A. R.: Progressive kyphosis following solid anterior spine fusion in children with tuberculosis of the spine. J. Bone Joint Surg., *57A*:1104, 1975.
20. Friedman, B.: Chemotherapy of tuberculosis of the spine. J. Bone Joint Surg., *48A*:451–474, 1966.
21. Ghobadi, F., Potenza, A. D., and DiBenedetto, A.: Spinal tuberculosis—treatment by debridement and anterior spine fusion. N.Y. State J. Med., *75*:1827, 1975.
22. Ghormley, R. K., and Bradley, J. I.: Prognostic signs in the x-rays of tuberculous spines in children. J. Bone Joint Surg., *10*:796–803, 1928.
23. Griffiths, D. L., Seddon, H. J., and Roaf, R.: Pott's Paraplegia. London, Oxford University Press, 1956.
24. Hadra, B. E.: Wiring the vertebrae as a means of immobilization in fractures and Pott's disease. Med. Times Register, *22*:423, 1891, reprinted in Clin. Orthop., *112*:4, 1975.
25. Henriques, C. Q.: Osteomyelitis as a complication of urology. Br. J. Surg., *46*:19–28, 1948.
26. Herlihy, W. F.: Revision of the venous system; the role of the vertebral veins. Aust. Med. J., *34*:661, 1947.
27. Herlihy, W. F.: Experimental Studies in the Internal Vertebral Venous Plexus. Essays in Biology, 151, 1948.
28. Hibbs, R. A.: An operation for progressive spinal deformities. N.Y. Med. J., *93*:1013, 1911.
29. Hippocrates: The Genuine Works of Hippocrates. Translated by F. Adams. London, The Sydenham Society, 1849.
30. Hodgson, A. R., and Stock, F. E.: Anterior spinal fusion. A preliminary communication on the radical treatment of Pott's disease and Pott's paraplegia. Br. J. Surg., *44(185)*:266–275, 1956.
31. Hodgson, A. R., and Stock, F. E.: Anterior spinal fusion. In Rob, C., and Smith, R. (eds.): Operative Surgery. London, Butterworths, 1960.
32. Hodgson, A. R., Stock, F. E., Fang, H. S. Y., and Ong, G. B.: Anterior spinal fusion. The operative approach and pathological fidings in 412 patients with Pott's disease of the spine. Br. J. Surg., *48*:172, 1960.
33. Hodgson, A. R.: Correction of fixed spinal curves. A preliminary communication. J. Bone Joint Surg., *47A(6)*:1221, 1965.
34. Hodgson, A. R., Yau, A. C. M. C., Kwon, J. S., and Kim, D.: A clinical study of 100 consecutive cases of Pott's paraplegia. Paraplegia, *5*:1–16, 1967.
35. Hodgson, A. R., Skinsnes, O. K., and Leong, C. Y.: The pathogenesis of Pott's paraplegia. J Bone Joint Surg., *49A*:1147–1156, 1967.
36. Hodgson, A. R., and Yau, A. C. M. C.: Vordere Operative Zugänge sur Wirbelsäule. Stuttgart, Georg. Thieme Verlag, 1969.
37. Hodgson, A. R., and Yau, A. C. M. C.: Anterior surgical approaches to the spinal column. In Recent Advances in Orthopaedics. London, Churchill, 1969.
38. Hodgson, A. R., Wong, W., and Yau, A. C. M. C.: X-ray Appearances of Tuberculosis of the Spine. Springfield, Ill., Charles C Thomas, 1969.
39. Hodgson, A. R.: Correction of spinal deformities. Proc. Le Roy. Abbott Soc., *2*:9, 1972.
40. Hodgson, A. R.: Infectious disease of the spine. In Rothman, R. M., and Simeone, F. A. (eds.): The Spine. Philadelphia, W.B. Saunders Co., 1975.
41. Hodgson, A. R., and Stock, F. E.: Anterior spine fusion for the treatment of tuberculosis of the spine. J. Bone Joint Surg., *42A*:295, 1960.
42. Hodgson, A. R., Stock, F. E., Fang, H. S. Y., and Ong, G. B.: Anterior spinal fusion—the operative approach and pathological findings in 412 patients with Pott's disease of the spine. Br. J. Surg., *48*:172–178, 1960.
43. Ito, H., Tsuchiya, J. and Asami, G.: A new radical operation for Pott's disease. J. Bone Joint Surg., *16*:499, 1934.

44. Jenkins, D. H. R., Hodgson, A. R., Yau, A. C. M. C., Dwyer, A. P., and O'Mahoney, G.: Stabilization of the spine in the surgical treatment of severe spinal tuberculosis in children. Clin. Orthop., 110:69, 1975.

45. Johnson, R. W., Hillman, J. W., and Southwick, W. O.: The importance of direct surgical attack upon lesions of the vertebral bodies, particularly in Pott's disease. J. Bone Joint Surg., 35A:17, 1953.

46. Jones, B. S.: The management of late onset Pott's paraplegia caused by a bony ridge. S. Afr. Med. J., 46:1664, 1972.

47. Kaplan, C. J.: Conservative therapy in skeletal tuberculosis—an appraisal based on experience in South Africa. Tubercle (London), 40:355–368, 1959.

48. Kondo, E., and Yamada, K.: End results of focal debridement in bone and joint tuberculosis and its indications. J. Bone Joint Surg., 39A:27–31, 1957.

49. Konstam, P. G., and Blesovsky, A.: The ambulant treatment of spinal tuberculosis. Br. J. Surg., 50:26–38, 1962.

50. Konstam, P. G., and Konstam, S. T.: Spinal tuberculosis in southern Nigeria, with special reference to ambulant treatment of thoraco-lumbar disease. J. Bone Joint Surg., 40B:26–32, 1958.

51. Kulowski, J.: Pyogenic osteomyelitis of the spine. An analysis and discussion of 102 cases. J. Bone Joint Surg., 18:343–364, 1936.

52. Martin, N. S.: Tuberculosis of the spine—a study of the results of treatment during the last twenty-five years. J. Bone Joint Surg., 52B:613, 1970.

53. Medical Research Council Working Party on Tuberculosis of the Spine: A controlled trial of ambulant out-patient treatment and in-patient rest in bed in the management of tuberculosis of the spine in young Korean patients on standard chemotherapy. A study in Masan, Korea. J. Bone Joint Surg., 55B:678–697, 1973.

54. Medical Research Council Working Party on Tuberculosis of the Spine: A controlled trial of plaster-of-Paris jackets in the management of ambulant out-patient treatment of tuberculosis of the spine in children on standard chemotherapy—a study in Pusan, Korea. Tubercle, 54:261–282, 1973.

55. Medical Research Council Working Party on Tuberculosis of the Spine: A controlled trial of débridement and ambulatory treatment in the management of tuberculosis of the spine in patients on standard chemotherapy. A study in Bulawayo, Rhodesia. J. Trop. Med. Hyg., 77:72–92, 1974.

56. Medical Research Council Working Party on Tuberculosis of the Spine: A controlled trial of anterior spinal fusion and débridement in the surgical management of tuberculosis of the spine in patients on standard chemotherapy—a study in Hong Kong. Br. J. Surg., 61:853–866, 1974.

57. Medical Research Council Working Party on Tuberculosis of the Spine: A five year assessment of controlled trials of in-patient and out-patient treatment of plaster-of-paris jackets for tuberculosis of the spine in children on standard chemotherapy. J. Bone Joint Surg., 58B:399, 1976.

58. Menard, V.: Etude Pratique sur le Mal de Pott. Paris, Masson et Cie, 1900.

59. Orell, S.: Chemotherapy and surgical treatment in bone and joint tuberculosis. Acta Orthop. Scand., 21:190–203, 1941.

60. Paus, B.: Treatment for tuberculosis of the spine. Acta Orthop. Scand., Suppl. 72, 1964.

61. Pott, P.: Remarks on That Kind of Palsy of the Lower Limbs Which Is Frequently Found to Accompany a Curvature of the Spine. London, J. Johnson, 1779.

62. Puig Guri, J.: The formation and significance of vertebral ankylosis in tuberculous spines. J. Bone Joint Surg., 29:136–148, 1947.

63. Rauch, R. N. L.: Spinal Caries: Surgical debridement versus radical resection and bone grafting. J. Bone Joint Surg., 57B:261, 1975.

64. Riska, E. B.: Spinal tuberculosis treated by antituberculous chemotherapy and radical operation. Clin. Orthop., 119:148, 1976.

65. Seddon, H. J.: Pott's Paraplegia—prognosis and treatment. Br. J. Surg., 22:769–799, 1935.

66. Seward, D. N. L.: Some problems in diagnosis and management of spinal tuberculosis. Med. J. Aust., 1:822, 1976.

67. Smith, T.: Tuberculosis. Paper presented at AAOS continuing education course, San Diego, Dec. 3, 1976.

68. Stevenson, F. H., and Manning, C. W.: Tuberculosis of the spine treated conservatively with chemotherapy—series of 72 patients collected 1949–1954, and followed to 1961. Tubercle (London), 43:406–411, 1962.

69. Swett, P. P., Bennett, G. E., and Street, D. M.: Pott's disease: The initial lesion, the relative infrequency of extension by contiguity, the nature and type of healing, the role of the abscess and the merits of operative and non-operative treatment. J. Bone Joint Surg., 22:815–823, 1940

70. Tuli, S. M.: Results of treatment of spinal tuberculosis by "middle-path" regime. J. Bone Joint Surg., 57B:13, 1975.

71. Tuli, S. M.: Treatment of neurological complications in tuberculosis of the spine. J. Bone Joint Surg., 51A:680–692, 1969.

72. Tuli, S. M.: Treatment of tuberculosis of the spine—a review. Indian J. Surg., 35:195–213, 1973.

73. Tuli, S. M. Brighton, C. T., Morton, H. E., and Clark, L. W.: Experimental induction of localized skeletal tuberculous lesions and accessibility of such lesions to antituberculous drugs. J. Bone Joint Surg., 56B:551–559, 1974.

74. Tuli, S. M., and Kumar, S.: Early results of treatment of spinal tuberculosis by triple drug therapy. Clin. Orthop., 81:56–70, 1971.

75. Tuli, S. M., Srivastava, T. P., Varma, B. P., and Sinha, G. P.: Tuberculosis of spine. Acta Orthop. Scand., 38:445–458, 1967.

76. Wilkes, L. L., and Colmers, R. A.: Tuberculous spondylitis. J. Med. Assoc. Ga., 65:9, 1976.

77. Wilkinson, M. C.: The treatment of tuberculosis of the spine by evacuation of the paravertebral abscess and curettage of the vertebral bodies. J. Bone Joint Surg., 37B:382–391, 1955.

78. Wilkinson, M. C.: Tuberculosis of the spine treated by chemotherapy and operative debridement. J. Bone Joint Surg., 51A:1331–1342, 1969.

79. Williams, N. E.: Spinal tuberculosis. Proc. R. Soc. Med., 68:545, 1975.

80. Yau, A. C. M. C., Hsu, L. C. S., O'Brien, J. P., and Hodson, A. R.: Tuberculous kyphosis treatment with spinal osteotomy, halo pelvic distraction and anterior and posterior fusion. J. Bone Joint Surg., 56A:1419, 1974.

# CONGENITAL HEART DISEASE
# AND SCOLIOSIS

## INTRODUCTION

There is a strong relationship between scoliosis and congenital heart disease. The incidence of "idiopathic-like" scoliosis in patients with congenital heart disease is 10 times that of idiopathic scoliosis in the population as a whole. In addition, patients with congenital scoliosis may have a coexistent congenital heart defect. The significant problems of patient management make this a relevant subject.

## LITERATURE REVIEW

Several authors have commented upon the increased incidence of scoliosis in patients with congenital heart disease.[1, 3, 4, 5, 7, 9, 10, 11] If these were all congenital scoliotics, we would

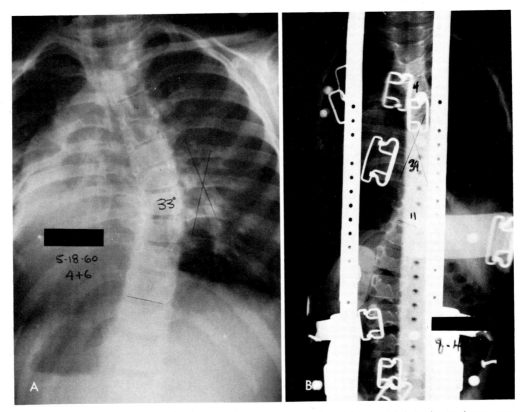

**Figure 23–48**   A, A four-year-old girl with coarctation of the aorta and an atrial septal defect. This 33 degree curve was noted on a chest x-ray. Note the cardiac enlargement. B, She was placed in a Milwaukee brace, but no correction was obtained. C, At age 8, her curve is noted to have reached 48 degrees. She was lost to orthopedic follow-up at this time. D, She was finally seen again for orthopedic care at age 14, having been under the care of pediatricians and cardiovascular surgeons in the interim. She had not worn her brace since age 8. The atrial septal defect was repaired at age 9. E, She was placed in halofemoral traction, and the primary thoracic curve was corrected from 92 degrees to 54 degrees. Her lumbar curve, originally secondary, is now a major curve also. It was corrected from 72 degrees to 52 degrees. F, One year post-fusion, her curves measure 57 degrees and 50 degrees. She had no complications during or following surgery.

*Illustration continued on the opposite page*

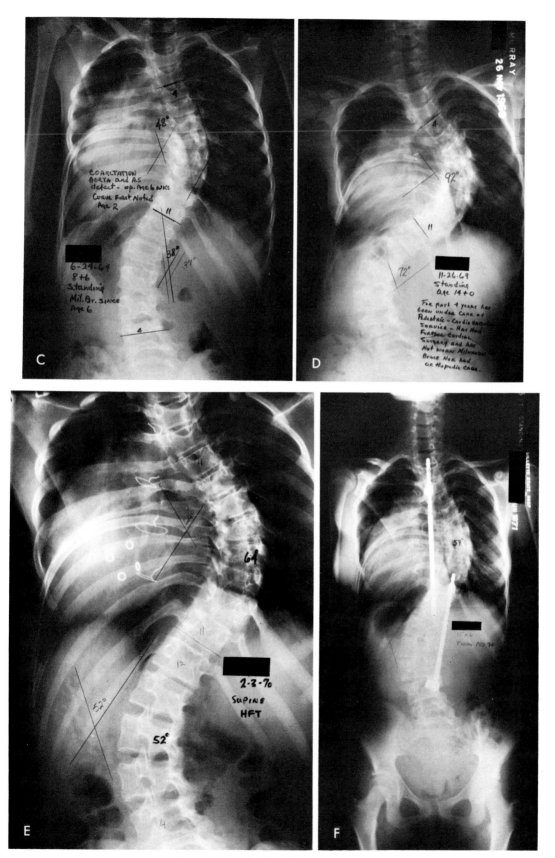

**Figure 23–48** *See legend on opposite page.*

not be very surprised. However, most of these scoliotics have an idiopathic type curvature. By this it is meant that there are no visible vertebral anomalies and no curve at birth, and the patterns of curvature as well as the behavior of the curve are quite similar to idiopathic scoliosis.

The reader is referred to the excellent paper by Reckles and co-workers from the Mayo Clinic,[8] who have analyzed this problem in detail. They found the incidence of congenital heart defects among the adolescent scoliosis population was 5 per cent, a figure 10 times greater than the incidence of congenital heart disease in the population at large. The incidence of idiopathic-like scoliosis with curves greater than 20 degrees among patients with congenital heart defects (followed for at least 10 years after cardiac surgery) was 8.5 per cent. This is 10 times greater than the population at large. These same authors found no significant correlation between scoliosis and sex, type of cardiac anomaly, size of heart, side of heart, side of aortic arch, cyanosis, age at surgery, number and type of surgical incisions, number and side of ribs removed, or number and type of surgical procedures.

Luke and McDonnell[4] reviewed 3540 patients with congenital heart disease. There were 850 with cyanotic heart disease. Of these, 51 (6 per cent) had scoliosis. There were 2690 with noncyanotic heart disease. Of these, 22 (0.8 per cent) had scoliosis. They felt that there was definitely a strong correlation with cyanotic heart disese. They found no correlation with the side of the aortic arch or the side of the thoracotomy and the side of the scoliosis. There was no relationship between the severity of cyanosis and the severity of the curve.

Roth et al.[9] reviewed 500 consecutive patients in the heart clinic at Boston Children's Hospital. Scoliosis of greater than 10 degrees was noted in 12 per cent, and scoliosis greater than 20 degrees in 4.6 per cent. There was a 28.4 per cent incidence in those with cyanotic heart disease versus 8.7 per cent in those with noncyanotic heart disease. The lower the arterial oxygen saturation, the greater was the incidence of scoliosis. The highest incidence, however, was in patients with simple coarctation, 30 per cent of whom had curves of 10 degrees or more[7] (35 out of 115). Forty per cent of the males and 26 per cent of the females with coarcta-

tion had scoliosis. Twenty-eight curves were between 10 and 19 degrees. Six curves were between 20 and 29 degrees, and only one curve was severe.

Zorab[12] has noted that electrocardiographic abnormalities indicate true heart conditions and cannot be attributed to alterations of the thorax by the curve.

Thus, in summary, there is a high incidence of idiopathic type scoliosis in patients with congenital heart disease. There is probably a strong correlation with cyanotic heart disease.

## TREATMENT

Because the patient with congenital heart disease is usually under treatment by the medical profession, there should be no difficulty in early detection of the scoliosis. Scoliosis should be sought in all chest x-rays in these patients (Fig. 23–48). If a curve of 10 degrees or more is noted, consultation with an orthopedist knowledgeable about scoliosis should be obtained. Progressive curves of 15 degrees or more and established curves of 20 degrees or more should be treated aggressively by bracing in the growing child. One should be even more aggressive about starting brace treatment early in these children because a) we have the feeling that the larger curves do less well in braces than do the usual idiopathic, and b) the surgical risks may be much higher.

Children with congenital heart disease, especially those with cyanotic heart disease, are slow to reach the end of growth. Treatment must continue until skeletal growth is complete, no matter what the chronologic age. The techniques of bracing are no different from those used with the idiopathic scoliosis (see Chapter 15).

A patient with congenital heart disease should not be denied adequate scoliosis surgery. However, surgical treatment presents special hazards and problems. Bunch[2] pointed out that patients with cyanotic congenital heart disease may have "functional thrombocytopenia" with low normal platelet counts, normal Factor VIII, and decreased Factor V. Congenital heart patients tolerate variations in fluid replacement poorly during surgery, so the volumes must be precisely measured. A central venous pressure catheter is strongly recommended along with controlled monitoring of blood gases. For patients with heart block or other arrhythmias, a transvenous pacemaker can be extremely valuable.

Surgery of congenital heart patients should always be undertaken in an institution capable of performing such monitoring activity, in terms of both equipment and personnel. The principles of surgery are the same as for the patient with idiopathic scoliosis.

## References

1. Beals, R. V., Kenney, K. H., and Lees, M. H.: Congenital heart disease and idiopathic scoliosis. Clin. Orthop., 89:112–116, 1972.
2. Bunch, W. H., and Komp, D. M.: Surgical correction of scoliosis in a child with hemostatic abnormalities secondary to congenital heart disease. Clin. Orthop., 89:139–142, 1972.
3. Jordan, C. E., White, R. I., Fisher, K. C., Neill, C., and Dorst, J. P.: The scoliosis of congenital heart disease. Am. Heart J., 84:463–469, 1972.
4. Luke, M. J., and McDonnell, E. J.: Congenital heart disease and scoliosis. J. Pediatr., 73:725–733, 1968.
5. Marisaki, N.: Spinal scoliosis associated with congenital heart disease. J. Japn. Orthop. Assoc., 38:699–700, 1964.
6. Nilsen, N. Ö.: Anomalies in derivatives from the visceral arches combined with congenital heart defects. Scand. J. Thorac. Cardiovasc. Surg., 3:211–214, 1969.
7. Poitras, B., Rosenthal, J., and Hall, J.: Scoliosis and coarctation of the aorta. J. Pediatr., 86:476–477, 1975.
8. Reckles, L. N., Peterson, H. A., Bianco, A. J., and Weidman, W. H.: The association of scoliosis and congenital heart disease. J. Bone Joint Surg., 57A:449–455, 1975.
9. Roth, A., Rosenthal, A., Hall, J. E., and Mizel, M.: Scoliosis and congenital heart disease. Clin. Orthop., 93:95–102, 1973.
10. White, R. I., Jordan, C. E., Fisher, K. C., Lampton, L., Neill, C., and Dorst, J. P.: Skeletal changes associated with adolescent congenital heart disease. Am. J. Roentgenol., 116:531–538, 1972.
11. Wright, W. D., and Niebauer, J. J.: Congenital heart disease and scoliosis. J. Bone Joint Surg., 38A:1131–1136, 1956.
12. Zorab, P.: The cardiac aspects of scoliosis. Scoliosis Research Society, 1973.

# SCOLIOSIS AND CONGENITAL LIMB DEFICIENCY

## INTRODUCTION

Although isolated case reports had appeared earlier, such as that by Epps,[1] scoliosis in association with congenital upper limb deficiency was not recognized as an entity until the report by Makley and Heiple in 1970.[2] The authors of this book have also noted the strong relationship between congenital upper limb deficiency (complete or partial) and an idiopathic type scoliosis.

## INCIDENCE

In the review by Makley and Heiple there were 27 patients with major limb deficiencies. There were 18 patients with radial hemimelia, of whom 9 had scoliosis, and 7 of the 9 had an idiopathic type scoliosis. There were 6 patients with ulnar hemimelia, 4 of whom had scoliosis, and all 4 were idiopathic. Three patients had amelia or phocomelia, and 2 had scoliosis, both idiopathic. Thus, the incidence of *significant* scoliosis was 48 per cent. Five patients underwent spine fusion. Congenital anomalies were *not* noted at surgery.

Makley and Heiple also found no increased incidence of scoliosis in minor limb anomalies such as syndactylism or thumb hypoplasia. Congenital anomalies of the upper extremities, especially Sprengel's deformity (congenital elevation of the scapula) are frequently associated with congenital scoliosis. Such congenital scolioses may or may not be a problem, and for these, the reader is referred to Chapter 7.

## TREATMENT

These curves may appear at any time during growth but have a strong tendency to develop in the infantile (0 to 3) and juvenile (3 to 10) years. Because of the many years

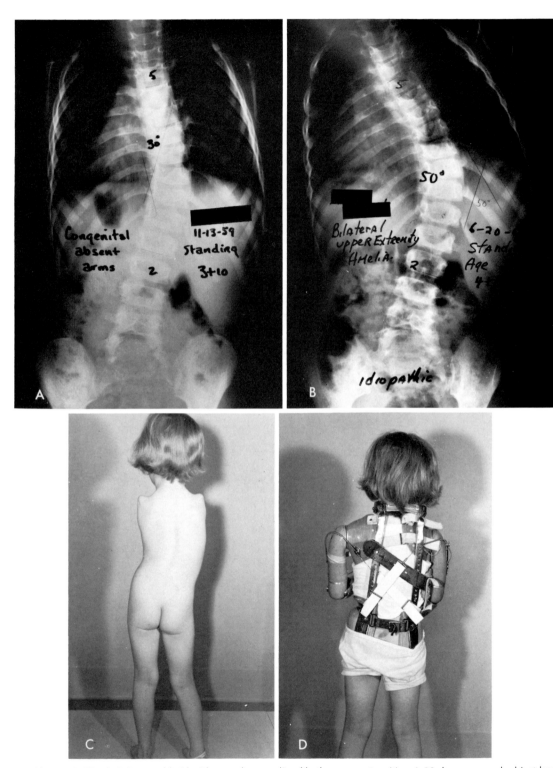

**Figure 23–49** *A,* A 3-year-old girl with complete amelia of both upper extremities. A 30 degree curve had just been noted. There were no anomalous vertebrae. No treatment was given. *B,* Seven months later, the curve had progressed to 50 degrees. A Milwaukee brace was applied. *C,* A photograph at age 4 years, 5 months. *D,* A photograph at age 6 showing the Milwaukee brace plus bilateral upper extremity prostheses.

*Illustration continued on the opposite page*

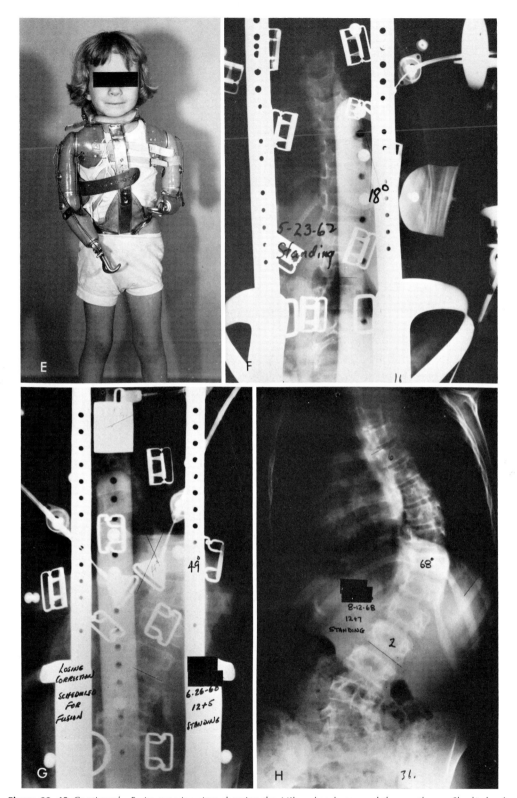

**Figure 23–49** *Continued E,* An anterior view showing the Milwaukee brace and the prostheses. She had voluntary control over both elbow joints and both terminal devices. *F,* An x-ray at age 6 showing excellent control of the curve at 18 degrees. *G,* She did well until age 12 when the curve relentlessly began increasing despite full-time brace use. This curve increase coincided with her growth spurt. *H,* An x-ray out of the brace showed increase to 68 degrees. Fusion was obviously necessary.

*Illustration continued on the following page*

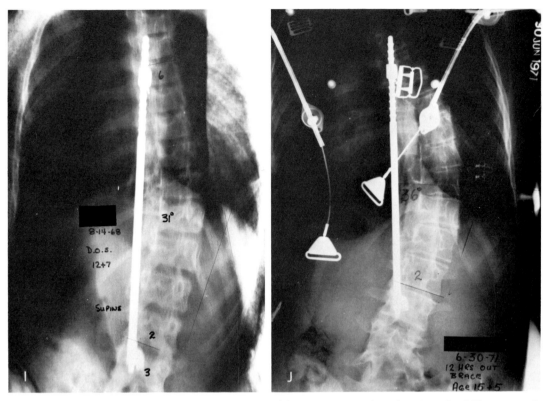

**Figure 23–49** *Continued* *I*, Standard instrumentation and fusion were carried out from T5 to L3. *J*, Three years after fusion and now age 15, the fusion is solid and the curve measures 26 degrees. At age 21 she is employed in a bank and is self-supporting. She requires assistance only in donning her prostheses each morning.

of growth remaining, very severe curves can occur if not treated.

There has been a disturbing tendency to avoid treating the curve because of the limb deficiency problem. All too often the statement is made, "The child can't tolerate too many gadgets, and the hand is most important." or "Torso motions are needed for the prosthesis, therefore we mustn't apply a spine brace." Such philosophies have frequently resulted in severe curve progression and a short, deformed child with poor pulmonary function and reduced self-image superimposed on the arm problem. In addition, such curves require surgical fusion, which may indeed be necessary but which may take away some needed torso movement.

We feel the spine must be vigorously treated. For thoracic curves (the usual problem), a Milwaukee brace is recommended (Fig. 23–49). Progressive curves of 20 degrees or more in the growing child must be braced to prevent further progression. Curves of 60 degrees or more cannot be braced and should be fused.

In the authors' experience, there has been an excellent benefit from the Milwaukee brace in its ability to control the scoliosis for many years (until the growth spurt), but fusion has seldom been altogether avoided (Fig. 23–50).

Since the pattern of scoliosis in these patients is identical to idiopathic scoliosis, the reader is referred to Chapter 6.

### References

1. Epps, C. H.: Upper extremity limb deficiency with concomitant infantile structural scoliosis. Inter-Clinic Information Bulletin, *5(2)*:1–9, Nov., 1965.

2. Makley, J. T., and Heiple, K. G.: Scoliosis associated with congenital deficiencies of the upper extremity. J. Bone Joint Surg., *52A*:279–287, 1970.

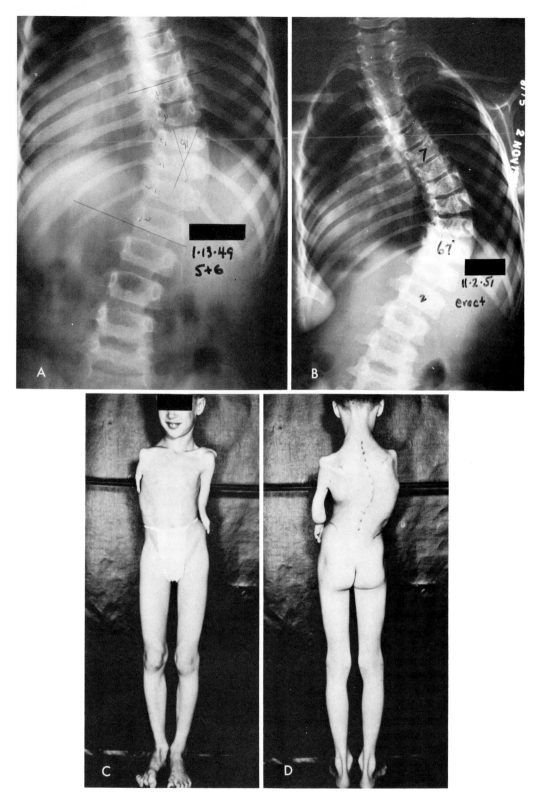

**Figure 23–50**  *A,* A five-year-old male with a 40 degree right thoracic scoliosis. No treatment was given. *B,* At age 8, his curve had increased to 67 degrees. Such increase should never be permitted. *C,* A photograph at age 8 showing the single digit at shoulder level on the right and a single digit at elbow level on the left. He was an accomplished toe-user. *D,* A posterior photograph at age 8 to show the scoliosis. He went on to fusion later but should have been braced when first noted at age 5.

**645**

# THORACIC CAGE DEFECTS AND CONTRACTURES WITH SCOLIOSIS

Three types of thoracogenic scolioses occur: those secondary to thoracoplasty, those secondary to empyema treatment by rib resection and drainage, and those due to resection of the thoracic wall for malignancy. Thoracogenic scoliosis has been recognized as a complication of major chest wall surgery for many decades.

## THORACOPLASTY

In the early years of the present century, thoracoplasty was an accepted method of treating pulmonary tuberculosis. As a result of massive rib resections and collapsing of the upper chest wall during growing years, the spine would curve to a varying degree toward the side of the rib resection. Factors within the thorax such as scarring on the opposite side producing contractural forces would add to the deformity. These curvatures were seldom severe. Since thoracoplasties are no longer done, spine curvatures of this etiology are mainly of historical interest. They are alike in causing scoliosis in the growing child but are productive of different varieties of contractures (Fig. 23–51).

## EMPYEMA

Thoracogenic scoliosis of a severe degree was a common result of empyema treated by rib resection and prolonged pleural drainage. Pleural and lung scarring frequently followed drainage of the purulent exudate, and the resultant spine curvature not only was severe but also was almost totally resistant to cast correction. During the decades before antibiotics we encountered a number of these. The severe lung scarring and thoracic deformity most often led to death from cardiopulmonary failure in adult years. The deformity was nearly always severe when the patient reached our scoliosis center, and our attempts at cast correction

and spine fusion were then failures. As in all infections, early drainage of the purulent exudate usually resulted in a relatively rapid cure, and scoliosis did not occur. The patients who came to our attention in the early days of our interest in scoliosis had severe scoliosis as a result of the massive scarring of the pleura and lung and had deformities that were always concave to the side opposite the involved lung. Fusion of ribs about the empyema fistula added to the contracture.

## RESECTION OF CHEST WALL

Thoracogenic scoliosis from defects in the thoracic wall may be the direct result of resection of large portions of the wall from local resection of malignancy. The scoliosis may result from a combination of thoracic wall resection coupled with radiation therapy. The convexity of the curve is to the side of the resected chest wall, and when performed early in life, the curvature is progressive and must be fused. It is not amenable to brace treatment except possibly when the curve is just beginning. A Milwaukee brace may temporarily control progression. Early fusion is the best answer to scoliosis resulting from chest wall resections. (Fig. 23–52).

Delay in treating progressive curves creates problems in pseudarthrosis. Most resections of the chest wall for malignancies are also treated with radiation. The vertebral bodies show the results of irradiation, becoming sclerotic and relatively avascular; additional problems in obtaining a solid fusion are created by poor skin coverage (Fig. 23–53).

Scoliosis secondary to chest wall resections is not common, but will create problems if progression is permitted to occur. As in all forms of scoliosis, early treatment by fusion gives the best results. The spine always curves toward the side of the chest wall defect.

*Text continued on page 652*

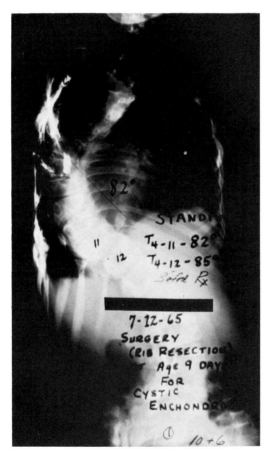

**Figure 23–51** M.E., age 10+6. Scoliosis resulting from total resection of left ribs at age 9 days for cystic enchondroma. The opacities represent attempted covering with foil. A severe curve developed which was not improved after several years' treatment with a Milwaukee brace. Her pulmonary function and scarring made surgical treatment of the scoliosis impossible. This patient died at age 20 of pulmonary complications.

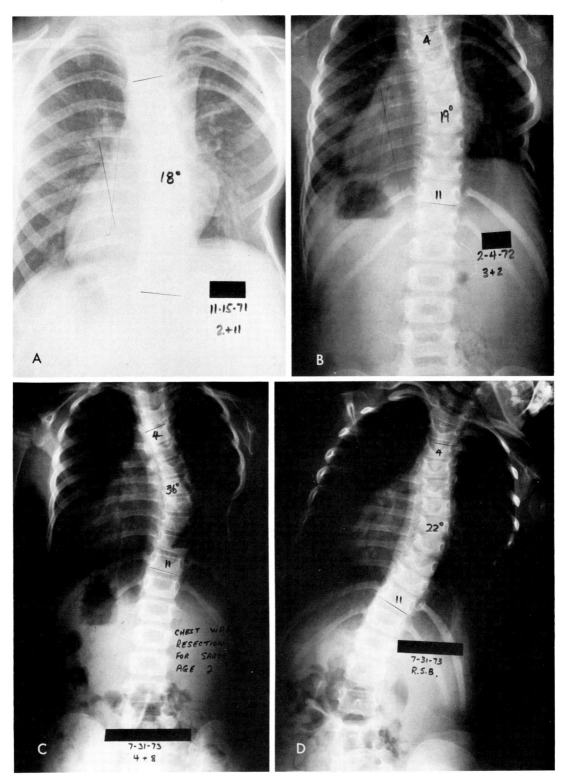

**Figure 23–52** *See legend on opposite page.*

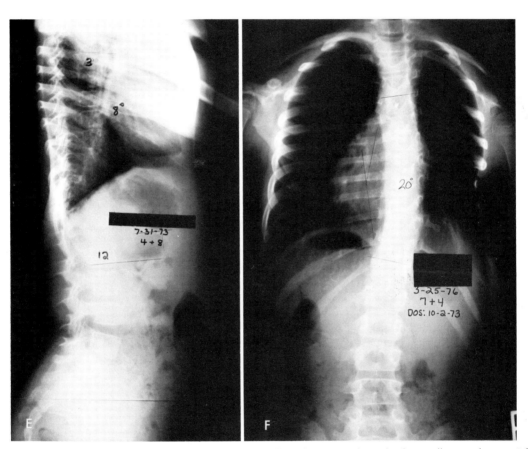

**Figure 23–52** *A*, M.P., age 2+11, 11/15/71. Thoracic scoliosis beginning after right chest wall removal at age 2 for sarcoma, *B*, M.P., age 3+2, 2/4/72. Chest wall defect with missing ribs clearly evident. The curve apex is toward the chest wall defect. *C*, M.P., age 4+8, 7/31/73. Curve increasing, with deformity more evident. *D*, M.P., 7/31/73. Marked structural nature of curve shown on R.S.B. film. *E*, M.P., 7/31/73. Lateral view shows 8 degrees kyphosis. *F*, M.P., age 7+4, 3/25/76. Spine fused at age 4+11. Good correction obtained and maintained at 20 degrees 3 years postoperatively.

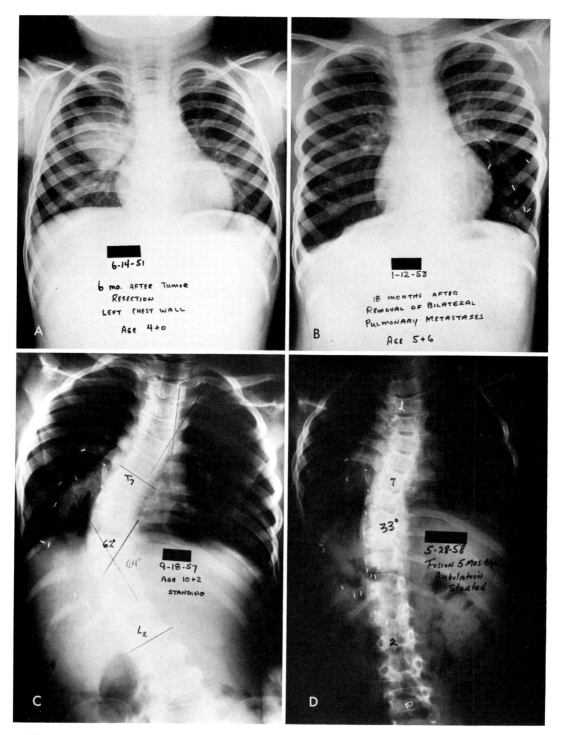

**Figure 23–53**  *A,* R.S., age 4, 6/14/51. Tumors under scapula noted at age 3½. Resection included two ribs, chest wall muscles, intercostal muscles, and pleura. The tumor was diagnosed as a rhabdomyosarcoma. *B,* R.S., age 5+6, 1/12/53. Metastasis to right lower lobe, resected 1951 (4 months after first operation). Further chest wall resection plus wedge resection of small tumor nodule left lower lobe. Radon seeds implanted 1951 and 1961. *C,* R.S., 9/18/57. Treatment begun at age 10+2 for severe thoracic scoliosis, apex to resected chest wall. In 1952 had recurrent nodule left chest wall and further resection done, including paravertebral muscles. *D,* Fusion T3–L4 and cast correction. A pseudarthrosis developed with loss of correction, which was recorrected and the defect repaired on 4/28/59. The vertebral bone was hard and avascular.

*Illustration continued on the opposite page*

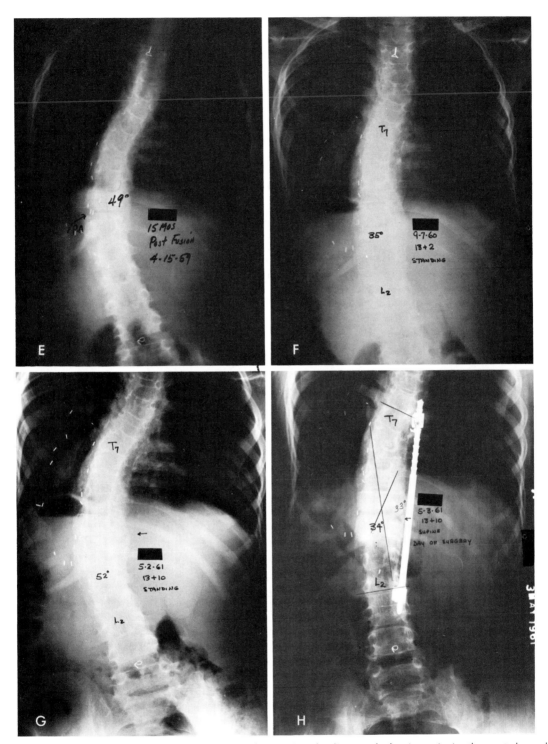

**Figure 23–53** *Continued   E,* R.S., 4/15/59. Loss of correction after first pseudarthrosis repair. Another central pseudarthrosis is visible. *F,* R.S., age 13+2, 9/7/60. Fusion appeared solid and correction good. *G,* R.S., age 13+10, 5/2/61. A persistent pseudarthrosis is again visible in the same area with loss of correction. *H,* R.S., age 13+10, 5/18/61. Newly acquired Harrington instrumentation used to treat the pseudarthrosis loss. Repair again performed.

*Illustration continued on the following page*

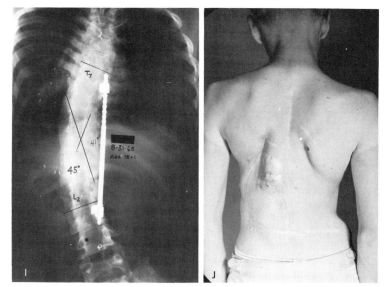

**Figure 23–53** *Continued*  *I*, R.S. 8/31/65. Fusion now solid with minimal loss of correction 4 years after last repair. *J*, Appearance excellent, 1964. No further loss of correction. In 1977 patient was still in good health with no further loss of correction.

### References

1. Alexander, J.: Postoperative management of thoracoplastic patients. Am. Rev. Tuberc. 61:57, 1950.
2. Dwork, R. E., Dinken, H., and Hurst, A.: Post-thoracoplasty scoliosis. Arch. Phys. Med., 32:722, 1951.
3. Winter, R. B., and Tongen, L. A.: A malignant chest wall sarcoma with bilateral pulmonary metastasis. A 15 year survival after multiple radical local excision and resection of bilateral pulmonary metastasis and a successful treatment of scoliosis secondary to tumor surgery. Surgery, 62:374–378, 1967.

# SCOLIOSIS SECONDARY TO BURNS

The reports of burn contractures producing scoliosis are so rare that a search of the literature has not revealed any such reference. The contractures occur as a result of neglected treatment of severe deep burns, allowing scar contracture on one side of the body to mechanically pull the spine into a lateral curvature. The concavity of the curve is invariably toward the side of the burn contracture (Fig. 23–54).

The burn contracture, if located anteriorly, may give rise to a progressive kyphosis.

If properly treated from onset of burn contractures, scoliosis can be avoided. Release of contracture with skin grafting will usually result in marked improvement. If treatment is not too long delayed, the scoliosis or kyphosis will respond to the Milwaukee brace after adequate surgical release of the contracture (Fig. 23–55).

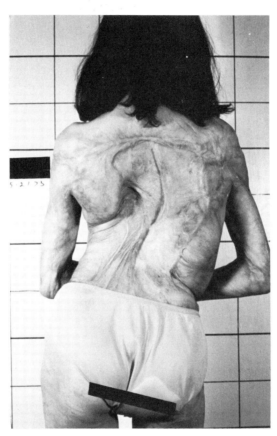

**Figure 23–54** A patient from Brazil demonstrating a severe scoliosis from neglected care of a severe burn with contracture on the left side. The concavity is on the side of the contracture. No follow-up was available.

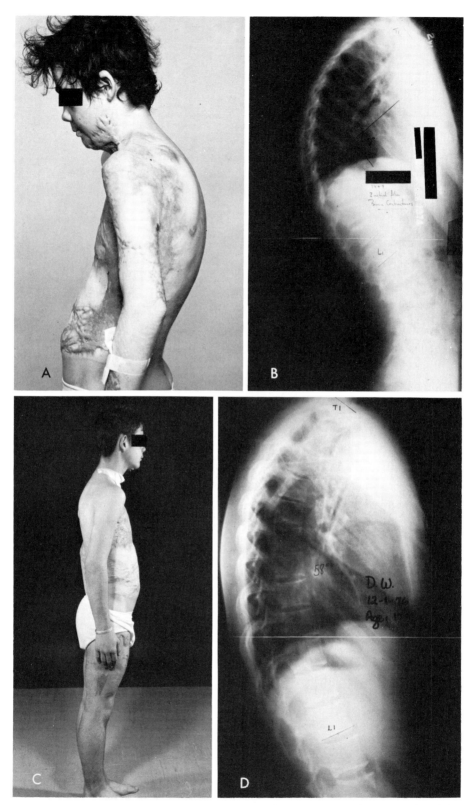

**Figure 23–55**  *A*, D.W. An example of a kyphosis from a severe burn contracture of anterior neck and chest treated by scar release plus skin grafting and the use of a Milwaukee brace. The kyphosis was completely overcome without spine surgery. *B*, A 90 degree kyphosis caused by the burn contracture. *C*, D.W., age 17. End result of surgical release of burn contractures, skin grafts, and Milwaukee brace treatment. *D*, D.W., age 17. Lateral x-ray showing kyphosis reduced from 90 to 58 degrees.

# LORDOSIS SECONDARY TO LUMBAR PERITONEAL SHUNTING PROCEDURES

## INTRODUCTION

This relatively uncommon condition is fortunately becoming less common since neurosurgeons have virtually abandoned the lumbar peritoneal shunting procedure for hydrocephalus. Multiple lumbar laminectomies, coupled with arachnoid adhesions and laminary scarring, may lead to a progressive lumbar lordosis. This progressive lumbar lordosis tends to be rigid and may reach severe proportions. Efforts to treat the condition by conventional orthopedic means, i.e., posterior release of the contracted tissues, Harrington instrumentation, and posterior spine fusion, have led to a high frequency of catastrophe. The scarred and adherent nerve roots do not tolerate the stretching, and neurologic deficits have been reported frequently.

## REVIEW OF THE LITERATURE

In 1970, King and Hall reported five cases.[1] The first three had been treated by posterior exposure, Harrington instrumentation, and posterior fusion. Two of the three had neurologic problems secondary to nerve stretching. These neurologic complications were permanent. Of these three patients, two were males who had surgery at age 14 and 16. One patient had a 160 degree lordosis corrected to 104 degrees, the second a 172 degree lordosis corrected to 103 degrees. Both of these patients suffered significant degrees of paralysis due to the procedure. The third patient, a 19 year old female, had the same procedure at age 12. Her lordosis was less severe, 105 degrees, and was corrected to 78 degrees. This is the single patient who did not develop postoperative paralysis.

The authors then developed a new approach, an anterior closing wedge osteotomy. They felt this approach was better because it shortened the "long" side (convexity) of the curve rather than attempting to stretch the contracted and scarred concavity of the curve. Two patients were operated by this technique; one male and one female, both age 15. One was corrected from 140 degrees to 78 degrees.

The amount of correction given to the second patient was not reported. Neither of these patients had any neurologic deficit. The technique reported was a transperitoneal approach to the midlumbar spine going between the aorta and vena cava. Because of the severe hyperlordosis, the spine tends to protrude anteriorly, and the vena cava falls to the right while the aorta falls to the left. This allows exposure between the bifurcation of the aorta below and the renal artery above. Two intervertebral discs and corresponding wedges of an end-plate of the vertebral bodies were removed. No internal fixation was used. Postoperatively, the patients were treated in balanced skeletal traction with the hips flexed 90 degrees and knees flexed 90 degrees with pins through the distal femur suspending the patient with the buttocks off the bed. Sufficient bony healing had occurred by six to eight weeks that a cast could be applied and the traction discontinued. Final healing was accomplished in six months.

Kushner et al.[2] reported a follow-up of patients with lumbar peritoneal shunts. Of the 27 without myelomeningocele, 13 had scoliosis, and 6 of these had increased lumbar lordosis. Severe arachnoiditis was noted on exploration and at autopsy.

Steele and Adams reported a patient with a severe lumbar hyperlordosis.[3] The patient was treated using a combination of anterior closing wedge osteotomy and posterior fusion without instrumentation. The patient was corrected by suspension from an overhead frame in a two-part cast with gradual correction of the lordosis by positioning of the two portions of the cast. The patient had no neurologic complications and ended treatment with an excellent result.

The reports dealing with treatment of this problem thus emphasize the hazards of posterior correction and fusion with Harrington distraction instrumentation. The adherent nerve roots do not tolerate traction, and neurologic complications are frequent. Anterior disc excision and osteotomy with closure by some type of flexion technique thus prevent neurologic complications and promote a rapid bony union.

## PERSONAL EXPERIENCE

Five patients with lumbar hyperlordosis secondary to lumbar peritoneal shunting procedures have been seen by the authors. The first of these patients was treated by the posterior approach with Harrington instrumentation and fusion. She suffered severe neurologic deficit with only partial recovery. This was done prior to the reports of Hall and Steele (Fig. 23–56).

After hearing the reports by King and Hall, the subsequent cases treated here were done by anterior disc excision and closing wedge osteotomy. Two of the patients had pure lumbar lordosis and were treated by the technique as described by Hall (Fig. 23–57). Neither had any neurologic deficit related to their treatment. The fourth patient seen here had been treated previously elsewhere by posterior fusion without instrumentation. This was accomplished without neurologic complications. She was seen here because of a postlaminectomy kyphosis due to the proximal extension of the laminectomy beyond the thoracolumbar junction. This was treated by anterior and posterior fusions without complication. The fifth patient treated here had an associated scoliosis in addition to the lumbar lordosis and was treated by anterior surgery using a Dwyer instrumentation from L1 to L4.

*Text continued on page 660*

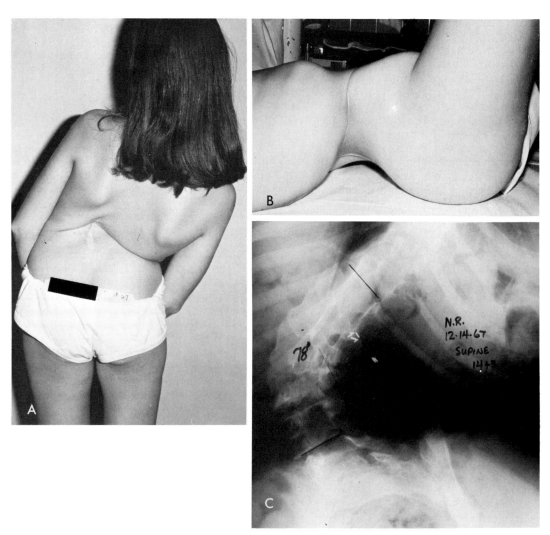

**Figure 23–56**　*See legend on opposite page.*

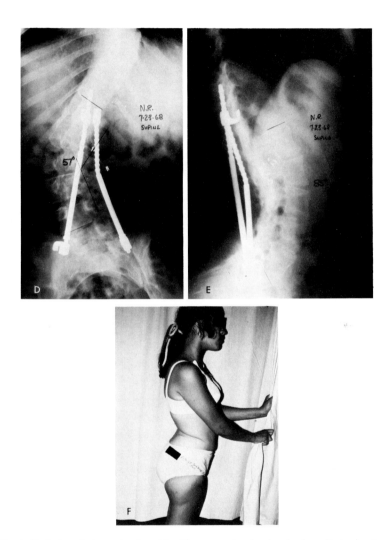

**Figure 23–56**  *A,* Posterior photograph of a girl with progressive lumbar lordoscoliosis due to a lumbar peritoneal shunting procedure for hydrocephalus. *B,* Lateral photograph with the patient in femoral pin suspension prior to surgery. *C,* AP x-ray prior to surgery. *D,* AP x-ray following surgery. *E,* Lateral x-ray following posterior Harrington instrumentation and spine fusion. She suffered severe but not total neurologic deficit following this procedure. *F,* Lateral standing photograph 19 months following surgery. She had a partial recovery from her paralysis. She is cosmetically improved but functionally worse.

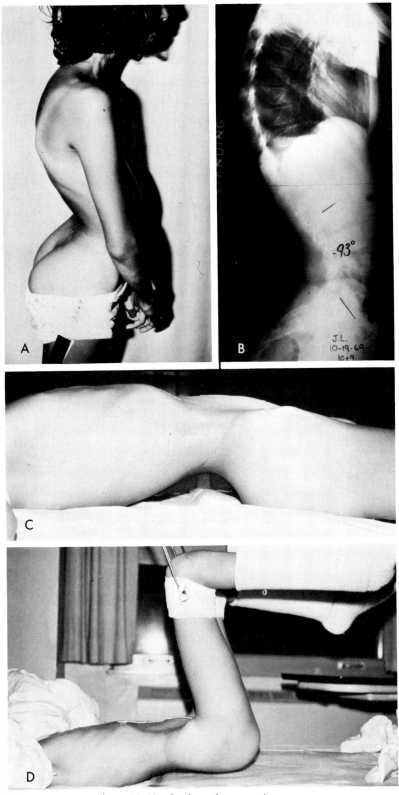

**Figure 23–57** *See legend on opposite page.*

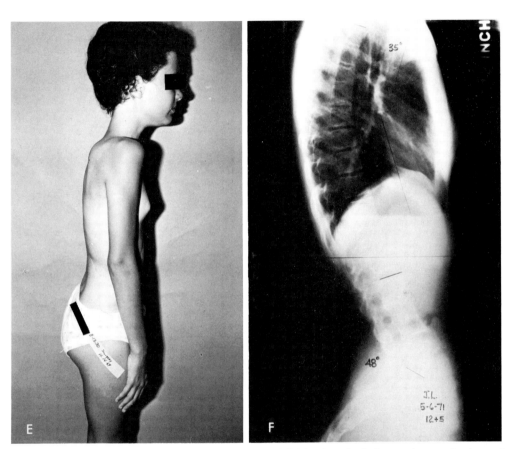

**Figure 23–57**   *A,* Lateral standing photograph of a patient with lumbar hyperlordosis secondary to a lumbar-peritoneal shunting procedure for hydrocephalus. *B,* Lateral standing x-ray showing the increased lordosis of 93 degrees at age 10. *C,* Lateral photograph in the operating room under general anesthesia. The lumbar spine protrudes against the anterior abdominal wall. There was *no* hip flexion contracture. *D,* Lateral photograph five days following anterior wedge disc removal. Note the improved lumbar lordosis. This suspension was maintained for six weeks, then a cast was applied for five months. *E,* Lateral photograph one year postoperatively. *F,* Lateral x-ray showing correction to a normal lumbar lordosis two years post-op. She reappeared at age 18 with an extruded L4–L5 disc with acute foot drop. The curve had not changed from this x-ray.

## SUMMARY

Lumbar peritoneal shunting procedures in childhood are associated with a high incidence of progressive lumbar lordosis. Scoliosis may or may not be present. This is a structural deformity and cannot safely be corrected by posterior stretching operations owing to the dense arachnoid adhesions. The optimal treatment appears to be: 1) Prevention of the problem by avoidance of lumbar peritoneal shunting procedures; 2) If a curvature has developed, anterior disc excision and anterior closing wedge osteotomy is the procedure of choice in order to prevent catastrophic neurologic damage.

### References

1. King, J. D., and Hall, J. E.: Hyperlordosis following lumboperitoneal shunts. Scoliosis Research Society, Toronto, 1970.
2. Kushner, J., Alexander, E., Davis, C., and Kelly, D.: Kyphoscoliosis following lumbar subarachnoid shunts. Neurosurg., 34:783, 1971.
3. Steele, H. H., and Adams, D. J.: Hyperlordosis caused by the lumboperitoneal shunt procedure for hydrocephalus. J. Bone Joint Surg., 54A:1537, 1972.

# Appendix

# EXERCISE ROUTINES

The following is an outline of the exercise routines that we have found helpful in managing patients with spinal deformities.* The exercise program encompasses routines for 1) postural exercises, 2) exercises to maintain spinal flexibility, 3) Milwaukee brace exercises for scoliosis, 4) Milwaukee brace exercises for kyphosis, 5) exercises to be done in the TLSO brace, 6) home program, post surgery, 7) program for postoperative patients kept on bed rest, and 8) an information handout that we routinely distribute to our brace patients.

## I
## POSTURAL EXERCISES

All exercises are done 10 times daily except #5, which is done 40 times. All exercises should be done on a firm surface (i.e., floor) and done slowly.

### Abdominal and Trunk Strengthening Exercises

1. Pelvic tilt supine with your knees flexed. Hold to count of five—relax.
   A. Force the small of your back onto the floor by tightening your abdominal muscles.
   B. Avoid lifting buttocks off floor or pushing with feet.
   C. Breathe regularly. Keep your head and shoulders relaxed and on the floor.
2. Pelvic tilt, supine with your knees straight. Repeat A, B, and C.
3. Pelvic tilt, standing—correct standing and walking posture (Fig. A–1).
   A. Practice standing with your back against the wall (heels approximately 3 inches from wall).
   B. Relax your knees; tilt your pelvis. Emphasis is on strong abdominal tightening with buttocks tucked under.
   C. Keep shoulders back—breathe regularly.
   D. Stand tall! Tuck your chin in, stretch yourself *up* and *back*, maintaining the pelvic tilt.
   E. Walk, holding the tilt. Make this posture a habit. Use a full-length mirror to check your posture.
4. Partial "sit-ups" maintaining the pelvic tilt. Up slowly, hold position with head, back, and shoulders square to count of five and slowly return to starting position (Fig. A–2).
   Progressive positions—all positions start with the pelvic tilt.
   A. Knees extended, elbows straight—reach toward your knees.
   B. Knees flexed, elbows straight—reach toward your knees.
   C. Knees flexed with your arms across your chest—reach toward your knees.
   NOTE: Your feet can initially be stabilized by a parent or under a stable object. Progress to a partial sit-up without feet stabilization.

---

*Furnished with the help of the Physical Therapy Department, Fairview Hospital, Minneapolis, Minnesota.

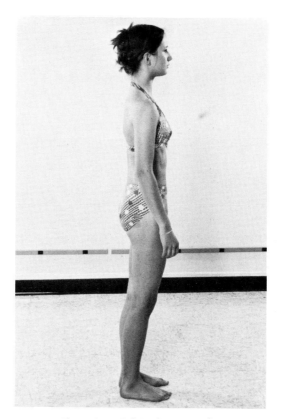

**Figure A-1**   Pelvic tilting—standing.

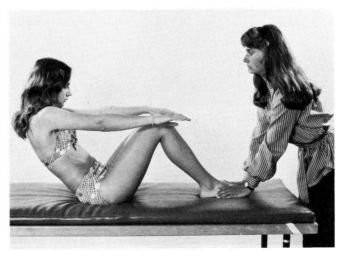

**Figure A-2**   Partial sit-ups, maintaining pelvic tilt.

### Back Strengthening Exercises

1. Back extension while lying on abdomen. Hold position to five—relax. Do 40 times.
   A. Place pillow under waist to help prevent sway back. Place towel under forehead.
   B. Arms straight down by your sides with palms down.
   C. Tilt your pelvis, and hold the tilt throughout the exercise.
   D. Pinch your shoulder blades together, rolling your shoulders back.
   E. Raise your head and arms up approximately 1 inch.
   F. Keep your chin tucked in and stretch your neck so that your head is away from your shoulders; eyes on the floor.

## II
## STRETCHES TO MAINTAIN OR INCREASE FLEXIBILITY

### Pectoral Stretch

1. Stand facing doorway, elbows at shoulder level with forearms supported against outside of door casings. Lean through doorway. Count to 10, repeat 10 times.
2. Stand 12 to 18 inches away from and facing a corner, with feet 12 inches apart. Place one hand at shoulder level on each wall. Tilt and lean forward. Count to 10, repeat 10 times.

### Hamstring Stretch (Fig. A-3)

1. Stand facing a chair or object of similar height. Place one leg on chair and bend forward until you feel a pull in the back of the leg. Bounce down as far as you can, keeping the knee straight. Repeat 10 times for each leg.
2. Lie on back, facing wall. Raise both legs and rest them on wall. Keeping knees straight, slide buttocks toward wall. Remain in this position 5–10 minutes.
3. Lying on back, manually raise one leg, maintaining both straight, to a vertical position. Hold 10 seconds; repeat 10 times.

**Figure A-3** Hamstring stretch.

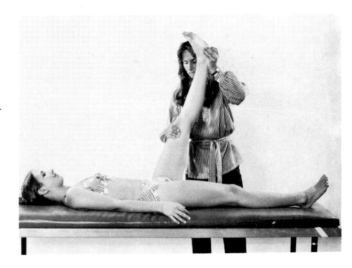

### Hip Flexor Stretch

1. Lie on back, with buttocks and back supported by table and legs left unsupported off edge of table. Draw both knees to chest. Hold one knee toward chest with hands, and allow the leg to be stretched to hang unsupported over the edge of table. Maintain position 5–10 minutes.
2. Assume a semi-crouch running position, with the leg to be stretched straight behind. Bounce 5 times, repeat 10 times.

### Low Back Stretch (Fig. A–4)

1. Lie on back with both legs straight out. Bring both knees toward sides of the chest as far as you can, hold 5 seconds, and straighten. Repeat _____ times.
2. Sit tailor fashion with hands behind neck and elbows straight out. Tilt, curl forward until you feel a pull in the low back. Bounce down 5 times as far as you can without losing tilt, then straighten trunk. Repeat 10 times. Stretch should be felt in the low back.

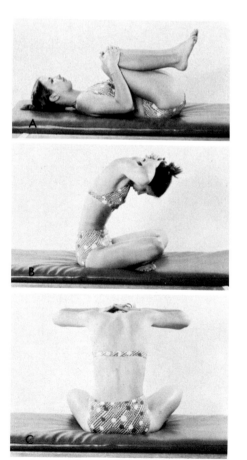

**Figure A–4**   Back stretching exercises.

### Upper Back Stretch

1. Sit tailor fashion with hands behind neck and elbows straight out. Tilt, curl at head and neck, as if to touch top of head to feet. Bounce. Repeat 10 times. Stretch should be felt in upper back. ESPECIALLY INDICATED WITH THORACIC LORDOSIS.

## III
## MILWAUKEE BRACE EXERCISES

### Scoliosis

Exercises 1 through 6 are done ten times once a day. Exercises 7 and 8 are to be *done many times a day.* Exercises should be done on a firm surface (i.e., floor) and done slowly.

*ABDOMINAL AND TRUNK STRENGTHENING EXERCISES* (Fig. A–5)

1. Pelvic tilt supine with your knees flexed. Hold to count of five—relax.
    A. Force the small of your back onto the floor by tightening your abdominal muscles.
    B. Avoid lifting buttocks off floor or pushing with feet.
    C. Breathe regularly. Keep your head and shoulders relaxed and on the floor.
2. Pelvic tilt, supine with your knees straight. Repeat A, B, and C.
3. Pelvic tilt, standing—correct standing and walking posture (Fig. A–6)
    A. Practice standing with your back against the wall (heels approximately 3 inches from wall).
    B. Relax your knees; tilt your pelvis. Emphasis is on strong abdominal tightening with buttocks tucked under.
    C. Keep shoulders back—breathe regularly.
    D. Stand tall! Tuck your chin in, stretch yourself *up* and *back* in the brace.
    E. Walk, holding the tilt. Make this posture a habit. Use a full-length mirror to check your posture.
4. Partial "sit-ups" maintaining the pelvic tilt. Curl forward slowly, hold position for count of five and slowly return to starting position. This exercise is always done out of the brace.
    Progressive positions—all positions start with pelvic tilt.
    A. Knees extended, elbows straight—reach toward your knees.

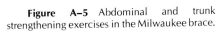

**Figure A–5** Abdominal and trunk strengthening exercises in the Milwaukee brace.

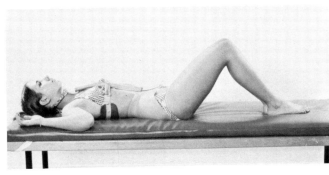

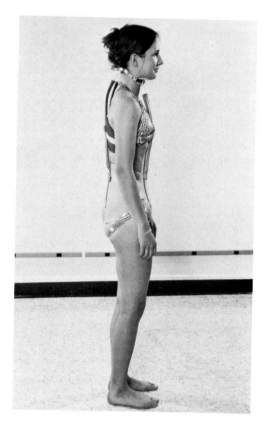

**Figure A-6** Pelvic tilt—standing in Milwaukee brace.

B. Knees flexed, elbow straight—reach toward your knees.

C. Knees flexed with your arms across your chest.

NOTE: Your feet can initially be stabilized by a parent or under a stable object. Progress to a partial sit-up without feet stabilization.

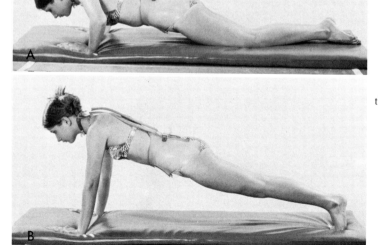

**Figure A-7** Push-ups with pelvis tilted, in the Milwaukee brace.

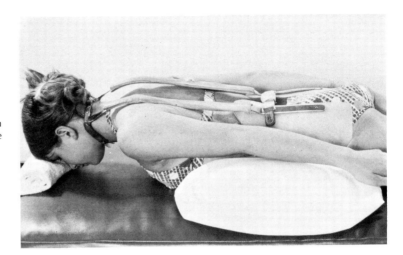

**Figure A–8** Back extension while lying on the abdomen in the Milwaukee brace.

5. Push-ups with pelvis tilted (modified on knees or regular). When doing a modified push-up, avoid sway back and coming up to a crawl position. In the "up" position, the head, shoulders, and knees are in straight alignment with one another (Fig. A–7).
6. Back extension while lying on abdomen. Hold position to count of five—relax (Fig. A–8).
   A. Place pillow under waist to help prevent sway back; place towel roll under forehead.
   B. Arms straight down by your sides with palms down.
   C. Tilt your pelvis, and hold the tilt throughout the exercise.
   D. Pinch your shoulder blades together, rolling your shoulders back.
   E. Raise your head and arms up about 1 inch.
   F. Keep your chin tucked in and stretch your neck so that your head is away from your shoulders; eyes on the floor.

*ACTIVE CORRECTIONAL EXERCISES*

The following exercises are always done in the brace. Your therapist will designate how many times each exercise is to be done.
7. Derotation Breathing—filling out "thoracic valley" and reducing rib hump (Fig. A–9).
   A. Stand and position your arms so that your elbows are forward and at shoulder level. Hold onto anterior upright with both hands.
   B. Tilt your pelvis and hold throughout exercise.
   C. Inhale deeply, expanding backward against the posterior uprights with your chest wall. The thoracic pad will engage your rib hump and derotate your spine. Emphasize filling out of your thoracic valley. "Arch like a cat." Your low back should be well against the back of the pelvic girdle as your thoracic area is against the posterior uprights. Respiration should be slow both in inhalation and in exhalation.

   Do exercise _____ times/day.

8. Shift—active correction of major curve(s) (Fig. A–10).

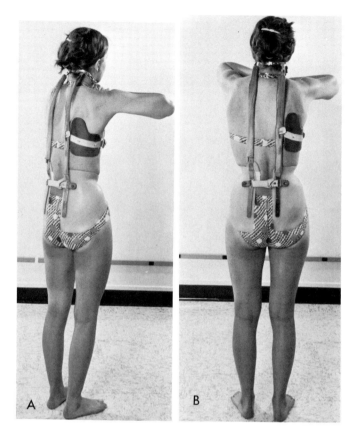

**Figure A–9**  Derotational breathing.

A. Initially practice with your hands on your hips. Use a mirror. Progress to arms down at your sides.
B. Tilt the pelvis.
C. "Shift" away from pad, and hold corrected position to count of five. Avoid sway back and twisting of your body. Your head and shoulders should be in straight alignment with your body. The shift is a lateral (side) movement.

Do exercise _____ times/day.

If you are wearing the brace full-time or are out 2 to 4 hours, the following applies for your exercises:
All exercises are done daily in the brace except #4, which is always done out of the brace.
If you are wearing the brace for more than 4 hours during the day, the exercises are done daily—in and out of the brace on alternate days.
If you are wearing the brace only at night, all exercises are to be done out of the brace with the exception of #7 and #8, which are to be done in the brace. Exercises #7 and #8 are always done in the brace, and #4 is always done out of the brace.

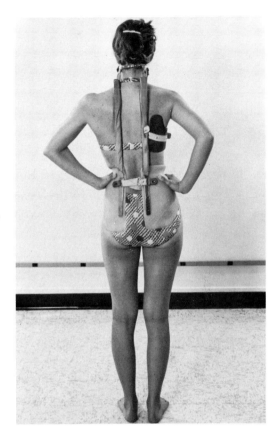

**Figure A–10**  Active correction of the major curvature by thoracic shifting in the Milwaukee brace.

# IV
# MILWAUKEE BRACE EXERCISES

## Kyphosis

All exercises are done 10 times daily except #6, which is done 40 times daily. All exercises should be done on a firm surface (i.e., floor) and done slowly.

### ABDOMINAL AND TRUNK STRENGTHENING EXERCISES

1. Pelvic tilt, supine with your knees flexed. Hold to count of five—relax.
    A. Force the small of your back onto the floor by tightening your abdominal muscles.
    B. Avoid lifting buttocks off floor or pushing with feet.
    C. Breathe regularly. Keep your head and shoulders relaxed and on the floor.
2. Pelvic tilt, supine with your knees straight. Repeat A, B, and C.
3. Pelvic tilt, standing—correct standing and walking posture.
    A. Practice standing with your back against the wall (heels approximately 3 inches from wall).
    B. Relax your knees; tilt your pelvis. Emphasis is on strong abdominal tightening with buttocks tucked under.
    C. Keep shoulders back—breathe regularly.
    D. Stand tall! Tuck your chin in, stretch yourself *up* and *back* in the brace, maintaining the pelvic tilt.

   E. Walk, holding the tilt. Make this posture a habit. Use a full-length mirror to check your posture.
4. Partial "sit-up" maintaining the pelvic tilt. Up slowly, hold position with head, back, and shoulders square to count of five, and slowly return to starting position.
   Progressive positions—all positions start with the pelvic tilt.
   A. Knees extended, elbows straight—reach toward your knees.
   B. Knees flexed, elbows straight—reach toward your knees.
   C. Knees flexed with your arms across your chest—reach toward your knees.
   NOTE: Your feet can initially be stabilized by a parent or under a stable object. Progress to a partial sit-up without feet stabilization.
5. Push-ups with pelvis tilted (modified on knees or regular).
   When doing a modified push-up, avoid sway back and coming up to a crawl position. In the "up" position, the head, shoulders, and knees are in straight alignment with one another.

## BACK STRENGTHENING EXERCISES

6. Back extension while lying on abdomen. Hold position to five—relax. Do exercise 40 times every day.
   A. Place pillow under waist to help prevent sway back; place towel under forehead.
   B. Arms straight down by your sides with palms down.
   C. Tilt your pelvis and hold the tilt throughout the exercise.
   D. Pinch your shoulder blades together, rolling your shoulders back.
   E. Raise your head and arms up approximately 1 inch.
   F. Keep your chin tucked in and stretch your neck so that your head is away from your shoulders; eyes on the floor.

If you are wearing the brace full-time or you are out 2 to 4 hours, all exercises are done in the brace daily.

If you are out of the brace for more than 4 hours during the day, the exercises are done daily—in and out of the brace on alternate days.

**V**

**TLSO EXERCISES**

Exercises 1 through 4 are done ten times daily. Exercises should be done on a firm surface (i.e., floor) and done slowly.

### Abdominal and Trunk Strengthening Exercises

1. Pelvic tilt supine with your knees flexed. Hold to count of five—relax.
   A. Force the small of your back onto the floor by tightening your abdominal muscles.
   B. Avoid lifting buttocks off floor or pushing with feet.
   C. Breathe regularly. Keep your shoulders flat on the floor.
2. Pelvic tilt, supine with your knees straight. Repeat A, B, and C.
3. Pelvic tilt, standing—correct standing and walking posture.
   A. Practice standing with your back against the wall (heels approximately 3 inches from wall).

B. Relax your knees; tilt your pelvis. Emphasis is on strong abdominal tightening with buttocks tucked under.

C. Keep shoulders back—breathe regularly.

D. Stand tall! Tuck your chin in, stretch yourself *up* and *back* in the brace.

E. Walk, holding the tilt. Make this posture a habit. Use a full-length mirror to check your posture.

4. Partial "sit-up" maintaining the pelvic tilt. Curl forward slowly, hold position for a count of five, and slowly return to starting position. This exercise is always done out of the brace.

Progressive positions—all positions start with pelvic tilt.

A. Knees extended, elbows straight—reach toward your knees.

B. Knees flexed, elbows straight—reach toward your knees.

C. Knees flexed with your arms across your chest.

NOTE: Your feet can initially be stabilized by a parent or under a stable object. Progress to a partial sit-up without feet stabilization.

# VI

# PHYSICAL THERAPY HOME PROGRAM

## Postoperative Exercises for the Scoliosis/Kyphosis Patient

*BREATHING EXERCISES*

Breathing exercises are of extreme importance to the scoliosis or kyphosis patient who has had a spinal fusion. The rib deformity, caused by the scoliosis and the rotation (twisting) of the spine, directly influences the function of the lungs. The rib cage or chest wall, which encases the lungs, actually changes in size and shape. By the necessary application of a body cast, a person tends to not breathe deeply. With these two points in mind, one can more fully understand why much emphasis is placed on deep breathing exercises. It is important that the patient improve and maintain pulmonary function.

1. *Deep Breathing (Chest Breathing)*
   Breathe deeply, achieving maximum chest expansion. Start with the lower rib cage and progress to the middle ribs and finally the upper rib cage—all in one inhalation without stopping. Expand out completely against the cast (front, back, and sides) and into the front window. Slowly exhale, with gradual tightening of the abdominal muscles for complete exhalation. Breathing should be slow.
   A. Position: On back with knees bent.
   B. Breathe in through your nose.
   C. Breathe out through your mouth with a "ssss" sound.
   D. Do this exercise at least 10 times daily.

2. *Derotation Breathing (Filling out of the thoracic valley)*
   With scoliosis there is rotation of the vertebrae; thus, the ribs rotate as well because they are attached to the vertebrae. This causes a rib prominence in back on the side of the curvature (convexity) and rib depression on the opposite side (concavity). A window has been cut in your cast on the concave side where the ribs are depressed and have formed a "thoracic valley." Breathing into the area of the concavity (window) assists in derotation of the vertebrae and ribs. As one inhales deeply, the rib prominence on the convex

side is held stationary by the cast, while the depressed ribs of the concavity are free to move out into the window—thus, derotation occurs. *YOU CAN ASSIST IN CORRECTING YOUR DEFORMITY* with the following derotation exercises:

A. *Back Lying*
    1) Knees bent, arms across chest.
    2) Breathe deeply *back* into the window.
    3) Arch your back against the cast as you inhale.
    4) Emphasis is on inhalation; breath slowly.
    5) You should feel your back go firmly against the bed/floor through the back window.
    6) Do this exercise at least 10 times daily.

B. *Side Lying*
    1) Lie on side opposite window with a firm pillow under your side. Support the head with a pillow.
    2) Straighten the top leg in line with the body and raise the top arm slightly forward of the head. The leg and arm on the floor are flexed.
    3) Breathe deeply *back* into the *window*.
    4) A hand may be placed in the back window so that the patient can feel where he/she is to expand.
    5) Arch your back against the cast as you inhale.
    6) Emphasis is on inhalation; breathe slowly.
    7) The back window should fill completely as the spine and ribs derotate.
    8) Do this exercise at least 10 times daily.

C. *Standing*
    1) Face the wall with feet 12 to 18 inches away from the wall.
    2) Position the arms so that the elbows are flexed and at shoulder level. Put hands on wall.
    3) Breathe deeply *back* into the *window*.
    4) A hand may be placed in the back window so that the patient can feel where he/she is to expand.
    5) Arch your back against the cast as you inhale.
    6) Emphasis is on inhalation; breathe slowly.
    7) The back window should fill completely as the spine and ribs derotate.
    8) Do this exercise at least 10 times daily.

## ABDOMINAL STRENGTHENING EXERCISES

During the time you are wearing your postoperative cast, your trunk is primarily supported by the cast. Consequently, your abdominal muscles become extremely weak if they are not exercised. The following exercises are designed to maintain and improve the strength of the abdominal muscles.

    ***Progressive Abdominal Exercises***

1. *Abdominal setting* with the knees flexed. Tighten abdominal muscles and hold to count of five—relax. Breathe normally.

    Start with _____ times and increase to 10 times.

2. *Single leg lifts* with one knee flexed and one leg straight on floor. Hold tight with abdominals and flex the "straight" leg at the knee and hip so that the

thigh is vertical and the knee is flexed to 90 degrees. Hold position to count of five and return to starting position. Repeat with other leg.

Start with _____ times and increase to 10 times.

3. Double leg lifts with knee flexed. Avoid arching in low back—"sway back." Hold tight with abdominals, and slowly lift legs so that the thighs are vertical and the knees are flexed to 90 degrees. Hold position to count of five and return to starting position.

   Start with _____ times and increase to 10 times.

4. *Single leg*
   A. Straight leg raising
   B. Bicycle

   Start with _____ times and increase to 10 times.

5. *Double leg*
   *A. Bicycle*

   Start with _____ times and increase to 25 times.

6. *Partial sit-up*
   A. Upside-down chair for assistance (legs straight).
   B. One or two pillows for assistance (legs straight).
   C. Legs straight—arms in front.
   D. Legs flexed—arms in front.
   Progress from A to D. Once you can do A 10 times well, progress to B, etc. When you are able to do 10 sit-ups (C or D) well, you may discontinue exercises #1 through #5.

7. *Push-ups* are started as soon as you can tolerate them. Start with a modified push-up on your knees. Work toward 10 times daily.

8. Practice walking with your abdominals "set" and standing tall—head up and out of your cast.

The previous exercises, as marked by your physical therapist, are to be done every day at home. During the first month, exercise twice a day, then once a day until you return for your cast change. Your exercises will be checked by a physical therapist when you return for your cast change.

## VII
## PHYSICAL THERAPY HOME PROGRAM

### Spinal Fusion Patients on Bed Rest

*BREATHING EXERCISES*

Breathing exercises are of extreme importance to the scoliosis and/or kyphosis patient who has had a spinal fusion and must remain on bed rest. Activity is important to the function of the lungs. When a person is not able to be active (on bed rest), breathing exercises must be done to improve and maintain good function of the lungs. Pulmonary function is directly influenced by the rib deformity, which is caused by the scoliosis and/or kyphosis and the rotation (twisting) of the spine. The rib cage, or chest wall, which encases the lungs, actually changes in size and shape. By the necessary application of a body cast, a person tends to not breathe deeply. With these three points in mind, one can more fully understand why much emphasis is placed on deep breathing exercises.

1. *Deep Breathing (Chest Breathing)*

   Breathe deeply, achieving maximum chest expansion. Start with the lower rib cage and progress to the middle ribs and finally the upper rib cage—all in one inhalation without stopping. Expand out completely against the cast (front, back, and sides) and into the front window. Slowly exhale with gradual tightening of the abdominal muscles for complete exhalation. Breathing should be slow.

   A. Position: On back with knees bent.

   B. Breathe in through your nose.

   C. Breathe out through your mouth, making a "ssss" sound.

   Exercise _____ times/day for 10 minutes.

2. *Deep Breathing (Abdominal or Diaphragmatic Breathing)*

   Put your hands on your stomach/abdomen. As you inhale deeply, your abdomen should come up, and as you exhale it goes down or flattens. With this kind of breathing, there should not be any movement of the chest wall.

   A. Position: On back with knees bent. Hands on stomach/abdomen.

   B. Breathe in through your nose.

   C. Breathe out through your mouth with a "ssss" sound.

   Exercise _____ times/day for 10 minutes.

3. *Blow Bottles*

   Gradually work toward moving all the water from one bottle to another one in one exhalation. Exhalation may be somewhat more forceful than in the previous two exercises. The respiration still should be slow.

   A. Position: Back or on your side.

   Exercise _____ times/day for 10 minutes.

## ARM EXERCISES

1. *Elbow Extension (Triceps)*

   A. Elbow straight overhead.

   B. Keep elbow pointed at ceiling.

   C. Straighten and bend elbow _____ times with _____ weight.

   D. Repeat A, B, and C with other arm.

   Exercise _____ times/day.

2. *Elbow Flexion (Biceps)*

   A. Arm straight on bed.

B. Bend and straighten elbow _____ times with _____ weight.
C. Repeat A and B with other arm.

Exercise _____ times/day.

3. *Shoulder Flexion*
   A. Arm straight down by your side.
   B. Keep arm straight.
   C. Raise arm up over head _____ times with _____ weight.
   D. Repeat A, B, and C with other arm.

Exercise _____ times/day.

4. *Shoulder Rotation*
   A. Arms straight out from your side.
   B. Bend both elbows to 90 degrees (right angle).
   C. Roll shoulders forward (palms down on bed).
   D. Roll shoulders backward (palms up).

Exercise _____ times _____ times/day.


*LEG EXERCISES*

1. *Knee Flexion and Extension*
   A. Bring knees individually up toward chest.
   B. Return down to straight leg position.

Exercise _____ times each leg _____ times/day.

2. *Knee Extension (Strengthening Quadriceps)*
   A. Support knee in bent position.
   B. Straighten and bend the knee with weight on ankle.

Exercise _____ times with _____ weight (R), _____ weight (L).

Exercise _____ times/day.

   NOTE: If the patient has a cast that includes the thigh or one or both legs, move him/her so that the knees are at the edge of the bed and can bend freely. *Rest the feet on a chair or stool.*

3. *Straight Leg Raising*
   A. Keep leg straight and lift up with weight on ankle.
   B. Return to starting position.

Exercise _____ times with _____ weight (R), _____ weight (L).

Exercise _____ times/day.

4. *Hip Abduction*
   A. Keep legs straight.
   B. Spread legs apart and bring them together (do individually or together).

Exercise _____ times _____ times/day.

5. *Hip Rotation*
   A. Keep legs straight.
   B. Roll legs in, then out.

   Exercise _____ times _____ times/day.

6. *Ankle Exercises*
   A. Move feet up and down (pumping motion).
   B. Move feet in a circular motion — both directions.

   Exercise _____ times _____ times/day.

7. *Gluteal Setting (Buttock Muscles)*
   A. Pinch buttocks together.
   B. Count to five and relax.

   Exercise _____ times _____ times/day.

8. *Abdominal Setting*
   A. Tighten the abdominal (tummy) muscles.
   B. Count to five and relax.

   Exercise _____ times _____ times/day.

9. *Hamstring Muscle Stretching (only if indicated)*
   A. One leg flat on bed.
   B. Have someone *gently* raise opposite leg up, keeping knee straight.
   C. Pull should be felt in back of knee.

   Exercise _____ times _____ times/day.

The exercises that have been marked by your physical therapist are to be done every day at home. Your exercises will be checked when you return to the hospital for your cast change.

## SCOLIOSIS/KYPHOSIS AND YOUR SPINAL BRACE
## INFORMATION FOR PATIENT

The day that your doctor orders your brace, you go to the Orthotics Lab and have a mold taken of your frame. This will be done by putting a thick wrapping of plaster around your torso. After the plaster hardens, it will be taken off and used to tailor-make your new brace. Physical therapy exercises will also be given to you that day so that you can work on them during the time the brace is being fabricated.

### When Will You Get Your Brace?

It normally takes two to three weeks to complete your brace after the mold has been taken. When the brace is ready, the Orthotics Lab will notify the doctor's secretary, and she will contact you so that you may come in on the next clinic day.

Brace fittings start in the morning and may take anywhere from two to six hours. After the Orthotics Lab has fitted the brace on you, you will return to the Scoliosis Clinic so that your doctor may examine you in the brace. Any necessary adjustments will then be requested by him, and you will return to the Orthotics Lab to have his orders carried out. It may take several adjustments before the doctor is satisfied that you are getting the best correction possible in your brace.

On the day of the brace fitting, you will also go to physical therapy. It is important that you learn those exercises that you must do in the brace the very same day you get your new brace. Your therapy appointment will be scheduled for you by the secretary, and the clinic personnel will inform you of your appointment when you arrive to see the doctor.

### What Clothing Can You Wear?

You can wear any clothing that you wish. You should wear a pair of loose fitting jeans or slacks that will enable you to wear your new brace comfortably. You may need a larger size; "skin tight" pants or jeans will be impossible to put on over the brace. An undershirt, T-shirt, or body shirt, preferably one that has no seams (tube type), must be worn under your brace. If you wish, you may use only the bottom part of an undershirt, cutting away just under the sleeves. This is the only clothing that should be worn under the brace. Underpants should be worn on the outside of the brace. If you perspire heavily, you should change the T-shirt or body shirt twice a day.

### How Do You Take Care of Your Brace?

You can learn to put the brace on by yourself. To put the brace on, hold it by the posterior uprights and spread it open. Place one shoulder and arm through at a time. Then secure the neck ring by tightening the screw. Lift the brace up and tighten the girdle to the mark designated by the doctor. After tightening, push the brace down to fit snugly into your waistline. The first few times you put your brace on you will need someone to tighten it to the correct mark for you, but after you have become accustomed to how it should fit, you will be able to tighten the straps yourself. If it is loose it will ride down, putting pressure on the hip bones and making the skin red and sore. If the hip bones become sore, lift the brace as though applying it and tighten the strap still more. DO NOT LOOSEN THE GIRDLE BECAUSE OF SORE HIPS. After a big meal it is permissible to let it out a little, but do not forget to tighten it to the mark on the belt after about an hour. You will soon learn that the pelvic girdle is comfortable only when it is snug.

Projecting metal will be hard on any clothes that you wear. Do not use moleskin or other sticky adhesives on the brace. The uprights and screws may be covered by plastic or leather held with Velcro. These may be obtained from your orthotist.

The care of the brace is simple. The longevity of the brace depends greatly upon the cleanliness of your skin and the brace. The polypropylene pelvic section (and pads, if made of plastic) should be washed daily inside and out with mild soap and warm water.Saddle soap can be used to clean the leather pads. Dry thoroughly before putting the brace on again. This will prevent any build-up of body odors. Keep screws tight throughout the entire brace. Use coverings (plastic or leather) for the uprights and outriggers. Do not leave the brace exposed to extreme heat, as it may lose its shape. If repairs are needed, or if you feel that the brace is becoming much too small for you to wear at all, contact your doctor or the Orthotic Lab where your brace was made, before it is beyond repair.

Holding pads are placed to maintain the most effective correction of the curves. Their position depends upon x-ray findings. The pads will be checked about once every three to four months by your orthopedic surgeon and their position changed only at his direction. Your orthopedic surgeon may order your brace to be lengthened if it becomes too short owing to your growth or changes in the curve. Adjustments should never be made without his permission.

## Care of the Skin

The brace should be removed daily for a bath and replaced within an hour. After bathing, dry well, and rub the "pressure area" under the pelvic girdle and holding pads with rubbing alcohol. Pay particular attention to the areas that are red. The alcohol will help to toughen your skin and prevent skin breakdown. When the skin is dry, dust lightly with powder or cornstarch for a soothing effect and to help prevent itching. If the skin does become blistered or open, apply a dry nonadhesive Telfa dressing, which can be obtained from the local drugstore. Never use a greasy ointment, creams, Band-Aids or 4 × 4 dressings. Notify your doctor immediately.

## Physical Therapy Exercises: For Scoliosis

You will be given specific corrective exercises to be carried out in your brace. These are listed on the instruction sheet that will be given to you by a physical therapist. It is important to do them correctly. The exercise program is designed to 1) decrease lumbar lordosis (sway back), 2) decrease the major curve and/or list, 3) decrease the rib prominence and fill out the thoracic valley, 4) increase the strength of the trunk musculature, 5) promote good posture, and 6) stretch out soft tissue tightness. Since the brace acts as a support for the trunk muscles, their strength may decrease owing to non-use. Therefore, the exercise program should be carried out daily.

## Physical Therapy Exercises: For Kyphosis

You will be given specific corrective exercises to be carried out in your brace. These are listed on the instruction sheet that will be given to you by a physical therapist. It is important to do them correctly. The exercise program is designed to 1) decrease lumbar lordosis (sway back), 2) increase the strength of the back extensors for maintenance of the correction obtained by the brace, 3) increase the strength of the trunk musculature, 4) promote good posture, and

5) stretch out soft tissue tightness. Since the brace acts as a support for the trunk muscles, their strength may decrease owing to non-use. Therefore, the exercise program should be carried out daily.

A physical therapist will check your exercises at the time of your clinic visits.

You should never feel soreness of your jaw or pressure on your teeth. Do not rest on the throat mold. Plan your study posture so that you look forward instead of downward. Portable easels are sometimes used to make it easier to write or hold a book. Prism or mirror glasses may be helpful. Avoid continued pressure on your throat or chin.

### Activities in the Brace

Your brace may be somewhat uncomfortable at first. During the first two or three days you may lie down without the brace on for an hour a couple of times a day to help you become adjusted to the brace. Always remember to put the brace back on after the hour's rest. After a few days, you should be wearing the brace the required amount of time the doctor has prescribed for you.

After you have worn the brace for a few days, you *should* resume all ordinary physical activities. *Increase rather than diminish your activity, because the brace is more effective when you are active.* A physical education program is desirable, but trampoline, vigorous gymnastics, and contact sports must be omitted. In the brace, the movements of your torso will be selectively limited. If you are as active as you should be, the screws in your brace will tend to loosen. They should be tightened as needed.

If you are tired, particularly when riding in a car for a long time, lie down in a comfortable position. If your back feels cramped or stiff, do your posture exercises. When resting on a bed, a soft one is sometimes more comfortable than a firm one. Either is satisfactory. Most patients find it easiest to sleep on their side. Firm or hard chairs are more comfortable to sit in than soft low chairs.

When the curve is partially corrected, the brace may be removed for swimming. Only flat dives from the pool edge are permitted. When you are not actually in the water, lie down on the edge of the pool for a rest. *Do not* sit at the side of the pool until the brace has been put on again within an hour or two as instructed. Please ask your physician about what specific instructions he may have for you regarding swimming or any other special activities in which you may desire to partake.

The length of time that you must wear the brace will depend upon the maturity of your bones. Some teenagers develop more rapidly than others. When you are nearly mature you will be weaned by gradually increasing the time out of the brace. Soon you may attend school without it. Eventually you will continue with the exercises but will wear the brace only at night.

# INDEX

Page numbers in *italics* indicate illustrations. Page numbers followed by t indicate tables.

**681**